Protocols for Gene Transfer in Neuroscience

Dedication

P.R.L. dedicates this book to Maria, for her unqualified and enthusiastic support in the face of mounting laboratory and family pressures; to Elijah who, by substantially reducing the time P.R.L. used to sleep at night, paradoxically taught an owl how to concentrate and get the best out of the hours of daylight.

L.W.E. dedicates this book to Kathy, whose never-ceasing support and understanding keeps the candle burning at both ends.

Protocols for Gene Transfer in Neuroscience

Towards Gene Therapy of Neurological Disorders

Edited by

P.R. Lowenstein
Molecular Medicine Unit, The University of Manchester, UK

and

L.W. Enquist
Department of Molecular Biology, Princeton University, USA

JOHN WILEY & SONS
Chichester · New York · Brisbane · Toronto · Singapore

National 01243 779777
International (+44) 1243 779777

Other Wiley Editorial Offices

John Wiley & Sons, Inc., 605 Third Avenue,
New York, NY 10158-0012, USA

Jacaranda Wiley Ltd, 33 Park Road, Milton,
Queensland 4064, Australia

John Wiley & Sons (Canada) Ltd, 22 Worcester Road,
Rexdale, Ontario M9W 1L1, Canada

John Wiley & Sons (Asia) Pte Ltd, 2 Clementi Loop #02-01,
Jin Xing Distripark, Singapore 0521

Library of Congress Cataloging-in-Publication Data

Protocols for gene transfer in neuroscience : towards gene therapy of neurological disorders / edited by P.R. Lowenstein and L.W. Enquist.
p. cm.
Includes bibliographical references and index.
ISBN 0-471-95766-6 (comb bound pbk. : alk. paper)
1. Nervous system—Diseases—Gene therapy. I. Lowenstein, P.R. (Pedro R.) II. Enquist, L.W. (Lynn W.)
[DNLM: 1. Central Nervous System Diseases—therapy. 2. Gene Therapy. 3. Gene Transfer—laboratory manuals. 4. Viruses—genetics—laboratory manuals. WL 300 P967 1995]
RC350.G45P76 1995
616.8′0442—dc20
DNLM/DLC
for Library of Congress 95–45487
CIP

British Library Cataloguing in Publication Data

A catalogue record for this book is available from the British Library

ISBN 0-471-95766-6

Typeset from the editor's disks in 10/11½pt Times by Vision Typesetting, Manchester
Printed in Great Britain by Bookcraft (Bath) Ltd, and bound by James Burn Binders, Oxford
This book is printed on acid-free paper responsibly manufactured from sustainable forestation, for which at least two trees are planted for each one used for paper production.

Contents

Section 4: Protocols for Gene Delivery Using Herpes Simplex Virus-1 Vectors

Section 4 Part A: Protocols for Gene Delivery Using Helper-dependent Herpes Simplex Virus-1 Vectors

Section 4 Part B: Protocols for Gene Delivery Using Helper-independent Herpes Simplex Virus-1 Vectors

Section 5: Protocols for Gene Delivery Using Cells

Section 6: Protocols for *in vivo* Application of Gene Transfer Methods

Protocols: By Chapter

Protocols from Chapter 6. Use of Fowl Plague, Vesicular Stomatitis and Semliki Forest Viruses to Study the Mechanisms of Neuronal Membrane Polarity

Protocols from Chapter 7. Gene Transfer into the Central and Peripheral Nervous System Using Adenoviral Vectors

Protocols from Chapter 8. The Use of Adenovirus Vectors to Transfer Genes to Identified Target Brain Cells *in vitro*

Protocols from Chapter 9. Adeno-associated Virus Vectors for Gene Transfer

Protocols from Chapter 11. Herpes Simplex Virus-1 Amplicons

Protocols from Chapter 22. Replication-competent Viral Therapy of Tumors in the Central Nervous System

Protocols from Chapter 23. Osmotic Blood–brain Barrier Disruption Methodologies for Global Delivery of Genetic Vectors to the Brain

Protocols from Chapter 24. Pseudorabies Virus: A Tool For Tracing Neuronal Connections

Protocols from Chapter 25. Tracing Connected Neurons with Herpes Simplex Virus Type 1

Protocols from Chapter 26. Immune Responses to Viruses: Practical Implications for the Use of Viruses as Vectors for Experimental and Clinical Gene Therapy

Protocols: By Application

Transfection Protocols

Protocols for the Selection of Cell Clones Expressing Transfected Transgenes

Protocols for the Short-term Study of Promoter Activity in Neural Cells

Generating and Growing Viral Recombinants

Adenovirus

Adeno-associated Virus

Herpes Simplex Virus-1

Retrovirus

Semliki Forest Virus

Pseudorabies Virus

Titering Viral Recombinants

Adenovirus

Adeno-associated Virus

Intratumor Administration

Disruption of Blood–Brain Barrier

Cell Transplantation: Gene Delivery, Bone Marrow and Tumors

Use of Viral Vectors *in vitro*

Expression of Transgenes During *in vitro* Latency

Biochemical Methods

Histochemical and Biochemical Enzyme Assays

Immunocytochemical Procedures

Trans-synaptic Tracing of Neuronal Connections

Assessing the Immune Response to Viral Vectors

Contributors

Timothy E. Allsopp *Department of Veterinary Pathology, University of Edinburgh, Summerhall, Edinburgh, EH9 1QH, UK*
Tel: 0131 650 6160 Fax: 0131 650 6160 Email:tallsopp@lab0.vet.ed.ac.uk

Derek Bain *University of Manchester, School of Medicine, Department of Medicine, Molecular Medicine Unit, Room 1.302, Stopford Building, Manchester M13 9PL, UK*
Tel: 0161 275 5670 Fax: 0161 275 5672

Jeffrey S. Bartlett *Gene Therapy Center and Department of Pharmacology, School of Medicine, University of North Carolina at Chapel Hill, CB #7352, Chapel Hill, NC 27599-7352, USA*
Tel: 919 966 0905 Fax: 919 966 0908 Email: jbart@med.unc.edu

Peter Bergold *Department of Pharmacology, SUNY Downstate, NY, USA*

Andrew P. Byrnes *Department of Human Anatomy, South Parks Road, Oxford, OX1 3QX, UK*
Tel: 01865 272145 Fax: 01865 272420 Email: byrnesa@vax.ox.ac.uk

J. Patrick Card *Departments of Neuroscience and Psychiatry, 446 Crawford Hall, University of Pittsburgh, Pittsburgh, PA 15260, USA*
Tel: 412 624 6995 Fax: 412 624 9198 Email: card@bns.pitt.edu

Maria G. Castro *University of Manchester, School of Medicine, Department of Medicine, Molecular Medicine Unit, Room 1.302, Stopford Building, Manchester M13 9PL, UK*
Tel: 0161 275 5671 Fax: 0161 275 5672 Email:mgcastro@manchester.ac.uk

Harry M. Charlton *Department of Human Anatomy, South Parks Road, Oxford, OX1 3QX, UK*
Tel: 01865 272199 Fax: 01865 272420

Angel Cid-Arregui *Cell Biology Program, European Molecular Biology Laboratory, Postfach 10.2209, Meyerhofstrasse 1, D-69012 Heidelberg, Germany*
Tel: 49 6221 387321 Fax: 49 6221 387306 Email: cid@embl-heidelberg.de

David T. Curiel *Gene Therapy Program, Comprehensive Cancer Center, 1824 6th Avenue South, Room WTI 620, Birmingham, AL 35294-3300, USA*
Tel: 205 934 8627 Fax: 205 975 7476

Meltsje J. de Hoop *Cell Biology Program, European Molecular Biology Laboratory, Postfach 10.2209, Meyerhofstrasse 1, D-69012 Heidelberg, Germany*
Tel: 49 6221 387321 Fax: 49 6221 387306

Neal A. DeLuca *Department of Molecular Genetics and Biochemistry, University of Pittsburgh School of Medicine, Pittsburgh, PA 15261-2072, USA*
Tel: 412 648 8105 Fax: 412 624 8997

K. Dobrenis *Sidney Weisner Laboratory of Genetic Neurological Disease, Department of Neuroscience, Rose F. Kennedy Center for Research in Mental Retardation and Human Development, Albert Einstein College of Medicine, Bronx, NY 10461, USA*
Tel: 718 430 4025 Fax: 718 430 8821

Lynn W. Enquist *Department of Molecular Biology, Princeton University, Princeton, NJ 08544, USA*
Tel: 609 258 2415 Fax: 609 258 1035 Email: lenquist@molbiol.princeton.edu

Alberto L. Epstein *Centre de Génétique Moléculaire et Cellulaire, CNRS - UMR 106 - Université Claude Bernard Lyon, 143 boulevard du 11 Novembre 1918, 69622 Villeurbanne Cedex, France*
Tel: 33 72 43 13 25 Fax: 33 72 44 05 55 Email: epstein@biomserv.univ-lyon1.fr

Howard J. Federoff *Department of Neurology, University of Rochester Medical Center, Box 673, 601 Elmwood Avenue, Rochester, NY 14642, USA*
Tel: 716 273 4851 Fax: 716 442 6646 Email:hfed@medinfo.rochester.edu

Lawrence Feldman *Department of Microbiology and Immunology, UCLA School of Medicine, Center for the Health Sciences, 10833 Le Conte Avenue, Los Angeles, CA 90024-1747, USA*
Tel: 310 206 1014 Fax: 310 206 3865 Email: lfeldman@microimmun.medsch.ucla.edu

Niza Frenkel *Department of Cell Research and Immunology, Tel Aviv University, Tel Aviv 69978, Israel*
Tel: 972 3 6407166 Fax: 972 3 6422046 Email: frenkeln@ccsg.tau.ac.il

Theodore Friedmann *Departments of Pediatrics and Center for Molecular Genetics, School of Medicine, University of California at San Diego, La Jolla, CA 92093-0634, USA*
Tel: 619 534 4268 Fax: 619 534 1422 Email: tfriedmann@ucsd.edu

Fred H. Gage *Laboratory of Genetics, The Salk Institute, La Jolla, CA 92037, USA*
Tel: 619 453 4100 Fax: 619 597 0824

Henrik Garoff *Department of Biosciences at Novum, Karolinska Institute, S 141 57 Huddinge, Sweden*
Tel: 46 8 608 9125 Fax: 46 8 774 5538 Email: insig@thon.csb.ki.se

Joseph C. Glorioso *Department of Molecular Genetics and Biochemistry, University of Pittsburgh School of Medicine, Pittsburgh, PA 15261-2072, USA*
Tel: 412 648 8105 Fax: 412 624 8997 Email: joe@server1.mgen.pitt.edu

Ian Gordon *Department of Human Anatomy, South Parks Road, Oxford, OX1 3QX, UK*
Tel: 01865 272145 Fax: 01865 272420 Email: ian.gordon@human-anatomy.ox.ac.uk

Ruth A. Harris *University of Glasgow, Institute of Virology, Church Street, Glasgow, G11 5JR, UK*
Tel: 0141 339 8855, ext. 4635/4630 Fax: 0141 337 2236

Philippe Horellou *Laboratoire de Génétique Moléculaire de la Neurotransmission et des Processus Dégénératifs, C9923, CNRS, 91198 Gif sur Yvette, France*
Tel: 1 69 82 35 80, Fax: 1 69 07 50 31

William D. Hunter *Molecular Neurosurgery Laboratory, Georgetown Brain Tumor Center, Department of Neurosurgery, Georgetown University Medical Center, 3800 Reservoir Road NW, Washington DC 20007, USA*
Tel: 202 687 4972 Fax: 202 687 3744 Email: whunte02@gumedlib.dml.georgetown.edu

D.R. Stuart Jamieson *University of Glasgow, Institute of Virology, Church Street, Glasgow, G11 5JR, UK*
Tel: 0141 339 8855, ext. 4635/4630 Fax: 0141 337 2236

Koji Kajiwara *Department of Human Anatomy, South Parks Road, Oxford, OX1 3QX, UK*
Tel: 01865 272145 Fax: 01865 272420 Email: koji.kajiwara@human-anatomy.ox.ac.uk

Jill Lang *Department of Human Anatomy, South Parks Road, Oxford, OX1 3QX, UK*
Tel: 01865 272145 Fax: 01865 272420 Email: lang@vax.ox.ac.uk

David S. Latchman *Department of Molecular Pathology, University College London Medical School, The Windeyer Building, Cleveland Street, London, W1P 6DB, UK*
Tel: 0171 380 9343 Fax: 0171 387 3310

Gildas Le Gal La Salle *Institut Alfred Fessard, Unité propre de recherche 2212, CNRS, 91198 Gif sur Yvette Cedex, France*
Tel: 1 69 82 34 28 Fax: 1 69 07 05 38 Email: legal@iaf.cnrs-gif.fr

Peter Liljeström *Department of Biosciences at Novum, Karolinska Institute, S-141 57 Huddinge, Sweden*
Tel: 46 8 608 9133 Fax: 46 8 774 5538 Email: peli@cbt.ki.se

P.R. Lowenstein *University of Manchester, School of Medicine, Department of Medicine, Molecular Medicine Unit, Room 1.302, Stopford Building, Manchester M13 9PL, UK*
Tel: 0161 275 5672 Fax: 0161 275 5672 Email: lowenstein@man.ac.uk

J.C. MacMillan *Queensland Clinical Genetics Service, Royal Children's Hospital, Herston 4029, Brisbane, Australia*
Tel: 61 7 3253 1686 Fax: 61 7 3253 1987

Jacques Mallet *L.G.N., C.N.R.S., Bâtiment Cervi, 5e Étage, Hôpital de la Pitié, Salpêtrière, 83 Boulevard de l'Hôpital, 75013 Paris, France*
Tel: 33 1 42 17 75 32 Fax: 33 1 42 17 75 33

Robert L. Martuza *Molecular Neurosurgery Laboratory, Georgetown Brain Tumor Center, Department of Neurosurgery, Georgetown University Medical Center, 3800 Reservoir Road NW, Washington DC 20007, USA*
Tel: 202 687 4972 Fax: 202 687 3744

Mary McMenamin *Department of Human Anatomy, South Parks Road, Oxford, OX1 3QX, UK*
Tel: 01865 272145 Fax: 01865 272420 Email: mary.mcmenamin@human-anatomy.ox.ac.uk

E. Morrison (deceased) *University of Manchester, School of Medicine, Department of Medicine, Molecular Medicine Unit, Room 1.302, Stopford Building, Manchester M13 9PL, UK*
Tel: 0161 275 5670 Fax: 0161 275 5672

Bhaskar Mukherjee *Department of Medicine, Albert Einstein College of Medicine, 1300 Morris Park Avenue, Bronx, New York, NY 14061, USA*

Peter K. Mulderry *MRC Brain Metabolism Unit, Royal Edinburgh Hospital, Morningside Park, Edinburgh, EH10 5HF, UK*
Tel: 0131 537 6527 Fax: 0131 537 6110 Email: mulderry@castle.ed.ac.uk

Leslie L. Muldoon *Department of Cell and Developmental biology, Oregon Health Sciences University, 3181 SW Sam Jackson Park Road L-603, Portland, OR 97201-3098, USA*
Tel: 503 494 5626 Fax: 503 494 5627 Email: muldoonl@ohsu.edu

C.A. Murray *University of Manchester, School of Medicine, Department of Medicine, Molecular Medicine Unit, Room 1.302, Stopford Building, Manchester M13 9PL, UK*
Tel: 0161 275 5670 Fax: 0161 275 5672

Edward A. Neuwelt *Department of Neurology, Division of Neurosurgery and Department of Biochemistry and Molecular Biology, Oregon Health Sciences University, 3181 SW Sam Jackson Park Road L-603, Portland, OR 97201-3098, USA*
Tel: 503 494 5626 Fax: 503 494 5627 Email: neuwelte@ccmail.ohsu.edu

Theo D. Palmer *Laboratory of Genetics, The Salk Institute, La Jolla, CA 92037, USA*
Tel: 619 453 4100 Fax: 619 597 0824

Michel Perricaudet *Institut Gustave Roussy, Unité associée 1301, CNRS, 39 rue Camille Desmoulins, 94805 Villejuif Cedex, France*
Tel: 1 45 59 44 90 Fax: 1 45 59 40 90

Chris M. Preston *MRC Virology Unit, Institute of Virology, Glasgow, G11 5JR, UK*
Tel: 0141 339 8855, ext. 4635/4630 Fax: 0141 337 2236 Email: cpreston@vir.gla.ac.uk

Samuel D. Rabkin *Molecular Neurosurgery Laboratory, Georgetown Brain Tumor Center, Department of Neurosurgery, Georgetown University Medical Center, 3800 Reservoir Road NW, Washington DC 20007, USA*
Tel: 202 687 8047 Fax: 202 687 3046 Email: rabkins@medlib.georgetown.edu

Frédéric Revah *Rhône-Poulenc Rorer, Centre de Recherche Vitry-Alfortville, 13 quai Jules Guesde, 94403 Vitry sur Seine Cedex, France*
Tel: 1 45 73 85 11 Fax: 33 1 45 73 77 96

Jean Jacques Robert *Laboratoire de Génétique Moléculaire de la Neurotransmission et des Processus Dégénératifs, C9923, CNRS, 91198 Gif sur Yvette, France*
Tel: 1 69 82 35 80 Fax: 1 69 07 50 31

J. Rowe *University of Manchester, School of Medicine, Department of Medicine, Molecular Medicine Unit, Room 1.302, Stopford Building, Manchester M13 9PL, UK*
Tel: 0161 275 5670 Fax: 0161 275 5672

Jackie Russell *MRC Virology Unit, Institute of Virology, Glasgow, G11 5JR, UK*
Tel: 0141 339 8855, ext. 4635/4630 Fax: 0141 337 2236 Email: c/o cpreston@vir.gla.ac.uk

Richard Samulski *Gene Therapy Center and Department of Pharmacology, School of Medicine, University of North Carolina at Chapel Hill, CB #7352, Chapel Hill, NC 27599-7352, USA*
Tel: 919 962 3285 Fax: 919 966 0907 Email: rjs@med.unc.edu

Mark S. Sands *Department of Pathobiology, School of Veterinary Medicine, University of Pennsylvania, 300 Spruce Street, Philadelphia, PA 19104-6008, USA*
Tel: 215 898 2324 Fax: 215 573 2162

Ronit Sarid *Department of Cell Research and Immunology, Tel Aviv University, Tel Aviv 69978, Israel*
Tel: 972 3 6407166 Fax: 972 3 6422046 Email: rntsrd@ccsg.tau.ac.il

A.F. Shering *University of Manchester, School of Medicine, Department of Medicine, Molecular Medicine Unit, Room 1.302, Stopford Building, Manchester M13 9PL, UK*
Tel: 0161 275 5670 Fax: 0161 275 5672

Roderic L. Smith *Department of Neurology, University of Colorado Health Sciences Center, Denver, CO, USA*

M.A. Thrall *Department of Pathology, College of Veterinary Medicine and Biomedical Sciences, Colorado State University, Fort Collins, CO 80523, USA*
Tel: 970 491 7508 Fax: 970 491 0603 Email: mthrall@vines.colostate.edu

P. Tomasec *University of Manchester, School of Medicine, Department of Medicine, Molecular Medicine Unit, Room 1.302, Stopford Building, Manchester M13 9PL, UK*
Tel: 0161 275 5670 Fax: 0161 275 5672

Gabriella Ugolini *Laboratoire de Génétique des Virus, CNRS, F-91198 Gif sur Yvette, France*
Tel: 33 1 69 82 37 69 Fax: 33 1 69 82 43 08

Emmanuelle Vigne *Institut Gustave Roussy, Unité Associée 1301, CNRS, 39 rue Camille Desmoulins, 94805 Villejuif Cedex, France*
Tel: 1 45 59 44 90 Fax: 1 45 59 40 90

Alison Vine *Department of Human Anatomy, South Parks Road, Oxford, OX1 3QX, UK*
Tel: 01865 272145 Fax: 01865 272420 Email: amvine@vax.ox.ac.uk

S.U. Walkley *Sidney Weisner Laboratory of Genetic Neurological Disease, Department of Neuroscience, Rose F. Kennedy Center for Research in Mental Retardation and Human Development, Albert Einstein College of Medicine, Bronx, NY 10461, USA*
Tel: 718 430 4025 Fax: 718 430 8821 Email: walkley@aecom.yu.edu

Christine L. Wilcox *Department of Microbiology, Colorado State University, Fort Collins, CO 80523, USA*
Tel: 303 491 2552 Fax: 303 491 1815 Email: cwilcox@vines.colostate.edu

Gavin W.G. Wilkinson *Department of Medicine, University of Wales College of Medicine, Tenovus Building, Heath Park, Cardiff, CF4 4XX, UK*
Tel: 01222 745215 Fax: 01222 745003 Email: wmdgww@cardiff.ac.uk

John H. Wolfe *Department of Pathobiology, School of Veterinary Medicine, University of Pennsylvania, 300 Spruce Street, Philadelphia, PA 19104-6008, USA*
Tel: 215 898 2324 Fax: 215 573 2162 Email: jhwolfe@pobox.upenn.edu

Kathryn J. Wood *Nuffield Department of Surgery, University of Oxford, John Radcliffe Hospital, Oxford, OX3 9DU, UK*
Tel: 01865 221300 Fax: 01865 63545 Email: kathryn.wood@nds.ox.ac.uk

Matthew J.A. Wood *Department of Human Anatomy, South Parks Road, Oxford, OX1 3QX, UK*
Tel: 01865 272145 Fax: 01865 272420 Email: mjwood@vax.ox.ac.uk

Xiao Xiao *Gene Therapy Center and Department of Pharmacology, School of Medicine, University of North Carolina at Chapel Hill, CB #7352, Chapel Hill, NC 27599-7352, USA*
Tel: 919 962 1221 Fax: 919 966 1313 Email: xxi@med.unc.edu

Takahito Yazaki *Departments of Neurosurgery and Physiology, School of Medicine, Keio University, 35 Shinanomachi, Shinjuku-ku, Tokyo 160, Japan*
Tel: 81 3 3353 1211, ext. 2613 Fax: 81 3 3357 5445

Preface

Why this book was commissioned

The brain and the cells that compose it have always presented unique challenges to any kind of outside interventions, including drug delivery, surgical procedures and the genetic manipulation of its constituent cells. These challenges include the blood–brain barrier, the cranium and the terminal differentiated state of neurons. This book was commissioned because new technology is rapidly developing to overcome these hurdles. Although the special problems relating to drug delivery and surgical procedures such as transplantation, and the targeting of genes to the brains of transgenic animals, are treated in detail elsewhere, this book represents the first compilation of the practical aspects of gene manipulation in the nervous system.

A variety of procedures have been developed during the last 5 years that enable delivery of genes directly to the brain or specifically into neurons and glial cells. Not surprisingly, such techniques are variations on themes commonly used in virology, biochemistry, molecular and cell biology. This volume presents the ways in which these techniques can be used by the neuroscience community. We have collected 151 procedures and techniques used in molecular neuroscience and present them as practical step-by-step protocols, coupled to the theoretical background needed for a neuroscientist to understand, adapt and expand the technology as needed.

Classical pharmacology taught that cell functions could not be altered, but this dogma is being rewritten. With gene transfer technology we can introduce almost any desired function into a given target cell. This technology has raised the prospect of gene therapy or molecular medicine and with it new strategies for combating the wide range of diseases that continue to afflict mankind. As this book testifies, there are many ways to transfer genes into neurons and the brain. We hope to provide the tools and background so that neuroscientists can explore this exciting technology in their own systems.

We cover a variety of gene delivery technologies in this book, ranging from manipulation of isolated cells to direct introduction of genes into the nervous system of animals. Several gene delivery techniques are described in detail, including direct DNA delivery, use of viral vectors and use of transduced cells. We present methods for *ex vivo* technology, in which a patient's cells are isolated, manipulated in culture and then returned to the patient. This methodology can be employed to deliver genes encoding soluble diffusible factors, such as neurotransmitters (e.g. dopamine) or growth factors (e.g. nerve growth factor or other neurotrophins) to the brain. Such an approach involves first inserting the new gene (the transgene) into a suitable expression system that may include a non-neuronal cell such as a fibroblast or bone marrow precursor, and using a virus to infect cells in culture. The cells carrying the transgene can be either transplanted directly into the brain or infused into the bloodstream, from where the cells can repopulate the CNS. We also present methods for direct *in vivo* gene delivery, in which new genes are placed directly into affected target neurons *in vivo*. In such cases, neurotropic viruses or DNA conjugates are used to infect the desired resident brain cells including highly specialized neurons, astroglial cells, oligodenroglial cells and endothelial cells.

What we wanted to achieve

Our goal was to provide a manual describing the "how to" of gene transfer into the brain and its resident cells. The manual is not for people who already know "how to", but rather for neuroscientists who are not accustomed to gene transfer technology but who can see the power of the methods. We have provided not only methods, but also brief theory and hints on troubleshooting. Our idea was to guide the experienced laboratory leader as well as the beginning graduate student into use of the new technology of gene delivery to the brain.

To provide the latest technology, we must of necessity present a "work in progress". Our book is not meant to be a definitive list of the final protocols in the field. We have compiled the latest techniques from the top gene delivery laboratories and what has emerged is a study of science in action. For example, we present several variations of a single protocol showing how different laboratories have solved a common problem in different ways. We hope that by seeing the variations on technical themes neuroscientists can find solutions to their own particular problems. Thus, this is a book not of prescriptions, but of choices. It was intended to be interactive and to evolve. One way we have chosen to catalyse this interaction is to provide a contact name for each particular technology described so that queries can be addressed directly to those actively working on the problems. As more neurobiologists use gene transfer technology, we hope that these methods will evolve and prosper.

How to use this book

This book is meant to be kept close to the bench. To that end, we have provided several forms of indexing to enable rapid perusal and location of a given technique or topic. For more detailed reading, the book is organized into chapters, with theory, detailed troubleshooting notes and references accompanying the specific protocols described in each chapter. The list of protocols is indexed numerically as well as in a thematic series grouped according to intended use. Finally, the index will enable the reader to search for individual words independent of the chapter location, intended use or description.

Pedro R. Lowenstein
Lynn W. Enquist

Acknowledgments

Although not linked by practical aspects, this book is linked in spirit to the conference "Gene Transfer into Neurons: Towards Gene Therapy of Neurological Disorders" (*Gene Therapy* **1,** Supplement 1, 1994) organized in Cardiff in 1993. That conference could not have happened without the encouragement and boldness of Tony Parsons who, sadly, is not with us any more to see the long-term fruits that grew from the magic seeds he sowed in 1992.

P.R. Lowenstein wishes to thank Fabian Appel, Colin Hyman, Hanno Koppel, Tim Jacob and Allan Stone for their friendship and undisputed support. In the laboratory Derek Bain, the late Ewan Morrison, Carol Murray, Andy Shering and Peter Tomasec critically reviewed many of the protocols and the laboratory team (Phil Blenning, Zoe Forrest, Carol Murray, the late Ewan Morrison, Jo Rowe, Tom Southgate and Kirsten Stewart) kept the excitement going during this venture. P.R.L. is currently supported by the Lister Institute of Preventive Medicine, The Wellcome Trust, The Royal Society and BBSRC.

L.W. Enquist extends special thanks to Alan Robbins, Mary Whealy and Logan House, whose special potions, technical prowess and enthusiasm kept his laboratory running. He is indebted to long-term collaborators Pat Card and Richard Miselis, who introduced him to neurobiology, and to Joan Dubin who helped him practice neurovirology in his own laboratory. Paul Husak, Anita Knapp-Ryseck, Marlies Eldridge and Rob Townley at the Princeton laboratory provided critical review of many of the protocols. During its initial stages, L.W.E. was supported by the Dupont Merck pharmaceutical company and is currently supported by the National Institutes of Neurological Diseases and Stroke.

CHAPTER 1

A Personal Perspective of Gene Therapy and the Nervous System

THEODORE FRIEDMANN

Departments of Pediatrics and Center for Molecular Genetics, School of Medicine, University of California at San Diego, La Jolla, CA 92093-0634, USA. Tel: 619 534 4268; Fax: 619 534 1422; Email: tfriedmann@ucsd.edu

One of the principal motivations for the study of the molecular genetics of cancer, degenerative disease or disorders of the central nervous system (CNS) lies in the urgency to move concepts and tools of modern molecular biology into therapy. This is particularly true for investigators with clinical training. Until the mid 1960s the common approach was to translate the language of biochemistry and cell biology into therapy by designing small organic chemicals as pharmacological agents—there were only limited possibilities at that time for any other approaches to therapy, especially for those based on genetic mechanisms.

The development of the powerful tools of molecular biology in the mid 1960s brought a sense of change. Work in a number of laboratories was aimed at interfering with disease pathogenesis, not at the level of the metabolic pathways that resulted from an underlying defect but rather directly at the underlying genetic defects. Although the pharmacological attack on disease was effective in some cases, it was of little use in many other disorders because the target of such an approach was the consequence of the symptoms of a defect rather than the defect itself.

The concept of gene therapy arose in the late 1960s and early 1970s and was based on the hope that methods would become available to correct genetic defects by introducing wild-type versions of defective alleles into cells. Despite the fact that there were few, if any, ideas on how genes could be introduced into cells, there were encouraging hints in the literature that solutions were on the horizon. For instance, it was known that the DNA tumor viruses SV40 and polyoma interfered with normal cellular replication and actively converted normal cells into malignant cells by introducing viral "transforming" genes into normal cells in a permanent, heritable fashion. The job description of these agents was to act as transducing agents to introduce foreign, albeit deleterious, genetic information into cells. It was not too much of a leap to imagine exploiting such a virus to carry potentially therapeutic genes into cells to correct a disease phenotype.

My interests in gene therapy were the result of being in the right place at the right time. I was working at the NIH in the late 1960s, first in the protein laboratory of Christian Anfinsen, and then in the human genetics laboratory of Jay Seegmiller. The enzyme defect for Lesch–Nyhan disease had just been described by Jay Seegmiller and his colleagues as a single gene defect in the X-linked HPRT locus. This disorder is a striking disease, involving a form of apparent mental retardation, choreoathetosis, uncontrolled movements, hyperuricemia leading to gout and renal destruction as well as a very strange self-mutilation behavior. What caught my attention was that

Protocols for Gene Transfer in Neuroscience: Towards Gene Therapy of Neurological Disorders
Edited by P.R. Lowenstein and L.W. Enquist

this complex physical and behavioral phenotype resulted from a genetically simple deficiency of the enzyme HPRT. My good fortune was to interact with John Subak-Sharpe from Glasgow, a visiting scientist at the NIH. We began intense discussions about what this novel biochemical marker meant, both as a tool and as a genetic defect. I recall a particular evening discussion, during which it became clear to us that HPRT could be a marker that would enable us to test the fundamental hypothesis of gene therapy—that one might imagine introducing a normal HPRT gene into a defective cell and determine if that gene could correct the disease phenotype. We thought that HPRT would be particularly useful because methods had been devised to select both for and against cells expressing HPRT in tissue culture. It was conceptually straightforward to expose HPRT-negative Lesch–Nyhan cells to whole cellular DNA from the normal human cell and to determine if the defective cells could pick up the normal DNA and express HPRT. We looked at that question by pulse labeling with radioactive hypoxanthine and by trying to select presumably corrected cells in HAT medium. Much to our delight we found, at a very rare frequency, cells that were unquestionably expressing normal HPRT because they were able to incorporate hypoxanthine after exposure to the foreign DNA. Unfortunately, the study ended there because we had little idea of how to make this process orders of magnitude more efficient. This would have required isolation of the HPRT gene or cDNA, a task that was not feasible at the time because the tools of recombinant DNA had not yet been developed. It seemed then that our only option was to take advantage of the work of Renato Dulbecco and his colleagues by transforming viruses to transduce foreign DNA into the cell in a stable heritable fashion.

Emboldened by our success with HPRT I took a leave of absence from the NIH and went to Dulbecco's laboratory with the intention of trying to take apart a polyoma virus capsid, stuff it with foreign DNA, and then use this "pseudo-virus" to deliver DNA into cells. In the course of that work we learned much about the structure and genetic organization of the model virus polyoma, but we never found ways to stuff new DNA into the virus capsid. Perhaps the most valuable effect of that work came when R. Roblin and I examined the generic problem of the feasibility of human gene therapy and prepared a paper that was published in *Science* in 1972.

In that review we looked at the possibility of using transforming viruses to introduce foreign genes into cells in a stable, permanent way. We identified some of the technical issues involved in developing methods of gene therapy for human disease and pointed to technical and ethical issues that are as relevant today as they were then. For example, we suggested that methods were needed for delivering genes specifically to the appropriate tissue, for ensuring that those foreign genes were regulated in an appropriate way, and for understanding the potential for an immune response to a foreign gene. We were also concerned about the inadvertent (not the deliberate) modification of the germline. What we had in mind, really, was a genetic attack on classical Garrod/Mendelian genetic disease—the inborn errors of metabolism—involving simple restoration of a gene encoding one of these enzymes by augmenting the defective cell genome with a normal gene that would correct the metabolic defect.

We were directed and focused in our thinking of inborn errors. The genetic components of many other kinds of human disease had not then been characterized, and we did not envision application of gene therapy concepts to diseases such as most forms of cancer, cardiovascular disease and neurological diseases. We *did* envision two general approaches to the restoration of a genetic defect. One idea was to remove cells from a patient with a genetic defect, manipulate them *in vitro* by introducing a therapeutic gene and then return the genetically modified and corrected cells to the patient at a site appropriate to restore a genetic function. Our second idea was to correct the defect *in vivo*—to deliver a piece of genetic information directly into the patient and correct the defect *in situ*. At the time we could not imagine the many technical, practical, legal and fundamental problems that remained to be articulated and resolved.

Our ideas about the feasibility of human gene therapy remained theoretical and out of reach until the early 1980s, when a single technical innovation—the development of the retroviral vectors—emerged to catalyse the field. Until then the subject of human gene therapy was almost a scientific embarrassment and unrealistic wishful thinking; not quite respectable. However, as a result of intense efforts in the 1970s to understand the molecular biology of retroviruses, three groups (those of Weinberg, Scolnik and Temin) independently developed in 1981 and 1982 methods by which retroviruses could be modified to carry foreign (and perhaps therapeutic) genes.

For the first time we had a truly efficient gene transfer reagent to work with, which opened an enormous number of experimental doors. Suddenly it became feasible to examine gene transfer into a large number of potential target cells, including bone marrow stem cells, hepatocytes, endothelial and epithelial cells. Disease models for gene therapy began to flourish because, by that time, more diseases were being characterized genetically and therapeutic genes were becoming available.

While the general field of gene therapy exploded in the early 1980s and optimism prevailed, we began to think that some diseases of the central nervous system might be amenable to genetic attack—something most of us had thought impossible because of the physiological inaccessibility of the brain and the numbing complexity of cell interactions in the CNS.

Initially we were encouraged because some diseases of the CNS, such as phenylketonuria or galactosemia, are principally defects of an easily accessible organ such as the liver, and not the brain. Retroviral mediated gene therapy could therefore be considered because this approach would focus on modification of hepatocyte function. We also began to think about modifying CNS function by genetic manipulation of the bone marrow and repopulating part of the central nervous system with microglial cells derived from bone marrow. We thought that such an approach might offer a therapy for, for example, Hurler's disease, Maroteaux–Lamy disease and adrenoleukodystrophy.

What other methods of genetic attack on disorders of the CNS seem possible today? I can imagine three general approaches. In the first, cells, native or genetically engineered, might be introduced directly into the CNS to act as a localized or a global "factory" for a therapeutic gene product. The cells might include fibroblasts, glia, or even human CNS precursor stem cells able to engraft normally in the CNS to provide gene products such as neurotransmitter components, trophic or tropic factors or other functions absent in the diseased CNS. The second approach would be to remove cells from the patient, modify them genetically *in vitro* and then graft the modified cells into the CNS. In the third approach a viral vector or other gene delivery vehicle might be used to introduce a gene into specific diseased regions of the CNS.

Some years ago, Rusty Gage and I began studies at the University of California at San Diego on several models of CNS disease that might be approached by *ex vivo* genetic modification. Rusty is interested in CNS grafts and in CNS plasticity. Both of us were aware of the emerging models based on the protective action of nerve growth factor (NGF) on degeneration of cholinergic neurons. Our approach was to develop cells for grafting that expressed large amounts of NGF and to test the hypothesis that such cells could rescue neurons that were deprived of their supply of NGF by specific brain lesions. We made lesions in rat fimbria fornix, the pathway connecting the cholinergic neurons of the basal forebrain with their source of NGF in the hippocampus. As long as this pathway is intact the cells remain intact and function normally but lesions in the fimbria fornix interrupt the supply of NGF and the cells in the forebrain degenerate. These cholinergic cells are known to play an important role in memory and are anatomically and functionally analogous to the cholinergic neurons that degenerate in humans with Alzheimer's disease.

We were encouraged by the knowledge that infusion of NGF into this lesion was effective in salvaging forebrain cholinergic neurons from degeneration, so we posed the very simple question: "could these NGF-deprived cells be saved by introducing cells that had been transduced with a retroviral vector expressing NGF, rather than introducing NGF itself into the lesion?"

We used a simple retrovirus vector with the 5′ long terminal repeat driving NGF and a Rous sarcoma virus long terminal repeat internal promoter driving the G418 resistance marker. We used this vector to transduce primary rat fibroblasts to G418 resistance and then to screen for colonies that expressed NGF. Genetically modified cells expressing maximal amounts of NGF were grafted into the brains of lesioned rats. We were gratified to find that the introduction of genetically modified non-neuronal cells can indeed affect a CNS phenotype. A control graft containing cells that had been transduced with an irrelevant gene (luciferase) to one side of a lesioned brain had no effect on the massive degeneration of cholinergic neurons caused by the lesion and NGF deprivation. Cells on the non-lesioned side were, of course, normal. However, when we grafted fibroblasts transduced *ex vivo* by the retroviral vector expressing NGF we found that the NGF-transduced cells prevented degeneration of the cholinergic neurons.

This paradigm suggested that the phenotype of these cells, and perhaps of other cells in the

CNS, may be modified by engrafting genetically manipulated cells to provide a therapeutic gene product. The degeneration of cholinergic brain cells of sufferers of Alzheimer's disease may be prevented by therapy of this nature. Several clinical studies are currently testing the possibility that delivery of pure NGF to the brains such patients might modify the progression of the disease. If this proof of principle is established, grafting of genetically engineered cells to deliver NGF or other trophic factors might be defensible. Similar approaches are being considered for Parkinson's disease, a disorder caused by the degeneration of the nigrostriatal pathway. The disease is currently treated with L-dopa, a precursor of the neurotransmitter dopamine. The enzyme tyrosine hydroxylase drives the rate-limiting step in the synthesis of dopa and the expression of a virally delivered TH transgene might therefore be useful to restore dopamine function in brains of sufferers of Parkinson's disease.

Many issues remain to be resolved, including the survival of the grafted cells, the stable and regulated expression of the transgene, the potential for immune response to the transgene products and the issue of long-term safety of putting autologous non-CNS cells into the CNS. Progress is being made and I am sanguine about this approach to treating CNS disorders.

One particularly exciting area of research involves the concept of a universal donor cell for grafting into the CNS. While such cells are not yet available, they may be in the not too distant future. Connie Cepko, Chris Austin, Jack Price, Ron MacKay, M. Noble and Evan Snyder have, among others, been studying the potential for the genetic reconstitution and grafting of multipotential cells into the CNS that have the capability to participate in the developmental program of the brain. It is clear that the immortalization of these primary neurons with the avian *myc* oncogene, for instance, gives rise to a non-tumorigenic cell that can mature into multiple cell types and participate in the normal development of a rodent brain. These plastic cells therefore have the potential for restoring and correcting cytoarchitectural defects or for introducing new genes into the CNS.

A long-term interest of mine has been the development of vectors for direct delivery of therapeutic genes to the CNS. Jiing-Kuan Yee (my laboratory) has recently made a major improvement in the retroviral technology, which has increased our enthusiasm for this approach. Growing the current class of retrovirus vectors to high titer is challenging, to say the least: titers of 10^6 are rarely exceeded and titers of 10^7 are usually more than satisfactory. Furthermore, the current retrovirus vectors are labile and cannot really be concentrated by standard methods. Jiing-Kuan Yee has provided us with some solutions to this problem by employing a simple idea—the concept of pseudotypes. It is possible for retroviruses to exchange envelopes with other viruses by a process known as phenotypic mixing. Jiing-Kuan Yee thought that it would be useful to replace the labile retroviral envelope glycoprotein and replace it with a membrane protein from a more robust, unrelated virus such as vesicular stomatitis virus (VSV). He therefore constructed a retrovirus vector that had the VSV G protein in its envelope in place of the normal retrovirus envelope protein (a "pseudotype" virus), and found that it did not require retroviral receptors on the cell surface for cell entry. This virus uses the VSV G protein receptor, or receptors, for entry. The VSV G receptor seems to be much more broadly distributed than the retrovirus receptor, so Jiing-Kuan's vector has a markedly expanded host range which permits it to infect a very wide range of cells. As an example, these VSV pseudotype retroviruses efficiently infect cells of zebrafish and other fish, which will permit genetic and developmental studies in this and other previously inaccessible species. This virus is also very stable and can be concentrated by ultracentrifugation without any appreciable loss—in one round of concentration a 220-fold concentration, to titers a log or two higher than possible with most retroviral vectors, is possible. We have now obtained concentrations of well over 10^9 particles per ml by using a second concentration step. This approach to improved retroviral vectors is of fundamental importance for those of us interested in gene therapy because increased titer implies that *in vivo* delivery of therapeutic genes might become possible with this important class of vectors.

My laboratory has been exploring another type of virus vector for gene delivery to the CNS, based on the neurotropic human herpes virus herpes simplex type 1 (HSV-1). Paul Johnson has been exploring the use of HSV-1 vectors in the Lesch–Nyhan model. Our HSV-1 vectors are based on the prototype immediate early 3-deleted virus originally made by Roger Everett and the Glasgow group (The IE3 gene encodes a transcription regulator called variously ICP4 or

Vmw175). We realized early on that these HSV-1 IE3 deleted viruses, despite being replication defective, had a significant cytopathic effect and at high multiplicities of infection did significant damage to the infected cells. One interesting cytopathic effect was that, 6 h after infection, large areas of infected BHK cells' chromosomes unwound in a distinctive and reproducible fashion. Because the cytotoxicity of the vectors is caused by continued expression of other viral genes in the vectors, many laboratories are now engaged in engineering defined mutations in HSV-1 vectors to eliminate these cytopathic effects. The laboratories of Neal DeLuca and Joe Glorioso have shown that such an approach is feasible. Undoubtedly, the neurotropic property of the alpha herpesviruses will eventually be useful for gene therapy and for gene delivery to neurons in culture.

The adenoviruses and the adeno-associated viruses (AAV) provide yet another opportunity to use viruses as gene delivery vehicles for the CNS. Adenovirus vectors have been exploited by a number of groups, including those of Michel Perricaudet, Ron Crystal, Jim Wilson and Frank Graham, and AAV vectors have been pioneered particularly in the laboratories of Ken Burns, Tom Shenk, Nick Muzyczka and Jude Samulski. Considerable work has suggested that these vectors can express foreign genes in neurons and much work is being done on manipulating the factors that control the extent and level of foreign gene expression. One issue that must be understood is the cause and nature of the host immune response to viruses such as adenovirus, AAV and HSV-1. Many people have antibodies to these agents because they are naturally widespread in the population, and we do not know whether this will cause problems if these agents are used as gene delivery agents; nor do we know whether it will be possible to make a completely defective virus that does not cause cell damage. The goal with these viruses is to transduce enough cells to obtain a therapeutic effect without inducing an inflammatory or immune response to the viral antigens that are also injected. Much still needs to be done to control the transgene expression of these vectors and control their ability to produce immune responses in the infected host.

One exciting and urgent area of CNS gene therapy is the treatment of CNS tumors by killing tumor cells in the brain using gene delivery. The concept is quite straightforward and involves two key points: first, retroviruses can complete their life cycle only in mitotic cells—they cannot efficiently express themselves in non-dividing cells; second, ganciclovir is a specific anti-herpesvirus drug that kills only herpesvirus-infected cells because the herpes thymidine kinase (TK) gene, but not the cellular TK gene, is able to phosphorylate ganciclovir and convert it into a form that is able to block DNA replication in infected cells. The challenge is to introduce engineered producer cells that deliver a retroviral vector expressing the herpes TK gene directly into gliomas or other brain tumors. The retroviral vector should diffuse from the implanted producer cell and infect neighboring tumor cells. It should be unable to infect (and therefore to express the TK gene) in the post-mitotic cells (e.g. host neurons), but should be able to infect the replicating tumor cells and to express the TK gene in those cells. It is known that cells expressing the HSV TK gene can be killed by giving the patient ganciclovir. Results in animal models are quite encouraging but results of human clinical trials have so far been less definitive.

The use of transgenic mice as models for CNS disease is enabling us to test the basic tenets of gene therapy with some rigor. My laboratory has a long-standing interest in Lesch–Nyhan disease, a particularly difficult disease to study. Thanks largely to the work of Hyder Jinnah, who is now doing clinical work at Johns Hopkins University, we have new understanding and tools for studying this most unusual disease. Surprisingly, when the gene for HPRT is deleted from the mouse (producing a "knock out mouse"), the animals demonstrate no aberrant neurological phenotype. However, a behavioral abnormality can be induced in these mice by exposing them to amphetamine, an agent known to release dopamine from the striatum. Normal animals treated with amphetamine go through an excitatory, hyperactive phase which resolves quickly. This activity is easily monitored and quantitated. Animals deficient in HPRT respond very differently—they get so excited that they are paralyzed and sit down grooming themselves excessively. They exhibit a marked hyperactivity and excessive grooming behavior that results in a slower, biphasic pattern of response. Knock out mice have an abnormal biochemical phenotype similar to that in the Lesch–Nyhan affected human: both have an over-active *de novo* purine pathway and defects in their CNS dopamine pathways.

THE FUTURE

The concepts and tools of human gene therapy matured markedly over the last decade and are now widely accepted by medical, molecular genetic, ethics and public policy communities. The introduction of genetic material into cells to complement genetic defects or to augment aberrant metabolic pathways will come to play a role in the therapy of many kinds of human disease, not only in the relatively uncommon classical inborn errors of metabolism but also in the more universal disorders such as cancer, atherosclerosis and coronary artery disease and even in infectious diseases such as AIDS. Most investigators consider disorders of the central nervous system (CNS) to be relatively unattractive targets for genetic therapy because, more than most other organs, the CNS has seemed inaccessible to genetic manipulation and to be less forgiving of interference with established pathways, normal or aberrant, than most other organs. Adding to the complexities of genetic manipulation of the CNS is the fact that the brain is a highly compartmentalized organ in which the functions of a set of cells in one region can affect the functions of many cells in many other regions. Furthermore, post-mitotic neurons—presumably the appropriate target cells for treatment of many CNS diseases—cannot be infected by the retroviruses, which are well characterized gene transfer tools, because they require cell replication for growth. Despite these apparently discouraging features, recent studies have shown that some diseases and defects of the CNS *are* amenable to genetic approaches to therapy.

The field is in its infancy and major improvements are needed at every level. The rapidity at which advances are being made seems to ensure that the role of gene transfer in the arsenal of neuroscientists in general, and in the treatment of some diseases and defects of the human CNS in particular, is likely to increase.

REFERENCES

Burns J.C., Friedmann T., Driever W., Burrascano M. and Yee X.-K. Vesicular stomatitis virus G glycoprotein pseudotyped retroviral vectors—concentration to very high titer and efficient gene transfer into mammalian and nonmammalian cells. *Proc. Natl Acad. Sci. USA* 1993; **90:** 8033–8037.

Culver K.W., Vickers T.M., Lamsam J.L., Walling H.W. and Seregina T. Gene therapy for solid tumors. *Br. Med. Bull.* 1995; **51:** 192–204.

Friedmann T. A brief history of gene therapy. *Nature Genetics* 1992; **2:** 93–98.

Friedmann T. and Roblin R.R. Gene therapy for human genetic disease? *Science* 1972; **175:** 949–955.

Glorioso J.C., Goins W.F., Fink D.J. and De Luca N. Herpes-simplex virus vectors and gene-transfer to brain. *Dev. Biol. Stand.* 1994; **82:** 79–87.

Graham F.L. and Prevec L. Manipulation of adenovirus vectors, in *Gene Transfer and Expression Protocols*, ed E.J. Murray, Humana Press, pp.109–128, 1991.

Kotin P.M. Perspectives for the use of adeno-associated virus as a vector for human gene therapy. *Hum. Gene Therapy* 1994; **5:** 793–801.

Rosenberg M.B., Friedmann T., Robertson R.C., Tuszynski M., Wolff J.A., Breakfield X.O. and Gage F.H. Grafting genetically modified cells to the damaged brain—restorative effects of NGF expression. *Science* 1988; **242:** 1575–1578.

Sambrook J., Westphal H., Srinivasan P.R. and Dulbecco R. The integrated state of viral DNA in SV40 transformed cells. *Proc. Natl Acad. Sci. USA* 1968; **60:** 1288–1293.

Shimotohno K. and Temin H. Formation of infectious progeny virus after insertion of herpes-simplex thymidine kinase gene into DNA of an avian retrovirus. *Cell* 1981; **26:** 67–77.

Snyder E.Y. Grafting immortalized neurons to the CNS. *Curr. Opin. Neurobiol.* 1994; **4:** 742–751.

Tabin C.J., Hoffman J.W., Goff S.P. and Weinberg R.A. Adaptation of a retrovirus as a eukaryotic vector transmitting the herpes-simplex virus thymidine kinase gene. *Mol. Cell Biol.* 1982; **2:** 426–436.

Wei C., Gibson M., Spear P.G. and Scolnick E.M. Construction and isolation of a transmissible retrovirus containing the *src* gene of Harvey murine sarcoma-virus and the thymidine kinase gene of herpes-simplex virus type-1. *J. Virol.* 1981; **39:** 935–944.

Wolff J.A., Fisher L.J., Xu L., Jinnah H.A., Langlais P.J., Iuovne P.M., O'Malley K.L., Rosenberg M.B., Shimohama S., Friedmann T. and Gage F.H. Grafting fibroblasts genetically modified to produce L-dopa in a rat model of Parkinson disease. *Proc. Natl Acad. Sci. USA* 1989; **86:** 9011–9014.

Yee X.-K., Miyanohara A., La Porte P., Bouic K., Burns J.C. and Friedmann T. A general method for the generation of high-titer, pantropic retroviral vectors—highly efficient infection of primary hepatocytes. *Proc. Natl Acad. Sci. USA* 1994; **91:** 9564–9568.

SECTION 1

Protocols for Gene Delivery to Cultured Cells Using Physical Methods

CHAPTER 2

Calcium-phosphate, DEAE-dextran Coprecipitation, and Electroporation to Transfer Genes into Neuronal and Glial Cell Lines

M.G. Castro, J. Rowe, E. Morrison, P. Tomasec, C.A. Murray, A.F. Shering and P.R. Lowenstein

University of Manchester, School of Medicine, Department of Medicine, Molecular Medicine Unit, Room 1.302, Stopford Building, Manchester M13 9PL, UK. Tel: 0161 275 5671 Fax: 0161 275 5672; Email: mgcastro@manchester.ac.uk

1 INTRODUCTION

Introducing genes into neurons could provide useful information on the molecular and biochemical mechanisms which underlie neuronal function. For example, we can introduce mutations into specific genes and study the effects of these mutations in a neuronal environment using gene transfer techniques. Much information on neuronal function can be gained by using neuronal cell lines as targets for the introduction of genetic material. This approach has been used successfully to study sodium channels (Schever et al., 1990), acetylcholine (Claudio et al., 1987) and 5-HT receptors (Julius et al., 1989) and post-translational processing of neuropeptide precursors, (proopiomelanocortin: Nöel et al., 1989), procorticotrophin-releasing hormone (Castro et al., 1991) and proenkephalin (Lindberg et al., 1991).

We have studied the intracellular trafficking and post-translational processing of neuropeptide precursors. We are currently using procorticotrophin-releasing hormone (proCRH) as a model neuropeptide precursor. This is synthesized within the parvocellular neurons of the hypothalamic paraventricular nucleus (Castro et al., 1992; Swanson et al., 1983) and is cleaved at pairs of basic amino acids to generate the neuropeptide CRH(1-41) (Castro et al., 1991). One of the main physiological roles of CRH(1-41) is the modulation of the endocrine response to stress (Antoni, 1986; Castro, 1993). It has also been identified in cortical neurons and is widely distributed in cells of both the central and the peripheral nervous systems. The level of expression of CRH in the hypothalamus is very low, and any biochemical or biological studies on this precursor molecule have proven to be very difficult. The problems of low expression and instability can be overcome using gene transfer techniques.

Another possible approach to understanding neuropeptide processing is to transfect non-neuronal cells. Thus, expression of proCRH in cells which do not possess a regulated secretory pathway, and therefore lack the enzymes that are primarily responsible for the endoproteolytic processing of proneuropeptides within the regulated secretory pathway of neurons, can constitute a good source of the intact precursor molecule for studies of its biological activity. We are using CHO-K1 cells to express high levels of unprocessed proCRH, which we then use to

Protocols for Gene Transfer in Neuroscience: Towards Gene Therapy of Neurological Disorders
Edited by P.R. Lowenstein and L.W. Enquist

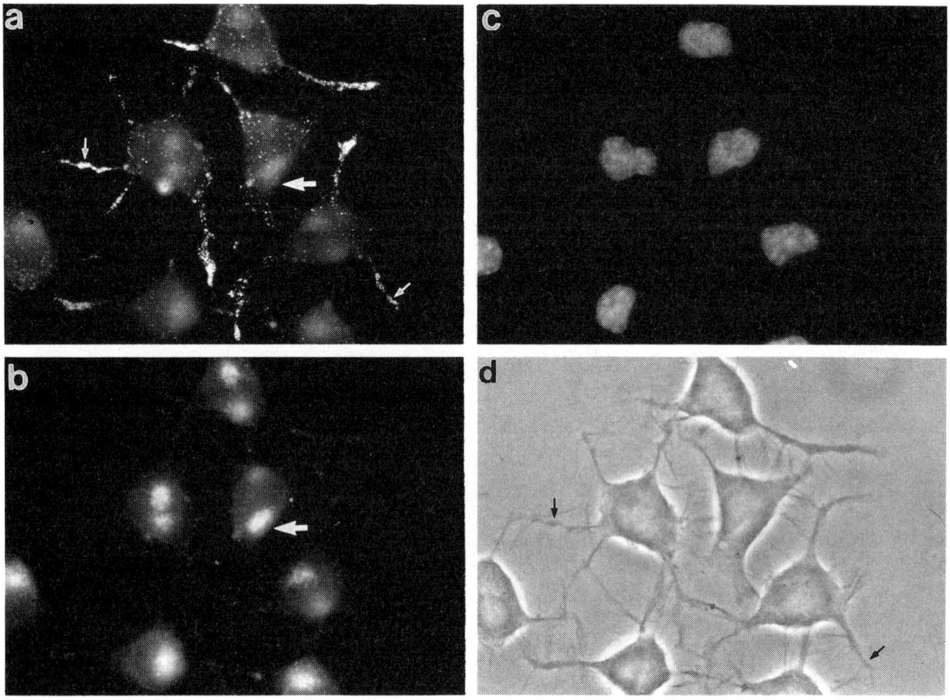

Figure 2.1 Localization of immunoreactive corticotrophin-releasing hormone (IR-CRH) within stably transfected Neuro 2A cells using immunofluorescence techniques. Neuro 2A cells were transfected using pGWH1/rat pre-proCRH cDNA and selected for expression of guanine phosphoribosyl transferase. (a) Stably transfected Neuro 2A cells immunostained with the CRH-specific antibody M2; (b) the same cells stained with fluorescently labeled wheat germ agglutinin (WGA), a histochemical marker for the Golgi apparatus; (c) the cells stained with the DNA-specific dye DAPI to indicate the position of nuclei; (d) phase-contrast image of the same cells. Note the accumulation of IR-CRH along the cellular processes and also at the tips of the processes

examine the putative mitogenic role of the precursor molecule (Castro et al., 1995; Morrison et al., 1995).

In this chapter we shall describe the transfection techniques used in our laboratory to transfect neuronal, glial and fibroblast cell lines. The cells which have been successfully transfected using the methods described below are Neuro 2A, a mouse neuroblastoma cell line (ECACC no. 89112104) (Fig. 2.1); NG115, a mouse neuroblastoma/rat glioma hybrid (ECACC no. 87032003); AtT20 D16V, a mouse corticotrophic tumor cell line (ECACC no. 87021902); CHO-K1, derived from Chinese hamster ovary epithelial cells (ECACC no. 85051005) (Fig. 2.2) and COS-7, a fibroblast cell line derived from African green monkey kidney cells transformed by SV40 (ECACC no. 87021302).

Until recently, it was not possible to use gene transfer techniques for neuronal cells in primary culture because appropriate transfer vectors, which would allow gene transfer into post-mitotic cells, were not available. This has been made possible by the use of viral vectors—herpes simplex type 1, adenovirus and retrovirus vectors.

The methods for introducing foreign genes into cells can be grouped into five main classes:

(1) direct introduction of cloned DNA by microinjection;
(2) use of viral vectors such as herpes simplex type I and adenovirus;
(3) use of carrier systems such as lipofection;

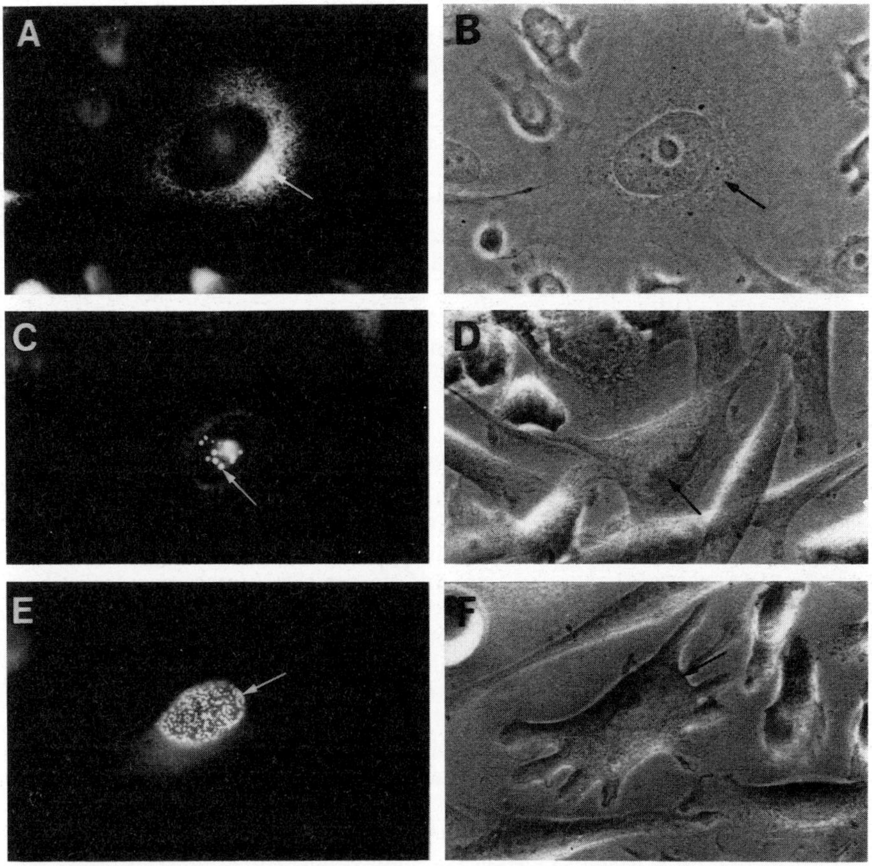

Figure 2.2 Immunoreactive CRH staining patterns in CHO-K1 cells stably transfected with the rat pre-proCRH cDNA. Cells in A, C and E were immunostained with the CRH(1-41)-specific antibody 3B3; B, D, and F are phase-contrast photographs of the cells shown in A, C and E, respectively. (A) transfected CHO-K1 cell displaying the strong perinuclear (arrow) and reticular cytoplasmic immunoreactive CRH staining seen in most transfected cells; (C) transfected CHO-K1 cell displaying large CRH-immunoreactive foci within the nucleoplasm (arrow); (E) transfected CHO-K1 cell displaying small CRH-immunoreactive dots throughout the nucleus. The regions indicated by white arrows in A, C, and E are indicated by black arrows in B, D, and F. (Modified from Morrison et al., 1995)

(4) formation of complexes between DNA and chemical agents such as calcium phosphate or DEAE–dextran;
(5) use of physical methods such as electroporation.

This chapter focuses on the last two categories; the first three classes are reviewed elsewhere in this book.

2 MATERIALS AND EQUIPMENT

2.1 Calcium Phosphate-mediated DNA Transfection

(1) Cells to be transfected at 80% confluence in 75 cm^2 flasks.
(2) DNA stock (from Qiagen Maxi kit; Qiagen Ltd., Dorking, Surrey, UK) in sterile Tris–EDTA

pH 8.0 (10 mM Tris–HCl, 1 mM EDTA).

(3) 2 × Hepes-buffered saline (2 × HBS): Mix 8.18 g NaCl, 5.95 g Hepes and 0.2 g Na_2HPO_4 up to 500 ml distilled water. Adjust pH to 7.1 with approximately 6 ml 1 N NaOH (**The pH of this solution is critical**). Adjust the volume to 500 ml, filter sterilize (0.2 μm filter) and store at 4°C.

(4) 2 M $CaCl_2$. Filter sterilize and store at 4°C.

(5) 15% glycerol–HBS: Mix 15 ml glycerol, 50 ml 2 × HBS and 35 ml distilled water. Filter sterilize and store at 4°C.

(6) Non-selective growth medium: Mix 500 ml Dulbecco's modified Eagle's Medium, 50 ml horse serum, 25 ml newborn calf serum, 6 ml glutamine (100 mM), 6 ml 100 × non-essential amino acids and 6 ml 5000 U penicillin + 6 mg/ml streptomycin.

(7) 2M $CaCl_2$.

(8) Tissue culture media (see next section for details): complete growth medium; selection medium (containing suitable selection agent depending on the marker present in the expression vector); serum-free medium.

2.2 DEAE–dextran-mediated DNA Transfection

(1) COS-7 cells—available from the American Type Culture Collection (ATCC) or the European Collection of Animal Cell Cultures (ECACC).

(2) Dulbecco's modification of Eagle's medium (DMEM), containing 10% horse serum, glutamine at a final concentration of 2 mM, and 1% penicillin/streptomycin solution. This is a basal medium, and COS cells will grow happily in it. COS cells should also grow in supplemented (e.g. with sodium pyruvate, non-essential amino acids) culture medium.

(3) Petri dishes (100 mm) coated for tissue culture (for biochemical analysis), glass coverslips coated with poly-L-lysine in six-well tissue-culture plates (for immunocytochemistry).

(4) Sterile phosphate-buffered saline (PBS, Ca^{2+} and Mg^{2+} free).

(5) DEAE-dextran, 2.5 mg/ml in PBS, filter sterilized and stored at 4°C.

(6) 100 mM chloroquine in PBS. Filter sterilize and store at −20°C in 100 μl aliquots in foil-covered tubes (it is light sensitive).

! CAUTION: CHLOROQUINE IS TOXIC !

(7) Filter-sterilized DMSO (requires solvent-resistant 0.2 μm syringe filters). Store at −20°C in 5 ml aliquots.

(8) Supercoiled plasmid DNA in Tris–EDTA buffer pH 7.4 or sterile water. An adequate concentration to use is 1 μg/μl.

2.2.1 For Immunocytochemical Analysis

(1) Ethanol-washed and air-dried glass coverslips.

(2) Poly-L-lysine dissolved in sterile filtered water at 1 mg/ml.

(3) DEAE transfection cocktail (each 100 mm Petri dish requires 4 ml cocktail): 3.2 ml PBS; 0.6 ml DEAE-dextran in PBS (final concentration 0.25 mg/ml) (McCutchan and Pagano, 1968; Al-Moslih and Dubes, 1973; Oprian et al., 1987; Morrison et al., 1992); Plasmid DNA to a concentration of 5 μg/dish. This cocktail is easily scaled up for multiple plates or down for smaller dishes. Mix by gentle inversion—do not vortex to avoid shearing the plasmid DNA. Warm to 37°C.

2.3 Electric Field Mediated DNA Transfection (Electroporation)

(1) Cells to be transfected in logarithmic phase of growth in non-selective growth medium. This requires approximately 10^7 cells per transfection.

(2) Suitable electroporator (from Bio-Rad, Hoefer, etc.). Models differ according to the electricity mains supply in the country of use—refer to the relevant catalog for details.

(3) Sterile PBS without Ca^{2+} or Mg^{2+} (or Ham F12 media: SEE SECTION 4.4.2).

(4) DNA in sterile Tris–EDTA, pH 8.0.

(5) Non-selective growth medium.
(6) Serum-free medium.
(7) Sterile electroporation cuvettes (0.4 cm) (Bio-Rad).

2.4 Selection for Cells Expressing the Neomycin-resistance Gene

(1) G418: dissolve at 100 mg/ml in PBS. Filter sterilize and store at −20°C in 0.5 ml aliquots.

! G418 IS TOXIC—HANDLE WITH CARE !

(2) Non-selective growth medium (DESCRIBED IN 2.1, ABOVE).

2.5 Selection for Cells Expressing the Glutamine Synthetase Gene

2.5.1 Stock Solutions for GMEM-S Medium

(1) Double-distilled water, autoclaved in 400 ml aliquots.
(2) 10× Glasgow MEM without glutamine and tryptose phosphate broth (Gibco 042-02541). Store at 4°C.
(3) 7.5% sodium bicarbonate (Gibco 043-05080). Store at 4°C.
(4) 100× non-essential amino acids (NEAA) (Gibco 043-01140). Store at 4°C.
(5) 100× glutamate and asparagine (G+A): Mix 600 mg L-glutamic acid with 600 mg L-asparagine (Sigma). Make up to 100 ml in distilled water and sterilize by passing through a 2 μm filter (Nalgene). Store at 4°C.
(6) 100 mM sodium pyruvate (GIBCO 043-01360).
(7) 50× nucleosides:

35 mg adenosine
35 mg guanosine
35 mg cytidine
35 mg uridine
12 mg thymidine

(each from Sigma). Make up to 100 ml with distilled water, filter sterilize and store at −20°C in 10 ml aliquots.

(8) Dialysed FCS (GIBCO 014-06300). Heat-inactivate at 56°C for 30 min and store at −20°C.
(9) Penicillin–streptomycin at 5000 units/ml (P/S; GIBCO 043-05070).
(10) 100 mM L-MSX (Sigma). Prepare a solution of 18 mg/ml in PBS. Filter sterilize and store at −20°C in 1 ml aliquots.

! MSX IS TOXIC–HANDLE WITH CARE !

2.5.2 Stock Solutions for GMEM-Met Medium

(See stock solutions for GMEM-S medium, above).

100× methionine: dissolve 600 mg methionine in 100 ml distilled water. Filter sterilize and store at 4°C.

2.5.3 Media Preparation

(1) GMEM-S medium: Add the following in the order given and filter sterilize using a 500 ml, 0.2 μm filter unit (Nalgene).

Water	400 ml
10× GMEM	50 ml
Sodium bicarbonate	18.1 ml
NEAA	5 ml
G+A	5 ml
Sodium pyruvate	5 ml

Nucleosides	10 ml
Dialysed FCS	50 ml
Penicillin–streptomycin	5 ml

(2) GMEM-Met medium: Add the following in the order given and filter sterilize using a 500 ml, 0.2 μm filter unit (Nalgene).

Water	410 ml
10 × GMEM	50 ml
Sodium bicarbonate	18.1 ml
NEAA	5 ml
Sodium pyruvate	5 ml
Methionine	5 ml
Dialysed FCS	50 ml
G+A	1 ml
Penicillin–streptomycin	5 ml

The glutamate and asparagine concentrations are reduced to 100 μM each, nucleosides are omitted and the methionine concentration is increased to 500μM, compared with GMEM-S.

2.6 Selection for Cells Expressing the Guanine Phosphoribosyl Transferase (*gpt*) Gene

(1) 50 × H-T supplement (GIBCO 043-01065H).
(2) 50 × Xanthine: Prepare a solution of 12.5 mg/ml in 0.2 M NaOH. Filter sterilize and store at −20°C.
(3) 50 × Mycophenolic acid: Prepare a solution of 500 μg/ml in 0.1 M NaOH. Filter sterilize and store at −20°C.

! CAUTION: MYCOPHENOLIC ACID IS TOXIC !

(4) 50 × Aminopterin: Prepare a solution of 0.1 mg/ml in distilled water. Filter sterilize and store at −20°C.

! EXTREME CARE: AMINOPTERIN IS A POISON !

(5) 1 M HCl.
(6) Dulbecco's MEM with 0.11 g/l sodium pyruvate.
(7) 100 mM Glutamine.
(8) Dialysed fetal calf serum.

2.6.1 Media Preparation

Add the following in the order given and filter sterilize using a 500 ml, 0.2 μm filter unit (Nalgene).

Dulbecco's MEM (with 0.11 g/l sodium pyruvate)	86.5 ml
H-T supplement	2 ml
50 × Xanthine	2 ml
50 × Mycophenolic acid	2 ml
Dialysed FCS	5 ml
Aminopterin	2 ml
1 M HCl (to return the phenol red pH indicator to the normal orange-red color)	600 μl
Glutamine	0.5 ml

2.7 Isolation of Clonal Cell Lines of Stably Transfected Cells

(1) Tissue culture Petri dishes, 35 mm diameter.
(2) Sterile filter paper squares (Whatman no. 1 paper), 3 mm^2.
(3) Sterile forceps.
(4) 1 × Trypsin–EDTA solution (Sigma).
(5) Sterile PBS without Ca^{2+} or Mg^{2+}.
(6) Non-selective growth medium (SEE UNDER 2.1, ABOVE).

3 THE PROTOCOLS

Protocol #1: Vector Preparation for Physical Transfection Methods

(1) Grow bacteria harboring the expression vector overnight in 400 ml culture containing the appropriate antibiotic.
(2) Harvest bacteria and isolate the plasmid DNA using the Qiagen Maxiprep kit, following the manufacturer's instructions.
(3) Resuspend the isolated DNA at 0.5 mg/ml in sterile water or sterile Tris–EDTA pH 8.0.

Protocol #2: Preparation of Cells for Transfection

(1) Keep cells growing exponentially in non-selective growth medium without allowing them to reach confluency before transfection.
(2) The day before transfection, trypsinize the cells.
(3) Keep all solutions at 37°C in a water bath.
(4) Remove the media from the flasks by aspiration and add 1 ml of 1 × trypsin (25 cm^2 flask), or 2 ml for a 75 cm^2 flask.
(5) Return the flask to the incubator for 1–2 min.
(6) Examine the cells under an inverted microscope: they should exhibit a rounded appearance.
(7) Dislodge the cells from the flask by gentle shaking. If the cells remain adherent, return the flask to the incubator for a further minute.
(8) When the cells have been dislodged, add 10 ml of serum-containing medium (10% horse serum) to stop trypsin digestion and pipette the cell suspension up and down in order to disrupt any clumps (**avoid making bubbles**).
(9) Count the cells and replate them onto 10 cm Petri dishes at 10^6 cells per dish in 10 ml non-selective growth medium.

Protocol #3: Calcium Phosphate-mediated DNA Transfection

(1) Day 1: Bring the 2 × HBS and 2 M $CaCl_2$ solutions to room temperature.
(2) In a sterile tube, mix 62 μl 2 M $CaCl_2$ and 10 μg supercoiled DNA. Bring the volume to 0.5 ml with sterile Tris–EDTA, pH 8.0. This must be done for **each** dish to be transfected—always include a mock transfection solution in which Tris–EDTA is added instead of the DNA.
(3) Add 0.5 ml 2× HBS to a second sterile 15 ml tube.
(4) Form a precipitate, by adding the DNA in $CaCl_2$ to the 2× HBS solution **very slowly**, dropwise with continuous agitation.
(5) Immediately vortex the mixture for 10 s. The precipitate should have a fine-grained translucent appearance.
(6) Wash the cells in serum-free medium by aspirating off the existing medium, adding 10 ml serum-free medium and reaspirating immediately.
(7) Add the calcium phosphate–DNA precipitate, together with 1 ml serum-free medium, to the cells and return the dish to the incubator.
(8) Incubate the dishes at 37°C for 3.5–4 h, rocking them occasionally to ensure that they do not dry out.
(9) Remove the calcium phosphate–DNA precipitate from the cells by aspiration.
(10) Add 3 ml 15% glycerol–HBS to each dish and incubate at 37°C for 1.5 min.
(11) Add 10 ml serum-free medium and immediately remove by aspiration.
(12) Add 10 ml complete non-selective growth medium and return the dish to the incubator.
(13) After 24 h incubation, replace the medium with 10 ml selection medium.
(14) Feed with the appropriate selective medium (SEE PROTOCOL #7) after 4 days, and continue feeding until all the cells in the mock transfection are dead. Resistant colonies should appear in the transfected dishes after 2–3 weeks.

Protocol #4: DEAE Transfection Method

(1) On the day of the procedure prepare 4 ml of DEAE transfection cocktail per 100 mm Petri dish to be transfected.
(2) Remove the tissue culture medium from the dish by aspiration, rinse the cells once in prewarmed PBS and add the DNA cocktail to the dish. Spread evenly by tilting the dish and incubate at 37°C for 30 min. Tilt the plate occasionally to ensure that it is evenly covered and that the cells do not dry out.
(3) Without removing the DNA cocktail, add 8–10 ml prewarmed culture medium containing 100 μm chloroquine to each dish. Swirl gently to mix. If the dish is too small, remove some of the cocktail to accommodate the chloroquine/media mixture. Incubate the cells at 37°C for 2.5–3 h.
(4) Remove the supernatant by aspiration and add 4 ml prewarmed tissue culture medium containing 10% DMSO to each plate.
(5) Incubate at room temperature for 2.5 min (no longer), then remove the supernatant by aspiration and wash twice in 10 ml prewarmed culture medium.
(6) Add 10 ml culture medium to each plate and incubate at 37°C. Use the transfected culture within 72 h. It is important to prepare all the final solutions at the same time on the day of the transfection (store the chloroquine/medium in a dark container). After 48–72 h of incubation, both the culture medium and the cell extracts can be harvested for biochemical analysis.

Protocol #5: DEAE Transfection Method Followed by Immunocytochemical Analysis

(1) Grow cells on poly-L-lysine coated coverslips in six-well plates (coating procedure is described immediately below).
(2) Place the sterilized coverslips in each well of the plate.
(3) Cover the glass coverslips with poly-L-lysine solution. Use only enough to just cover the coverslips—if the solution spills onto the base of the plate it may weld the coverslip to the plastic, which makes the later steps of the procedure very difficult.
(4) Leave at room temperature in a laminar flow cabinet for at least 4 h, or overnight. The poly-L-lysine solution may dry out, but this is not a problem.
(5) Wash the coverslips by adding 2 ml sterile water to each well. Ensure that the water reaches underneath the coverslips by gently lifting them with sterile forceps.
(6) Incubate the plate for 2 h at room temperature, then aspirate and repeat the washing process.
(7) After washing for the second time, add 1 ml culture medium to each plate. Ideally, the plates should now be left in an incubator at 37°C overnight or longer, but 2–3 h is sufficient if time is pressing. After about 5–7 days in the incubator the poly-L-lysine may begin to detach from the glass. This is visible under an inverted microscope and if it happens new coverslips must be prepared.
(8) Remove the culture medium by aspiration before adding the COS cell suspension to the plate. The cells must be in the exponential phase of growth on the day of transfection.

Transfection procedure

(1) Each well receives 1 ml of the DNA cocktail, so prepare cocktail in batches of 6 ml (4.8 ml PBS and 1.2 ml DEAE-dextran). Each six-well plate is approximately equivalent to one 100 mm Petri dish, so plasmid DNA is added at 5 μg per six-well plate.
(2) After the first incubation add 2–3 ml medium with chloroquine to each well, incubate for 2.5 h and then remove medium by aspiration.
(3) Add 1 ml 10% DMSO in medium to each well. Leave for 2.5 minutes, then remove by aspiration and wash twice with 2 ml culture medium per well.
(4) Process the cells for immunocytochemistry, preferably within 48 h of transfection—after this the cells deteriorate due to plasmid replication and concomitant cell lysis.

Fixation

(1) Wash the cells once in prewarmed PBS.
(2) Add 2 ml ice-cold freshly prepared 4% paraformaldehyde in 0.1 M PBS, pH 7.4, to each well for 20 minutes. Aspirate this solution and wash the cells four times (5 min each wash) in PBS.

We carry out most of our immunofluorescence staining protocol in the six-well plate, which is very convenient. For a detailed protocol of the immunofluorescence technique, see Lowenstein et al., 1994.

Protocol #6: Electroporation-mediated DNA Transfection

(1) Day 1: trypsinize the cells and seed into 175 cm^2 flasks. Leave overnight at 37°C in complete growth medium.
(2) Day 2: trypsinize the cells and spin down in a bench-top centrifuge at 1000 r.p.m. for 5 min. Cells should be in the logarithmic growth phase.
(3) Wash the cells in 10 ml sterile PBS. Count the cells using a hemocytometer and centrifuge again as in step 2.
(4) Resuspend the pellet to 1×10^7 cells/ml in ice-cold PBS (or Ham F12 media). The volume of cell suspension should not exceed 0.8 ml per transfection.
(5) Transfer 0.8 ml aliquots of cell suspension to separate tubes.
(6) Add 40 μg linearized DNA to each tube. **Always** include a mock transfection, in which no DNA is added.
(7) Incubate the cell–DNA suspension on ice for 15 min.
(8) Transfer the suspension to an electroporation cuvette (0.4 cm) and electroporate at 1000 V, 25 μF (for PBS) or 250 V, 960 μF (Ham F12 media).
(9) Immediately place the cuvette on ice for 15 min.
(10) Add the electroporated cell suspension to 30 ml complete growth medium.
(11) Distribute 10 ml of the resultant cell suspension into a 96-well tissue culture plate (100 μl/well).
(12) Mix 10 ml of the cell suspension with 10 ml non-selective growth medium and distribute into two 96-well tissue culture plates.
(13) Mix the remaining 10 ml cell suspension with 40 ml non-selective medium and distribute into five 100 mm Petri dishes (10 ml per dish).
(14) Return all the plates and dishes to the incubator and incubate for 24 h at 37°C, in an atmosphere of 5% CO_2.
(15) Day 3: feed the cells with selection medium.
(16) Feed the cells again after 4 days. Continue feeding every 4 days until the cells in the mock transfection are all dead, and resistant colonies appear in the transfected dishes (usually 2–3 weeks after transfection).

Protocol #7: How to Select Cell Clones Expressing Transfected Transgenes

Selection for Cells Expressing the Neomycin Resistance Gene

(1) Add G418 to the non-selective growth medium, to a final concentration of 1 mg/ml.
(2) Remove the culture medium from the transfected cells 1 day after transfection and add selective medium.
(3) Change selective medium every 4 days until discrete colonies appear.

Selection for Cells Expressing the Glutamine Synthetase Gene

(1) On the day after transfection remove the non-selective culture medium from the transfected cells by aspiration.
(2) Add GMEM-S medium (10 ml per dish) containing the minimum concentration of MSX which will result in the total cell death of wild-type cells.
(3) Change medium every 4 days until discrete colonies appear.

Selection for Cells Expressing the Guanine Phosphoribosyl Transferase (*gpt*) gene

(1) One day after transfection remove the non-selective growth medium from the transfected cells by aspiration.
(2) Add *gpt*-selective medium (10 ml/dish).

Protocol #8: How to Isolate Clonal Cell Lines of Stably Transfected Cells

(1) Examine the transfected cell colonies under an inverted microscope. Mark the colonies to be picked using a marker pen on the underside of the dish.
(2) In a sterile laminar flow hood, add 2 ml non-selective growth media to as many 35 mm dishes as there are colonies to be picked, and label each dish clearly. (We usually pick 12–18 colonies from each transfection.)
(3) To a separate 35 mm dish add 2 ml 1 × trypsin–EDTA solution. Transfer the filter paper squares to this dish and allow them to soak.
(4) Wash the transfected cells twice by aspirating the culture medium and adding 10 ml (calcium/magnesium-free) PBS.
(5) Using sterile forceps, lay one trypsin-soaked filter paper square on top of each selected colony and return the dish to the incubator at 37°C for 1 min.
(6) Remove the filter paper squares from the colonies and place immediately into separate 35 mm dishes containing non-selective growth media. Swirl each dish gently to detach the cells from the filter paper, and place the dish in the incubator overnight at 37°C.
(7) After 24 h incubation, examine the cells under the inverted microscope to look for cell survival and attachment and select the cells using the appropriate selection media.
(8) Feed the cells every 4 days until 50–60% confluent. At this point the cells need to be transferred to larger culture vessels (e.g. 12.5 cm^2 flasks (Falcon)). To do this follow the cell trypsinization protocol detailed at the beginning of this section (SEE PAGE 15), using 200 μl trypsin and adding 1.8 ml growth medium after trypsinization.

4 NOTES AND TROUBLESHOOTING

4.1 On Protocol #1: Vector Preparation

The Qiagen method uses an anion-exchange column to bind plasmid DNA from cell lysates and to allow effective washing out of contaminants before plasmid elution. This method is faster than CsCl purification and avoids the use of toxic chemicals such as phenol and ethidium bromide. Yields are good (0.5–1 mg plasmid DNA from 500 ml overnight cultures, depending on the plasmid) and the DNA is suitable for a wide variety of molecular biology manipulations.

Circular plasmid DNA, purified once by CsCl density gradient centrifugation, may also be used. The plasmid DNA preparation should be checked to ensure that it is free of chromosomal DNA and RNA.

Electroporation is more efficient if linearized DNA is used. The restriction enzyme used in the linearization must be one that cuts only once, and it must not cut within an important part of the vector (e.g. the inserted gene, the promoter sequence or the selectable marker). Between 20 and 40 μg of linear DNA should be used per transfection. DNA can be used in restriction buffer, provided that the buffer is sterile (maximum volume 0.2 ml). Alternatively, the DNA may be ethanol-precipitated and resuspended in 100 μl sterile distilled water. Linearization may be checked by running a few microliters on an 0.8% agarose gel containing ethidium bromide.

! CAUTION: ETHIDIUM BROMIDE IS HAZARDOUS !

4.2 On Protocol #3: Calcium Phosphate-mediated DNA Transfection

4.2.1 General Considerations

The calcium phosphate-mediated DNA transfection technique was pioneered by Graham and Van der Eb in 1973. Since then many other methods have been used to overcome some of the disadvantages associated with this technique which are described below (Morgan et al., 1986;

Brash et al., 1987; Chen and Okayama, 1987; Appel et al., 1988). Calcium phosphate coprecipitation of DNA remains the most popular technique because it is effective for a wide range of cell types, is simple to perform and is low cost.

4.2.2 Critical Factors for Successful Experiments

Several issues have proven critical for the success of transfections using this technique.

(1) Efficiency of gene transfer depends on the amount of DNA used; 10–20 μg/100 mm dish has been quoted as optimum (Graham and Bacchetti, 1983) but the optimum concentration varies between cell types and must be determined empirically.
(2) The physical condition of the calcium phosphate–DNA precipitate plays a key role. Luckily it can be assessed visually! It should be a hazy white suspension (Graham and Van der Eb, 1973; Wigler et al., 1979; Graham and Bacchetti, 1983). If the precipitated DNA sinks to the bottom of the tube it must be purified by phenol extraction before preparing another precipitate.
(3) The time of incubation of the cells with the precipitate can be varied from 4 to 7 h.
(4) The pH of the HBS used to prepare the precipitate is critical.
(5) The quality of the cells is important. Use **only** cells in the logarithmic growth phase (Graham and Bacchetti, 1983; Rippe et al., 1990).
(6) Treatment of cells with DMSO or glycerol facilitates DNA uptake. The concentration of these reagents (usually 10–20%) and the treatment time needs to be optimized for specific cell lines.
(7) Circular DNA is more effective than linear DNA.
(8) The rate at which the precipitate is formed is important. Precipitation should be performed slowly, drop by drop, while bubbling air through the forming precipitate.

4.2.3 Problems, Limitations and Troubleshooting

The calcium phosphate technique also has its drawbacks—cytotoxicity associated with prolonged exposure, low efficiency and an inability to transfect certain cell types, such as those grown in suspension culture (Pohl et al., 1991). Results obtained using this technique are qualitatively reproducible although there is a great quantitative variability, for example in the number of transfected cells, from one experiment to another.

4.3 On Protocol #4: DEAE-dextran-mediated DNA Transfection, and Protocol #5: DEAE Transfection Method Followed by Immunocytochemical Analysis

4.3.1 General Considerations

These methods are ideally suited for experiments in which only transient expression of transfected genes is required, for example to produce a peptide that can then be tested in a biological assay. The cell line of choice for transient transfection assays is COS-7, an African Green Monkey kidney fibroblast cell line. The techniques are mostly used when there is a need for quick, reproducible results—for example in the rapid characterization of newly cloned cDNAs. A prime example from the point of view of a neuroscientist might be the expression of a receptor cDNA in COS cells. To check whether the adenylate cyclase-linked receptor cloned is functional transfect the COS cells with the cDNA in an appropriate expression vector, wait a day or two then treat the cells with the specific ligand for the receptor and measure the increase in intracellular cAMP.

We have used the COS system (1) for characterizing specific antibodies to the corticotrophin-releasing hormone receptor via both Western blots of transiently transfected cell extracts and immunocytochemistry of cells on coverslips; (2) to study the trafficking and processing of neuropeptide precursors within the constitutive secretory pathway, as COS cells lack a regulated secretory pathway and; (3) to study the biosynthetic pathway and constitutive activation of the CRH receptor. Other examples of the use of this system include the expression of pituitary adenylate cyclase-activating protein (PACAP) (Ohkubo et al., 1992) and studies on the degradation of nuclear proteins (Tsuneoka and Mekada, 1992).

The use of transient transfection systems has a number of advantages over using stable transfection assays:

- COS cells are extremely easy to look after in tissue culture because they grow rapidly and are very hardy. This allows experiments to be planned and carried out very quickly.
- The technique is simple, fast and very reliable.
- The COS system is designed to express high levels of recombinant proteins.

This last point is perhaps the most important when studying the molecular and biochemical properties of receptors and neuropeptide precursors which are expressed at relatively low levels *in vivo*. COS cells were immortalized using replication-deficient SV40, a double-stranded DNA tumor virus which integrates into the host genome. These viruses cause tumors, primarily through the expression of a viral protein referred to as the "large T antigen". This protein is responsible for the replication of the SV40 genome, as well as interacting with cellular components to cause cell immortalization. In COS cells the integrated SV40 genome lacks the viral origin of replication and is therefore incapable of replication (Gluzman, 1981); however, it still produces large amounts of large T antigen and this is exploited by the expression vectors used for COS transfections. These vectors carry a functional SV40 origin of replication (Tsui et al., 1982) in addition to having the usual features of a eukaryotic expression vector (except perhaps a selectable marker). After transfection into COS cells the vector interacts with large T antigen and is rapidly replicated, increasing the copy number of the cloned cDNA in the transfected cell. Very large yields of recombinant protein may therefore be obtained for up to 3 days after transfection, after which time the transfected cells die. In conclusion, if you wish to express large amounts of recombinant proteins fast the COS system could be your system of choice.

This is a very robust technique, and few problems will be experienced even if the incubation times quoted in Section (3) are not strictly followed. We usually achieve transfection efficiencies of 10–15%, as measured by immunofluorescence.

During routine tissue culture do not allow the COS cells to become confluent before splitting them, especially before setting up a transfection, because they form monolayers which are very resistant to trypsinization and will tend to detach in sheets or clumps. This makes it difficult to seed the plates with a well-dispersed cell suspension. Clumpy cultures are no good for immunocytochemistry, and they decrease the transfection efficiency.

Because of the nature of the transfection technique, the appearance of cell debris is inevitable. If, however, cells are detaching on a large scale before transfection or up to 72 hours after transfection either change your supplier of tissue culture plastics or serum or change your coverslip supplier. German glass is reputed to be the best.

Coverslips can also be washed in chromic acid, followed by distilled water, and then baked; this may improve the adherence of poly-L-lysine to the glass.

Generally speaking, the better the quality and the fresher the preparation of DNA and reagents, the better the results of transfection will be.

4.4 On Protocol #6: Electroporation-mediated DNA Transfection

4.4.1 General Considerations

Electroporation is becoming popular for the introduction of exogenous DNA into a wide variety of cells (Potter et al, 1984; Fromm et al., 1985). The first requisite for the acquisition of exogenous DNA by a cell, using electroporation, is the formation of hydrophilic pores in the cell membrane (Knutson and Yee, 1987; Neuman, 1989; Xie et al., 1990). Alternatively, DNA could be taken into the cells as a result of the electrostimulated formation of endosome-like vesicles (Chernomordik et al., 1990). Unlike calcium phosphate–DNA coprecipitation, in which DNA entering the cell is taken into phagocytic vesicles, electroporated DNA remains free in the cytosol and nucleoplasm (Potter, 1988). Such molecules are ultimately transported to the nucleus by as yet undefined mechanisms, and a subset of these molecules is stably integrated into the host chromosomes.

Linearized DNA is more efficient in allowing for the generation of recombinant cells than supercoiled or nicked circular DNA (in contrast to the calcium phosphate-mediated transfection technique). This could be one of the reasons why lower mutation frequencies are observed for electroporated DNA than with DNA introduced into cells by the calcium phosphate–DNA coprecipitation method (Toneguzzo et al., 1988).

Six key parameters influence the success of the electroporation method:

- The strength of the electrical field.
- The duration of the current pulse.
- The shape of the current pulse.
- The conductivity of the electroporation buffer.
- The DNA concentration.
- The cell concentration.

The control of the first three parameters is a function of the electroporator used. We have successfully used the Bio-Rad Gene Pulser apparatus (catalog number 165-2078).

4.4.2 Advantages

Advantages associated with the electroporation method include

- Ease of operation
- It may be used for both stable and transient transfection procedures
- It works with cells in suspension as well as with attached cells
- The conditions are reproducible
- The number of DNA molecules transfected is controllable.

One important technical difference between electroporation and other transfer methods is that the number of cells required is considerably higher for electroporation.

Some cell lines may be sensitive to high voltages and thus different electroporation buffers should be tested and/or used. For example, the use of Ham F-12 media at 250 V, 960 μF may give higher transfection frequencies than using PBS at 1000 V, 25 μF. The conditions must be manipulated to suit the cell line used. Optimal transfection is usually obtained at about 40–70% cell viability.

4.5 On Protocol #7: How to Select Cell Clones Expressing Transfected Transgenes

4.5.1 Selection for the Glutamine Synthetase Gene

A number of cells have endogenous glutamine synthetase (GS) activity, which allows them to grow in glutamine free medium, and the level of methionine sulfoximine (MSX) required to kill non-transfected control cells, including those which have amplified the endogenous GS genes, should be determined empirically. Transfection of a GS minigene expressed from the SV40 late promoter (Cockett et al., 1990) confers resistance to high levels of MSX.

In our hands, neuronal and glial cell lines (Neuro2A and NG115) are **not** successfully selected using this method because they express high levels of endogenous GS. However, AtT20 cells (anterior pituitary tumor cells) have been successfully selected using this method.

For cells which express high levels of endogenous GS the alternative medium GMEM-Met (in which the methionine concentration is increased) may be used. The MSX is partially detoxified via the methionine catabolism pathway and if the methionine concentration levels are raised this pathway becomes saturated, which increases the cytotoxicity of the MSX. However, some cells do not grow as well in this medium as in GMEM-S, and this should be determined empirically for each cell line to be transfected. GMEM-Met medium is useful in reducing the concentration of MSX needed to select cells with very high levels of endogenous GS activity.

4.6 On Protocol #8: How to Isolate Clonal Cell Lines of Stably Transfected Cells

4.6.1 Isolation of Clonal Cell lines of Stably Transfected Cells

As soon as colonies of cells begin to appear in the transfected dishes they must be isolated to ensure that pure clones of stably transfected cells are generated. Each clone will contain cells with the foreign DNA integrated into the same genomic site.

ACKNOWLEDGMENTS

This work was supported by project grants from the BBSRC (SERC: Biological Sciences) to M.G.C. and P.R.L. and from the BBSRC (Chemicals and Pharmaceuticals Directorate) to M.G.C. C.A.M is supported by a studentship from the BBSRC (SERC: Biological Sciences). We also wish to acknowledge the support our laboratories received from the Wellcome Trust, the Medical Research Council, the Welsh Scheme for the Development of Health and Social Research, the Royal Society, the Sir Halley Stewart Trust, the Nuffield Foundation and the Department of Physiology, University of Wales College of Cardiff. The expression vectors carrying the GS selectable marker were generously provided by doctors M. Cockett and C. Bebbington, Celltech Ltd., Slough, UK, and the expression vector carrying the gpt selectable marker by Dr J. Devine, British Biotechnology Ltd., Headington, Oxford, UK. We would also like to thank Professor V. Crunelli for his support and encouragement, Mrs M. Treloar and Mrs C. Hayes for their skilful secretarial assistance, Mr Bob Jones for outstanding photographic support and Mr Phil Blanning for excellent technical support.

REFERENCES

Al-Moslih, M.I. and Dubes, G.R. 1973. The kinetics of DEAE-Dextran-induced cell sensitization to transfection. *J. Gen. Virol.* **18:** 189–193.

Antoni, F.A. 1986. Hypothalamic control of adrenocorticotrophin secretion: advances since the discovery of 41-residues corticotrophin-releasing factor. *Endocrinol. Rev.* **7:** 351–378.

Appel, J.D., Fasey, T.M., Kohtz, D.S., Kohtz, J.D. and Johnson, E.M. 1988. Asbestos fibers mediate transformation of monkey cells by exogenous plasmid DNA. *Proc. Natl Acad. Sci. USA.* **85:** 7670–7674.

Brash, D.E., Reddel, R.R., Quanrund, M., Yang, K., Farrell, M.P. and Harris, C.C. 1987. Strontium phosphate transfection of human cells in primary culture: stable expression of the simian minus 40 large-T-antigen gene in primary human bronchial epithelial cells. *Mol. Cell Biol.* **7:** 2031–2034.

Castro, M.G. 1993. Effects of corticotrophin-releasing factor and arginine–vasopressin on proopiomelanocortin (POMC) RNA levels, release and storage of adrenocorticotrophin from mouse anterior pituitary cells. *Comp. Biochem. Physiol.* **104(A):** 105–112.

Castro, M.G., Brooke, J., Bullman, A., Hannah, M., Glynn, B.P. and Lowry, P.J. 1991. Biosynthesis of corticotrophin-releasing hormone (CRH) in mouse corticotrophic tumour cells expressing the human proCRH gene: intracellular storage and regulated secretion. *J. Mol. Endocrinol.* **7:** 97–104.

Castro, M.G., Lowry, P.J. and Lowenstein, P.R. 1992. Antibodies to neuropeptide precursors expressed as fusion proteins in *E. coli*: Their use to examine neuropeptide biosynthetic pathways, intracellular trafficking and physiological activities. *Int. J. Biochem.* **24(6):** 847–860.

Castro, M.G., Tomasec, P., Morrison, E., Murray, C.A., Hodge, P., Blanning, P., Linton, E., Lowry, P.J. and Lowenstein, P.R. 1995. Mitogenic effects and nuclear localisation of procorticotrophin-releasing hormone expressed within stably transfected fibroblast cells (CHO-K1). *Mol. Cell Endocrinol.* **107:** 17–27.

Chen, C. and Okayama, H. 1987. High-efficiency transformation of mammalian cells by plasmid DNA. *Mol. Cell Biol.* **7:** 2745–2752.

Chernormordik, L.V., Sokolov, A.V. and Budber, V.G. 1990. Electrostimulated uptake of DNA by liposomes. *Biochem. Biophys. Acta* **1024:** 179–183.

Claudio, T., Green, W.N., Hartman, D., Hayden, D. and Paupson, H.L. 1987. Genetic reconstitution of functional acetylcholine receptor channels in mouse fibroblasts. *Science* **238:** 1688–1694.

Cockett, M.I., Bebbington, C.R. and Yarranton, G.T. 1990. High level expression of tissue inhibitor of metalloproteinases in Chinese Hamster ovary cells using glutamine synthetase gene amplification. *Bio/Technology* **8:** 662–667.

Fromm, M.E., Taylor, L.P. and Wallot, V. 1985. Expression of genes transferred into monocot and dicot plants by electroporation. *Proc. Natl Acad. Sci. USA* **82:** 5824–5829.

Gluzman, Y. 1981. SV40 transformed simian cells support the replication of early SV40 mutants. *Cell* **23:** 175–182.

Graham, F.L. and Bacchetti, S. 1983. DNA mediated gene transfer of drosophila hsp 70–cat hybrid gene in

Aedes cells induced by heat shock. *Som. Cell Mol. Genet.* **11:** 371–377.

Graham, F.L. and Van der Eb, V. 1973. A new technique for the assay of infectivity of human adenovirus 5 DNA. *Virology* **52:** 456–467.

Julius, D., Livelli, T.J., Jessel, T.M. and Axel, R. 1989. Ectopic expression of the serotonin 1c receptor and the triggering of malignant transformation. *Science* **244:** 1057–1062.

Knutson, Y.C. and Yee, D. 1987. Electroporation: parameters affecting transfer of DNA into mammalian cells. *Analyt. Biochem.* **164:** 44–52.

Lindberg, I., Shaw, E., Finley, J., Leone, D. and Deininger, P. 1991. Post-translational modifications of rat proenkephalin overexpressed in Chinese Hamster Ovary cells. *Endocrinology* **128:** 1849–1856.

Lowenstein, P.R., Morrison, E.E., Bain, D., Shering, A.F., Banting, G., Douglas, P. and Castro, M.G. 1994. Polarized distribution of the trans-golgi network marker TGN38 during the *in vitro* development of neocortical neurons: effects of nocodazole and brefeldin A. *Eur. J. Neurosci.* **6:** 1453–1465.

McCutchan, J.H. and Pagano, J.S. 1968. Enhancement of the infectivity of simian virus 40 deoxyribonucleic acid with diethylaminoethyldextran. *J. Natl Cancer Inst.* **41:** 351–356.

Morgan, T.L., Maher, V.M., McCormick, J.J. 1986. Optimal parameters for the polybrene-induced DNA transfection of diploid human fibroblasts. *In Vitro Cell. Dev. Biol.* **22:** 317–319.

Morrison, E., Lowenstein, P.R., Tomasec, P., Hodge, P., Linton, E., Devine, J., Lowry, P.J. and Castro, M.G. 1992. Intracellular compartmentalization of procorticotrophin-releasing hormone. *Biochem. Soc. Trans.* **21:** 47S.

Morrison, E., Tomasec, P., Linton, E.A., Lowry, P.J., Lowenstein, P.R. and Castro, M.G. 1995. Expression of biologically active procorticotrophin-releasing hormone (proCRH) in stably transfected CHO-K1 cells: characterisation of nuclear proCRH. *J. Neuroendocrinol.* **7:** 263–272.

Neuman, E. 1989. The relaxation hysteresis of membrane electroporation. In: *Electroporation and Electrofusion in Cell Biology*. Neuman, E., Gowers, A.E. and Jordan, C.A., eds. New York: Plenum Press, pp.61–82.

Nöel, G., Zollinger, L., Laliberte, F., Rossart, E., Crine, P. and Boileau, G. 1989. Targeting and processing of pro-opiomelanocortin in neuronal cell lines. *J. Neurochem.* **52:** 1050–1057.

Ohkubo, S., Kimura, C., Ogi, K., Okazaki, K., Hosoya, M., Onda, H., Miyata, A., Arimura, A. and Fujino, M. 1992. Primary structure and characterisation of the precursor to human pituitary adenylate cyclase activating polypeptide. *DNA Cell Biol.* **11:** 21–30.

Oprian, D.D., Molday, R.S., Kaufman, R.J. and Khorana, H.G. 1987. Expression of synthetic bovine rhodopsin gene in monkey kidney cells. *Proc. Natl Acad. Sci. USA.* **84:** 8874–8878.

Pohl, H.L., Burn, T.C. and Tenen, D.G. 1991. Optimization of transient transfection into human myeloid cell lines using a luciferase reporter gene. *Exp. Hematol.* **19:** 1038–1041.

Potter, H. 1988. Electroporation in biology: methods, applications, and instrumentation. *Analyt. Biochem.* **174:** 361–373.

Potter, H., Weir, L. and Leder, P. 1984. Enhancer-dependent expression of human K immunoglobulin genes introduced into mouse pre-B lymphocytes by electroporation. *Proc. Natl Acad. USA.* **81:** 7161–7165.

Rippe, R.A., Brenner, D.A. and Leffert, H.L. 1990. DNA-mediated gene transfer into adult rat hepatocytes in primary culture. *Mol. Cell Biol.* **10:** 689–695.

Schever, T., Auld, V.J., Boyd, S., Offord, J., Dunn, R.D. and Catterall, W.A. 1990. Functional properties of rat brain sodium channels expressed in a somatic cell line. *Science* **247:** 854–858.

Swanson, L.W., Sawchenko, P.E., Rivier, J. and Vale, W.W. 1983. Organisation of ovine corticotrophin-releasing factor immunoreactive cells and fibres in the rat brain: An immunocytochemical study. *Neuroendocrinology* **36:** 165–186.

Toneguzzo, F., Keating, A., Lilly, S. and McDonald, K. 1988. Electric field-mediated gene transfer and patterns of integration in lymphoid cells. *Nucleic Acid Res.* **16:** 5515–5532.

Tsui, L.-C., Breitman, M.L.K., Siminovitch, L. and Buchveld, M. 1982. Persistence of freely replicating SV40 recombinant molecules carrying a selectable marker in permissive simian cells. *Cell* **30:** 499–508.

Tsuneoka, M. and Mekada, E. 1992. Degradation of a nuclear localised protein in mammalian COS cells, using *Escherichia coli* β-galactosidase as a model protein. *J. Biol. Chem.* **267:** 9107–9111.

Wigler, M., Sweet, R., Kee Sim, G., Wold, B., Pellicer, A., Lacey, E., Hamiatis, T., Solverstein, S. and Axel, R. 1979. Transformation of mammalian cells with genes from prokaryotes and eukaryotes. *Cell* **16:** 777–785.

Xie, T.D., Sun, L. and Tsoung, T.Y. 1990. Study of mechanisms of electric field-induced DNA transfection I. DNA entry by surface binding and diffusion through membrane pores. *Biophys. J.* **58:** 13–19.

CHAPTER 3

Gene Transfer into Post-mitotic Neurons in Culture by Microinjection

PETER K. MULDERRY AND TIMOTHY E. ALLSOPP*

MRC Brain Metabolism Unit, Royal Edinburgh Hospital, Morningside Park, Edinburgh EH10 5HF, UK. Tel: 44-(0)-131-537-6527; Fax: 44-(0)-131-537-6110; Email:mulderry@castle.ed.ac.uk

**Department of Veterinary Pathology, University of Edinburgh, Summerhall, Edinburgh EH9 1QH, UK. Tel: 0131 650 6160; Fax: 0131 650 6160; Email: tallsopp@lab0.vet.ed.ac.uk*

1 INTRODUCTION

The developing vertebrate nervous system generates an exuberance of post-mitotic neurons of varying phenotypes. A proportion of these are subsequently eliminated during a period of naturally occurring programmed cell death (apoptosis). These two phases of development play a large part in shaping the functional characteristics of the mature nervous system. Although a certain amount is known about the cellular interactions (often involving soluble neurotrophic factors) that determine neuronal phenotype and survival, the intracellular mechanisms regulating expression of specific genes or advancement of the cell death program remain poorly understood. Information on these mechanisms is likely to be important for the design and targeting of gene therapies intended to alleviate neurodegenerative diseases and other neurological disorders. The study of proteins involved in neuronal apoptosis and neuron-specific gene expression is therefore an important part of experimental neurobiology.

To study the function of a particular neuronal protein, one may wish to express artificially the protein of interest or to suppress activity of the endogenous protein by using antisense or dominant negative mutant strategies. Alternatively, one may wish to study mechanisms regulating expression of a particular gene by use of a reporter gene under the control of promoter sequences from the gene of interest. While the creation of transgenic or homozygous null-mutant animals can provide an *in vivo* assessment of gene function, many questions concerning specific genes in a specific neuronal type can be more conveniently answered by transient transfection of neurons in primary culture. This has particular relevance in the case of "knock-out" experiments, in which culture systems allow the gene of interest to be disabled at a time chosen by the experimenter rather than being absent through all preceding stages of development.

The method we favor for transfection of post-mitotic neurons in primary culture is microinjection of plasmid DNA expression vectors directly into individual neurons. We have used this technique successfully to study the function of specific proteins in neuronal apoptosis and the function of neuropeptide gene promoters in both embryonic and mature vertebrate peripheral

Protocols for Gene Transfer in Neuroscience: Towards Gene Therapy of Neurological Disorders
Edited by P.R. Lowenstein and L.W. Enquist

neurons in culture (Allsopp et al., 1993a,b; Mulderry et al., 1993; Dobson et al., 1994). Microinjection might initially appear to be time-consuming and relatively ineffective in terms of the number of neurons that can be transfected, but the efficiency of transfection (the proportion of injected cells successfully transfected) is high and the technique offers distinct advantages over other methods of transfection. Although herpesvirus, adeno-associated virus, or adenovirus vectors offer the possibility of long-term expression of transgenes in post-mitotic neurons, the relatively short-term transient transfection offered by microinjection is often sufficient for assessment of functions such as apoptosis. Microinjection avoids the considerable investment in special facilities and time required for preparation of viral vectors, requiring only relatively simple plasmid constructs that can be grown up in *Escherichia coli*. It also avoids the possible interference with cellular functions that may be caused by uncharacterized parts of the viral genomes (McLorie et al., 1991; Chou and Roizman, 1992; White et al., 1992) and the possibility that efficiency of viral infection may depend on the type or condition of the neurons to be transfected. Nevertheless, microinjection remains "neurotropic" in that it can target expression vectors specifically into neurons, something that is not possible with other non-viral transfection methods such as calcium phosphate/DNA coprecipitation or bulk/scrape loading (Gabellini et al., 1992; Jiao et al., 1992; Borasio et al., 1993). Furthermore, microinjection avoids the use of potentially toxic reagents and is capable of introducing DNA directly into the nucleus. Finally, microinjection has the unique distinction that it is equally capable of delivering RNA, proteins or membrane-impermeant drugs and is therefore an invaluable technique in experimental cell biology generally. Its value as a method for gene transfer into neurons should be viewed in this light.

Recent developments have seen the standardization of techniques for the production, storage and handling of injection capillaries as well as the automation of microinjection procedures (Ansorge and Pepperkok, 1988; Pepperkok et al., 1988) so that injections may now be quickly and reproducibly made in large numbers, allowing bulk biochemical analysis of whole populations of injected cells.

In this chapter we discuss the use of manual and automated microinjection systems for transient transfection of neurons in culture. Microinjection has, however, also been employed to transfect neurons in invertebrate whole animal preparations *in vivo* (Kaang et al., 1993). Although production of transgenic animals by microinjection of cloned DNA into fertilized mammalian egg cells (Murphy and Hanson, 1987) has obvious relevance to the subject of gene transfer into neurons and to gene therapy, the apparatus and techniques used are different from those employed for injection into mammalian somatic cells, including neurons, and are not discussed here. Likewise, we do not discuss the special methods used for microinjection into *Xenopus* oocytes (Hitchcock et al., 1987) or the ionophoretic injection techniques often used in conjunction with electrophysiological studies (Purves, 1981).

2 MATERIALS AND EQUIPMENT

2.1 Neuronal Culture Equipment and Media

In addition to standard materials and equipment for primary cell culture (SEE SECTION 4, PAGE 30), the following items are required for microinjection.

(1) Tissue culture media buffered for CO_2 incubators (culture medium) and room air (injection medium). Media also contain required neurotrophic factors.
  - Ham's F14 salt preparation containing $NaHCO_3$ (24 mM), penicillin (60 mg/l) and streptomycin (100 mg/l) for neuronal cultures.
  - Ham's F12 preparation for room air medium (both pH 7.6).
  - Media for chicken neurons are supplemented with 10% heat-inactivated horse serum and 5% heat-inactivated fetal calf serum.
  - Media for mouse neurons are supplemented with defined medium additives (Bottenstein and Sato, 1979) minus insulin and transferrin.
  - Culture medium for adult rat DRG neurons is supplemented with 4% Ultroser G (Gibco), reduced to 0.5% during injection.

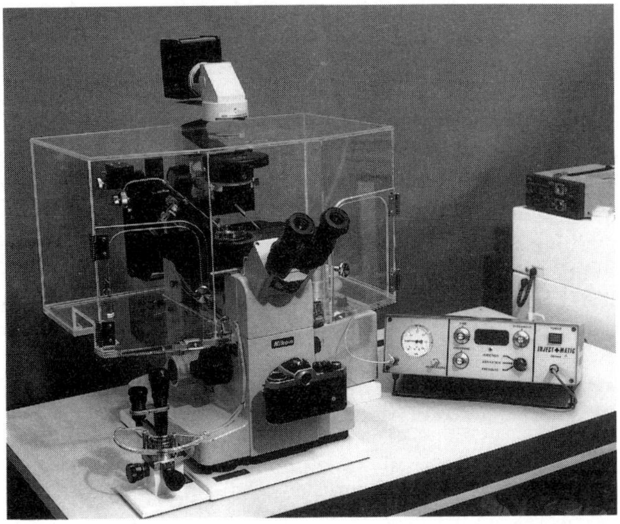

Fig. 3.1 Equipment for the microinjection of neurons using a manual remote micromanipulator, configured for a left-handed operator. The microscope stands on an antivibration platform supported by foam balls. The coarse manipulator controls are situated on the illumination support of the microscope, within the incubation chamber. Fine manipulator movements are performed by oil hydraulics and linked by tubing to the remote joystick (to the left of the microscope). Movement of the injection capillary in the axial direction is controlled by the "T" unit attached to the stalk of the joystick. Pressure is supplied by the electric pump situated to the right of the microscope

(2) Plasticware.
- Plain 35 mm or 60 mm diameter plastic tissue-culture dishes (for assay of neuronal apoptosis).
- Glass coverslips (13 mm diameter) or 35 mm dishes with wells 10 mm in diameter, 1 mm deep molded into the base (Greiner, Germany) for assay of gene promoter activity.

(3) Poly-DL-ornithine (0.5 mg/ml in 0.15 M borate buffer, pH 8.7) and laminin (20 μg/ml in phosphate-buffered saline) for coating dishes and coverslips.

2.2 Pressure Microinjection Equipment

(1) Inverted microscope with a high-power (40 ×) long working distance phase-contrast objective (for use during microinjection) and lower powered objectives (for initial positioning of the injection capillary) and an extra long working distance condenser that will not obstruct access by the injection capillary.
(2) Heated microscope headstage incubation chamber (optional, SEE SECTION 4, PAGE 30).
(3) Anti-vibration base plate or table (optional, SEE SECTION 4, PAGE 30).
(4) Micromanipulator.
(5) Pneumatic pressure control system.
(6) Injection capillaries.

2.3 Solutions for Injection

(1) Plasmid DNA containing cDNA insert, purified on CsCl gradients (stored frozen at 1 mg/ml; ideal ratio of absorbance at 260 nm to that at 280 nm of 1.8).
(2) Fluorescently labeled (FITC or RITC) dextran (mol. wt. 20 000) for checking injection technique.

(3) Injection buffer for diluting the above (Ca^{2+} and Mg^{2+}-free phosphate-buffered saline or 10 mM Tris–HCl, pH 7.4), sterilized by passing through a 0.2 μm pore filter.
(4) Microloader tips (Eppendorf) and pipette for back-filling injection capillaries.

3 THE PROTOCOLS

Protocol #9: Setting up the Equipment for Intracellular Microinjection

(1) Warm culture and injection media to 37°C. If using a microscope headstage incubator, place a container of water into the chamber to minimize evaporation of medium while injecting.
(2) Dilute DNA for microinjection to the desired concentration (SEE SECTION 4, PAGE 30) in injection buffer (20 μl diluted DNA should be sufficient for a full day's injecting).
(3) Centrifuge the DNA solution in a benchtop centrifuge for 5 min at 13 000 r.p.m. to remove any sediment.
(4) Fill a capillary with 1–2 μl DNA solution. As soon as the injection capillary has been filled, fit it onto the capillary holder on the micromanipulator (the micromanipulator should be set to its highest position). If using Eppendorf femtotips, remove the protective cover first by holding the capillary vertically (tip downwards) and loosening the cover until it drops off. Set the angle of the micromanipulator head correctly for axial injections (45°) and lower it until the tip just enters the medium in the culture dish. Do not delay getting the tip into the medium, as it is likely to become blocked if it spends too long in the air.
(5) Place the capillary in the injection holder attached to the manipulator (SEE SECTION 4.2.2, PAGE 32). Lower the capillary close to the bottom of the dish using coarse controls. Center the tip of the capillary in the middle of the field of view (use the built-in photographic reticule in the microscope)—this is crucial to establish the central point of reference for the capillary tip while injecting under high power. Switch to high-power magnification (40 ×) and lower the capillary using the fine controls on the joystick until the capillary is approximately 40–50 μm from the bottom, just clear of the cells.
(6) Check the flow characteristics by applying pressure and looking for Schlieren patterns in the medium or movement of debris. Alternatively, use a fluorescent dye in the injection solution and view with fluorescence optics. If using commercial capillaries (femtotips) a steady discharge should be apparent. Capillaries that you have pulled yourself will probably require opening (see next step).
(7) Use the fine micromanipulator to exert vertical downward movement of the capillary tip. Concomitant with this movement, drag the capillary across the culture dish by moving the joystick towards you; the capillary moves from top to bottom of the field of view. Some physical displacement of the capillary tip occurs. A tiny piece of glass should be removed from the tip, visible as a dark speck. Check the flow characteristics as described in Step 6. If flow is excessive, start over with a new capillary.

Protocol #10: Assay of Protein Function in Neuronal Apoptosis Using Delivery of Genes by Manual Microinjection

(1) Using a sterile scalpel blade, score a square (1 cm^2) in the center on the inside of the culture dish. Divide the square into four equal quadrants.
(2) Using warmed medium, wash the dish and remove the plastic debris formed from scoring the dish. To do this, tilt the dish on its side and, while dripping medium (approx. 10 ml) from the top, remove medium from the bottom by aspiration. This will not remove viable neurons.
(3) Replace culture medium with supplemented injection medium (10 ml) and place the dish on the microscope. It is not necessary to resupplement trophic factors at this stage, as the neurons will survive for the time period of injection and are washed again at the end of injection.
(4) Briefly estimate the density of cells in each quadrant and choose two adjacent quadrants that contain approximately 50–100 neurons each. With experience, this should be the number that can be injected within 60–75 min. Do not be tempted simply to inject the quadrants with the greatest number of neurons—this could be very time-consuming.

(5) Rotate the dish so that the squares to be injected are on the side furthest from the manipulator. This is to ensure that the capillary holder does not touch the side of the dish when neurons at the edge of the quadrant are injected.
(6) Position a filled injection capillary tip (SEE SECTION 4.3.2, PAGE 33) in the center of the first quadrant to be injected using dark field optics, with the injection capillary in the center of field of view (use the photo reticule as a guide).
(7) Switch to the 40 × objective, focus on the bottom of the dish and move to the top left-hand corner of the quadrant. Lower the capillary tip using fine micromanipulator control. "Open" the capillary tip as described above if necessary.
(8) Move across the quadrant to locate the first neuron. The capillary tip should always be kept approximately 30–50 μm above the bottom of the dish and in the center of the reticule. Move the nucleus and the neuron below the tip. Lower the tip vertically until it just touches the nucleus. If solution is flowing (pressure approx. 20 kPa), a slight indentation should appear as the tip just touches the nucleus.
(9) Using the fine control for movement along the capillary axis (fourth dimension), penetrate the nucleus with a short forward and downward movement of the tip followed by a rapid backward and upward movement.
(10) Pass methodically across and through the quadrant, using the reticule as an area marker, and inject all neurons within the area.
(11) After injecting both quadrants, raise the capillary with the coarse manipulator. Remove the holder from the manipulator, replace the dish lid and mark the two quadrants that were injected.
(12) Wash the dish with warm injection medium (about 10 ml). Replace the medium with 5 ml of supplemented culture medium and return the dish to the CO_2 incubator.
(13) Assay the effects on apoptosis, as described in Section 4.3.8.

Protocol #11: Assay of Gene Promoter Activity Using Delivery of Genes by Automated Injection

(1) If neurons have been grown on glass coverslips, transfer the coverslip from the culture well to a plain 35 mm diameter culture dish containing 2.5 ml injection medium. (Coverslips can be lifted out of wells easily using two pairs of fine forceps or a pair of forceps and a fine hypodermic needle.) If neurons are in 10 mm wells, aspirate the growth medium and replace with injection medium. Transfer the dish to the microscope stage.
(2) Fill the injection capillary, open it and position it above the cells as described above.
(3) Set the automatic injection system to give an injection pressure of approximately 20 kPa and holding pressure at about 7 kPa. Set the injection time to 0.5 s and turn on the axial injection setting.
(4) Position the injection capillary tip immediately over a medium-sized neuron (Fig. 3.2A).
(5) Lower the injection tip slowly until it just starts to depress the cell membrane. Under phase-contrast optics this can be seen as a brightening of the membrane in the area immediately surrounding the tip. Set the height limit for injection (Fig. 3.2B).
(6) Lift the tip of the injection capillary clear of the cell and lower the height limit by 5 μm (Fig. 3.2C).
(7) Press the injection button. The injection capillary should move to the correct position for axial injection, enter the cell, inject some solution and return to its original position (Fig. 3.2D–F).
(8) If the injection capillary fails to enter the neuron, if it enters the cell but no sign of injection is seen, or if it bursts or gouges the cell it will be necessary to reset the height limit, reset the injection pressure or replace the injection capillary (SEE SECTION 4.3.7).
(9) If the first injection is made successfully, continue to make injections without resetting the height limit or injection pressure for as long as they appear satisfactory—perhaps as many as 10 cells. When these settings fail to make effective injections, reset the height limit or injection pressure. Keep the holding pressure at approximately one-third of the injection pressure.
(10) Assay reporter gene expression (SEE SECTION 4.3.11).

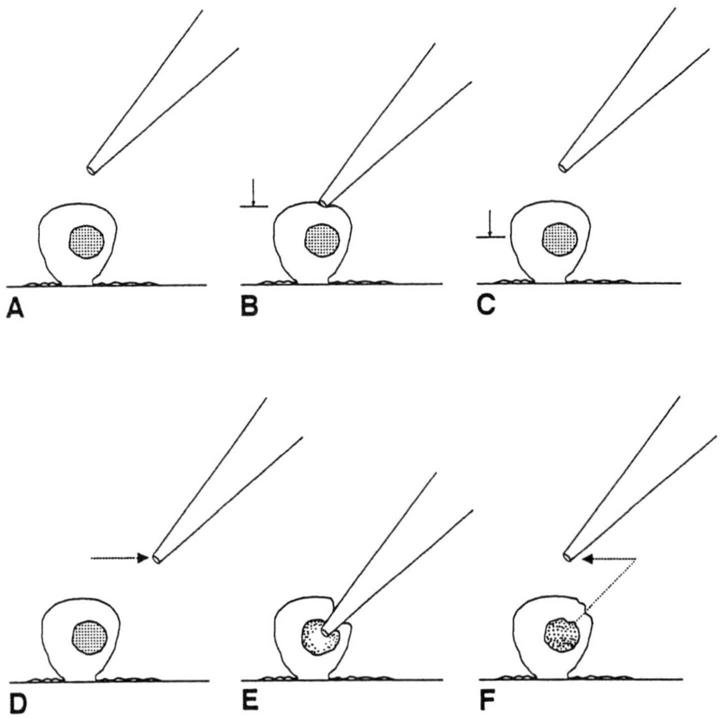

Figure 3.2 Cartoon representation of microinjection into adult rat DRG neurons using the Eppendorf automated microinjection system. (A) The tip of the injection capillary is positioned directly over a neuron. (B) The tip is lowered until contact with the cell is made. The height limit is set. (C) The tip is raised just clear of the neuron. The height limit is lowered by 5 μm. (D) The injection switch is pressed. The micromanipulator automatically moves the capillary to the correct position for axial injection. (E) Injection. The capillary penetrates the cell and fluid is ejected. (F) The capillary is withdrawn from the cell and returns to the starting position. Note that, although a nuclear injection is shown here, the large volume of cytoplasm surrounding the nucleus and cell movement due to the shape of DRG neurons means that consistently making injections into the nucleus is virtually impossible and, in practice, most injections are into the cytoplasm. Other cell types with a flatter morphology or less perinuclear cytoplasm may permit a much higher frequency of intranuclear injection

4 NOTES AND TROUBLESHOOTING

4.1 On Materials and Methods: Cell Culture of Autonomic Neurons

4.1.1 Neuronal Culture

Sensory and parasympathetic neurons from embryonic chick and mouse and adult rat DRG neurons are prepared for culture as described elsewhere (Davies, 1988a,b; Lindsay et al., 1991; Allsopp et al., 1993a,b) and are grown on dishes or coverslips precoated with polyornithine and laminin. For studies on the effects of cellular proteins on neuronal apoptosis, low-density neuronal cultures (approximately 400–600 neurons/cm^2) of embryonic chicken or mouse neurons are grown on 60 mm diameter culture dishes. For assay of promoter activity, adult rat DRG neurons are grown on glass coverslips at 8000–10 000 neurons per coverslip or in 10 mm diameter wells at 5000–7000 neurons per well. The choice is determined by whether one wants to assess reporter gene expression by immunocytochemical means (use coverslips) or by biochemical assay (use wells). If using coverslips, these should be washed in 1 N hydrochloric acid, rinsed in tissue culture grade water and sterilized by autoclaving or baking before use for cell culture. As attachment is rapid on laminin, neurons can be ready for microinjection within 4–6 h of plating. Usually, however, they are left overnight before attempting injection.

4.2 On Protocol #9: Setting up the Equipment for Intracellular Microinjection

4.2.1 Pressure Microinjection Equipment

Inverted Microscope

It is useful for the inverted microscope to be equipped with a mercury vapor light source and filters for epifluorescence optics that can be used to monitor delivery of solutions containing fluorescent dyes.

Headstage Incubation Chamber

The heated microscope headstage incubation chamber may be unnecessary if the injection experiment can be completed quickly. We have not experienced any problems in allowing adult rat DRG cultures to cool to room temperature for periods of up to 40 min.

Antivibration Tables

Although sophisticated antivibration tables are commercially available, it is not difficult to arrange effective damping of vibration using readily available materials (Purves, 1981) and in many cases a heavy bench of sturdy construction standing on a solid floor will provide adequate insulation.

Micromanipulator System

A manual micromanipulator system, consisting of a coarse three-dimensional manipulator mounted on the illumination support of the microscope and a joystick-controlled oil hydraulic micromanipulator system (e.g. Narishige) with four degrees of movement (x, y, z and axial) attached to the coarse manipulator, will allow very effective injection into neurons. Alternatively, microprocessor-controlled micromanipulator systems capable of making automated injections are available. The Eppendorf microprocessor-controlled micromanipulator automatically makes timed axial injections at a height set by the user. Thus, once a suitable injection height is set, it is necessary only to position the tip of the injection capillary over the cell and press a foot switch to make an injection automatically. Although this system can make many injections very rapidly, the proportion of ineffective injections due to failure to introduce DNA into the cell or physical damage to the cell is likely to be higher than with a manual system, especially when cells are of variable size. Nevertheless, we have used the Eppendorf automatic system successfully to inject rat DRG neurons. Whatever type of micromanipulator system is chosen, it is essential that it should be capable of making axial movements of the injection capillary.

Pressure System

The pressure system can be an electric pump, gas cylinder or institutional pressurized air supply. The pressure control system should be capable of providing fine control over pressure applied to the injection capillary. Typically, a pressure of 10–100 kPa will be required to eject fluid from the injection capillary into the cell at a reasonable rate. A simple pressure control system can apply this injection pressure continuously, whether the injection capillary is in a cell or not. Some injection systems use pulsed pressure for injections and a lower holding pressure (5–20 kPa) between injections just sufficient to prevent culture medium entering the pipette tip by capillary action. This type of arrangement may help to achieve greater consistency of injection volume between individual injections, especially when using an automated micromanipulator (Ansorge, 1982). Another feature, useful for dislodging material accumulated on the injection capillary tip and for removing blockages, is the ability to apply a pulse of relatively high pressure (a few hundred kilopascals) to the injection capillary. Pressure control units possessing all these features as well as the ability to coordinate injection pressure pulses with automated movements of the micromanipulator are made by Eppendorf.

4.2.2 Setting up the Injection Equipment

Before starting any injection experiments, be prepared to devote hours to performing these initial adjustments to the microscope, micromanipulator and capillary to ensure that the subsequent repetitive neuronal microinjections are frustration-free and that, on the day of experimentation, valuable time is not wasted.

The manipulator needs to be attached to the microscope and the joystick positioned for left-handed or right-handed operation. Lengthy periods are to be spent looking down the oculars so it is essential that equipment is ergonomically positioned and adjusted.

Some effort must be made to minimize vibration of the injection capillary, as this may cause increased damage to the cells during injection. The microscope should be placed on an antivibration slab on a table separate from the routine work bench. The laboratory floor should preferably be solid concrete. The microscope should, ideally, be dedicated for microinjection and be in a room that can be maintained at a constant comfortable ambient temperature (air conditioning is helpful). If using a heated headstage incubator, check that it maintains a steady 37°C.

If you intend to make your own injection capillaries, determine the heating and pulling conditions required to give the optimum tip shape and initial flow characteristics for microinjection (the manufacturer of the puller should be able to offer advice concerning the initial starting parameters to pull injection capillaries). When viewed at high magnification (40 × objective) the tip of the injection capillary appears dark, shimmers slightly and the visible extremity is 2–3 μm in diameter. To permit the continuous discharge of a DNA solution the tip requires "opening" (SEE PROTOCOL #9). This procedure is difficult and requires practice. However, it is not usually necessary if using the Eppendorf ready-made injection capillaries.

4.2.3 Injection Capillaries

For injection into vertebrate neuronal cells, capillaries with a tip diameter of less than 1 μm are required. Suitable capillaries can be made with a microelectrode puller (e.g. Campden Instruments Model 753 moving coil puller). A device that permits the operator to adjust heating times and pulling force is really all that is required, although an additional prepull stage is an advantage. Capillary glass tubes (Narishige) with internal glass fiber (for back-filling the injection capillary with DNA solution), size 1 × 90 mm are used. Commercial microinjection capillaries (femtotips) are made by Eppendorf. These have a tip diameter of 0.5 ± 0.2 μm and are supplied sterile and RNAse free in individually sealed packs. We have used these successfully for microinjection into rat DRG neurons. A recent review by Proctor (1992) describes in detail all aspects of the manufacture, handling and storage of capillaries for pressure injection into mammalian cells.

4.2.4 Preparing Glass Coverslips

To prepare these wash 13 mm diameter coverslips in 1 N hydrochloric acid for 2 h with occasional agitation. Rinse extensively in tissue culture grade water and then sterilize by autoclaving in a covered beaker of water or wrap in foil and bake in an oven.

4.2.5 Choice of Promoter or Reporter Gene

For studies on the function of ectopically expressed proteins viral promoters can be used to generate high levels of constitutive expression in neurons. Promoters that drive expression in sensory neurons are (with most effective first): cytomegalovirus long terminal repeat (LTR), Rous sarcoma virus 3′ LTR, SV40 early promoter, murine Moloney leukemia virus LTR. However, the most suitable promoter should be determined empirically for each specific application.

For gene promoter studies, *lacZ* is probably the most versatile reporter gene, as discussed in Section 4.3.11 PAGE 37. However, for analysis of reporter gene expression at the single cell level, luciferase or fluorescent protein reporter genes (Chalfie et al., 1994) may offer very attractive solutions to problem of reporter gene assay in single cells.

4.2.6 Best Method of Purifying DNA for Microinjection

We have used both CsCl density gradient and ion-exchange column (e.g. Qiagen) methods for purifying plasmid DNA for microinjection. Purification on CsCl gradients is relatively time consuming and involves the use of ethidium bromide, which is carcinogenic and teratogenic. However, on balance, this method is recommended over the use of columns as DNA prepared by the latter method may contain extraneous matter that might increase the risk of blockage of the injection capillary.

4.2.7 Injection Buffer

Some authors favor phosphate buffers for microinjection, on the grounds that they are more physiological (Graessmann et al., 1980; Graessmann and Graessmann, 1983; Proctor, 1992), but we have found that phosphate buffers offer no obvious increase in transfection efficiency and are associated with more frequent blockage of the capillary tip, possibly due to salt precipitation within the capillary. Some cell types may be more tolerant than others of non-physiological buffers, however, and testing buffers of different compositions is recommended when first attempting microinjection into a given type of cell. We normally omit EDTA from stock solutions of DNA used for microinjection, although we have not found the presence of 1 mM EDTA to have any significant effect on reporter gene expression in DRG neurons.

4.3 On Protocol #10: Assay of Protein Function in Neuronal Apoptosis Using Delivery of Genes by Manual Microinjection, and Protocol #11: Assay of Gene Promoter Activity Using Delivery of Genes by Automated Injection

4.3.1 Risk of Contamination

It is a not uncommon belief that leaving culture dishes open to unfiltered air will inevitably result in infection with yeast or fungi and that elaborate precautions are required to prevent contamination of cultures exposed during microinjection procedures. However, our experience is that contamination need not be feared if the simple precaution of replacing the medium used for microinjection with fresh sterile medium immediately following injection is taken.

4.3.2 Filling Capillaries

We back-fill injection capillaries using microloader tips on a standard laboratory hand pipettor. However, they can also be filled by capillary action from the tip (Proctor, 1992). Do not push the microloader tip right into the shaft of the capillary tip as this prevents air from escaping, leaving bubbles which block the tip, and can deposit flakes of plastic into the DNA solution.

4.3.3 Intranuclear Injection

It is safe to assume that the nucleus is the best site within the cell for efficient transcription from the expression construct. Furthermore, the nuclear membrane is more resistant than the cytoplasmic membrane to the physical trauma of injection. Injections should therefore be made into the nucleus if at all possible. For cells with large volumes of perinuclear cytoplasm (e.g. mature DRG neurons) this is best done using manual injection. The nucleus should swell slowly and the residence time of the capillary within the nucleus should be no more than 1 s. Despite the advantages of nuclear injection, we find that cytoplasmic injection can be relied upon to transfect a substantial proportion of cells and can therefore be used if nuclear injections are too difficult.

4.3.4 How Much DNA Should be Injected?

It is important to understand that the quantity of DNA injected varies considerably between individual injections because of the difficulty of controlling the volume of solution injected. Minaschek et al. (1989) describe the use of fluorescently labeled protein to measure injection volume into non-neuronal cells and report a five-fold variation in injection volume between individual injections, which they attribute to differences in cytoplasmic viscosity. Although methods for estimating the average volume injected have been suggested (Graessmann et al., 1980) these are likely to be subject to considerable error. Further complications are added by the fact that the characteristics of individual injection capillaries vary so much. The properties of individual injection capillaries can change with time due to accumulation of small quantities of cellular debris or slight damage to the tip. Thus, any estimate of the volume injected can only be very approximate.

Because of the difficulty of controlling injection volume, any attempt to vary the quantity of DNA injected should always be made by altering the concentration of the DNA solution, not by altering the injection volume. The ratio between the average number of DNA molecules injected in two series of injections can then be quite accurately known. Using the *lacZ* reporter gene driven by constitutive promoters, we have found that expression of injected constructs reaches maximum when the concentration of the injected DNA is approximately 100 μg/ml. This is therefore a good starting concentration when investigating a new construct. Assuming that the volume injected (large enough to be seen but not large enough to burst the cell) lies between 10% and 100% of the total cell volume, this corresponds to between 10^3 and 10^4 plasmid copies per cell for adult rat DRG neurons.

4.3.5 What can be done if the Injection Capillary does not Open or Becomes Blocked?

If dragging the capillary across the surface of the dish does not open it, try again after slightly increasing the angle of the injection holder to the bottom of the dish. Also increase the amount of vertical movement with the micromanipulator (and downward force onto the capillary tip) when the capillary is being dragged. The capillary should initially appear exactly horizontal as viewed down the microscope, so that movement of the joystick brings the capillary from the top of the viewing field to the bottom. If the DNA solution still does not flow, there may be an air bubble in the capillary shaft, or it may be clogged with sediment in the DNA solution. The remedy is to use a new, filled capillary. Accumulation of cellular debris may also cause the capillary to block during use. The blockage is sometimes cleared by applying a pulse of high pressure. If this does not work, try raising and lowering the tip through the meniscus of the medium a few times. Finally, try bumping the capillary tip against the bottom of the dish by very gently tapping the micromanipulator or by dragging it against the bottom of the dish as described above. If all this fails to reopen the tip or if it is chipped and the flow after reopening is uncontrollably high, replace the capillary.

If a whole series of capillaries very quickly become blocked, it may be due to impurities in the DNA solution. Try centrifuging the solution again or diluting it more. In extreme cases, it may be necessary to prepare fresh DNA (SEE SECTION 4.2.6, PAGE 33).

Another reason for repeated blocking could be the shape of the injection capillaries. Blocking can occur more frequently if the capillary remains very narrow for too great a distance away from the tip.

4.3.6 Optimizing Transfection Efficiency

If transfection efficiency seems low, inject fluorescently labeled dextran to determine whether the problem is due to failure to introduce DNA into the cell or because the cells are being killed by the trauma of injection. These problems are likely to be more prominent when using an automatic microinjection system. Examine the cells for fluorescence immediately after injection. If many cells do not appear to contain fluorescent material, check that the injection capillary is successfully penetrating the cells and use a different height limit for injection if necessary. Also try increasing the average injected volume by increasing the pressure or injection time. If many neurons are being killed by injection, because they burst immediately or die later, make sure that you use only injection capillaries with fine tips and immediately replace any that suffer physical damage in use. Also try to reduce the average injection volume by using lower injection pressure or shorter injection time. For adult rat DRG neurons injected using the Eppendorf automatic microinjection system, we have found that 60–80% of the injected neurons survive after 2 days and that 50–65% of the survivors (i.e. approximately 40% of the injected neurons) contained detectable quantities of the injected fluorescent material.

4.3.7 Problems Setting the Eppendorf Automated Microinjection System

When adjusting the Eppendorf automatic microinjection system for automatic injection into neurons a number of common problems can arise. If the procedures described in Section 3 have been followed but effective injections still cannot be achieved, the following notes may help.

The Tip Does not Move

This probably means either that no height limit for injection has been set or that the tip is already at the set limit. Reset the height limit as described.

The Capillary Tip Moves but Does not Enter the Cell

The height limit for injection has been incorrectly set too high (reset the height limit), or the capillary tip was not directly above the cell at the start of its movement (check positioning by varying the focus), or it was so far above the cell that it did not have time to reach the cell within the allowed time. The set injection time is measured from the moment the capillary starts its movement to the moment it starts its withdrawal from the cell. It is therefore important that the starting height should be consistent. The easiest way to achieve this is to set the starting height so that it is just clear of the cells.

The Injection Capillary Enters the Cell but the Cell is Gouged or Ruptured

Gouging can result from capillary entry being vertical rather than axial or from a blunt capillary tip. Check that the injection mode has been set to axial and, if gouging persists, change the injection capillary. If the membrane is ruptured the flow rate is too high. It may be possible to achieve a satisfactory rate by reducing the pressure. However, if this cannot be achieved even when the pressure is reduced to 5 kPa, then the tip diameter is probably too large and the injection capillary should be replaced. Reducing the injection time is rarely a satisfactory solution because of the difficulty of achieving consistent injection with very short injection times. We always keep the injection time constant and adjust only the pressure to achieve satisfactory injections.

The Tip Enters the Cell but no Sign of Injection is Seen

If no sign of fluid ejection can be seen, even when the high pressure is applied to the capillary, then it is almost certainly blocked (See Section 4.3.5).

The Tip Spends too little Time in the Cell for the Experimenter to Determine whether Injection has been Made

Either the injection time has been set too short or the starting level is too high (see above).

4.3.8 Assays of Protein Function in Neuronal Apoptosis by Manual Microinjection

Neurons from the peripheral nervous system are microinjected with expression constructs containing constitutively active promoters. The ability of the encoded proteins to affect neuronal apoptosis is analysed in short-term viability assays (1–6 days), determined in the presence or absence of specific trophic factors. In assays of apoptosis, approximately 70–90% of neurons may die within 24 h when deprived of suitable trophic factors. All injections for assay of apoptosis should be performed on the same day and within 24 h of initial plating. Part of the culture dish (approximately 400 cells) should be subdivided into two separate populations, one for injection and the remainder considered as an uninjected control.

An inherent feature of the manual microinjection technique is that only a small percentage of neurons in the dish are transfected. Manual injection is time consuming and requires patience and a certain degree of manual coordination. The experimenter should aim initially to inject four dishes in a 6-h period. This includes a cell count for each dish approximately 2 h after injection to determine the initial sizes of the injected and uninjected neuronal populations and time required for the preparation and injection of other dishes. More than 85% of neurons should survive the trauma of intranuclear injection. The more experienced operator should deal with 6–8 dishes in a day (6–8 hours). This should be sufficient to permit the analysis of several variables in one experiment, each variable being assessed in duplicate dishes.

As there is considerable size variation among neurons from the peripheral nervous system, manual injection might be preferred to an automatic injection system. With manual control, movement of the injection capillary in the axial direction can be more reliable, as the automatic device assumes each neuron to be a uniform distance from the bottom of the culture dish.

4.3.9 Assay of Gene Promoter Activity by Automated Injection

To assay gene promoter activity, we make enough injections to assay reporter gene expression directly in whole culture extracts. Neurons are plated on small glass coverslips or in shallow culture wells of small surface area. A small plating area permits a large number of injections to be made rapidly and allows extraction into a small volume so that concentrated extracts can be made for reporter gene assay. Although it might appear preferable to plate a few hundred neurons and make injections into all of them, rather than plate several thousand and transfect a fixed number (as we do), it is extremely difficult in practice to obtain consistent numbers of neurons in each well or coverslip when plating very small numbers of cells, and the method we use results in greater consistency. In our assays non-specific background signal from the excess of untransfected cells is low.

Because reporter plasmid expression may depend on the length of time the cells have been in culture at the time of injection, as well as the period between injection and assay, all the injections necessary for a given experiment should be made on the same day. We usually make injections into 350 DRG neurons on each coverslip or well. With experience, this can be completed in 30–45 min. Three replicate coverslips or wells are used for each plasmid or set of culture conditions. Allowing for time spent in preparation, transferring cultures to and from the incubator, replacing injection capillaries and so on, one can realistically expect to process 9–12 coverslips or wells in the course of a single working day.

When using the Eppendorf automatic system, one aims to set the injection height at a level that will be suitable for the "average" cell. A number of injections can then be made simply by positioning the tip of the injection capillary above each cell in turn and pressing the foot switch. Because adult rat DRG neurons possess a large volume of cytoplasm surrounding the nucleus, and because their high profile off the culture substrate means that they invariably move as the injection capillary penetrates the cell, it is virtually impossible to consistently make injections into the nuclei of these cells when using the automatic injection system. Although most of the injections are therefore cytoplasmic and the efficiency of transfection may not be as high as it would be if all the injections were made into the nucleus, at least 15% of the injections can result in effective transfection. The large number of injections made means that the level of transfection is consistent from one experiment to another.

Move across the coverslip in a series of parallel lines, spaced far enough apart that cells are not injected twice. It is important that every neuron that comes into the field of view should receive an injection, to eliminate the possibility of unconscious bias for or against neurons of any special appearance. It is easier to avoid accidentally injecting the same cells twice if the photography reticule is in place during injection and if injections are made only into those cells lying within the rectangle.

For replicate experiments with any given reporter construct, make exactly the same number of injections on each coverslip. We stop at 350: this is enough to average out the variation in individual injections and can be completed within a reasonable time.

4.3.10 Analysis of Exogenous Gene Expression

When using microinjection to study the function of ectopically expressed proteins, methods suitable for analysis of small numbers of cells are needed to assay expression of the transgene. Reverse-transcriptase polymerase chain reaction (RT-PCR) potentially allows detection of exogenous gene expression in a very small number of cells, albeit at the mRNA level. This analysis is restricted to those circumstances in which primers can be used to distinguish the exogenous gene from any homologous endogenous gene. For example, primers are designed to distinguish between the ectopic expression of a rat protein and the endogenous chicken protein in microinjected chicken neurons (Allsopp et al., 1993a) or if primers are designed to recognize a unique artificially introduced and in-frame "tag" nucleotide sequence in the exogenous gene. Quantitative analysis of expression can be obtained using competitive PCR. The target mRNA produced by the expression construct is coamplified with a run-off transcript from a cDNA that has additional bases inserted between the primer annealing sites. A known amount of this template is added as an internal standard (Wyatt and Davies, 1993).

Immunocytochemistry can be used to detect expression of the ectopically expressed protein in individual neurons. In addition, immunocytochemistry can be used to show that the expressed protein is appropriately processed and distributed within the neuron. However, detection of exogenous protein expression is restricted to those circumstances in which species-specific antibodies can be used to distinguish exogenous from endogenous protein expression (Allsopp et al., 1993a,b) or to situations in which constructs are used to produce epitope-tagged proteins. Immunocytochemistry can also be used to detect reporter gene expression where colocalization with some endogenous protein needs to be studied. However, it is unlikely to be as sensitive as methods based on the enzymatic properties of the reporter gene product (SEE SECTION 4.3.11). In combination with computer-based image analysis, immunofluorescence may be used for quantitative assay of ectopic gene expression in single cells (Pepperkok et al., 1993).

4.3.11 Assay of Reporter Gene Expression

A total of 350 injections transfects enough neurons for expression of *lacZ* or *CAT* reporter genes to be assayed directly by biochemical assay. Measurement of β-galactosidase enzymic activity can be made using the fluorogenic substrate methylumbelliferyl-β-D-galactopyranoside (MUG) in a simple assay (Mulderry et al., 1993) and CAT protein concentrations can be measured using a commercially available ELISA kit (Dobson et al., 1994). The non-specific background contribution from uninjected cells is sufficiently low in both these assays for reporter gene expression to be assayed readily, even in the presence of a large excess of uninjected cells.

lacZ expression can also be visualized easily by staining with the chromogenic β-galactosidase substrate X-Gal (5-bromo-4-chloro-3-indolyl-β-D-galactopyranoside). This is an extremely sensitive method for the detection of β-galactosidase expression in transfected cells. It can be used to assess transfection efficiency, but the opacity of the reaction product means that it is not suitable for quantitative evaluation of *lacZ* expression at the single cell level, nor for colocalization of reporter gene expression with endogenous genes. However, fluorogenic β-galactosidase substrates are available that can be used with living cells and whose reaction products are retained within the cell (Zhang et al., 1991). The use of such substrates in conjunction with a quantitative fluorescent imaging system could allow quantitative assay of *lacZ* expression in individual transfected cells.

ACKNOWLEDGMENTS

This work was supported by the MRC and the Wellcome Trust. We would like to thank our colleagues, particularly Professor A.M. Davies, Doctors A.J. Harmar, K. Chapman, J. Quinn and J. Morrow, Mr S. Dobson and Mrs V. Lyons for their help, support and advice and Sean Earnshaw for photography.

REFERENCES

Allsopp, T.E., Robinson, M., Wyatt, S. and Davies, A.M. (1993a). Ectopic trkA expression mediates a NGF survival response in NGF-independent sensory neurons but not in parasympathetic neurons. *J. Cell Biol.* **123:** 1555–1566.

Allsopp, T.E., Wyatt, S., Paterson, H.F. and Davies, A.M. (1993b). The proto-oncogene *bcl-2* can selectively rescue neurotrophic factor-dependent neurons from apoptosis. *Cell* **73:** 295–307.

Ansorge, W. (1982). Improved system for capillary microinjection into living cells. *Exp. Cell Res.* **140:** 31–37.

Ansorge, W. and Pepperkok, R. (1988). Performance of an automated system for capillary microinjection into living cells. *J. Biochem. Biophys. Meth.* **16:** 283–292.

Borasio, G.D., Markus, A., Wittinghofer, A., Barde, Y.-A. and Heumann, R. (1993). Involvement of ras p21 in neurotrophin-induced response of sensory, but not sympathetic neurons. *J. Cell Biol.* **121:** 665–672.

Bottenstein, J. and Sato, G. (1979). Growth of a rat neuroblastoma cell line in serum-free supplemented medium. *Proc. Natl Acad. Sci. USA* **76:** 514–517.

Chalfie, M., Tu, Y., Euskirchen, G., Ward, W.W. and Prasher, D.C. (1994). Green fluorescent protein as a marker for gene expression. *Science* **263:** 802–805.

Chou, J. and Roizman, B. (1992). The $\gamma_1$34.5 gene of herpes simplex virus I precludes neuroblastoma cells from triggering total shutoff of protein synthesis characteristic of programmed cell death in neuronal cells. *Proc. Natl Acad. Sci. USA* **89:** 3266–3270.

Davies, A.M. (1988a). Neurotrophic factor bioassay using dissociated neurons, in: *Nerve growth factors* (R.A. Rush, ed.), J. Wiley (Chichester). pp. 95–109.

Davies, A.M. (1988b). The trigeminal system: an advantageous experimental model for studying neuronal development. *Development* **103:** 175–183.

Dobson, S.P., Quinn, J.P., Morrow, J.A. and Mulderry, P.K. (1994). The rat vasoactive intestinal polypeptide cyclic AMP response element regulates gene transcriptional responses differently in neonatal and adult rat sensory neurons. *Neurosci. Lett.* **167:** 19–23.

Gabellini, N., Minozzi, M.-C., Leon, A. and Dal Toso, R. (1992). Nerve growth factor transcriptional control of C-FOS promoter transfected in cultured spinal sensory neurons. *J. Cell. Biol.* **118:** 131–138.

Graessmann, A., Graessmann, M. and Mueller, C. (1980). Microinjection of early SV40 DNA fragments and T antigen. *Meth. Enzymol.* **65:** 816–825.

Graessmann, M. and Graessmann, A. (1983). Microinjection of tissue culture cells. *Meth. Enzymol.* **101:** 482–492.

Hitchcock, M.J.M., Ginns, E.I. and Marcus-Sekura, C.J. (1987). Microinjection into Xenopus oocytes: Equipment. *Meth. Enzymol.* **152:** 276–284.

Jiao, S., Ascadi, G., Jani, A., Felgner, P.L. and Wolff, J.A. (1992). Persistence of plasmid DNA and expression in rat brain cells *in vitro*. *Exp. Neurol.* **115:** 400–413.

Kaang, B.-K., Kandel, E.R. and Grant, S.G.N. (1993). Activation of cAMP-responsive genes by stimuli that produce long-term facilitation in *Aplysia* sensory neurons. *Neuron* **10:** 427–435.

Lindsay, R.M., Evison, C.J. and Winter, J. (1991). Culture of adult mammalian peripheral neurons, in: *Cellular neurobiology—a practical approach* (J. Chad and H. Wheal, eds), IRL Press (Oxford). pp. 3–17.

McLorie, W., McGlade, C.J., Takayesu, D. and Branton, P.E. (1991). Individual adenovirus E1B proteins induce transformation independently but by additive pathways. *J. Gen. Virol.* **72:** 1467–1471.

Minaschek, G., Bereiter-Hahn, J. and Bertholdt, G. (1989). Quantitation of the volume of liquid injected into cells by means of pressure. *Exp. Cell Res.* **183:** 434–442.

Mulderry, P.K., Chapman, K.E., Lyons, V. and Harmar, A.J. (1993). 5′-Flanking sequences from the rat preprotachykinin gene direct high-level expression of a reporter gene in adult rat sensory neurons transfected in culture by microinjection. *Mol. Cell. Neurosci.* **4:** 164–172.

Murphy, D. and Hanson, J. (1987). The production of transgenic mice by the microinjection of cloned DNA into fertilized one-cell eggs, in: *DNA cloning, a practical approach* (D.M. Glover, ed.), IRL Press (Oxford). vol. 3, pp. 213–248.

Pepperkok, R., Herr, S., Lorenz, P., Pyerin, W. and Ansorge, W. (1993). System for quantitation of gene expression in single cells by computerized microimaging: Application to *c-fos* expression after microinjection of anti-casein kinase II antibody. *Exp. Cell Res.* **204:** 278–285.

Pepperkok, R., Zanetti, M., King, R., Delia, D., Ansorge, W., Philipson, L. and Schneider, C. (1988).

Automatic microinjection system facilitates detection of growth inhibitory mRNA. *Proc. Natl Acad. Sci. USA* **85:** 6748–6752.

Proctor, G.N. (1992). Microinjection of DNA into mammalian cells in culture: theory and practice. *Meth. Mol. Cell. Biol.* **3:** 209–231.

Purves, R.D. (1981). *Microelectrode methods for intracellular recording and ionophoresis.* Academic Press (London).

White, E., Sabbatini, P., Debbas, M., Wold, W.S.M. and Kusher, D.I. (1992). The 19-kilodalton adenovirus E1B transforming protein inhibits programmed cell death and prevents cytolysis by tumour necrosis factor. *Meth. Mol. Cell. Biol.* **12:** 2570–2580.

Wyatt, S. and Davies, A.M. (1993). Regulation of expression of mRNAs encoding the nerve growth factor receptors p75 and *trkA* in developing sensory neurons. *Development* **119:** 635–647.

Zhang, Y.-Z., Naleway, J.J., Larison, K.D., Huang, Z. and Haugland, R.P. (1991). Detecting *LacZ* gene expression in living cells with new lipophilic, fluorogenic β-galactosidase substrates. *FASEB J.* **5:** 3108–3113.

CHAPTER 4

Methods for Gene Transfer Using Adenovirus–Polylysine–DNA Complexes

DAVID T. CURIEL

Gene Therapy Program, Comprehensive Cancer Center, 1824 6th Ave South, Room WTI 620, Birmingham, AL 35294-3300, USA. Tel: 205 934 8627; Fax: 205 975 7476

1 INTRODUCTION

Strategies have been developed to accomplish gene delivery via the receptor-mediated pathway (Wu and Wu, 1988; Cotten et al., 1990; Wagner et al., 1990, 1991, 1992b; Zenke et al., 1990; Curiel et al., 1991, 1992; Wu et al., 1991; Citro et al., 1992; Rosenkranz et al., 1992; Zatloukal et al., 1992; Ferkol et al., 1993). As cells possess endogenous pathways for internalization of macromolecules, the utilization of these pathways for the purpose of DNA delivery represents a strategy which potentially allows certain practical advantages. In this regard, these pathways can be highly efficient—for example, internalization of the iron transport protein transferrin can be thousands of molecules per minute per cell (Huebers and Finch, 1987; Thortensen and Romslo, 1990). Such pathways thus represent a potentially efficient physiologic method to transport nucleic acids across the cell membrane. To accomplish gene transfer via receptor-mediated endocytosis, a vehicle must be derived that allows DNA entry into these cellular pathways.

Molecular conjugate vectors have been derived for this purpose, consisting of two linked functional domains: (1) a DNA-binding domain, to transport the DNA as part of the vector complex; (2) a ligand domain to target a cellular receptor allowing entry of the conjugate–DNA complex via the receptor-mediated endocytosis pathway. For incorporating DNA into the vector complex binding must be achieved in a non-damaging, reversible manner. For this linkage, an electrostatic association between the binding domain and the nucleic acid is accomplished. To achieve this, the DNA-binding domain comprises a polycationic amine, such as poly-L-lysine, which can associate with the negatively charged DNA in an electrostatic, non-covalent manner. Entry of the vector complex through a receptor-mediated pathway is achieved using a ligand for the target cell—this may be a cell surface receptor ligand, an antireceptor antibody, or other agent which allows specific association with target cell membranes.

The interaction of the DNA with its binding domain serves not only to attach it to the molecular conjugate vector but also to condense it into a compact circular toroid (Wagner et al., 1991). In this configuration the ligand domain is presented on the exterior of the complex. By virtue of its surface location the ligand is free to recognize its target receptor on the cell surface membrane. After binding the ligand domain, the conjugate–DNA complex is internalized by the receptor-mediated pathway. In this schema, after internalization the complex is initially located within the cellular endosomes, and then may deliver its DNA to the target cell nucleus, where expression of

Protocols for Gene Transfer in Neuroscience: Towards Gene Therapy of Neurological Disorders
Edited by P.R. Lowenstein and L.W. Enquist

the transported genes may occur. Alternatively, the complex may be degraded in the lysosomes. Optimally, DNA delivery to the nucleus permits heterologous gene expression.

Delivery of genes by the receptor-mediated pathway offers certain features and potentials (Zatloukal et al., 1992; Cotten et al, 1993):

- large amounts of the conjugate vector can be prepared
- toxicity associated with target cell membrane perturbation is circumvented; thus the potential exists to administer the vector on a repetitive or continuous basis
- the marked plasticity of the system allows the potential to derive a vector with the properties of cell-specific targeting; that is, through choice of the ligand, domain cells possessing receptors for that ligand may be targeted, allowing this vector system to be used for gene therapy applications requiring cell-specific delivery of therapeutic genes
- the molecular conjugate vector system is devoid of viral gene elements: it would thus also be devoid of the potential safety hazards deriving from the presence of viral gene sequences and functions.

Gene delivery by receptor-mediated endocytosis was first described by Wu and Wu (1988),who selectively targeted hepatocytes using a receptor unique to this cell type. Hepatocytes possess receptors for recognition and clearance of asialoglycoproteins; these receptors are constituents of a high-efficiency internalization pathway that is relatively specific to hepatocytes. Asialoorosomucoid, a physiologic ligand for this receptor, was chemically conjugated to poly-L-lysine. The resulting conjugates formed complexes with DNA which could be shown to accomplish gene delivery specifically through the asialoglycoprotein receptor of hepatocytes. Utilizing this schema, Wu and colleagues were able to achieve selective delivery to hepatocytes *in vitro* and *in vivo* in a rodent model (Wu and Wu, 1988; Wu et al., 1991; Wilson et al., 1992).

Utilizing similar strategies other workers have developed a molecular conjugate system for delivering DNA through the transferrin internalization pathway (Wagner et al., 1990; Zenke et al., 1990). Transferrin is internalized by receptor-mediated endocytosis as part of a recycling pathway (Thortesen and Romslo, 1990). The transferrin receptor is expressed ubiquitously but is relatively enriched in proliferative and hematopoietic cells (Huebers and Finch, 1987). Gene transfer could also be accomplished through this pathway.

Gene delivery via receptor-mediated endocytosis has been described using antibodies directed against the polymerized IgA receptor (Ferkol et al., 1993) and using ligand systems employing folate, gp 120 and surfactant protein B (Baatz et al., 1994).

Thus, the receptor-mediated schema of gene delivery has been developed for an increasing number of gene transfer applications to capitalize on the potential to achieve non-toxic cellular entry and cell-specific gene delivery.

Despite the many potential advantages of receptor-mediated gene delivery, the efficacy of molecular conjugate vectors has been variable (Cotten et al., 1990; Zatloukal et al., 1992). For many target cells, even though the requisite cell surface receptor is present, gene transfer via the corresponding internalization pathway has not resulted in efficient expression of transferred genes—although the internalized complexes have been demonstrated within cellular endosomes (Zenke et al., 1990). This finding suggests that the inefficient gene expression is not related to initial binding and internalization steps, but reflects events occurring after entry of the complex into the cell. If the conjugate–DNA complex is entrapped within cellular endosomes, the internalized DNA cannot access the nucleus for gene expression. Consistent with this concept, it has been reported that treatment of cells with selected lysosomotropic agents can significantly augment gene expression in conjugate-transfected cells (Cotten et al., 1990). This suggests that loss of conjugate–DNA complexes through cellular degradation may be etiologic of their inability to achieve nuclear localization (and thus expression of transferred genes).

Taken together, these findings illustrate a fundamental flaw of the receptor-mediated gene transfer strategy as initially conceptualized: although the molecular conjugate vector possesses an efficient mechanism to achieve cellular internalization, it lacks a specific mechanism to escape entrapment within the endosome, which limits effective gene transfer and expression. If the molecular conjugate vector possessed an endosome escape mechanism the DNA internalized might not target to cellular pathways that destroy it. This effect could have a favorable outcome on overall efficiency of gene transfer.

In developing methods to overcome endosome entrapment of conjugate–DNA complexes the entry mechanisms of certain viruses were studied. The initial step in cellular entry of both enveloped and non-enveloped viruses involves binding to a specific cellular receptor. In a subset of these viruses internalization after binding occurs via receptor-mediated endocytosis (Pastan et al., 1986; Kielian and Jungerwirth, 1990). Once inside the cell, these viruses employ specific mechanisms to allow their genetic material to escape endosomes so that the viral life cycle may be completed in the cell nucleus or cytosol. Viral entry thus possesses certain parallels to the entry of molecular conjugate vectors: like the conjugate vector, viruses may possess specific and efficient receptor-mediated entry mechanisms. However, in contrast to conjugate vectors, after internalization viruses possess mechanisms that allow them to escape entrapment within cell vesicles.

It was hypothesized that this property of certain viruses could be exploited to overcome endosome entrapment of the conjugate–DNA complex, and thus facilitate gene transfer. Previous studies had linked viral entry to enhanced cellular uptake of various macromolecules. Fernandez-Puentes and Carrasco (1980) used both enveloped and non-enveloped virus to show augmented cellular internalization of macromolecules. Although these studies did not delineate the mechanistic basis for this phenomenon, or distinguish between membrane bound or fluid phase molecules, the link between viral uptake and enhanced cellular entry of heterologous molecules was clearly established.

FitzGerald et al. (1983) developed a system of anti-tumor therapeutics based on delivery of ligand–toxin chimeras via receptor-mediated endocytosis. Entrapment of the chimeric toxin molecule in the cellular endosome limited tumoricidal efficacy but this limitation could be overcome by codelivery of adenovirus with the toxin. FitzGerald et al. showed that the virus colocalized with the conjugate during internalization and that the adenovirus's ability to disrupt cellular endosomes allowed ingress of the conjugate into the cytosol, where its activity was potentiated.

This effect is mediated by viral capsid proteins and is independent of viral gene expression. In this regard, the entry cycle of the adenovirus has been partially elucidated (Chardonnet and Dales, 1970; Svensson and Persson, 1984; Pastan et al., 1986). The virus first attaches to the target cell by binding to a specific cell surface receptor. This receptor has not yet been characterized, but its presence has been established by functional studies and it appears to be expressed in a ubiquitous manner. The adenovirus accomplishes this initial binding step using a specific capsid protein named fiber. Once bound to the cellular recognition receptor, uptake is facilitated by subsequent binding of specific viral capsid regions to cellular proteins which act as uptake "triggers" (Wickham et al., 1993). The virion is then localized within cellular endosomes. The virus then acidifies the endosome, disrupting it, and escapes from the cell vesicle system. Studies using cellular targets with defective acidification of their endosomes, or augmenting the endosomal pH of otherwise normal cells, have shown that these changes limit adenovirus propagation (Seth et al., 1984). Importantly, replication-defective adenovirus strains may still complete the principal entry steps as well as wild-type viruses. Based on these findings, it has been suggested that acidification of the endosome alters the conformation of certain capsid proteins (Seth et al., 1984; Pastan et al., 1986), which allows the virion to interact with the endosome membrane in such a way as to disrupt the vesicle. It is the capsid proteins that mediate the effect of endosome disruption—viral gene expression is not an essential feature of this process.

Based upon this concept, we hypothesized that adenovirus entry could be exploited to aid the internalized conjugate–DNA complex to escape endosomes. In this schema, the provision of endosome disruption functions would be expected to augment the overall gene transfer efficiency mediated by the molecular conjugates. To test this hypothesis, transferrin–polylysine–DNA complexes containing a firefly luciferase reporter plasmid DNA were codelivered with the replication-defective adenovirus *dl*312 to HeLa cells. This use of the replication-defective adenovirus provided a convenient means of separating the possible effects mediated by viral entry and viral gene expression, as this adenovirus strain is defective in its gene expression secondary to a genomic deletion in the E1A/B early viral gene regions (Jones and Shenk, 1979). We noted that as input of adenovirus increased there was a corresponding increase in the level of luciferase gene expression (Curiel et al., 1991) up to a level of luciferase gene expression more than 2000 times that observed when the conjugates were used without virus. Significantly, the amount of virus required to achieve these augmented levels of gene expression corresponded to the number of receptors for the adenovirus on the target cell (Defer et al., 1990). The characteristics of receptor-mediated endocytosis facilitation by this route were saturable, as would be expected in a receptor-limiting context.

To determine the mechanism of the virus's ability to augment gene transfer mediated by molecular conjugates, virus entry was uncoupled from virus-mediated endosome disruption by mild heat treatment of the adenovirus (Defer et al., 1990). Additionally, mild heat treatment does not affect the structural integrity of the adenoviral genome. By selectively removing the viral endosome disruption capacity, its contribution to adenovirus-mediated augmentation of molecular conjugate gene transfer could be ascertained. In these experiments, heat treatment completely abrogated the ability of the virus to augment the conjugate's gene transfer capacity, confirming that it is specifically the viral property of endosomolysis that contributes to its capacity to augment the conjugate's gene transfer capacity. This furthermore underscores the fact that it is the molecular conjugate vector's lack of an endosome escape mechanism that represents its principal limitation to achieving efficient gene transfer to target cells.

The augmented levels of net gene expression accomplished by adenoviral augmentation of molecular conjugates are consistent with increased gene expression in a transfected cell subset or with an increase in the number of cells transfected. To distinguish between these possibilities, HeLa cells were transfected with transferrin–polylysine conjugates containing a β-galactosidase reporter gene (Cotten et al., 1992). Cells transduced with the complexes alone demonstrated a transduction frequency of less than 1% but when adenovirus was added as a facilitator more than 95% of the HeLa cells expressed the β-galactosidase reporter gene. Thus, adenoviral augmentation of conjugate-mediated transfer significantly enhanced the frequency of transfection. To demonstrate this further, limiting dilutions of transferrin–polylysine–luciferase DNA complexes were delivered to cells with or without adenovirus. In the presence of adenovirus, the same levels of heterologous gene expression were noted as when two orders of magnitude more DNA were delivered without adenoviral augmentation (Curiel et al., 1991). Thus, the virus appears to confer a high level of efficiency on the process of DNA delivery mediated by molecular conjugates. This phenomenon has been observed in a variety of cell types treated in this manner. Additionally, certain cell types which appeared refractory to transferrin–polylysine-mediated gene transfer were less so if adenovirus was codelivered (Curiel et al., 1991).

Selective exploitation of adenoviral entry features is possible because adenoviral capsid proteins mediate the endosome disruption step of viral entry. In this regard, expression of the viral genome is not required to facilitate molecular conjugate entry. In this context, steps may be undertaken to remove viral gene elements while sparing the capacity of the capsid to accomplish cell vesicle disruption; for example, ultraviolet light alone and in combination with psoralen abolishes viral infectivity while retaining the virus's ability to facilitate molecular conjugate-mediated gene transfer (Cotten et al., 1992). Employing this methodology, it is possible to render the adenoviral genome inactive in two complementary manners: genetic deletion of the adenoviral genome and physical inactivation of the adenoviral genome. This is in marked contradistinction to recombinant viral vectors, in which the integrity of viral gene elements is crucial to gene transfer efficacy, as the heterologous sequences are contained in the context of the parent viral genome. For recombinant viral vectors it is thus not possible to more completely inactivate viral gene elements.

DNA delivery by this method is very flexible. The polylysine component of the molecular conjugate interacts with DNA in a sequence-independent manner. Thus, DNA of any design can be incorporated into the conjugate–DNA complex and delivered for transfection purposes. Because the heterologous DNA is not packaged into a virion capsid, the amount of DNA that may be delivered is not limited by the corresponding packaging constraints. Using this approach, DNA plasmids of up to 48 kb have been delivered (Cotten et al., 1992). The fact that the heterologous sequences are not incorporated into a viral genome minimizes the possibility of interactions among the distinct regulatory regions.

The utility of the adenovirus in facilitating DNA entry in the *trans* configuration suggested that it might also be possible to accomplish this with the adenovirus functioning in *cis*. As molecular conjugates are functionally limited by their lack of an endosome escape mechanism, and because adenovirus possesses such a mechanism, it seems logical to incorporate the adenovirus into the configuration of the molecular conjugate vector. The first technical barrier to achieving this was the problem of attaching the adenovirus to the polylysine–DNA binding moiety: attaching moieties to the adenoviral capsid could perturb the capsid proteins involved in adenoviral binding and entry. The adenoviral proteins "fiber" and "penton base" are thought to be of major importance in the entry steps (Seth et al., 1984; Pastan et al., 1986) but protein "hexon" is thought to function as "scaffolding" of the capsid, and is thus less important in viral entry processes.

Therefore, the most favorable site on the adenovirus to which to link the polylysine–DNA complex was hexon, and antibodies directed toward the hexon protein were used to achieve such a link. First, the hexon gene of the adenovirus was isolated, then specific mutations were introduced into the hexon gene to create a region coding for a heterologous epitope. The gene sequence that was altered corresponded to a region of the hexon protein known to be present on the exterior surface face of the virus. It was thus possible to generate a chimeric adenovirus with the heterologous epitope localized in a manner to permit non-neutralizing interaction with a monoclonal antibody specific for it.

Once the chimeric adenovirus was created, attachment could be carried out using the antibody specific for the heterologous epitope. When condensed with DNA, the resulting toroid possessed surface-localized immunoglobin capable of recognizing the heterologous epitope on the chimeric virus.

When linking the polylysine-DNA-binding moiety to the adenovirus exterior, specific steps were undertaken to avoid perturbing adenoviral capsid proteins involved in endosome disruption. It has been shown that these specific steps are not obligatory for functional incorporation of the adenovirus into the configuration of the molecular conjugate vector: Wagner et al. (1992b) demonstrated that DNA–polylysine complexes may be attached to the adenoviral capsid enzymatically, employing transglutaminase and by exploiting the biotin–streptavidin interaction, using streptavidin–polylysine conjugates in conjunction with biotin-labeled adenovirus; Cristiano et al. (1993) have also shown that adenovirus and polylysine may be linked directly utilizing the heterobifunctional cross-linking agent EDC. This is an extremely easy method of constructing this vector and we presently employ a variation of this methodology. Adenovirus conjugates derived by these methods possess activity profiles comparable to complexes employing immunologic methods of attachment.

Adenovirus in the linked configuration is capable of significantly higher levels of gene expression than those obtained by free viral facilitation. This probably reflects the different pathways of DNA delivery in the two different contexts. In free adenovirus facilitation of molecular conjugates, the virus enhances gene transfer by disrupting cell vesicles to allow ingress of the conjugate–DNA complex into the cytosol but the internalized complex possesses no specific mechanism to achieve localization in the nucleus after cell entry. In contrast, in the linked configuration, after endosome disruption, the complex possesses the additional capacity to localize to the nuclear pore, based on the adenoviral moiety's capacity to do so (Greber et al., 1993). In this situation, the overall dynamics of gene transfer are more favorable for expression of the heterologous genes. Thus, adenovirus in the linked configuration provides the important entry features of cell vesicle disruption and nuclear localization of the delivered DNA.

In the adenovirus–polylysine–DNA complex configuration, the adenovirus moiety was incorporated to function as an endosome disrupter but it also represents the sole ligand domain of the molecular conjugate. The relative gene transfer efficiency of this vector might be determined by the relative tropism of the adenovirus for a given cellular target. This is indeed the case: HeLa and KB cells, cells with a relatively high number of surface receptors for adenovirus, are highly susceptible to gene transfer by this vector system. In contrast, cells such as HBE1 and MRC-5, with relatively fewer cell surface receptors for adenovirus, have a correspondingly lower susceptibility to gene transfer by the adenovirus–polylysine–DNA complexes (Curiel et al., 1992). Strategies have been developed to determine whether the adenovirus could be employed as an endosomolysis agent in conjunction with an alternative ligand: this would presumably overcome the limitation of adenoviral receptor targeting of the adenovirus–polylysine–DNA complexes.

The derivation of the "combination complexes" was thus undertaken. Vector construction involves the sequential addition of adenovirus, linker antibody–polylysine conjugate, DNA, followed by a second ligand–polylysine conjugate to form a complex containing multiple independent functional domains: a ligand domain to target specific cell subsets, an endosomolysis domain to enhance overall gene transfer efficiency by accomplishing cell vesicle escape, and a DNA binding domain.

The combination complexes were delivered to HeLa cells, a cellular target with receptors for both adenovirus and the alternative ligand (in this case transferrin). The combination complexes mediated even further augmentation of gene expression (Curiel et al., 1992), which was greater than an additive effect of transferrin–polylysine and adenovirus–polylysine would predict. This suggests that effectively there is an element of cooperativity related to the ability of the complexes to accomplish DNA delivery because these complexes are capable of entering cells by both the transferrin and the adenovirus internalization pathways.

To establish this concept, the combination complexes were delivered to cellular targets relatively poor in adenovirus receptors, such as the HBE1 cell line, which is refractory to transduction with adenovirus–polylysine–DNA complexes. When transfected with the combination complexes, however, levels of gene expression comparable to those seen in HeLa cells were noted in HBE1 cells. The complexes probably enter the cell through non-adenoviral pathways, demonstrating the utility of providing a second ligand in the complex design.

Once it became known that high-efficiency gene delivery could be achieved by including an endosomolytic domain into the design of the molecular conjugate, alternative strategies were developed to incorporate this functional attribute. There are many reasons for eliminating intact adenovirus from the conjugate configuration: the incorporated virion possesses the capacity to function as an alternate ligand domain, potentially undermining the desired property of cell-specific targeting; additionally, although the adenoviral genome is inactivated, its presence represents a potential safety concern. Attempts have been made to isolate the portion of the adenoviral capsid which mediates cell vesicle disruption for inclusion into the molecular conjugate design. However, these attempts have not been successful, possibly reflecting the fact that adenovirus-mediated cell vesicle disruption is a complicated process, requiring the coordinated actions of multiple capsid components (E. Wagner, personal communication). This also bears negatively upon attempts to utilize recombinant capsid components deriving from adenovirus. Cotten et al. (1993) have recently employed a xenotropic adenovirus for this purpose. The adenoviral strain CELO was demonstrated to perform as an endosomolysis agent at functional levels comparable to human serotypes but it is relatively difficult to prepare large amounts of this virion.

The optimal endosome disruption agent would be a synthetic product—circumventing any issues associated with virus or viral products. To this end, Wagner et al. (1992a) have explored the utility of synthetic viral peptides with fusogenic properties. Inclusion of these peptides into the molecular conjugate structure can be demonstrated to augment gene transfer efficiencies, but the levels of augmentation observed are far inferior to those observed with intact adenovirus. Thus, for the present, the intact adenovirus provides the most effective means of conferring upon molecular conjugate vectors the capacity to achieve cell vesicle escape and thus to accomplish high-efficiency gene delivery.

In combination complexes multiple independent domains are incorporated to provide multiple independent functions. These functions operate in a concerted manner to facilitate overall gene transfer. The incorporation of the adenovirus provides the important functional attribute of cell vesicle escape for the complex but by virtue of its binding capacity through its fiber protein, it provides an alternative ligand domain for the complex. This alternative source of binding undermines the capacity to achieve cell-specific targeting, one of the theoretical attributes of the molecular conjugate vector system. Thus, it would be desirable to exploit the endosomolytic capacity of the adenovirus without allowing it to behave as an alternative ligand.

One way of doing this is to block adenoviral binding using an antibody specific for the cell receptor binding domain of the adenoviral fiber protein (Michael et al., 1993). Such an antibody was derived by immunization with purified adenoviral fiber protein and screening for antibodies with neutralizing capacity. The capacity of the antibody to block adenoviral binding and internalization was first established, then it was determined whether the antibody's blockade of adenoviral entry could destroy the ability of free adenovirus to facilitate molecular conjugate-mediated gene transfer. The antifiber antibody was indeed found to remove the ability of the adenovirus to facilitate molecular conjugate-mediate gene transfer, confirming that cellular entry of the virus is crucial to its capacity to augment conjugate-mediated gene delivery.

The next step was to derive combination complexes which incorporate adenovirus precoated with antibody against the fiber protein (to block entry via adenoviral receptor pathways). It was suggested that the "adenovirus-blocked" complex could still enter via the pathway of the alternative ligand, transferrin, and the virus would still be able to mediate endosomolysis. When analysed, the use of binding-incompetent virus did not decrease the overall levels of gene transfer observed, which indicated that fiber binding was not required for the virus to mediate endosome disruption. Thus, the processes of adenoviral binding and endosome disruption are not functionally linked. It is therefore theoretically possible to construct a molecular conjugate vector in which the adenovirus moiety is incorporated exclusively in the capacity of an endosomolytic agent, and does not function as a competition ligand.

Removal of the adenovirus moiety as a potential competitor ligand enhances the overall specificity of the conjugate vector for a given target cell. However, there are other sources of non-specific binding within the conjugate design as well as the adenovirus. For example, certain cells bind to polylysine–DNA complexes in a non-specific manner (Cotten et al., 1993). In these cases, when non-ligand–polylysine–DNA complexes are codelivered to cells with adenovirus, they may accomplish levels of gene transfer comparable to ligand–polylysine complexes. This represents another factor potentially undermining the cell-specific binding capacity of the vector.

This non-specific association between polylysine and the target cell surface is on an electrostatic basis, so it was hypothesized that by neutralizing the charge differential this non-specific attachment would be reduced. To this end, yeast tRNA, a negatively charged polynucleotide, was employed to treat polylysine-condensed DNA. This treatment significantly reduced the non-specific binding mediated by the polylysine–DNA complex (Michael and Curiel, 1994). To determine whether the tRNA interfered with specific ligand–polylysine internalization, transferrin–polylysine–DNA complexes were treated in a similar manner and analysed for their capacity to achieve binding and internalization when codelivered with adenovirus. The tRNA did not interfere with specific ligand–polylysine gene transfer. Thus, maneuvers capable of reducing non-specific cell binding of the polylysine component of the ligand–polylysine complexes may be employed without affecting the specific receptor-mediated endocytosis uptake of ligand–polylysine complexes. This has the potential to enhance the cell specificity of the conjugate vector.

Various methods of eliminating potential sources of non-specific binding may be employed in the molecular conjugate to achieve cell-specific gene delivery. The specificity of the molecular conjugate is determined by its ligand domain, which dictates the cellular binding of the vector. Ligands employed may be physiologic, as in the case of asialoglycoprotein and transferrin, or may be a synthetic mimic of a physiologic ligand. Wagner et al. (1992b) have targeted the asialoglycoprotein receptor using an asialoglycoprotein mimic.

Anti-receptor antibodies have also been used (Curiel et al., 1994) with anti-IgG immunoglobulin serving as ligand for cell-surface immunoglobulins for targeting B lymphocytes. The use of viral proteins with specific affinity for cell-type markers has also been demonstrated by targeting CD4 human lymphocytes with HIV gp120–ligand conjugates. In these instances, ligands were employed to direct molecular conjugate vectors into pathways which were known to be associated with efficient cellular internalization. We thought that it might also be possible to target conjugates employing ligands which do not bind to characterized cellular internalization pathways. Batra et al. (1995) have developed molecular conjugates exploiting the utility of cell surface–lectin interactions for vector targeting and found that lectins could facilitate effective gene delivery mediated by molecular conjugates. In this instance, cell surface binding of the lectin–polylysine–DNA complex appeared sufficient to induce a level of cellular internalization permissive of effective gene delivery. Thus, targeted molecular conjugate vectors may be designed to exploit characterized cellular receptor-mediated endocytosis pathways. Additionally, in some instances the employment of ligand moieties possessing cell binding affinity may be sufficient to allow functionally relevant internalization of the conjugate–DNA complex.

The design of adenovirus–component molecular conjugate vectors represents a unique manner of exploiting viral entry features to achieve gene delivery. This strategy is distinct from the design of recombinant viral vectors. In the instance of recombinant viral vectors, the overall entry mechanism of the virus is exploited to achieve gene delivery through incorporation of the foreign gene into the virus genome but for the adenovirus–component molecular conjugate vectors, viral entry features are exploited to facilitate gene transfer in a highly selective manner. This possibility arises from the fact that the capacity of the adenovirus to achieve entry is an intrinsic property of its capsid proteins. This mechanism may thus be incorporated into a vector system whereby the viral gene elements are obviated. The vector design that derives from this strategy results in a system with potential advantages related to utility and safety. Furthermore, the development of a vector system with the engineered capacity to achieve cell-specific gene delivery is in conceptual accord with the concept of a "targetable-injectable" vector (Morgan and Anderson, 1993). The further development of the capacities within the present vector design may allow the achievement of a vector system possessing many of the attributes of this proposed vector ideal.

2 MATERIALS AND EQUIPMENT

(1) Cell culture medium: Dulbecco's Modified Eagle's Medium (DMEM) supplemented with 10% heat-inactivated fetal calf serum (FCS) and penicillin/streptomycin is used for routine cultivation of tissue culture cells. For particular experiments, this medium is modified (SEE SECTION 3).
(2) CsCl, density 1.33: dissolve CsCl in 5 mM HEPES, pH 7.3 (454.2 mg/ml).
(3) CsCl, density 1.45: dissolve CsCl in 5 mM HEPES, pH 7.3 (609.0 mg/ml).
(4) HBS solution: 20 mM HEPES, pH 7.3, plus 150 mM NaCl.
(5) Poly-L-lysine solution: 500 mg poly-L-lysine (Sigma P-2636) dissolved in 50 ml HBS and pH adjusted to 7.3. The final volume is brought up to 84 ml with HBS and the reagent stored in 500 μl aliquots at -20°C.
(6) Poly-L-lysine (pL) solution: poly-L-lysine (Sigma P-2636) dissolved to 1 mg/ml in HBS stock and stored in 500 μl aliquots at -20°C. This reagent is distinct from the reagent prepared in the previous step, which is used in the chemical linkage protocol (Protocol #14).
(7) EDC: dissolve 1 g EDC powder (Pierce #2280G) in 4.0 ml distilled water at time of use and store at 4°C. Any unused solution should be discarded immediately after use. Unused EDC powder should be stored at -20°C.
(8) Viral preservation medium: Combine 1 ml 1 M Tris, pH 8.0, 2 ml 5 M NaCl and 0.1 g bovine serum albumin (BSA). Bring volume up to 50 ml and mix until BSA is dissolved. Add 50 ml glycerol, filter sterilize and store at 4°C.
(9) Appropriate plasmid DNA containing gene(s) of interest should be purified on CsCl gradient for best results. Removal of endotoxin may also be beneficial.

3 THE PROTOCOLS

Protocol #12: Large-scale Preparation of Adenovirus

(1) Grow 293, HeLa or W162 cells to roughly 80% confluence in 20 75-cm^2 flasks (approx. 10^7 cells/flask) in DMEM/10% fetal calf serum with penicillin and streptomycin.
(2) Remove medium.
(3) Dilute seed viral stock in 100 ml DMEM/2% heat-inactivated fetal calf serum ("2% FCS medium") and add 5 ml to each flask. Viral stock should contain 10^{10}–10^{11} viral particles to achieve a multiplicity of infection of 100–1000 viral particles per cell.
(4) Incubate 1–2 h at 37°C, in an atmosphere of 5% CO_2.
(5) Add 10 ml complete medium to each flask (DMEM/10% fetal-calf serum/penicillin and streptomycin).
(6) Incubate for 48–72 h, 37°C, 5% CO_2 atmosphere until prominent cytopathic effect is seen in cells.
(7) Decant cells and medium from flasks into 50 ml capped centrifuge tubes.

(8) Spin down at 1000 r.p.m. for 10 min at 4°C.
(9) Remove supernatant by aspiration and resuspend combined cell pellets in 20 ml 2% FCS medium.
(10) Freeze–thaw four times (may use a 37°C bath alternating with a dry ice/ethanol bath).
(11) Spin down at 4000 r.p.m., 20 min, 4°C. Harvest supernatant and save at 4°C while setting up gradients.
(12) Prepare a discontinuous CsCl gradient in a Beckmann SW28 tube: first add 20 ml CsCl density 1.33 and then add 10 ml layer of CsCl density 1.45.
(13) Overlay gradient with 5 ml viral cell lysate and centrifuge at 18 000 r.p.m. for 90 min, 20°C. Virus will make visible bands in the middle of the gradient.
(14) Harvest lowest opalescent band by puncturing tube with a needle/syringe and collecting approximately 2 ml.
(15) Dilute solution 1:1 with 5 mM HEPES, pH 7.3.
(16) Prepare a discontinuous CsCl gradient in a Beckmann SW41 tube: 4 ml CsCl density 1.33 followed by a layer of 4 ml CsCl, density 1.45.
(17) Overlay with the diluted virus prepared in step 15.
(18) Spin at 25 000 r.p.m. for at least 18 h at 20°C.
(19) Harvest lower band in minimal volume.
(20) Use virus directly for chemical coupling to poly-L-lysine (Protocol #14) or preserve by diluting one part virus solution with five parts viral preservation medium and store in 50–100 μl aliquots at −70°C.

Protocol #13: Determination of Adenovirus Concentration

(1) Mix 100 μl of adenovirus solution with 900 μl 1 × Tris–EDTA, pH 7.8.
(2) Determine absorbance at 260 nm: 1 unit equals approximately 10^{12} viral particles per ml.

Protocol #14: Chemical Linkage of Adenovirus and Poly-L-lysine

(1) Prepare virus as described in Protocol #12.
(2) After the second spin (step 11), resuspend virus in CsCl density 1.33 to a final volume of 2.5 ml.
(3) Load onto PD10 column (Pharmacia) pre-equilibrated with HBS.
(4) Elute with 2 ml HBS.
(5) Resuspend in HBS to final volume 3.6 ml.
(6) Linkage reaction: to 3.6 ml virus, add 0.4 ml poly-L-lysine and 0.04 ml EDC.
(7) Incubate on ice 4 h.
(8) Mix well with 8 ml CsCl density 1.45.
(9) Centrifuge at 25 000 r.p.m. for 18 h in an SW41 tube.
(10) Harvest opalescent band.
(11) Dilute with viral preservation medium to achieve a concentration of 1×10^{11} particles/ml and divide into 100 μl aliquots.
(12) Store at −70°C.

Protocol #15: Preparation of Adenovirus–polylysine–DNA Complexes

This protocol will prepare 6.0 μg DNA (enough for the transfection of about 1×10^6 cells). The protocol may be scaled up or down, as required.

(1) Add 100 μl adenovirus–polylysine (EDC-linked AdpL at 1×10^{11} particles/ml) to 6.0 μg plasmid DNA in 200 μl HBS, pH 7.3.
(2) Incubate 30 min at room temperature.
(3) Add 4.0 μl pL solution in 200 μl HBS or 6.0 μl human transferrin–polylysine (Serva; 1 mg/ml) in 200 μl HBS.
(4) Incubate for 30 min at room temperature.

(5) Add the complex produced to cells that are in half of the normal culture volume in 2% FCS medium.
(6) Incubate 60 min at 37°C.
(7) Add half the final volume of media with FCS to bring final FCS concentration to a maintenance level appropriate for that cell line.

4 NOTES AND TROUBLESHOOTING

For certain applications, adenovirus–component molecular conjugate vectors are ideal in their present, unmodified, form. For example, they are highly efficient transfection reagents for many *in vitro* applications. In addition to mediating high-efficiency gene transfer in transformed human cells, they are able to mediate high-efficiency gene transfer in primary cell cultures of various tissue types. This is of significance in *ex vivo* transduction of cells that are to be retransplanted after transfection with the gene of interest.

Another important property of the molecular conjugate design is its ability to deliver large DNA constructs, which often cannot otherwise be done in many recombinant viral systems. This may allow the use of specific promoter elements to achieve specificity of gene expression. In addition to delivering large genes efficiently, it is also possible to deliver multiple DNA constructs simultaneously.

Despite their efficacy *in vitro*, their efficacy *in vivo* has been idiosyncratic. Gao et al. (1993) have shown that molecular conjugate vectors are able to mediate gene transfer in the airway epithelium of cotton rats but observed gene transfer was not as efficient as would be expected from the efficacy observed *in vitro*. This is due to the instability of molecular conjugates *in vivo*. The polylysine component of the conjugates is a target of humoral factors after *in vivo* delivery (E. Wagner; personal communication).

As one basis of conjugate instability is understood, several steps may be taken to address this problem. The polylysine component is the primary locus of conjugate instability *in vivo*, and it is therefore logical that replacing the polylysine–DNA binding moiety with some other DNA-binding component may overcome this limitation. An alternative strategy would be to directly link the DNA to the ligand using cross-linking reagents or with a high affinity biotin–streptavidin linkage.

In addition, a conceptually distinct strategy that is presently being developed seeks to mask the polycation component of conjugates using "stealthing" procedures.

Methods for enhanced *in vivo* gene delivery complex formation have been reported which give acceptable efficiencies of gene transduction. For example, Perales et al. (1994) have shown that by optimizing ionic conditions during complex formation it is possible to deliver conjugate–DNA complexes with a more compact, discrete size. These complexes have been reported to achieve efficient, targeted gene delivery after systemic vector administration. These methodologies may therefore circumvent the limitations to gene delivery *in vivo* noted in earlier studies.

ACKNOWLEDGMENTS

The author wishes to express his gratitude to his coworkers Frosty Loechel and Sharon Michael at the University of Alabama at Birmingham, Raj Batra and Ling Gao at the University of North Carolina, Chapel Hill and Matt Cotten and Ernst Wagner at the Institute of Molecular Pathology in Vienna, Austria.

REFERENCES

Baatz, J.E., Bruno, M.D., Ciraolo, P.J., Glasser, S.W., Stripp, B.R., Smyth, K.L., Korfhagen, T.R. (1994). Utilization of modified surfactant-associated protein B for delivery of DNA to airway cells in culture. *Proc Natl Acad Sci USA* **91:** 2547–2551.

Batra, R.K., Johanning, F.W., Wagner, E., Garver Jr., R.I., Curiel, D.T. (1995). Receptor-mediated gene delivery employing lectin-binding specificity. *Gene Ther* **1:** 255–260.

Chardonnet, Y., Dales, S. (1970). Early events in the interaction of adenoviruses with HeLa cells. 1. Penetration of Type 5 and intracellular release of the DNA genome. *Virology* **40:** 462–477.

Citro, G., Perrotti, D., Cucco, C., et al. (1992). Inhibition of leukemia cell proliferation by receptor-mediated uptake of c-myb antisense oligodeoxynucleotides. *Proc Natl Acad Sci USA* **89:** 7031–7035.

Cotten, M., Wagner, E., Birnstiel, M.L. (1993). Receptor mediated transport of DNA into eukaryotic cells. *Methods Enzymol* **217:** 618–644.

Cotten, M., Lange-Rouault, F., Kirlappos, H., et al. (1990). Transferrin-polycation-mediated introduction of DNA into human leukemic cells: Stimulation by agents that affect the survival of transfected DNA or modulate transferrin receptor levels. *Proc Natl Acad Sci USA* **87:** 4033–4037.

Cotten, M., Wagner, E., Zatloukal, K., Phillips, S., Curiel, D.T., Birnstiel, M.L. (1992). High-efficiency receptor-mediated delivery of small and large (48 kilobase) gene constructs using the endosome-disruption activity of defective or chemically inactivated adenovirus particles. *Proc Natl Acad Sci USA* **89:** 6040–6098.

Cotten, M., Wagner, E., Zatloukal, K., Birnstiel, M.L. (1993). Chicken adenovirus (CELO virus) particles augment receptor-mediated DNA delivery to mammalian cells and yield exceptional levels of stable transformants. *J Virol* **67:** 3777–3785.

Cristiano, R.J., Smith, L.C., Kay, M.A., Brinkley, B.R., Woo, S.L. (1993). Hepatic gene therapy: Efficient gene delivery and expression in primary hepatocytes utilizing a conjugated adenovirus–DNA complex. *Proc Natl Acad Sci USA* **90:** 11548–11552.

Curiel, D.T., Agarwal, S., Wagner, E., Cotten, M. (1991). Adenovirus enhancement of transferrin–polylysine-mediated gene delivery. *Proc Natl Acad Sci USA* **88:** 8850–8854.

Curiel, D.T., Wagner, E., Cotten, M., et al. (1992). High efficiency gene transfer mediated by adenovirus coupled to DNA–polylysine complexes. *Hum Gene Ther* **3:** 147–154.

Curiel, T., Cook, D.R., Bogedain, C., Jilg, W., Harrison, G.S., Cotten, M., Curiel, D.T., Wagner, E. (1994). Efficient foreign gene expression in Epstein–Barr virus-transformed human B-cells. *Virology* **198:** 577–585.

Defer, C., Belin, M-T., Caillet-Boudin, M-L., Boulanger, P. (1990). Human adenovirus–host cell interactions: Comparative study with members of subgroups B and C. *J Virol* **64:** 3661–3673.

Ferkol, T., Kaetzel, C.S., Davis, P.B. (1993). Gene transfer into respiratory epithelial cells by targeting the polymeric immunoglobulin receptor. *J Clin Invest* **92:** 2394–2400.

Fernandez-Puentes, C., Carrasco, L. (1980). Viral infection permeabilizes mammalian cells to protein toxins. *Cell* **20:** 769–775.

FitzGerald, D.J.P., Padmanabhan, R., Pastan, I., Willingham, M.C. (1983). Adenovirus-induced release of epidermal growth factor and pseudomonas toxin into the cytosol of KB cells during receptor-mediated endocytosis. *Cell* **32:** 607–617.

Gao, L., Wagner, E., Cotten, M., Agarwal, S., Harris, C., Romer, M., Miller, L., Hu, P-C., Curiel, D. (1993). Direct in vivo gene transfer to airway epithelium employing adenovirus-polylysine-DNA complexes. *Hum Gene Ther* **4:** 17–24.

Greber, U.F., Willetts, M., Webster, P., Helenius, A. (1993). Stepwise dismantling of adenovirus 2 during entry into cells. *Cell* **75:** 477–486.

Huebers, H., Finch, C. (1987). The physiology of transferrin receptors. *Physiol Rev* **67:** 520–582.

Jones, N., Shenk, T. (1979). An adenovirus type 5 early gene function regulates expression of other early viral genes. *Proc Natl Acad Sci USA* **76:** 3665–3669.

Kielian, M., Jungerwirth, S. (1990). Mechanisms of enveloped virus entry into cells. *Mol Biol Med* **7:** 17–31.

Michael, S.I., Curiel, D.T. (1994). Strategies to achieve targeted gene delivery via the receptor-mediated endocytosis pathway. *Gene Ther* **1:** 223–232.

Michael, S.I., Huang, C-h., Romer, M.U., Wagner, E., Hu, P-c., Curiel, D.T. (1993). Binding-incompetent adenovirus facilitates molecular conjugate-mediated gene transfer by the receptor-mediated endocytosis pathway. *J Biol Chem* **268:** 6866–6869.

Morgan, R.A., Anderson, W.F. (1993). Human Gene Therapy. *Annu Rev Biochem* **62:** 191–217.

Pastan, I., Seth, P., FitzGerald, D., Willingham, M. (1986). Adenovirus entry into cells: Some new observations on an old problem. In *Virus Attachment and Entry into Cells*. Crowell, R.L., Lonberg-Holm, K. (eds). Washington, DC: American Society for Microbiology; 141–146.

Perales, J.C., Ferkol, T., Beegen, H., Ratnoff, O.D., Hanson, R.W. (1994). Gene transfer *in vivo*: sustained expression and regulation of genes introduced into the liver by receptor-targeted uptake. *Proc Natl Acad Sci USA* **91:** 4086–4090.

Rosenkranz, A.A., Yachmenev, S.V., Jans, D.A., et al. (1992). Receptor-mediated endocytosis and nuclear transport of a transfecting DNA construct. *Exp Cell Res* **199:** 323–329.

Seth, P., FitzGerald, D., Ginsberg, H., Willingham, M., Pastan, I. (1984). Evidence that the penton base of adenovirus is involved in potentiation of toxicity of Pseudomonas exotoxin conjugated to epidermal growth factor. *Mol Cell Biol* **4:** 1528–1533.

Svensson, U., Persson, R. (1984). Entry of adenovirus 2 into HeLa cells. *J Virol* **51:** 687–694.

Thorstensen, K., Romslo, I. (1990). The role of transferrin in the mechanism of cellular iron uptake. *Biochem J* **271:** 1–10.

Wagner, E., Zenke, M., Cotten, M., Beug, H., Birnstiel, M.L. (1990). Transferrin-polycation conjugates as carriers for DNA uptake into cells. *Proc Natl Acad Sci USA* **87:** 3410-3414.

Wagner, E., Cotten, M., Foisner, R., Birnstiel, M.L. (1991). Transferrin–polycation–DNA complexes: The effect of polycations on the structure of the complex and DNA delivery to cells. *Proc Natl Acad Sci USA* **88:** 4255–4259.

Wagner, E., Plank, C., Zatloukal, K., Cotten, M., Birnstiel, M.L. (1992a). Influenza virus hemagglutinin HA-2 N-terminal fusogenic peptides augment gene transfer by transferrin-polylysine-DNA complexes: Toward a synthetic virus-like gene-transfer vehicle. *Proc Natl Acad Sci USA* **89:** 7934–7938.

Wagner, E., Zatloukal, K., Cotten, M., et al. (1992b). Coupling of adenovirus to transferrin-polylysine/DNA complexes greatly enhances receptor-mediated gene delivery and expression of transfected genes. *Proc Natl Acad Sci USA* **89:** 6090–6103.

Wickham, T.J., Mathias, P., Cheresh, D.A., Nemerow, G.R. (1993). Integrins $\alpha_v\beta_3$ and $\alpha_v\beta_5$ promote adenovirus internalization but not virus attachment. *Cell* **73:** 30–319.

Wilson, J.M., Grossman, M., Cabrera, J.A., Wu, C.H., Wu, G.Y. (1992). A novel mechanism for achieving transgene persistence in vivo after somatic gene transfer into hepatocytes. *J Biol Chem* **267:** 11483–11489.

Wu, G.Y., Wu, C.H. (1988). Receptor-mediated gene delivery and expression in vivo. *J Biol Chem* **263:** 14621–14624.

Wu, G.Y., Wilson, J.M., Shalaby, F., Grossman, M., Shafritz, D.A., Wu, C.H. (1991). Receptor-mediated gene delivery in vivo. Partial correction of genetic analbuminemia in nagase rats. *J Biol Chem* **266:** 14338–14342.

Zatloukal, K., Wagner, E., Cotten, M., et al. (1992). Transferrinfection: A highly efficient way to express gene constructs in eukaryotic cells. *Ann NY Acad Sci* **660:** 136–153.

Zenke, M., Steinlein, P., Wagner, E., Cotten, M., Beug, H., Birnstiel, M.L. (1990). Receptor-mediated endocytosis of transferrin–polycation conjugates: An efficient way to introduce DNA into hematopoietic cells. *Proc Natl Acad Sci USA* **87:** 3655–3659.

SECTION 2

Protocols for Gene Delivery Using RNA Viruses

CHAPTER 5

Semliki Forest Virus Vectors for Gene Transfer

PETER LILJESTRÖM AND HENRIK GAROFF

Department of Biosciences at Novum, Karolinska Institute, S-141 57 Huddinge, Sweden.
Tel: 46 8 608 9133; Fax: 46 8 774 5538; Email: peli@cbt.ki.se

1 INTRODUCTION

In recent years interest has increased in the possibility of using RNA viruses as vectors for expression of heterologous genes. Vectors based on alphaviruses in particular have rapidly become popular and are currently used in diverse applications. Alphaviruses have several features that make them well suited as expression vectors:

- The RNA genome is infectious due to its positive polarity, i.e. naked genomic RNA is able to start an infection when introduced into the cytoplasm of a cell.
- The infecting RNA is self-replicating by coding for its own replicase, and this enzyme complex also caps all new RNA molecules.
- Replication is extremely efficient: over 10^5 RNA molecules and up to 10^8 molecules of the viral structural proteins may be produced per cell.
- Replication occurs exclusively in the cell cytoplasm and leads to rapid inhibition of host cell protein synthesis.
- Cytopathogenic effects in the infected cell arise late in infection, leaving an extensive time window during which a high expression level is combined with negligible morphological change.
- Alphaviruses also have a very broad host range and infect almost all animal cell types.

Alphavirus expression systems have been the subject of several recent reviews (Bredenbeek and Rice, 1992; Higgs et al., 1993; Liljeström, 1993, 1994; Rice, 1992; Schlesinger, 1993; Schlesinger et al., 1994).

Alphaviruses such as Semliki Forest virus (SFV) are small viruses composed of a single genomic RNA molecule enclosed in a nucleocapsid structure surrounded by an envelope containing the virus spike proteins (Schlesinger and Schlesinger, 1986, 1990). After entry into the host cell by receptor-mediated endocytosis (Marsh and Helenius, 1989; Lobigs and Garoff, 1990; Lobigs et al., 1990a; Salminen et al., 1992; Wahlberg and Garoff, 1992; Wahlberg et al., 1992; Bron et al., 1993), replication begins with the translation of the 5′ two-thirds of the genomic RNA to produce the viral replicase. This is responsible for production of genome-length negative strands that serve as templates for production of new positive strand genomes. The same replicase also recognizes an internal promoter on the minus strand to produce a smaller subgenome species that corresponds to the last one-third of the viral genome (Strauss and Strauss, 1986; de Groot et al., 1990; Takkinen et al., 1991; Sawicki and Sawicki, 1993; Lemm et al., 1994; Shirako and Strauss, 1994). The

Protocols for Gene Transfer in Neuroscience: Towards Gene Therapy of Neurological Disorders
Edited by P.R. Lowenstein and L.W. Enquist

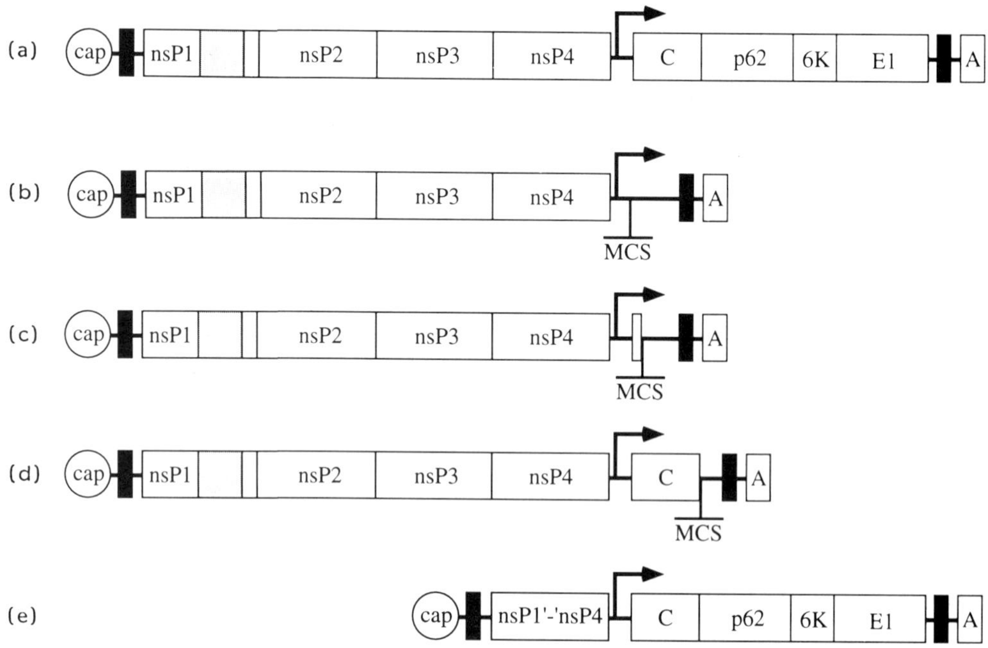

Figure 5.1 Replicons of the SFV expression system (see Liljeström and Garoff, 1991b, 1994; Berglund et al., 1993; Sjöberg et al., 1994; Suomalainen and Garoff, 1994, for technical details). The wild-type SFV genome (a) is a capped and polyadenylated positive-stranded RNA molecule 11512 nucleotides in length. The circle at the 5′ end denotes the cap structure, which is present on all RNAs. The black boxes close to the 5′ and 3′ ends denote the replication sequences used by the viral replicase. The A-box at the 3′ end denotes a poly-A stretch which is encoded by the genome itself. The stippled box in nsP1 is the packaging signal recognized by the capsid protein. nsP1–4 are the four replicase proteins made as a polyprotein, which self-cleaves to the individual polypeptides that form the replication complex. C is the capsid protein gene; p62, 6K and E1 are transmembrane proteins. The right-handed arrow denotes the promoter on the minus strand RNAs that is recognized by the viral replicase for transcription of the subgenomic RNA encoding the structural proteins or the heterologous sequences. MCS indicates a multiple cloning site. In pSFV1 (b) the complete coding sequence of the structural protein has been deleted and replaced by the polylinker region. Only a short stretch of the original untranslated sequence has been retained. In pSFV3 (c), the complete untranslated sequence and the initiating met codon of the capsid gene have been retained. Using this vector the heterologous insert is cloned in frame, which results in a slightly higher expression level than is usually obtained from pSFV1 constructs (depending on the individual translational initiation signals present in the insert sequence). In pSFVC (d) the upstream sequences, together with the complete capsid region, have been retained. Here, the insert is cloned in frame with the capsid protein. During translation, the protease moiety of the capsid protein will result in self-cleavage of the nascent chain, freeing the heterologous polypeptide. Because the first 100 or so bases of the capsid gene sequence function as a translational enhancer, significantly higher expression levels can be achieved using this vector. Helper 2 (e) encodes for all structural proteins of SFV but almost the complete replicase region has been deleted, including the packaging signal. The deletion flanking the remaining nsP sequences is indicated as nsP1′–′nsP4, the primes indicating the position of the deletion

subgenomic RNA encodes the structural proteins of the virus. The capsid protein is cytoplasmic and complexes with new genomic RNAs to form the nucleocapsid. The membrane proteins are translocated into the endoplasmic reticulum, where they heterotrimerize and then migrate to the cell surface (Wahlberg et al., 1989; Garoff et al., 1990; Lobigs et al., 1990b; Liljeström and Garoff, 1991a; Liljeström et al., 1991; Lusa et al., 1991). The budding of the virus out of the cell is driven by interactions between nucleocapsids and spike complexes at the plasma membrane (Suomalainen et al., 1992; Ekström et al., 1994; Zhao et al., 1994).

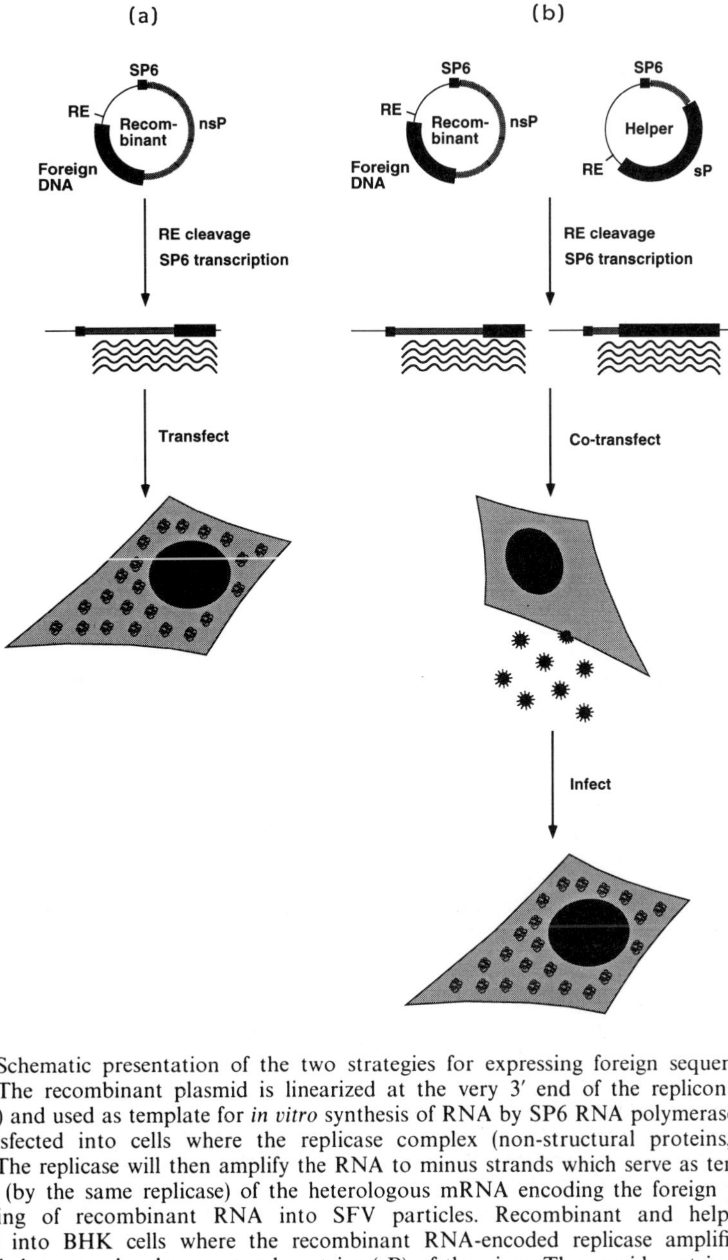

Figure 5.2 Schematic presentation of the two strategies for expressing foreign sequences with SFV vectors. (A) The recombinant plasmid is linearized at the very 3′ end of the replicon by restriction cleavage (RE) and used as template for *in vitro* synthesis of RNA by SP6 RNA polymerase. This RNA is directly transfected into cells where the replicase complex (non-structural proteins, nsP) is first synthesized. The replicase will then amplify the RNA to minus strands which serve as templates for the transcription (by the same replicase) of the heterologous mRNA encoding the foreign protein. (B) *In vivo* packaging of recombinant RNA into SFV particles. Recombinant and helper RNAs are cotransfected into BHK cells where the recombinant RNA-encoded replicase amplifies both RNA species. The helper encodes the structural proteins (sP) of the virus. The capsid protein packages only recombinant RNA molecules into nucleocapsids, because the helper RNAs lack a packaging signal (residing in the nsP1 gene). Assembly and budding of new recombinant SFV virions occurs at the cell surface through an interaction between cytoplasmically preformed nucleocapsids and the viral spike membrane proteins p62 and E1. The recombinant suicide particles are used to infect any type of animal cell, in which the scenario described in A occurs. As the infecting RNA lacks the SFV structural genes, new virions are not formed (non-productive replication)

A cDNA clone of the SFV genome was recently cloned (Liljeström, et al., 1991) and forms the basis for the expression vectors (Fig. 5.1). The use of these vectors allows an easy and quick way of expressing protein encoding sequences in almost any animal cell. We present two strategies for protein expression. In both cases the protein-coding sequence of interest is cloned into a plasmid vector, which subsequently is used to produce recombinant RNA *in vitro*. This RNA, which is of positive polarity, is transfected into cells where it is amplified by virtue of its self-encoded RNA replicase. The same replicase also produces a shorter RNA species that encode the protein-coding sequence of interest. Expression of the protein can be achieved in two ways. In the first strategy, the transfected cells are directly analysed for expression of the heterologous protein (Fig. 5.2A). The second strategy employs *in vivo* packaging of the RNA into SFV particles. For this, the recombinant RNA is cotransfected with a special helper RNA, which codes for the structural proteins needed for virus assembly (Fig. 5.2B). SFV particles carrying only recombinant RNA are formed, and are used to infect cells for analysis of protein expression.

When the helper is used to package recombinant RNA into infectious particles, recombination (strand-switching by the replicase) of the RNA species can occur (Geigenmüller-Gnirke et al., 1991; Weiss and Schlesinger, 1991; Berglund et al., 1993; Schlesinger et al., 1994). This could recreate a wild-type genome with production of SFV as a result. To remedy this, a safeguard was build into the helper system. Earlier studies had shown that one of the spike proteins (p62) needs to be proteolytically processed to its mature form in order for the assembled particles to be infectious (Salminen et al., 1992; Wahlberg and Garoff, 1992). Accordingly, a new helper molecule was constructed in which the spike-encoding gene was mutated to produce an uncleaved protein. As a result, the recombinant particles packaged *in vivo* incorporate the precursor form of the spike and are non-infectious. The virions may, however, be activated by brief treatment with protease. Should a recombination event occur during packaging, those particles can infect cells only once (after protease activation), because any new virions that may form after second round replication would contain the uncleaved form of the spike protein and be non-infectious thereby blocking further spread (Berglund et al., 1993). The safety of this system was also demonstrated in animal tests (Glasgow et al., 1991; Berglund, et al., 1993; Federal Register vol. 58 No 19, 1993; Glasgow et al., 1994).

2 MATERIALS AND EQUIPMENT

(1) DNA fragment of interest.
(2) pSFV1, pSFV3, pSFVC and pSFV3-lacZ (these plasmids can be obtained from Life Technologies Inc., Gaithersburg, MD, USA).
(3) SP6 RNA polymerase.
(4) rNTP mix (10 mM ATP, 10 mM CTP, 10 mM UTP, 5 mM GTP).
(5) m7G(5')ppp(5')G.
(6) RNAse inhibitor (e.g. RNasin).
(7) BHK-21 cells (available from American Type Culture Collection (ATCC) or European Catalogue of Animal Cell Cultures (ECACC)).
(8) Electroporator (e.g. BioRad).
(9) Electroporation cuvettes (0.4 cm).
(10) Lysis buffer.
(11) Optimem transfection buffer (Life Technologies).
(12) Lipofectin (Life Technologies).
(13) RNA spin columns Nu-Clean R50 (IBI).
(14) Isopropanol.
(15) TBE gel buffer for agarose gels: 50 mM Tris base, 50 mM H_3BO_3, 2.5 mM EDTA.
(16) 5 × TD solution: 20% Ficoll 400, 25 mM EDTA, pH 8.0, 0.05% bromophenol blue, 0.03% xylene cyanol.
(17) 10 × SP6 buffer: 400 mM Hepes–KOH, pH 7.4, 60 mM MgAc, 20 mM spermidine–HCl.
(18) Phosphate-buffered saline (PBS) without Mg^{2+} or Ca^{2+} (PBS−): 2.68 mM KCl, 1.47 mM KH_2PO_4, 136.8 mM NaCl, 8.0 mM $Na_2HPO_4 \times 7H_2O$, adjust pH to 7.0–7.2 with HCl,

autoclave 30 min and store at 4°C. PBS is also available commercially, for example from Gibco.

(19) BHK-21 medium: G-MEM (Gibco) 5% fetal calf serum, 10% tryptose phosphate broth, 20 mM Hepes, 2 mM glutamine, 0.1 U/ml penicillin (optional), 0.1 μg/ml streptomycin (optional).
(20) Starvation medium: Methionine-free MEM (Gibco), 2 mM glutamine, 20 mM Hepes.
(21) Chase medium: E-MEM (Gibco), 2 mM glutamine, 20 mM Hepes, 150 μg/ml unlabeled methionine.
(22) NP-40 lysis buffer: 1% NP-40 (use 10% stock), 50 mM Tris–HCl, pH 7.6, 150 mM NaCl, 2 mM EDTA.
(23) SDS lysis buffer: 1% SDS, 50 mM Tris–HCl, pH 7.4, 150 mM NaCl, 2 mM EDTA, 1 μg/ml PMSF.
(24) Z-buffer: 60 mM Na_2HPO_4, 40 mM NaH_2PO_4, 10 mM KCl, 1 mM $MgSO_4$, 40 mM 2-mercaptoethanol.
(25) ONPG (*o*-nitrophenyl-β-D-galactopyranoside) solution.
(26) Purified β-galactosidase.
(27) Xgal stain in PBS: 5 mM $K_4[Fe(CN)_6]$, 5 mM $K_3[Fe(CN)_6]$, 2 mM $MgCl_2$. Store refrigerated. At time of use, add Xgal (5-bromo-4-chloro-3-indolyl-β-D-galactopyranoside) to 1 mg/ml (stock in dimethylformamide).

3 THE PROTOCOLS

Protocol #16: Preparation of RNA *in vitro*

(1) Subclone the DNA fragment of interest into one of the SFV expression vectors and prepare purified plasmid DNA.
(2) Linearize the recombinant plasmid DNA by cutting with *Spe*I, phenol extract and ethanol precipitate the DNA. Resuspend the DNA in water to get a final concentration of 1.5 μg/5 μl.
(3) Set up *in vitro* transcription in a microcentrifuge tube by mixing, at room temperature, 5 μl each of linearized plasmid DNA, 10 × SP6 buffer, 50 mM DTT, 10 mM m7G(5′)ppp(5′)G and rNTP mix, 23 μl water, 1.5 μl RNasin (40 units) and 30 units of SP6 RNA polymerase.
(4) Incubate at 37°C for 60 min, then take 1 μl into 10 μl water, add 3 μl of DNA gel loading solution (5 × TD) and run sample on a 0.5% agarose gel to check the RNA for amount and uniformity in size. The RNA band should be defined (no smearing) and relatively thick (in comparison to the DNA bands). If necessary, RNA samples of known concentration can be run for comparison.
(5) Freeze the rest in aliquots at −80°C.

Protocol #17: Transfection of BHK Cells by Electroporation

(1) Grow BHK cells in a 75 cm² flask in 10 ml complete BHK medium (1–2 days).
(2) Aspirate medium and rinse cells once with PBS− buffer.
(3) To each 75 cm² flask, add 2 ml trypsin (0.5 mg/ml)-EDTA (0.2 mg/ml) in PBS− and incubate at 37°C until the cells detach (about 1 min), then briefly pipette cell solution back and forth to insure that a single-cell suspension is obtained (monitor by microscope). Stop trypsinization by adding 10 ml complete BHK medium.
(4) Harvest cells by centrifugation for 5 min at 400*g*, resuspend cells in 10–20 ml PBS−.
(5) Harvest cells as in step 4, and resuspend in PBS− to obtain 10^7 cells/ml.
(6) Transfer 0.8 ml cell suspension into an Eppendorf tube containing the RNA to be transfected, mix thoroughly by pipetting and transfer the mixture to a 0.4 cm electroporation cuvette. If you have many samples, and the cells have started to sediment in the cuvette before the pulse, press down the cap tightly and invert the cuvette once before giving the shock. A total of 5 μg RNA (about 10 μl transcription mixture) for 10^7 cells will give a transfection frequency close to 100%.
(7) Using a BioRad Gene Pulser, pulse twice at 850 V/25 μF at room temperature. The time constant after the pulse should be 0.4.

(8) Dilute transfected cells 20-fold in complete BHK medium and rinse the cuvette with the same medium to collect all cells. Transfer cells to tissue culture plates or flasks: it will take about 1 h for the cells to reattach to the dish.

Protocol #18: Transfection of Cells Using Lipofectin

(1) After transcription, dilute the mixture to 100 μl with water, then add 20 μl 3 M sodium acetate, pH 4.8.
(2) Add 72 μl of isopropanol at -20°C, mix and allow to stand on bench (room temperature) for 10 min.
(3) Microcentrifuge to pellet RNA, remove supernatant and rinse with 500 μl 75% ethanol. Spin down again, remove ethanol and dry. Resuspend pellet in transcription volume of 10 mM Tris–HCl, pH 7.5–0.1 mM EDTA.
(4) Grow cells on 35 mm plates to reach about 80% confluence. We usually use BHK-21 cells. Although Lipofectin can be applied for a wide variety of cells, the exact conditions may vary slightly. Parameters to be considered are final amounts of lipid and RNA, lipid:RNA ratio, and time of lipid–RNA administration.
(5) Remove medium and replace with 2 ml Optimem transfection buffer. Leave in incubator for 5–10 min while Step 6 is carried out.
(6) Mix 1 ml Optimem buffer with 9 μg Lipofectin and mix for 10 s. Add 2.3 μg purified RNA and mix again.
(7) Remove the Optimem buffer covering the cells, replace with the Lipofectin–RNA mixture and incubate at 37°C for 120 min, tilting the plate every 15 min. Up to 90% transfection frequencies can be obtained using Lipofectin. However, it is imperative that the transfection mixture covers the cells as evenly as possible at all times. Frequent tilting of plates is recommended for consistent results.
(8) Remove transfection mix, wash once with BHK medium. Finally replace with BHK medium and continue incubation for time required.

Protocol #19: Production of Recombinant SFV Particles and Determination of Stock Titer

(1) Prepare RNA by *in vitro* transcription from recombinant pSFV plasmid and from the Helper 2 plasmid.
(2) Mix the RNAs in a 1:1 ratio and transfect into BHK cells. Incubate 24 h at 37°C, 5% CO_2. (A 1:1 ratio of recombinant and helper RNAs simply means equimolar ratios.) In practice, equal amounts (in μl) of the transcription mixtures (or purified RNAs) can be used, as the transcription mixture was set up to contain a saturated amount of DNA (and thus promoter copies). Large deviations from a 1:1 ratio will lead to lower stock titers.
(3) Collect the medium, clarify, aliquot and freeze quickly on dry ice or in liquid nitrogen, store at -80°C.
(4) Thaw virus preparation on ice and add 1/20 volume of α-chymotrypsin (10 mg/ml in PBS containing 10 mM $MgCl_2$ and 20 mM $CaCl_2$) stock to virus preparation and incubate at room temperature for 30 min.
(5) Inactivate chymotrypsin by adding 0.5 volume of aprotinin (stock 2 mg/ml ready to use).
(6) Dilute activated virus preparation as appropriate in MEM containing 0.2% BSA and use solution to infect cells (see next protocol).

Protocol #20: Infection of Cells with SFV

(1) Use this protocol to infect BHK cells grown to 80–100% confluence on a 35 mm plate.
(2) Wash the cells thoroughly with PBS.
(3) Apply 500 μl of the virus solution to the cells and incubate at 37°C for 45–60 min.
(4) Remove virus solution, add 3 ml complete BHK medium (or other suitable medium) and continue incubation as required.

Protocol #21: Determination of Recombinant Semliki Forest Virus Stock Titer

(1) Grow cells on glass coverslips to about 70% confluence.
(2) Infect the cells with different dilutions of the recombinant virus stock (dilute in EMEM containing 0.2% BSA, 2 mM glutamine and 20 mM Hepes) as described in the previous protocol. Allow 7–15 h for expression of protein of interest.
(3) Rinse coverslips twice with PBS, then fix cells in methanol at −20°C for 5 min.
(4) Remove methanol and wash coverslips three times with PBS.
(5) Block non-specific binding by incubation at room temperature for 30 min with PBS containing 0.2% gelatin.
(6) Replace blocking buffer with same containing primary antibody and incubate at room temperature for 30 min.
(7) Wash three times with PBS, then bind secondary antibody as in Step 6.
(8) Wash three times with PBS and once with water, drain and let coverslip air dry.
(9) Mount on glass slide using 10–20 μl Moviol 4-88 containing 2.5% DABCO (1,4-diazobicyclo-[2.2.2]-octane) (the DABCO will reduce fading of FITC). Examine under a fluorescence photomicroscope.

Protocol #22: Analyses of Heterologous Protein by Metabolic Labeling of Cells

(1) Remove growth medium by aspiration and wash cells twice with 3 ml PBS prewarmed to 37°C, then overlay cells with 2 ml of starvation medium and incubate plates at 37°C (5% CO_2) for 30–45 min.
(2) Remove medium by aspiration and replace with 500 μl of the same containing 50–100 μCi/ml of ^{35}S-methionine, incubate for appropriate pulse time at 37°C.
(3) Remove pulse medium and wash cells once with 2 ml of chase medium, then overlay cells with 2 ml of chase medium and incubate for required chase time.
(4) Remove medium and wash cells with 3 ml ice-cold PBS, add 300 μl of lysis buffer and let stand on ice for 10 min.
(5) Resuspend cells and transfer solution into an Eppendorf tube, spin at 6000 r.p.m. for 5 min to pellet unbroken cells and nuclei. Transfer supernatant to a fresh tube and store at −80°C. If the protein product is pelleted, dissolve the pellet in SDS lysis buffer.
(6) Assay for protein expression by SDS-PAGE and autoradiography.

Protocol #23: Use of β-Galactosidase for Screening Gene Expression; Assay for β-Galactosidase

(1) Use 1 μl of the cell lysate (or about 200–300 cells) in NP-40 lysis buffer, and add Z-buffer to 400 μl.
(2) Incubate for 5 min at 37°C and then add 100 μl ONPG solution (4 mg/ml in Z buffer). Mix well by vortexing.
(3) Continue incubation until the sample obtains a yellow color, then stop the reaction by adding 500 μl of 1 M Na_2CO_3. Mix well.
(4) Measure the absorbance at 420 nm. A standard curve using purified β-galactosidase should be made to allow determination of actual amounts of the enzyme produced in the cell lysate. A standard series ranging from (e.g.) 0.2 to 50 ng β-galactosidase is usually suitable. Incubation time in the assay for these samples is around 15 min. The exact number of units per microgram will vary with preparation, but usually about 1 unit is found for every 3 μg protein.

Protocol #24: Use of β-Galactosidase for Screening Gene Expression; Screening of β-Galactosidase-Positive Cells

(1) Infect or transfect cells and allow for expression of β-galactosidase (usually overnight incubation, but 7 h is sufficient).

(2) Wash cells twice with PBS, then fix cells for 5 min using 2 ml of −20°C methanol, incubating the plate at −20°C during fixation.
(3) Wash cells three times with PBS at room temperature and then overlay with Xgal stain. Staining is usually very fast (within minutes), and is complete after 2–3 h at 37°C. Alternatively, you can leave the plates at room temperature overnight.
(4) Monitor positive (blue)/negative (white) cells using a stereomicroscope.

4 NOTES AND TROUBLESHOOTING

4.1 General Comments

The success of using the SFV expression system is highly dependent on the efficiency of RNA transfection. Using conditions described in Protocol #17 practically all BHK cells can be transfected. Similar conditions can probably be obtained in other cell types if the transfection efficiency is analysed as a function of voltage, capacitance, time constant of electrical pulse and number of pulses given. Under optimal conditions transfection with lipofectin also gives good results. Another factor of importance is the efficiency of a given cell type to support virus particle formation. This can be checked using wild-type SFV. The recombinant virus stock should be stored at −80°C after quick freezing in dry ice or liquid nitrogen. The activated stock cannot be stored frozen or for longer periods of time on ice. Thus, the stock should be activated just before infection.

It is anticipated that 10^7 BHK cells yield about 10^9–10^{10} infectious recombinant particles when cotransfected with recombinant and helper RNA and incubated for 24 hours. If about 5 infectious units are used per cell in an expression experiment then most of the newly synthesized polypeptide chains should represent heterologous protein products after about 4 h incubation. This means that the heterologous protein should be seen as the major band in SDS gel analysis of pulse-labeled cells that have been infected and incubated for more than 4 h. After a 20–25 h of incubation the heterologous protein product should represent the major protein in the cell. Thus, Coomassie Brilliant Blue staining of SDS gels in which infected cells samples have been analysed should reveal the heterologous protein as a major band if cells were incubated for 20–25 h or longer.

4.2 On Protocol #18: Transfection of Cells using Lipofectin

If lipofectin is used for transfection, the transcription mixture needs to be purified to remove the NTPs from the reaction mixture. This can be done either by isopropanol precipitation of the RNA or by gel filtration. In the latter case, any commercial spin column designed for this purpose will do (e.g. IBI Nu-Clean R50 gives good results). In such cases, follow the protocol provided by supplier. The protocol given is for purification by isopropanol precipitation, in which only DNA/RNA larger than 100 b(p) in length is precipitated. However, it is important that the precipitation step be performed at room temperature.

4.3 On Protocol #19: Production of Recombinant SFV Particles and Determination of Stock Titer

4.3.1 Production of Recombinant SFV Particles

Recombinant and helper RNAs are cotransfected into BHK cells by either protocol described above (Protocol #17 or #18). As a result of trans-complementation, recombinant RNAs are packaged into SFV particles which are released into the growth medium (Fig. 5.2). The virus produced is used to infect cells in culture to assay for expression of cloned sequences.

4.4 On Protocol #21: Determination of Recombinant Semliki Forest Virus Stock Titer

Owing to the lack of structural genes the recombinant virus cannot initiate more than one round of intracellular replication. Therefore, the titer of the packaged stock cannot be determined by conventional plaque assay, but is instead measured by indirect immunofluorescence. Different dilutions of the virus stock are used to infect cells, and heterologous protein expression detected by specific antibodies.

4.5 On Protocol #22: Analyses of Heterologous Protein by Metabolic Labeling of Cells

Metabolic labeling of cells can be done as soon as 4 h after transfection. However, in order to achieve maximum labeling of the protein of interest and to assure minimum labeling of host proteins, it is recommended that 7–9 h is allowed to elapse after transfection before the pulse is given. The protocol is given for 35 mm diameter tissue culture plates (80–100% confluent).

4.6 On Protocol #24: Use of β-Galactosidase for Screening Gene Expression; Screening of β-Galactosidase-Positive Cells

The pSFV3-lacZ vector (Liljeström and Garoff, 1991b) is suitable for checking expression and transfection efficiencies. One of the most convenient and fastest ways of screening for β-galactosidase expression is by direct staining with Xgal.

REFERENCES

Berglund, P., M. Sjöberg, G.J. Atkins, B.J. Sheahan, H. Garoff and P. Liljeström. 1993. Semliki Forest virus expression system: Production of conditionally infectious recombinant particles. *Bio/Technology* **11:** 916–920.

Bredenbeek, P.J. and C.M. Rice. 1992. Animal RNA virus expression systems. *Sem. Virol.* **3:** 297–310.

Bron, R., J.M. Wahlberg, H. Garoff and J. Wilschut. 1993. Membrane fusion of Semliki Forest virus in a model system: correlation between fusion kinetics and structural changes in the envelope glycoprotein. *EMBO J.* **12:** 693–701.

de Groot, R.J., W.R. Hardy, Y. Shirako and J.H. Strauss. 1990. Cleavage-site preferences of Sindbis virus polyproteins containing the non-structural proteinase. Evidence for temporal regulation of polyprotein processing *in vivo*. *EMBO J.* **9:** 2631–2638.

Ekström, M., P. Liljeström and H. Garoff. 1994. Membrane protein lateral interactions control Semliki Forest virus budding. *EMBO J.* **13:** 1058–1064.

Federal Register vol. 58 No 19, 9. 1993. Addition of Appendix D-LX to the NIH Guidelines Regarding Semliki Forest virus. *Hum. Gene Ther.* **5:** 401.

Garoff, H., D. Huylebroeck, A. Robinson, U. Tillman and P. Liljeström. 1990. The signal sequence of the p62 protein of Semliki Forest virus is involved in initiation but not in completing chain translocation. *J. Cell Biol.* **111:** 867–876.

Geigenmüller-Gnirke, U., B. Weiss, R. Wright and S. Schlesinger. 1991. Complementation between Sindbis viral RNAs produces infectious particles with a bipartite genome. *Proc. Natl Acad. Sci. USA* **88:** 3253–3257.

Glasgow, G.M., H.M. Killen, P. Liljeström, B.J. Sheahan and G.J. Atkins. 1994. A single amino acid change in the E2 spike protein of a virulent strain of Semliki Forest virus attenuates pathogenicity. *J. Gen. Virol.* **75:** 663–668.

Glasgow, G.M., B.J. Sheahan, G.J. Atkins, J.M. Wahlberg, A. Salminen and P. Liljeström. 1991. Two mutations in the envelope glycoprotein E2 of Semliki Forest virus affecting the maturation and entry patterns of the virus alter pathogenicity for mice. *Virology* **185:** 741–748.

Higgs, S., A.M. Powers and K.E. Olson. 1993. Alphavirus Expression Systems—Applications to Mosquito Vector Studies. *Parasitol Today* **9:** 444–452.

Lemm, J.A., T. Rümenapf, E.G. Strauss, J.H. Strauss and C.M. Rice. 1994. Polypeptide requirements for assembly of functional Sindbis virus replication complexes: a model for the temporal regulation of minus- and plus-strand RNA synthesis. *EMBO J.* **13:** 2925–2934.

Liljeström, P. 1993. Virally based transient expression systems. *Curr. Opin. Ther. Pat.* **3:** 375–402.

Liljeström, P. 1994. Alphavirus expression systems. *Curr. Opin. Biotechnol.* **5:** 495–500.

Liljeström, P. and H. Garoff. 1991a. Internally located cleavable signal sequences direct the formation of Semliki Forest virus membrane proteins from a polyprotein precursor. *J. Virol.* **65:** 147–154.

Liljeström, P. and H. Garoff. 1991b. A new generation of animal cell expression vectors based on the Semliki Forest virus replicon. *Bio/Technology* **9:** 1356–1361.

Liljeström, P. and H. Garoff. 1994. Expression of proteins using Semliki Forest virus vectors. In *Current*

Protocols in Molecular Biology. F.M. Ausubel, R. Brent, R.E. Kingston, D.D. Moore, J.A. Smith, J.G. Seidman and K. Struhl, eds. Greene Publishing Associates and Wiley Interscience, New York. 16.20.1–16.20.16.

Liljeström, P., S. Lusa, D. Huylebroeck and H. Garoff. 1991. *In vitro* mutagenesis of a full-length cDNA clone of Semliki Forest virus: the 6000-molecular-weight membrane protein modulates virus release. *J. Virol.* **65:** 4107–4113.

Lobigs, M. and H. Garoff. 1990. Fusion function of the Semliki Forest virus spike is activated by proteolytic cleavage of the envelope glycoprotein p62. *J. Virol.* **64:** 1233–1240.

Lobigs, M., J.M. Wahlberg and H. Garoff. 1990a. Spike protein oligomerization control of Semliki Forest virus fusion. *J. Virol.* **64:** 5214–5218.

Lobigs, M., H. Zhao and H. Garoff. 1990b. Function of Semliki Forest virus E3 peptide in virus assembly: Replacement of E3 with an artificial signal peptide abolishes spike heterodimerization and surface expression of E1. *J. Virol.* **64:** 4346–4355.

Lusa, S., H. Garoff and P. Liljeström. 1991. Fate of the 6K membrane protein of Semliki Forest virus during virus assembly. *Virology* **185:** 843–846.

Marsh, M. and A. Helenius. 1989. Virus entry into animal cells. *Adv. Virus Res.* **36:** 107–151.

Rice, C.M. 1992. Examples of expression systems based on animal RNA viruses: alphaviruses and influenza virus. *Curr. Opin. Biotechnol.* **3:** 522–532.

Salminen, A., J.M. Wahlberg, M. Lobigs, P. Liljeström and H. Garoff. 1992. Membrane fusion process of Semliki Forest virus II: Cleavage dependent reorganization of the spike protein complex controls virus entry. *J. Cell Biol.* **116:** 349–357.

Sawicki, D.L. and S.G. Sawicki. 1993. A second nonstructural protein functions in the regulation of alphavirus negative-strand RNA synthesis. *J. Virol.* **67:** 3605–3610.

Schlesinger, S. 1993. Alphaviruses—vectors for the expression of heterologous genes. *Trends Biotechnol.* **11:** 18–22.

Schlesinger, S., S. Makino and M.L. Linial. 1994. Cis-acting genomic elements and trans-acting proteins involved in the assembly of RNA viruses. *Sem. Virol.* **5:** 39–49.

Schlesinger, S. and M.J. Schlesinger. 1990. Replication of Togaviridae and Flaviviridae. In *Virology*. B.N. Fields and D.M. Knipe, eds. Raven Press, Ltd, New York. 697–711.

Schlesinger, S.S. and M.J. Schlesinger. 1986. *The Togaviridae and Flaviviridae*. Plenum Press, New York. 453.

Shirako, Y. and J.H. Strauss. 1994. Regulation of Sindbis virus RNA replication: uncleaved P123 and nsP4 function in minus-strand RNA synthesis, whereas cleaved products from P123 are required for efficient plus-strand RNA synthesis. *J. Virol.* **68:** 1874–1885.

Sjöberg, M.E., M. Suomalainen and H. Garoff. 1994. A significantly improved Semliki Forest virus expression system based on translational enhancer segments from the viral capsid gene. *Bio/Technology* **12:** 1127–1131.

Strauss, E.G. and J.H. Strauss. 1986. Structure and replication of the alphavirus genome. In *The Togaviridae and Flaviviridae*. S.S. Schlesinger and M.J. Schlesinger, eds. Plenum Press, New York. 35–90.

Suomalainen, M. and H. Garoff. 1994. Incorporation of homologous and heterologous proteins into the envelope of Moloney murine leukemia virus. *J. Virol.* **68:** 4879–4889.

Suomalainen, M., P. Liljeström and H. Garoff. 1992. Spike protein—nucleocapsid interactions drive the budding of alphaviruses. *J. Virol.* **66:** 4737–4747.

Takkinen, K., J. Peränen and L. Kääriäinen. 1991. Proteolytic processing of Semliki Forest virus-specific non-structural polyprotein. *J. Gen. Virol.* **72:** 1627–1633.

Wahlberg, J. and H. Garoff. 1992. Membrane fusion process of Semliki Forest virus I: Low pH-induced rearrangement in spike protein quaternary structure precedes virus penetration into cells. *J. Cell Biol.* **116:** 339–357.

Wahlberg, J.M., W.A. Boere and H. Garoff. 1989. The heterodimeric association between the membrane proteins of Semliki Forest virus changes its sensitivity to mildly acidic pH during virus maturation. *J. Virol.* **63:** 4991–4997.

Wahlberg, J.M., R. Bron, J. Wilschut and H. Garoff. 1992. Membrane fusion of Semliki Forest virus involves homotrimers of the fusion protein. *J. Virol.* **66:** 7309–7318.

Weiss, B.G. and S. Schlesinger. 1991. Recombination between Sindbis virus RNAs. *J. Virol.* **65:** 4017–4025.

Zhao, H., B. Lindqvist, H. Garoff, C.-H. von Bondsdorff and P. Liljeström. 1994. A tyrosine-based motif in the cytoplasmic domain of the alphavirus envelope protein is essential for budding. *EMBO J.* **13:** 4204–4211.

CHAPTER 6

Use of Fowl Plague, Vesicular Stomatitis and Semliki Forest Viruses to Study the Mechanisms of Neuronal Membrane Polarity

MELTSJE J. DE HOOP AND ANGEL CID-ARREGUI

Cell Biology Program, European Molecular Biology Laboratory, Postfach 10.2209, Meyerhofstr. 1, D-69012 Heidelberg, Germany. Tel: 49 6221 387321; Fax: 49 6221 387306; Email: cid@embl-heidelberg.de

1 INTRODUCTION

Combined use of primary cultures of neurons and enveloped viruses that bud preferentially from specific cellular domains has provided new insights into the mechanisms determining neuronal asymmetry (see de Hoop and Dotti, 1993). The technique for establishing primary cultures from rat embryo hippocampi, developed by Banker and coworkers (described in detail in Goslin and Banker 1991), offers several advantages over other neuronal cultures. Firstly, embryonic hippocampal cells in culture are able to differentiate, apparently in a way similar to that occurring *in vivo*. Secondly, these cultures are predominantly composed of a single cell type—pyramidal neurons. In addition, axons and dendrites may be easily distinguished in these cells by morphological, functional and molecular criteria.

On the basis of their ability to bud asymmetrically, several viruses have been used in the past two decades to study epithelial cell polarity (Rodriguez-Boulan and Sabatini, 1978) and more recently neuronal polarity (Dotti and Simons, 1990). Thus, the Fowl Plague Virus (FPV) buds exclusively from the apical membrane in epithelial cells and from axons, while the Semliki Forest Virus (SFV) and the Vesicular Stomatitis Virus (VSV) bud from the basolateral membrane and from dendrites. This parallelism led to the idea that polarized epithelial cells and hippocampal neurons may use similar mechanisms to generate polarity (Dotti and Simons, 1990). We describe here some of the methods that have proven useful in our studies on protein traffic in neurons.

2 MATERIALS AND EQUIPMENT

2.1 Analysis of Protein Traffic in Rat Hippocampal Neurons by Immunofluorescence Localization of Newly Synthesized Viral Glycoproteins

(1) Virus stocks (FPV, VSV, SFV, and recombinant SFV, SEE SECTION 4, PAGE 71).
(2) Cultures of hippocampal neurons.
(3) Phosphate-buffered saline (PBS).
(4) 10 × PBS (82 g NaCl, 4.3 g NaH_2PO_4–$2H_2O$ and 17.4 g Na_2HPO_4, in a final volume of 1 liter).

Protocols for Gene Transfer in Neuroscience: Towards Gene Therapy of Neurological Disorders
Edited by P.R. Lowenstein and L.W. Enquist

(5) Humid chamber (SEE SECTION 4.5, PAGE 73).
(6) Saponin solution (SEE SECTION 4.5, PAGE 73).
(7) Blocking solution (SEE SECTION 4.5, PAGE 73).
(8) Primary antibodies: Anti-synaptophysin (Boehringer Mannheim), monoclonal; anti-phosphorylated neurofilament heavy (NFH) (Affinity Research Products Ltd., Nottingham, UK), monoclonal; anti-Tau-1 (Boehringer Mannheim), monoclonal; anti-microtubule-associated protein 2 (Map2) (Boehringer Mannheim). (SEE SECTION 4.5, PAGE 73.)
(9) Lucifer yellow (dilithium salt, Sigma Chemical Co., St. Louis, MO) (SEE SECTION 4.5, PAGE 73).

2.2 Use of Sulfosuccinimidyl-6-(biotinamido) hexanoato (NHS-LC-Biotin) for Biochemical Analysis of Protein Traffic in Neurons Infected with SFV or SFV Expression Vector

(1) Wild-type and/or recombinant SFVs, prepared as described in SECTION 4.1.3, PAGE 72.
(2) Dulbecco's PBS and Ca/Mg-PBS: Dulbecco's PBS containing 1 mM $CaCl_2$ and 0.5 mM $MgCl_2$.
(3) Hank's Balanced Salt Solution (HBSS): 8.0 g NaCl, 0.4 g KCl, 0.14 g $CaCl_2$, 0.1 g $MgSO_4 \cdot 7H_2O$, 0.1 g $MgCl_2 \cdot 6H_2O$, 0.06 g $Na_2HPO_4 \cdot 2H_2O$, 0.06 g KH_2PO_4, 1.0 g glucose, 0.35 g $NaHCO_3$, made up to 1 liter with deionized water.
(4) ^{35}S-methionine labeling mixture prepared by diluting Expre^{35}S-^{35}S methionine® (Amersham) to 0.5 mCi/ml in HBSS.
(5) Biotin solution: Just before use, dissolve NHS-LC-Biotin (ImmunoPure®, Pierce) in Ca/Mg-PBS at a concentration of 1 mg/ml by sonicating 2–5 seconds in a water bath sonicator. Keep this solution on ice until use.
(6) GB solution: 0.1 M glycine, 0.3% BSA, in Ca/Mg-PBS. Store at −20°C.
(7) Lysis buffer: 2% Nonidet P-40, 0.2% SDS in PBS, supplemented with a cocktail of protease inhibitors composed of chymostatin, leupeptin, antipain and pepstatin A (Sigma) to a final concentration of (each) 10 μg/ml.
(8) NET buffer: 50 mM Tris pH 7.0; 200 mM NaCl; 1% Nonidet P-40 and 2 mM EDTA.
(9) 70% (v/v) Protein-A-sephγrose (Pharmacia) in NET buffer. Store at 4°C.
(10) 0.1 M Glycine adjusted to pH 3.0 with HCl.
(11) 1 M Tris–HCl, pH 9.0.
(12) 2× SDS-loading buffer: 100 mM Tris–HCl, pH 6.8; 4% SDS; 0.2% bromophenol blue; 20% glycerol. Dithiothreitol is added to a concentration of 200 mM from a 1 M stock just before use.
(13) STR buffer: 25 mM Tris, pH 7.5; 250 mM NaCl; 5 mM EDTA; 1% Triton X-100; 1% BSA and 0.5 mM PMSF. Prepare just before use.
(14) Streptavidin-agarose (Pierce), 50% slurry. Store at 4°C.
(15) Washing solutions: (a) 2% Nonidet P-40, 0.2% SDS, in PBS, (b) 1% Nonidet P-40 in PBS, (c) 0.1% Nonidet P-40, 0.5 M NaCl in PBS, (d) 50 mM Tris–HCl pH 7.5, 25 mM DTT and (e) 50 mM Tris–HCl, pH 7.5.
(16) PAGE reagents and solutions.
(17) 50% Methanol and 50% methanol/10% acetic acid.
(18) Entensify® (DuPont), solutions A and B.

3 THE PROTOCOLS

Protocol #25: Preparation of Paraformaldehyde Fixative

(1) Add 8 g paraformaldehyde powder to 60 ml water at 60–70°C in a fume hood and stir.
(2) Add a few drops of 1 N NaOH until the solution clears.
(3) Add 8 g sucrose and 10 ml 10× PBS.
(4) Add distilled water to a total volume of 100 ml.
(5) Filter and check pH (should be 7.3–7.4).

(6) Store in 5–10 ml aliquots at $-20°C$.
(7) When needed, thaw an aliquot and mix it 1:1 with 1 × PBS.
(8) Bring the diluted fixative to 37°C before use.

Protocol #26: Preparation of Mounting Medium

(1) Add 10 g Mowiol (Calbiochem-Novabiochem Corp.) to 40 ml PBS.
(2) Stir at room temperature at least overnight.
(3) Add 20 ml glycerol and stir for an additional 24 h.
(4) Check for precipitates by phase-contrast microscopy: if these are present, spin the viscous solution for 15 min at 10 000 r.p.m. in a Sorvall.
(5) Store 1 ml aliquots at $-20°C$.

Protocol #27: Viral Infections of Neuronal Cultures

(1) Dilute the virus in N2 medium (Bottenstein and Sato, 1992) to the appropriate multiplicity of infection (MOI) (SEE SECTION 4.3, PAGE 72).
(2) Drain coverslips with attached cells, one by one, quickly onto absorbent tissue paper.
(3) Place the cells facing up on a Parafilm sheet within the humid chamber.
(4) Quickly pipette the virus onto the coverslips: use 100 μl of diluted virus per 15 mm diameter coverslip.
(5) Close the humid chamber and incubate 1 h at 36.5°C/5% CO_2.
(6) During virus absorption, prepare the incubation wells by adding 2 ml of N2 medium, taken from the dish in which the cells were growing, to each well of a 12-well tissue culture dish (Costar). Bring the multiwell plate to the incubator.
(7) Take the coverslips out of the humid chamber and drain on absorbent tissue paper to remove non-absorbed virus.
(8) Place the infected cells into the multiwells containing prewarmed medium. Return the multiwell plate to the incubator (36.5°C/5% CO_2) to allow expression of the viral proteins.

Protocol #28: Fixation and Permeabilization of Cells

Methanol Fixation

(1) Transfer coverslips into wells containing methanol at $-20°C$ for 5 min.
(2) Wash with PBS.

Paraformaldehyde Fixation

(1) Transfer coverslips without any previous washing into dishes containing prewarmed 4% paraformaldehyde in PBS. Leave for 15–30 min at room temperature.
(2) Wash twice with PBS.
(3) Quench excess aldehyde with 50 mM NH_4Cl in PBS. Leave for 10 min.
(4) Wash twice with PBS.
(5) Permeabilize the cells by one of the methods described below.

Procedures for Permeabilization of Paraformaldehyde-fixed Cells

Triton X-100

(1) Incubate the coverslips for 10 min with 0.1% Triton X-100 in PBS.
(2) Wash twice with PBS.

Ethanol

(1) Dehydrate the coverslips sequentially in solutions of increasing concentration of ethanol: 25–50–70–90–95% (all in distilled water), at room temperature for 5 min in each solution.

(2) Incubate coverslips for 10 min in 100% ethanol.
(3) Rehydrate by incubating the coverslips in ethanol 95–90–70–50–25% in distilled water at room temperature for 5 min each.
(4) Wash twice in PBS.

Saponin

(1) Remove unfixed coverslips from incubation medium and submerge for 20–30 s in a small beaker containing 0.01% saponin solution.
(2) Fix cells immediately in 4% paraformaldehyde.

Protocol #29: Immunocytochemistry Procedures for Cells Grown *in vitro*

(1) Pipette 100 μl of blocking solution onto each coverslip and incubate for 1 h at room temperature or overnight at 4°C.
(2) Remove the blocking solution by aspiration.
(3) Add 50 μl of primary antibody diluted in 10% blocking solution in PBS, and incubate for 1 h at room temperature or overnight at 4°C.
(4) Wash three × 5 minutes at room temperature with PBS.
(5) Incubate with appropriate fluorochrome-conjugated secondary antibody, diluted in 10% blocking solution (in PBS), for 30–60 min at room temperature.
(6) Wash three × 5 minutes at room temperature with PBS.
(7) Quickly rinse in distilled water.
(8) Mount coverslips on glass slides as follows: place each coverslip, neurons facing down, onto a small drop (2–5 μl) of mounting medium on a clean glass slide. Press gently on the coverslip to remove air bubbles and to squeeze out excess mounting medium.

Protocol #30: Lucifer Yellow Labeling of Early and Late Endocytic Compartments

(1) Prewarm a few 100 μl drops of M2 medium containing lucifer yellow in a humid chamber in an incubator on a piece of Parafilm.
(2) Place coverslips containing neurons upside down on the prewarmed droplets containing lucifer yellow and incubate for 10–20 min at 37°C/5% CO_2. To stain early endocytic structures go to Step 3; to stain late endocytic structures go to Step 4.
(3) To stain early endocytic structures:
    (a) Wash the coverslips extensively (five or more times) with ice-cold HBSS containing 0.2% BSA.
    (b) Fix immediately with either 4% paraformaldehyde or 4% paraformaldehyde and 0.25% glutaraldehyde at room temperature for 20 min.
    (c) Wash three times with PBS. If using paraformaldehyde and glutaraldehyde fix go to Step 3d; if using only paraformaldehyde fix go to Step 3e.
    (d) Quench glutaraldehyde plus formaldehyde fixative by incubating the coverslips three times for 5 min each in 0.5 mg/ml sodium borohydride in PBS.
    (e) Quench excess paraformaldehyde by incubating coverslips in 50 mM NH_4Cl in PBS for 10 min.
    (f) Wash 2–3 times rapidly with PBS and proceed with the blocking step described in Protocol #29, Step 1, to combine the experiment with immunocytochemical labeling, or mount the coverslips following Protocol #29, Step 8.
(4) To stain late endocytic components:
    (a) Rinse coverslips quickly in prewarmed N2 medium.
    (b) Incubate in prewarmed N2 for 2–3 h at 37°C/5% CO_2.
    (c) Go to Step 3b.

Protocol #31: Visualization of the Internalization of Plasma Membrane Proteins

(1) Incubate living neurons for 10–20 min with N2 medium containing a specific antibody against the ectodomain of the protein of interest, diluted as for immunofluorescence, following the

procedure described in Protocol #30 for lucifer yellow.
(2) Rinse the cells quickly in cold N2 medium or HBSS.
(3) Fix cells with paraformaldehyde. If the antibody used is conjugated to a fluorochrome go to Step 4; if the antibody used is not conjugated with a fluorochrome go to Step 6.
(4) Mount cells onto coverslips (Protocol #29, Step 8).
(5) Examine cells under the fluorescence microscope.
(6) Proceed with Protocol #29. Immunocytochemistry Procedures, to detect the distribution of the unlabeled antibody.

Protocol #32: Immunofluorescent Labeling of Surface-exposed Antigens; Low Temperature Labeling

(1) Dilute the antibody in a small volume (approx. 100 μl) in ice-cold air-MEM (MEM containing 4 mM $NaHCO_3$, 10 mM Hepes-NaOH, 2 mM glutamine, 0.6% glucose, 11 mg/100 ml pyruvic acid, 2% FCS and 2% BSA, pH 7.3).
(2) Remove coverslips with attached neurons from the incubator and drain excess medium.
(3) Place coverslips with neurons facing down onto the antibody-containing droplets, and incubate for 30 min on ice.
(4) Rinse the coverslips quickly in ice-cold air-MEM.
(5) Fix coverslips in 4% paraformaldehyde.
(6) Wash coverslips with PBS, 2 × 5 min.
(7) Quench excess paraformaldehyde by incubating coverslips in 50 mM NH_4Cl in PBS for 10 min.
(8) Wash briefly twice with PBS.
(9) Pipette 100 μl of blocking solution onto each coverslip and incubate for 1 h at room temperature or overnight at 4°C.
(10) Remove the blocking solution by aspiration.
(11) Incubate with a fluorochrome-labeled species-specific antibody (diluted in 10% blocking solution in PBS) for 1 h to detect the surface-bound antibody.
(12) Wash coverslips in PBS, distilled water, mount and examine. (For details SEE PROTOCOL #29.)

Protocol #33: Immunofluorescent Labeling of Surface-exposed Antigens; Fixation without Permeabilization

(1) Fix coverslips for 20 min at room temperature, either in 8% paraformaldehyde in PBS or in 4% paraformaldehyde/0.25% glutaraldehyde in PBS.
(2) Wash twice for 5 min with PBS.
(3) Quench excess aldehyde by incubating the coverslips for 15 min at room temperature in 50 mM NH_4Cl in PBS (if fixed with 8% paraformaldehyde), or by incubating with three changes (5 min each) of 0.5 mg/ml freshly prepared sodium borohydride in PBS (if 4% paraformaldehyde and 0.25% glutaraldehyde was used for fixation).
(4) Wash three times (5 min each) with PBS.
(5) Block and incubate the coverslips with the primary antibody raised against the protein of interest as described in Protocol #29. As a control incubate a few coverslips with an antibody against an intracellular antigen such as Map2 (SEE SECTION 2, PAGE 65 AND SECTION 4).
(6) Wash, incubate with fluorochrome-labeled secondary antibody and mount as described in Protocol #29.

Protocol #34: Use of Sulfosuccinimidyl-6-(Biotinamido) Hexanoato (NHS-LC-Biotin) for Biochemical Analysis of Protein Traffic in Neurons Infected with SFV or SFV Expression Vector

Infections

(1) Infect neurons using the appropriate dilution of wild-type or recombinant SFV as described in Protocol #27.

(2) After 1 h remove the infection medium, add fresh N2 medium and incubate the cells for at least 2 h to allow replication of the viral genome and expression of the viral glycoproteins. In this time the newly synthesized viral proteins concentrate in the cell body.

Metabolic Labeling

(3) Use a Petri dish of 3 cm diameter, containing approximately 10^4 neurons for each experiment. Remove the medium into a sterile tube and keep it in the incubator at 37°C/5% CO_2.
(4) Wash twice with PBS and twice with HBSS at room temperature.
(5) Add 0.5 ml of labeling mixture containing ^{35}S-methionine and incubate at 37°C/5% CO_2 for 30 min.
(6) Wash once with Ca/Mg-PBS and once with HBSS.
(7) Chase by incubating 30 minutes at 37°C/5% CO_2 in the initial, prewarmed, N2 medium. During this time prepare the biotin solution.

Surface Labeling of Proteins with S-NHS-LC-Biotin

(8) Perform the following steps at 4°C: place the dish onto an ice-cold metal plate and wash twice with cold Ca/Mg-PBS.
(9) Add 0.5 ml of freshly made S-NHS-LC-Biotin and incubate on ice for 30 min.
(10) Wash twice with cold Ca/Mg-PBS.
(11) Add 1 ml of GB solution and let stand on ice for 10 min to remove the unbound biotin.

Lysis

(12) Wash twice with Ca/Mg-PBS.
(13) Add 0.2 ml of lysis buffer and incubate for 10 min on ice.
(14) Pipette up and down several times using an automatic pipette fitted with a tip cut approximately 0.5 cm from the end.
(15) Transfer lysate to a 1.5 ml microcentrifuge tube and spin at 14 000*g*, 4°C to remove cellular debris and insoluble material.
(16) Transfer lysate to a new tube and keep overnight, or longer, at −20°C.

Immunoprecipitation

(17) Thaw the lysate and add 0.7 ml NET buffer.
(18) Add the corresponding antibody. Vortex to mix.
(19) Let stand 2–4 h at room temperature.
(20) Add 45 μl of Protein-A-sepharose and incubate 1 h at room temperature while rotating tube end over end.
(21) Spin down for 5 s in a microcentrifuge. Remove the supernatant by aspiration and discard.
(22) Add 0.8 ml NET buffer.
(22) Incubate with rotation at room temperature for 10 min.
(24) Centrifuge for 30 s in a microcentrifuge and remove the supernatant by aspiration using a needle or yellow tip, into a trap attached to a vacuum pump.
(25) Repeat Steps 22–24 three times.
(26) Elute the immunoprecipitated protein from the beads with 40 μl of 0.1 M glycine, pH 3.0, resuspend gently and leave at room temperature.
(27) After 1–2 minutes add 10 μl 1 M Tris–HCl, pH 9.0 to neutralize.
(28) Add 50 μl 2× SDS-loading buffer (without dithiothreitol).
(29) Centrifuge briefly, take a 5 μl aliquot and keep it at −20°C to load in the gel (Step 40) next to the sample containing the biotinylated protein—this will serve as a control showing the total immunoprecipitated protein.
(30) Add 0.7 ml of STR buffer. Mix gently.

(31) Centrifuge 30 s and transfer the supernatant to a new tube. Discard pellet.
(32) Add 35 μl streptavidin-agarose.
(33) Incubate by rotating at room temperature for 3 h; alternatively, incubate overnight at 4°C.
(34) Centrifuge 5 s and remove the supernatant.
(35) Wash twice with 0.8 ml washing solution (a), twice with 0.8 ml washing solution (b) and twice with 0.8 ml washing solution (c). For each wash resuspend the agarose beads by inverting the tube several times, centrifuge 5 s and discard supernatant by aspiration, using a needle or yellow tip, into a trap connected to a vacuum pump.
(36) Resuspend in 0.8 ml of washing solution (d) and let stand for 5 min at room temperature. Remove supernatant as in Step 19.
(37) Resuspend in 0.8 ml washing solution (e). Remove supernatant as in Step 19, except that centrifugation should be extended to 30 s and the needle introduced deeply into the agarose pellet to remove as much buffer as possible.
(38) Elute the protein with 30 μl of 1 × SDS-loading buffer. Centrifuge 30 s and transfer supernatant to a new tube.

Polyacrylamide Gel Electrophoresis (PAGE)

(39) Use 1 μl from the samples obtained from Steps 29 and 38 to measure counts/min in a scintillation counter.
(40) Load 200–5000 counts/min (ideally 1000, in a volume of 5–15 μl) per lane of a 15 × 15 cm gel (1 mm thick) to separate the biotinylated proteins by SDS–PAGE. Boil samples for 3 min before loading.
(41) (3) When the electrophoresis is completed, soak the gel briefly in 50% methanol and then fix in 50% methanol/10% acetic acid by incubating for 20 min on a rocking platform.

Fluorography

(42) Incubate the gel consecutively in solutions A (20 min) and B (20 min) of Entensify (DuPont/Biotechnology Systems).
(43) Place the gel on filter paper, dry and expose overnight at −80°C to X-OMAT (Kodak) or equivalent film using intensifying screens.

4 NOTES AND TROUBLESHOOTING

4.1 Notes on Preparation of Virus Stocks

4.1.1 FPV

Virus stock is prepared as described by Matlin et al. (1981) and Matlin and Simons (1983, 1984). Briefly, the allantoic cavities of 11-day-old embryonated chicken eggs are infected with 3000 plaque-forming units (p.f.u.) and incubated at 37°C. After 24 h, the allantoic fluid is collected and the viruses concentrated by ultracentrifugation. The number of viruses is determined using plaque titration on MDCK cells. The viral hemagglutinin is sorted to the axon in hippocampal neurons (Dotti and Simons, 1990).

4.1.2 VSV

This virus is grown in BHK cells as described in detail by Matlin et al. (1982) and White et al. (1981). BHK cells, infected with VSV at 0.01 p.f.u./cell are incubated at 37°C/ 5% CO_2 for 20 h. The virus is then concentrated from the medium by ultracentrifugation. The concentration of viruses is determined by plaque titration (Matlin et al., 1982). The viral glycoprotein G (VSV-G) is sorted to the somatodendritic domain in hippocampal neurons (Dotti and Simons, 1990).

4.1.3 SFV

SFV stock is prepared as described by White et al. (1981). The viral E2 glycoprotein is sorted to the dendritic domain in hippocampal neurons (Huber et al., 1993).

4.1.4 Recombinant SFV

See Chapter 5 for protocols for production of recombinant SFV.

4.2 Notes on Hippocampal Cultures

Primary cultures of fetal rat hippocampal neurons are performed as described by Goslin and Banker (1991). Cells are plated onto either poly-L-lysine coated dishes (Nunc) or on poly-L-lysine covered glass coverslips (15 mm diameter). The medium used for culture is called N2 (Bottenstein and Sato, 1979). We routinely use N2 medium supplemented with basic fibroblast growth factor (Boehringer Mannheim) to a final concentration of 1 ng/ml.

4.3 On Protocol #27: Viral Infections of Neuronal Cultures

For recombinant SFV use a MOI of about 1–3: this means that the number of viruses per cell is 1–3. For non-recombinant SFV, an MOI of 10 is used. Cells are infected with FPV or VSV with a MOI of 80–100.

4.4 On Protocol #28: Fixation and Permeabilization of Cells

The protocols described above work for most antigens; however, the first time it is advisable to try different protocols to determine which one is best suited to visualize the protein of interest (consult also Harlow and Lane, 1988 and related bibliography).

4.4.1 Methanol Fixation

Very suitable to detect cytoskeleton-associated antigens. It will also lead to permeabilization of the cells.

4.4.2 Paraformaldehyde Fixation

This method requires further permeabilization of the cells.

4.4.3 Triton X-100 Permeabilized Cells

This method has a tendency to yield high nuclear background staining in immunofluorescence. If this is the case, the cells should be permeabilized with ethanol.

4.4.4 Ethanol Permeabilization

Coverslips can remain in the 70% ethanol solution for hours or even days.

4.4.5 Saponin Permeabilization

Performed before fixation. It results in a very strong permeabilization of cells, which can be useful when part of the protein of interest is present as a soluble pool that needs to be removed to allow detection of the membrane-bound pool, as is the case, for instance, for many small GTPases.

4.5 On Protocol #29: Immunocytochemistry Procedures for Cells Grown *in vitro*

4.5.1 *Humid Chamber*

A square plastic plate of 15 × 15 cm can be used for up to 12 coverslips. Place in it three sheets of wet filter paper and a sheet of Parafilm or equivalent plastic.

4.5.2 *Saponin Solution*

Always prepare fresh saponin solution. Dissolve saponin (Sigma) to a concentration of 0.01% (w/v) in PIPES-KOH (pH 6.8) with 5 mM EGTA and 1 mM $MgCl_2$.

4.5.3 *Blocking Solution*

Mix 2% fetal calf serum, 2% bovine serum albumin and 0.2% cold-water fish-skin gelatin (Sigma) in water. Store at −20°C.

4.5.4 *Primary Antibodies*

Synaptophysin is a component of synaptic vesicles. This antibody may therefore be used to identify axons and synaptic contacts in polarized neurons.

Phosphorylated neurofilament (heavy) is an axon-specific cytoskeleton-associated protein. Antibodies against this antigen yield an excellent axonal staining in polarized hippocampal neurons in culture.

The anti-Tau-1 antibody recognizes dephosphorylated Tau-1, which is associated with axonal microtubules (Mandel and Banker, personal communication).

Map2 is dendritic marker.

4.5.5 *Immunocytochemistry Procedures*

Block the cells before incubation with the first antibody to prevent non-specific binding of primary antibodies.

4.6 On Protocol #30: Lucifer Yellow Labeling of Early and Late Endocytic Compartments

Lucifer yellow is dissolved in methanol-acetone (2:1), dried under vacuum and redissolved to a concentration of 5–10 mg/ml in N2 medium containing 0.1% BSA.

Lucifer yellow is a fluorescent dye used to study fluid-phase endocytosis. Internalization for 1–15 min will mainly label early endosomes (see Fig. 6.1), while at longer incubation times late endosomes and lysosomes will also be labeled. The dye does not fix very well, and it is advisable to fix the cells with a combination of 4% paraformaldehyde and 0.25% glutaraldehyde.

Fixation with glutaraldehyde will lead to a better intracellular retention of lucifer yellow, but it may affect the antigenicity of the protein of interest.

Alternatively, internalization of transferrin or transferrin receptors can be used to label early endosomes. The transferrin receptor is a protein that binds iron-loaded transferrin and recycles between the plasma membrane and the early endosomes. It is therefore conveniently used as a marker for early endosomes. In polarized hippocampal neurons the transferrin receptor is found exclusively in the early endosomes present in the dendrites (Cameron et al., 1991; Parton et al., 1992). A monoclonal antibody against the rat transferrin receptor is commercially available (e.g. from Boehringer Mannheim). These antibodies might be useful for endosomal co-localization studies.

Early endosomes can also be labeled by adding fluorescent conjugated human transferrin (Molecular Probes) to the medium to a concentration of 50 μg/ml and incubating the cells at 37°C/5% CO_2 for 1 h. The human transferrin binds to the rat transferrin receptor. The signal can be enhanced if neurons are washed and incubated for a few hours in transferrin-free N2 medium before adding labeled transferrin to the medium.

4.7 On Protocols #32 and #33: Immunofluorescent Labeling of Surface-exposed Antigens

Interpretation of immunofluorescence results of plasma membrane proteins is often complicated by labeling of the internal pool of such protein. Two ways to circumvent this problem are described in the protocols.

4.7.1 Low-temperature Labeling

This is performed by incubating living cells with antibodies against the protein of interest at 4°C (low temperature blocks endocytosis and therefore prevents internalization of the antibodies). The major disadvantage is that neurons suffer from low-temperature incubations.

4.7.2 Fixation Without Permeabilization

It is possible to fix the cells in such a way that no permeabilization occurs. The reliability of this method depends on the integrity of the cells because unhealthy cells are permeabilized quite easily. Unfortunately, many antigens are sensitive to the conditions required for this fixation.

Surface accessibility may also be demonstrated biochemically by surface biotinylation of ^{35}S-labeled proteins (see corresponding protocol).

4.7.3 Further General Notes on Protocols #32 and #33

FPV, VSV and SFV should be handled following local safety regulations and all work should be done under appropriate containment.

The incubation time with primary and secondary antibodies is determined empirically. Better results might be obtained by incubating the cells overnight at 4°C or 37°C instead of the normal incubations of 30–60 min at room temperature or 37°C. However, there is no general rule for this, and you must determine the best conditions (incubation time, temperature, antibody dilution and volume) for your laboratory.

If double immunofluorescence is to be performed, better results are obtained when samples are processed as two successive single immunofluorescence experiments rather than when cocktails of primary and/or secondary antibodies are used.

The lucifer yellow staining can be followed in living cells; alternatively, internalized lucifer yellow can be detected by staining permeabilized cells with anti-lucifer yellow antibodies (Molecular Probes).

Horseradish peroxidase (HRP) may also be used as a fluid-phase marker to label endocytic compartments. It is added to the culture medium to a concentration of 10 mg/ml. Antibodies against HRP are commercially available (Sigma), allowing fluorescent detection of the internalized HRP.

Coverslips mounted in Mowiol do not need to be sealed, but Mowiol needs at least 1 h to set.

When performing "fixation without permeabilization" protocols no labeling should be seen in control cells incubated with an antibody against an intracellular antigen. Moreover, to be sure that lack of labeling with control antibodies is not due to loss of antigenicity of the corresponding intracellular protein caused by the harsh fixation conditions, the following controls should be introduced: (1) coverslips fixed and permeabilized with 4% paraformaldehyde followed by permeabilization with Triton X-100; and (2) coverslips fixed with 8% paraformaldehyde or 4% paraformaldehyde/0.25% glutaraldehyde and permeabilized as before. If the fluorescence observed in the coverslips of (2) is low compared with the coverslips processed in (1), the antigen is affected by the stronger fixation conditions and this protocol is inappropriate.

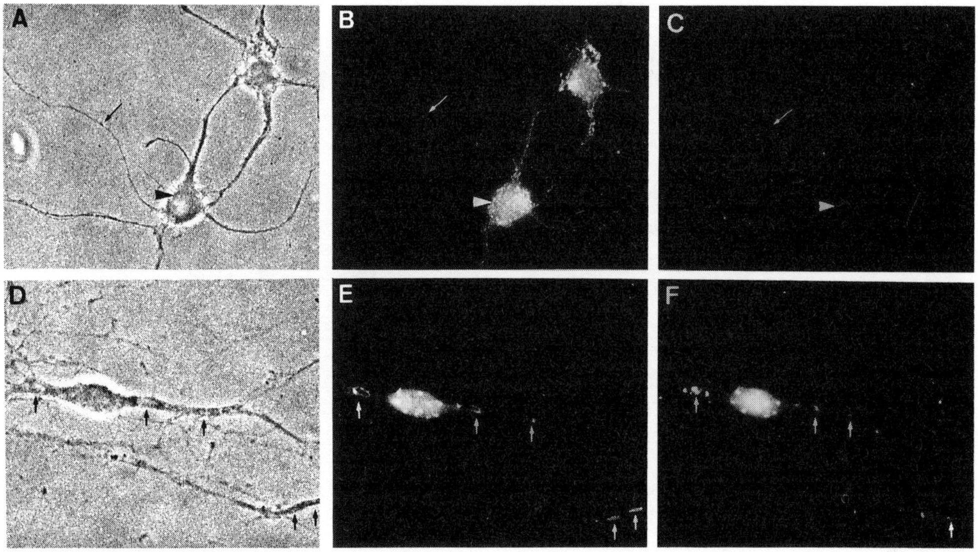

Figure 6.1 Colocalization of SFV-overexpressed rab5 and lucifer yellow: endocytic structures visualized in non-infected neurons (A, B and C) or neurons infected with a recombinant SFV encoding a dominant-positive mutant of Rab5 (Rab5Q79L) (D, E and F). Cells cultured on coverslips were incubated 7.5 h after infection with the fluid-phase ligand lucifer yellow for 15 min (SEE PROTOCOL #30), fixed with paraformaldehyde, permeabilized with Triton X-100, and stained with anti-rab5 antibodies diluted so that they detected the overexpressed (recombinant) protein but not the endogenous rab5 (de Hoop et al., 1994). A, D: phase contrast; B, E: lucifer yellow staining; C, F: detection of recombinant Rab5 by immunofluorescence. The arrows in A, B and C point to an axon and the arrowheads to endocytic vesicles (early endosomes) present in the cell body. Arrows in D, E and F point to neurites containing overexpressed Rab5a. Bar represents 10 μm

4.8 On Protocol #34: Use of Sulfosuccinimidyl-6-(biotinamido) Hexanoato (NHS-LC-Biotin) for Biochemical Analysis of Protein Traffic in Neurons Infected with SFV or SFV Expression Vector

NHS-LC-Biotin is a water-soluble biotin analog that binds very efficiently to proteins and peptides at neutral pH. Biotinylation has been used successfully to label selectively apical or basolateral membrane proteins in polarized epithelial cells such as MDCK, which form tight junctions *in vitro* (Sargiacomo et al., 1989; Le Bivic et al., 1990). It has also been used to detect secretory proteins at the surface of the neuroendocrine cell line P12 after stimulation of regulated secretion (Pimplikar and Huttner, 1992). In our laboratory we have used biotinylation to label newly synthesized SFV spike glycoproteins on the surface of neurons under specific conditions (Cid-Arregui et al., 1995) (see Fig. 6.2). Although the presence of these proteins and their location in the different neuronal domains can be easily shown by immunofluorescence, biotinylation offers a unique means to demonstrate that they are located at the cell surface. This technique can also be applied with the same efficiency to detect exogenous proteins expressed in neurons upon infection with recombinant SFV carrying the respective coding sequences (SEE CHAPTER 5 for details on the use of SFV-expression vectors).

4.8.1 ^{35}S-methionine Labeling Mixture

This solution can be used several times. If necessary, it may be stored at −20°C. In our experience, freezing and thawing this solution up to three times causes no significant degradation.

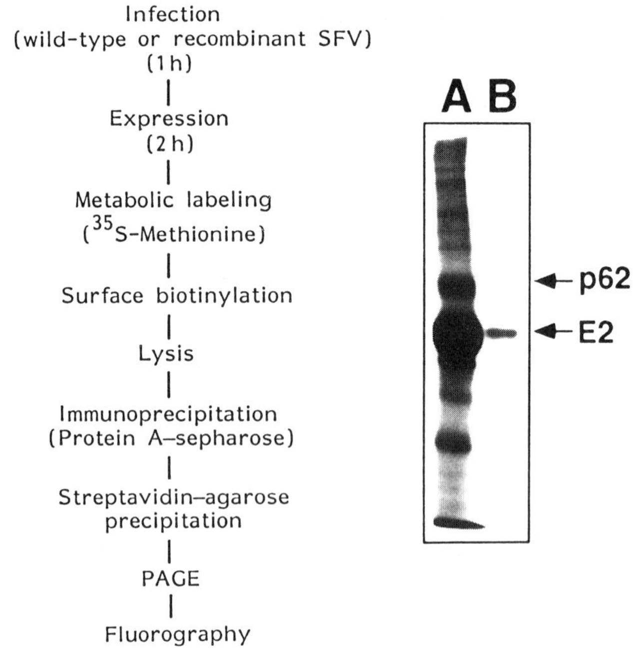

Figure 6.2 Detection of viral glycoproteins at the surface of rat hippocampal neurons infected with wild-type SFV. The scheme on the left summarizes the method described in detail in Part B. On the right a fluorograph of biotinylated E2 glycoprotein precipitated from SFV infected neurons is shown. Hippocampal neurons from a 14-day primary culture, maintained in a 3 cm diameter dish, were radioactively labeled with ^{35}S-methionine, surface biotinylated with NHS-LC-biotin and lysed as described (SEE PROTOCOL #34). The lysates were immunoprecipitated using a monoclonal antibody raised against the extracytoplasmic portion of the p62 and E2 SFV glycoproteins (Burke et al., 1983). The proteins were separated in a 10% polyacrylamide gel. Lane A: total immunoprecipitated protein. Lane B: biotinylated protein recovered with streptavidin-agarose

4.8.2 General Notes on Protocol #34

Media and materials in contact with virus must be decontaminated by treatment with formalin and autoclaved. Safety rules for handling ^{35}S should be followed. Whenever possible use plastic disposable material. The use of a biocontainment hood and incubator is advisable.

This method is very sensitive and can be scaled down for cells cultured on a single coverslip (15 mm diameter). In this case, special care should be taken to recover the cell lysate (Step 14) without any losses and elution from the streptavidin-agarose beads (Step 38) should be in 15 μl or less to facilitate loading of the whole sample volume in a single lane.

It is important to pipette media and buffers in and out of the dish carefully to avoid losing cells. If the volume of lysate recovered in Step 14 is lower than 150 μl repeat this step by adding another 50 μl of lysis buffer.

Steps 3–5 should be performed as quickly as possible to cause minimal stress to the cells. If more than one dish is going to be used, start infections at different times (e.g. at 15 min intervals) so that no more than one dish is out of the incubator when performing these steps.

To pipette Protein-A-sepharose and streptavidin-agarose, we recommend using yellow tips cut at 0.5 cm from the end to insure delivery of equal amounts in each tube.

If the antibody used for immunoprecipitation is a mouse monoclonal it may convenient to use Protein-G instead of Protein-A-sepharose beads (see Harlow and Lane, 1988).

Elution of the immunoprecipitate (Step 26) can also be performed with 1 × SDS-loading buffer. However, we obtain best results at low pH as described.

ACKNOWLEDGMENTS

We are grateful to Dr C.G. Dotti for his constant support and encouragement, Dr S.H. Pimplikar for his valuable advice concerning the biotinylation labeling and Mrs L. Meyn and H. Virta for excellent technical assistance. A.C.A. was funded by the Deutsche Forschungsgemeinschaft (SFB 317) and M. de H. was supported by a fellowship from the International Human Frontier Science Program Organization (LT118/92).

REFERENCES

Bottenstein, J.E. and Sato, G.H. (1979) Growth of a neuroblastoma cell line in serum-free supplemented medium. *Proc. Natl Acad. Sci. USA* **76:** 719–731.

Burke, B., Walter, C., Griffiths, G. and Warren, G. (1983). Viral glycoproteins at different stages of intracellular transport can be distinguished using monoclonal antibodies. *Eur. J. Cell. Biol.* **31:** 315–324.

Cameron, P.L., Südhof, T.C., Jahn, R. and De Camilli, P. (1991) Co-localization of synaptophysin with transferrin receptors: Implications for synaptic vesicle biogenesis. *J. Cell. Biol.* **116:** 151–164.

Cid-Arregui, A., Parton, R.G., Simons, K. and Dotti, C.G. (1995). Nocodazole-dependent transport, and Brefeldin A-sensitive processing and sorting of newly synthesized membrane proteins in cultured neurons. *J. Neurosci.* **15**: 4259–4269.

Dotti, C.G. and Simons, K. (1990) Polarized sorting of viral glycoproteins to the axon and dendrites of hippocampal neurons in culture. *Cell* **62:** 63–72.

Goslin, K. and Banker, G. (1991) Rat hippocampal neurons in low density cultures. In: G. Banker and K. Goslin (eds): *Culturing nerve cells.* p.251–281. MIT Press, Cambridge.

Harlow, E. and Lane, D. (1988) *Antibodies. A laboratory manual.* Cold Spring Harbor Laboratory, New York.

de Hoop, M. J. and Dotti, C. G (1993) Membrane traffic in polarized neurons in culture. *J. Cell. Sci.* **17:** 85–92.

de Hoop, M.J., Huber, L.A., Stenmark, H., Williamson, E., Zerial, M., Parton, R.G. and Dotti, C.G. (1994) The involvement of the small GTP-binding protein rab5a in neuronal endocytosis. *Neuron* **13:** 11–22.

Huber, L.A., de Hoop, M.J., Dupree, P., Zerial, M., Simons, K. and Dotti, C. (1993) Protein transport to the dendritic plasma membrane of cultured neurons is regulated by rab8p. *J. Cell. Biol.* **123:** 47–55.

Le Bivic, A., Sambuy, Y., Mostov, K. and Rodriguez-Boulan, E. (1990) Vectorial targeting of an endogenous apical membrane sialoglycoprotein and ovomorulin in MDCK cells. *J. Cell. Biol.* **110:** 1533–1539.

Matlin, K.S. and Simons, K. (1983) Reduced temperature prevents transfer of a membrane glycoprotein to the cell surface but does not prevent terminal glycosylation. *Cell* **34:** 233–243.

Matlin, K.S. and Simons, K. (1984) Sorting of an apical plasma membrane glycoprotein occurs before it reaches the surface in cultured epithelial cells. *J. Cell. Biol.* **99:** 2131–2139.

Matlin, K.S., Reggio, H., Helenius, A., and Simons, K. (1981) Infectious entry pathway of influenza virus in a canine kidney cell line. *J. Cell Biol.* **91:** 601–613.

Matlin, K.S., Reggio, H., Helenius, A and Simons, K. (1982) Pathway of vesicular stomatitis virus entry leading to infection. *J. Mol. Biol.* **156:** 609–631.

Parton, R.G., Simons, K. and Dotti, C.G. (1992) Axonal and dendritic endocytic pathways in cultured neurons. *J. Cell. Biol.* **119:** 123–137.

Pimplikar, S.W. and Huttner, W.B. (1992) Chromogranin B (Secretogranin I), a secretory protein of the regulated pathway, is also present in a tightly membrane-associated form in PC12 cells. *J. Biol. Chem.* **267:** 4110–4118.

Rodriguez-Boulan, E.J. and Sabatini, D.D. (1978) Asymmetric budding of viruses in epithelial monolayers: a model system for the study of epithelial polarity. *Proc. Natl Acad. Sci. USA* **75:** 5071–5075.

Sargiacomo, M., Lisanti, M., Graeve, L., Le Bivic, A. and Rodriguez-Boulan, E. (1989) Integral and peripheral protein composition of the apical and basolateral membrane domains in MDCK cells. *J. Membr. Biol.* **107:** 277–286.

White, J., Matlin, K. and Helenius, A. (1981) Cell fusion by Semliki Forest, Influenza, and Vesicular Stomatitis Viruses. *J. Cell. Biol.* **89:** 674–679.

SECTION 3

Protocols for Gene Delivery Using Adenoviruses and Adeno-associated Viruses

CHAPTER 7

Gene Transfer into the Central and Peripheral Nervous System Using Adenoviral Vectors

FREDERIC REVAH, PHILIPPE HORELLOU*, EMMANUELLE VIGNE†, GILDAS LE GAL LA SALLE‡, JEAN JACQUES ROBERT*, MICHEL PERRICAUDET† AND JACQUES MALLET§

Rhône-Poulenc Rorer, Centre de Recherche Vitry-Alfortville, 13 quai Jules Guesde, 94403 Vitry sur Seine Cedex, France. Tel: 1 45 73 85 11; Fax: 1 45 73 77 96.

**Laboratoire de Génétique Moléculaire de la Neurotransmission et des Processus Dégénératifs, C9923, CNRS, 91198 Gif sur Yvette, France. Tel: 1 69 82 35 80; Fax: 1 69 07 50 31.*

†Institut Gustave Roussy, Unité Associée 1301, 39 rue Camille Desmoulins, CNRS, 94805 Villejuif Cedex, France. Tel: 1 45 59 55 90; Fax: 1 45 59 40 90.

‡Institut Alfred Fessard, Unité Propre de Recherche 2212, CNRS, 91198 Gif sur Yvette Cedex, France. Tel: 1 69 82 34 28; Fax: 1 69 07 05 38; Email: legal@iaf.cnrs-gif.fr

§L.G.N., C.N.R.S., Bâtiment Cervi, 5e Étage, Hôpital de la Pitié, Salpêtrière, 83 Boulevard de l'Hôpital, 75013 Paris, France. Tel: 33 1 42 17 75 32; Fax: 33 1 42 17 75 33

1 INTRODUCTION

Classical pharmacotherapy for neurological disorders must cope with tight constraints specific to the nervous system. In particular, the blood–brain barrier prevents the passage of numerous macromolecules of therapeutic interest (including growth factors, cytokines, or enzymes participating in neurotransmitter synthesis) from the bloodstream into the brain. In general, the only method of delivering such components to the brain is by intracerebral injection, intraventricular injection into the cerebrospinal fluid, or infusion using osmotic pumps (Olson et al., 1992). These methods require complex neurosurgical procedures and, when coupled with the limited stability of the injected substance, the risks associated with such interventions (e.g. infection) clearly overwhelm their potential therapeutic benefits. As might be expected, implantation of a minipump also disrupts the patient's normal daily routine. Intracerebral neuronal grafts of embryonic brain cells have been proposed as an alternative to pharmacotherapy, and have been tested in the case of Parkinson's disease (Björklund and Stenevi, 1979; Perlow et al., 1979; Lindvall et al., 1990; Freed et al., 1992; Spencer et al., 1992; Widner et al., 1992). Although recent studies are promising, the general use of this type of therapy is hampered by the limited availability of embryonic tissues.

In theory, gene therapy should enable neurologists to overcome the problems raised by pharmacotherapy or grafting of embryonic cells. Indeed, gene transfer into a given brain structure should permit local and controlled expression and release of a therapeutic protein, ideally after a single administration. Gene transfer to the brain can be achieved either by direct transfer (*in vivo*

Protocols for Gene Transfer in Neuroscience: Towards Gene Therapy of Neurological Disorders
Edited by P.R. Lowenstein and L.W. Enquist

gene therapy) using an appropriate vector, or by intracerebral grafting of genetically engineered cells (*ex vivo* gene therapy: Horellou et al., 1990; Ushida et al., 1990; Fisher et al., 1991; Jiao et al., 1993). We and other workers have demonstrated the potency of recombinant adenovirus vectors for *in vivo* gene transfer in the brain (Akli et al., 1993; Bajocchi et al., 1993; Davidson et al., 1993; Le Gal La Salle et al., 1993). We have also shown that adenoviruses can be used for an *ex vivo* approach (Ridoux et al., 1994). Adenovirus was initially considered as an interesting candidate for neuronal gene therapy because, unlike retroviruses that require host DNA replication for infection, adenoviruses can infect post-mitotic terminally differentiated cells including neurons. This technology also has several advantages in terms of safety and simplicity of preparation.

1.1 Safety

Our recombinant adenoviruses are derived from type 5 adenovirus (Ad5), which has not been reported to be associated with oncogenicity in humans. The effects of wild-type adenovirus infection are well documented—more than 10 million patients have received live adenovirus tablets as an oral vaccine with no major side effects (Rubin and Rorke, 1988). Furthermore, adenovirus typically does not integrate into the genome, which limits the chances of insertional mutagenesis. Finally, adenovirus naturally moves towards the respiratory tract, which is of some importance in the context of gene therapy for the brain because wild-type viruses are rarely found in human brain (Kelsey, 1978). As a consequence, when a recombinant adenovirus defective for replication is injected into the brain there is little risk that the defect will be complemented or rescued by a resident wild-type virus. This may not be the case when using herpes simplex virus-1-based vectors, as this virus is neurotropic and a large proportion of the population is naturally infected by herpes viruses.

1.2 Production of Recombinant Viruses

The adenovirus genome is 36 kb, and is divided into early (mainly E1 to E4) and late (L1 to L5) regions, based on gene expression before and after viral DNA replication. The infection cycle includes a step of attachment to cell-specific receptors, internalization into endosomes, release into the cytoplasm by endosomolysis and translocation to the nucleus, where activation of the early regions is followed by DNA replication and activation of the late regions. No latent state has been described for adenoviruses. The transcription machinery and viral cycle of adenoviruses is relatively simple (one should stress **relatively**) compared with HSV-1-based vectors. This means that straightforward strategies for the production of replication-defective recombinant viruses can be developed. Such strategies involve deletion of early regions necessary for viral replication and replacement of part of these regions by the transgene of interest (SEE SECTION 3, PAGE 83). Helper viruses that could contaminate the preparations of recombinant virus are not required. The viruses described here can accommodate transgenes up to 7.5 kb in length, and can be obtained at titers as high as 10^{11}–10^{12} p.f.u./ml.

In spite of the advantages of adenovirus, and although the first results obtained using adenoviruses encoding β-galactosidase from *Escherichia coli* (AdβGal) for both *in vivo* and an *ex vivo* gene therapy approaches are promising, several issues remain to be solved before human applications can be implemented. These include the fine tuning of cell specificity, time course and levels of transgene expression. An understanding and way of circumventing the cytopathic effects of adenoviruses that can sometimes be observed (SEE SECTION 4, PAGE 87) are also necessary. Also, for *in vivo* gene therapy, the diffusion of the virus must be improved after stereotactic injection. Finally, gene delivery studies using recombinant adenoviruses in the CNS will undoubtedly benefit from current human clinical trials of gene therapy for cystic fibrosis using adenoviruses encoding the cystic fibrosis transmembrane regulator (CFTR). In particular, it will be invaluable to define the parameters required for safety with respect to the patient, the associated medical staff and the environment.

2 MATERIALS AND EQUIPMENT

Materials required for preparation of recombinant adenoviruses are listed below. Specific reagents needed for infection of neural cells *in vitro* or *in vivo* are detailed along with the particular protocol.

(1) Cell line and media: The 293 cell line is available from the ATCC and ECACC. Grow these cells in MEM supplemented with 7% fetal calf serum (FCS) heated to inactivate complement. We use MEM + 2% FCS for viral infection.
(2) Buffer A for dialysis: Tris 10 mM, pH 7.5; $MgCl_2$ 1 mM; NaCl 135 mM.
(3) Buffer B for dialysis: buffer A + 10% glycerol.
(4) Buffer C: Tris 10 mM, pH 7.5; EDTA 0.5 mM; SDS 0.5%; proteinase K 50μg/ml.
(5) Agar mix: Agar 2% 2 ml; MEM 2× 2 ml; FCS 80 μl.
(6) TD solution: NaCl 750 mM; KCl 50 mM; Tris 250 mM; Na_2HPO_4 10 mM. Adjust pH to 7.4.
(7) CsCl solutions: (a) density 1.25: 361.6 g/l of TD; (b) density 1.34: 512 g/l of TD; (c) density 1.4: 620g/l of TD.

3 THE PROTOCOLS

Protocol #35: Preparation of Adenovirus

Infection of 293 Cells

(1) Prepare dishes (10 cm diameter) of 293 cells that are 80–90% confluent 1 or 2 days before infection. We recommend using 50–120 dishes for a viral preparation.
(2) Remove the medium and add 1 ml of virus diluted in MEM + 2% FCS per 10 cm dish (0.5 ml/60 mm dish) at a multiplicity of infection (MOI) of 10 p.f.u./cell.
(3) Incubate 1 h at 37°C, gently rocking the plates every 20 minutes to evenly distribute the inoculum.
(4) Remove inoculum by aspiration and refeed with MEM + 2% FCS.
(5) Between 40 and 48 h later, gently harvest the infected cells: they appear rounded and begin to detach and float.
(6) Centrifuge infected cells for 10 min at 800*g*.
(7) Resuspend the cells in 5 ml of medium per 10^8 cells.
(8) Freeze and thaw three times to release virus from cells.
(9) Centrifuge at 3300*g* for 10 min to pellet cell debris. Collect the supernatant containing virus and store at −20°C.

Viral Stock: Preparation of Purified Virus or DNA

(1) Infect at least 5 × 10^8 cells as described above.
(2) Gently layer the crude virus supernatant on a preformed CsCl gradient (densities 1.4 and 1.25) in an ultracentrifuge tube.
(3) Centrifuge for 1 h at 180 000*g* and 18°C.
(4) Remove the dense band of virus with a needle and syringe. Note that many bands are usually visible, but the lighter ones correspond to empty capsids or immature virions.
(5) Apply the rescued virus on a layer of CsCl (density 1.34).
(6) Centrifuge for 18 h at 180 000*g* and 18°C.
(7) Collect the viral band as above.

Preparation of Purified Virus

(1) Dialyse the virus twice in a dialysis tubing in 1 l of buffer A for 1 h and once in buffer B for 2 h.
(2) Divide the virus into aliquots and store at −70°C.

! NEVER REFREEZE A THAWED ALIQUOT !

Preparation of DNA

(1) Precipitate the viral band for 30 min at −70°C with 2 volumes of water and 6 volumes of ethanol in Eppendorf tubes.
(2) Centrifuge 10 min at 15 000*g*.
(3) Resuspend the pellet in 0.5 ml buffer C. Incubate 1 h at 37°C.
(4) Extract twice with phenol and twice in chloroform:isoamyl alcohol (24:1).
(5) Precipitate with 2 volumes of ethanol. Centrifuge 10 minutes at 15 000*g*. Wash with 70% ethanol to remove traces of salt from the DNA precipitate.
(6) Resuspend the pellet in water, quantify the DNA and store in 5 μg aliquots at −20°C.

Protocol #36: Plaque Assay for Adenovirus

(1) Prepare 293 cells in 60 mm dishes 1 or 2 days before infection. They must be **just** confluent on the day of infection.
(2) Sequentially dilute the virus stock 1:10, to a final dilution of 10^{11}.
(3) Infect the plate following Protocol #35.
(4) One hour after infection, remove the inoculum and add 4 ml of agar mix. Add the agar very slowly to avoid detaching the cells.
(5) Add a new layer of agar every 4 days.

Protocol #37: Extraction of DNA from Adenovirus-infected Cells

This protocol (modified Hirt procedure: Gluzman and Van Doren, 1983) allows the rapid extraction of the viral DNA from infected cells. It is valid for use with infected 293 cells prepared in a 60 mm dish.

(1) As soon as the infected cells are rounded, collect them gently.
(2) Centrifuge 5 min at 300*g*, rinse with PBS, then centrifuge for a further 5 min at 300*g*.
(3) Resuspend the pellet in 360 μl of 1× Tris–EDTA, pH 8. Add 25 μl SDS (10%), 8 μl EDTA (0.5 M) and 4 μl proteinase K (20 mg/ml). Incubate 2 h at 37°C.
(4) Add 100 μl 5 M NaCl. Keep on ice for at least 3 h.
(5) Centrifuge at 15 000*g* for 1 h. **Thoroughly** harvest the supernatant.
(6) Extract once with phenol:chloroform:isoamyl alcohol (25:24:1). Precipitate with 2 volumes of ethanol.
(7) Centrifuge for 10 min at 15 000*g*. Wash with 70% ethanol and resuspend the pellet in 50 μl water containing 0.1 mg/ml RNAse.

Protocol #38: Construction of Recombinant Adenoviruses; Transfection Protocol

(1) Prepare 70% confluent 293 cells in 60 mm dishes.
(2) Digest 5 μg of the plasmid containing the desired DNA sequence with a restriction enzyme not contained in regions involved in interactions with the virus genome (see Fig. 7.1). The enzyme used will depend on the transgene sequence.
(3) Cut 5 μg of dl324 viral DNA to completion with *Cla*I (Thimmappaya et al., 1982).
(4) Cotransfect 293 cells with the digested DNA, following the calcium phosphate technique of Sambrook et al. (1989).
(5) At least 4 h after transfection, replace medium with fresh medium. Wait for the appearance of a cytopathic effect (CPE) 6–10 days after transfection. The cells become round and no longer adhere to the substrate, forming clusters.
(6) Collect the cells when the CPE is total. Freeze and thaw three times, then centrifuge for 10 min at 3300*g*.
(7) Prepare a six-multiwell plate of 70% confluent 293 cells.
(8) Infect the wells with 10% or 20% of the supernatant.
(9) As soon as the cells in the wells are rounded, apply the Hirt procedure on the contents. Digest each fifth of the DNA with appropriate restriction enzymes that will give a diagnostic pattern

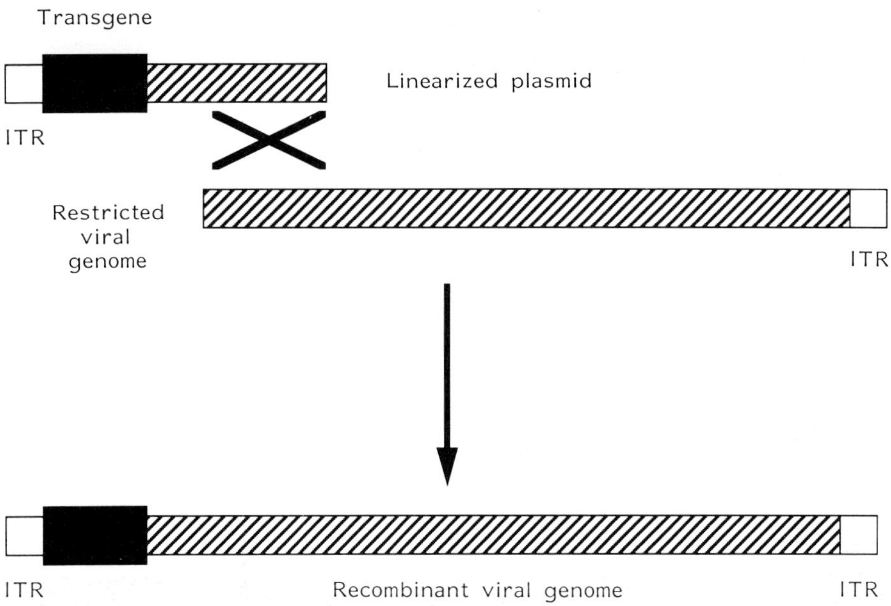

Figure 7.1 Homologous recombination in 293 cells generating a recombinant adenovirus deleted in E1 region

of fragments enabling unequivocal identification of the desired recombinant. If this is not successful, start again at Step 1 with newly thawed 293 cells.

Protocol #39: Construction of Recombinant Adenoviruses; Isolating Virus Plaques and Production of RAd Stock

(1) Prepare 293 cells in 60 mm dishes as for a plaque assay (Protocol #36).
(2) Dilute the supernatant obtained from Step 6 of Protocol #38 sequentially 1:10 to a final dilution of 10^9.
(3) Follow Protocol #36, Step 3–5. Plaques should appear 5–7 days after infection.
(4) Pick well isolated plaques by punching out agar plugs using a sterile Pasteur pipette, and resuspend each plug in 500 μl of MEM + 2% CSF. This can be stored at −20°C. Freeze and thaw three times.
(5) Prepare 12-multiwell plates of 20% confluent 293 cells. Infect each well with 250 μl of a plaque. Collect the contents of each well separately when cells are lysed. Freeze and thaw three times and centrifuge for 10 min at 3300*g*.
(6) Prepare six-multiwell plates of 80% confluent 293 cells. Infect each well with the supernatant obtained from Step 5.
(7) As soon as the cells in each well have become rounded, apply the Hirt procedure on its contents. Digest each fifth of the DNA with restriction enzymes chosen to clearly indicate whether the pattern is the one expected for the RAd. Choose the plaque with the desired DNA pattern.
(8) Amplify the chosen plaque until a viral stock is obtained. Purify this stock on CsCl gradients, as described in Protocol #35.
(9) Determine the stock titer by plaque assay. Titers are generally between 10^{10} and 10^{12} p.f.u./ml. Therefore dilutions from 10^1 to 10^{12} fold are required. Plaques may be counted 8–12 days after infection.

Protocol #40: Adenovirus-mediated Gene Transfer; General Protocol for *in vivo* CNS Gene Transfer in Adult Rats

(1) Use rats weighing about 180–250 g at the time of surgery.
(2) Anesthetize the animals. We suggest intraperitoneal injection of Equithesin (3 ml/kg). Equithesin is made up as follows: 16 ml pentobarbital, 5 ml chloral hydrate, 25 ml sodium sulfate (10 H_2O), 43 ml propane-1,2-diol, 10 ml ethanol.
(3) Shave the skin on the animal's head.
(4) Once deep anesthesia is obtained, fix the animal in a stereotactic frame (Kopf Instruments) through ear clips and jaw pieces.
(5) Make a longitudinal incision of about 0.5–1 cm with a scalpel. Pull aside the edges of the incision and gently expose the bone.
(6) Drill a hole with a dental drill at the appropriate coordinates, calculated either from the sutures of the skull or from a suitable atlas.
(7) Lower a Hamilton syringe (10 μl) attached to a holder through the burr hole into the target structure according to the appropriate coordinates.
(8) Connect the adapter to a special device for pushing the syringe and administer the solution over 10–30 min.
(9) Leave in place 5 min longer, then withdraw the syringe.
(10) Close the wound with thread, catgut or clips.

Protocol #41: *In vivo* CNS Gene Transfer in Adult Rats using Recombinant Adenovirus; Gene Transfer into the Striatum

(1) Dilute viral vector in PBS to 1.66×10^7 p.f.u./μl. Always keep virus on ice (4°C).
(2) Select the site(s) to be injected according to Protocol #40.
(3) Inject 9 μl of viral suspension stereotactically into nine sites in the striatum using a stainless steel cannula (external and internal diameter 0.28 mm/0.18 mm) at a rate of 0.5 μl/min by means of a microinjection pump (CMA/100; Carnegie Medicin, Stockholm, Sweden) at the following coordinates (toothbar set at zero).
   - (i–iii) A: + 1.8 mm; L: 2.5 mm; V: 5 mm/V: 4.6 mm/V: 4.2 mm
   - (iv–vi) A: + 0.6 mm; L: 2.0 mm; V: 5 mm/V: 4.6 mm/V: 4.2 mm
   - (vii–ix) A: + 0.6 mm; L: 3.2 mm; V: 5 mm/V: 4.6 mm/V: 4.2 mm.

This method has been used to express tyrosine hydroxylase in a rat model of Parkinson's disease (Horellou et al., 1994).

Protocol #42: Adenovirus-mediated Gene Transfer; *in vivo* Gene Transfer by Intraventricular Administration

(1) Connect a 35 cm long flexible catheter to a 23G needle and fix the needle on a stereotactic holder.
(2) Fill the whole system with a sterile solution (culture medium, for example).
(3) Connect a 10 μl Hamilton syringe to the end of the system and gently draw in air until it becomes visible about 1–2 mm into the catheter.
(4) Draw up the desired volume of adenovirus solution and connect the syringe.
(5) Lower the syringe into the lateral or third ventricle according to stereotactic coordinates.
(6) Disconnect the syringe. The liquid must go down to the bubble. If it does not, gently move the needle up or down along the frontal plane.

Protocol #43: Evaluation of Gene Transfer and Expression after *in vivo* Administration of Adenovirus Vectors

Perfusion, Fixation and Preparation of Brain Sections

(1) Kill rats at different times after inoculation of virus using intraperitoneal injection of 8 ml 6% sodium pentobarbital.

(2) Perfuse the animal through the heart with saline followed by freshly prepared 4% paraformaldehyde solution in 0.1 M phosphate buffer, pH 7.4.
(3) Remove the brain and post-fix it in the same fixative for about 2 h at 4°C.
(4) Incubate the fixed brain in 30% sucrose solution for about 2 days, until it sinks.
(5) Cut the brain into serial frozen sections of 30–40 μm in a frontal plane using a freezing microtome or a vibratome.
(6) Wash the sections with PBS.

Histochemistry

(1) Select sections for histochemical staining to reveal β-galactosidase activity using the substrate X-gal.
(2) Rinse the samples in PBS.
(3) Immerse sections in a solution containing 4 mM $K_3Fe(CN)_6$, 4 mM $K_4Fe(CN)_6$, 4 mM $MgCl_2$, and 0.2 mg/ml of the X-gal stain (5-bromo-4-chloro-3-indolyl-D-galactoside dissolved in *N,N*, dimethyl formamide at 20 mg/ml) in PBS for 3 h at 37°C.
(4) Wash sections several times in PBS.
(5) Mount on glass slides.
(6) Counterstain with 1% neutral red solution, and cover with a coverslip.

Immunohistochemistry

(1) Select sections for immunohistochemical detection of β-gal and place them in wells of a 24-well tissue culture plate.
(2) Rinse in PBS.
(3) Preincubate with 1% hydrogen peroxide for 30 min to block endogenous peroxidase activity.
(4) Incubate in 0.25% Triton-X100 in PBS+2% normal serum swine (NSS) for 2 h at room temperature.
(5) Incubate in anti-β-galactosidase antiserum (dilution: 1/800)(Cappel Rabbit IgG) in PBS+2% NSS overnight at 4°C.
(6) Rinse three times for 5 min each in PBS.
(7) Incubate in anti-rabbit antiserum (dilution: 1/200) in PBS+1% NSS for 1 h at room temperature.
(8) Wash several times in PBS (30 min total rinsing time).
(9) Add peroxidase anti-peroxidase from rabbit (dilution: 1/100) in PBS+1% NSS for 1 h at room temperature.
(10) Wash three times for 5 min each in PBS.
(11) Wash three times for 5 min each in Tris–HCl, pH 7.6.
(12) Incubate with diaminobenzidine (DAB: 310 mg DAB+0.7 g nickel sulfate+3 μl hydrogen peroxide in 30 ml Tris–HCl 0.05 M, pH 7.6) for 2–15 min.
(13) Wash sections several times in Tris–HCl, pH 7.6.
(14) Wash sections several times in PBS.
(15) Mount on glass slides and cover with a coverslip.

4 NOTES AND TROUBLESHOOTING

4.1 Safety Warning

Recombinant adenoviruses must be constructed and used under the appropriate confinement conditions in accordance with local regulations. In France RAds encoding growth factors, as well as animals inoculated with these viruses, must be handled in an airtight room equipped with an airlock, and under negative pressure. The atmosphere of the laboratory is filtered using an "absolute filter" before being discarded. The laboratory is equipped with a double-access autoclave. No material should exit the laboratory without being decontaminated. The research scientist must wear protective clothing, including an air mask and protective spectacles.

4.2 On *in vitro* Gene Transfer of Adenovirus into Neural and Non-neural Cells

We have successfully inoculated a variety of primary cell cultures including newborn rat superior cervical ganglia neurons, fetal rat cortical neurons, 15-day-old rat mesencephalic neurons, 8-day-old rat cerebellar granule neurons and newborn rat brain astrocytes. For each preparation, it is critical to determine the titer required to infect a significant percentage of cells without noticeable cytopathic effect. In addition, an initial series of experiments is necessary to optimize the duration of infection (from 24 h to several days) and the multiplicity of infection (p.f.u./cell) according to each cell type.

To infect cultures *in vitro* (for further details See Chapter 8, Page 93) remove the cell culture medium and save it. Add a thin layer of medium without serum, just sufficient to avoid drying. Next, add adenovirus at final MOI ranging of 1–1000 p.f.u./cell. After gentle rocking to distribute the virus inoculum, let the virus absorb for 30–60 min at 37°C (if insufficient time is allowed for absorption the infection will be suboptimal, but if too much time is allowed, a cytotoxic effect will be seen). Finally, add the reserved cell culture medium back to the culture.

The kinetics of transgene expression will vary depending on the cell type and the promoter driving the expression. For example, 48 h is usually sufficient to allow expression of β-galactosidase under the control of the LTR-RSV promoter.

4.2.1 Ex vivo *Gene Transfer*

Adenovirus is also a vector of choice for genetic manipulation of cells intended for subsequent transplantation into the nervous system. Most of the methods used for introducing DNA sequences into donor cells result in weak efficacy or transient gene expression after transplantation. In a recent paper we demonstrated that primary astrocytes cultured from brains of newborn rats are efficiently infected with adenovirus encoding the *E. coli lacZ* gene (Ridoux et al., 1994a). A large proportion of β-galactosidase-expressing cells survived after brain grafting and continued to express the transgene for prolonged period of time, at least 5 months.

Taken together, these results show that adenovirus-mediated gene expression is a particularly efficient vector for inducing long-lasting expression of a transgene in intracerebrally grafted nerve cells.

4.3 On Protocol #35: Preparation of Adenovirus

The recombinant adenoviruses (RAd) our team constructs are deleted for the E1 region which can be transcomplemented by the 293 cell line (Graham et al., 1977), and for the E3 region which is not required for *in vitro* replication. A plasmid carrying the following sequences (Fig. 7.1) is required to construct a RAd:

- the extreme left end of the genome (i.e. the inverted terminal repeat) and encapsidation sequences
- a polylinker, in which transgene sequences are introduced (inserts up to 7.5 kb)
- an Ad sequence allowing recombination with the viral genome

After cotransfection in 293 cells of this plasmid and the appropriately restricted viral genome (dl324), homologous recombination results in the expected RAd. We construct our RAds by using homologous recombination in 293 cells rather than ligation before transfection, because the adenovirus genome has few unique restriction enzyme sites.

4.4 On Protocol #40: Adenovirus-mediated Gene Transfer; General Protocol for *in vivo* CNS Gene Transfer in Adult Rats

4.4.1 Some General Considerations

Our current understanding of results obtained with adenovirus vectors for gene transfer into nerve cells enables us to outline some general properties and observations. Clearly the expected overall result is a compromise between different parameters. Therefore, before starting the experiments we suggest carefully defining the objective of the experiment. Generally there are at least five requirements for successful *in vivo* gene transfer and expression:

(1) A substantial number of transgene-expressing cells.
(2) Accurate targeting of the transgene to specific nerve cells.
(3) Precise anatomic localization of the infected cells.
(4) Lack of any cytotoxic or side effects (cell death, gliosis, inflammation, ventricle dilatation, etc.).
(5) Persistence of transgene expression over time (for prolonged periods—e.g. weeks or months).

It is difficult to fulfill all these requirements and experiments directed to this end are still rare in the literature. At present the final result is a subtle compromise between all requirements.

Following intracerebral inoculation of the viral vector AdRSVβgal the number and extent of cells expressing the transgene and the persistence of the expression depends on a number of parameters (SEE CHAPTER 26, PAGE 365). The most important are the titer of the virus stock, the diffusion of viral particles after injection, the volume injected and the target structure. As a general rule it is highly advisable to perform pilot studies to determine the pattern of infectability of the target structure.

The ability of adenovirus to infect nerve cells of the brain *in vivo* and to express a foreign gene has been demonstrated for a number of brain regions. However, detailed analysis of adenoviral infection has mostly focused on a limited set of high therapeutic interest: the hippocampus, the substantia nigra and the striatum (Fig. 7.2; see Plate I). Although the whole brain appears susceptible to infection, technical problems can make intracerebral gene transfer into specific structures or particular subregions difficult.

Adenovirus-mediated gene transfer and expression in nerve cells of the living brain can be achieved using various experimental procedures. These include direct stereotactic inoculation of the adenovirus vectors into selected brain structures, inoculation into the cerebral ventricles and targeting of the vector towards specific neurons using its capacity of retrograde transport (Le Gal La Salle et al., 1993; Ridoux et al., 1994b). These modalities of *in vivo* gene transfer using adenovirus vectors are detailed in the following sections and illustrated with the *LacZ* reporter gene encoding the *E. coli* enzyme β-galactosidase.

The delivery process must be optimized, checked and adapted case by case. The procedure described in this chapter serves as a general guideline for stereotactic administration of a given viral solution into a given structure.

4.4.2 **In vivo** ***Gene Transfer via Retrograde Transport***

One of the mechanisms used by adenovirus to enter the living brain is retrograde transport to cell bodies after being taken up at the nerve terminals. This mode of penetration can be used for the delivery of foreign genes into selected subsets of specific neuronal cell populations (Ridoux et al., 1994b). Evidence of retrograde transport was demonstrated in the nigrostriatal system. Dopaminergic neurons of the substantia nigra can be selectively infected and express a reporter gene after inoculation of the virus into the striatum. Examples of retrograde transport were also reported for other neuronal systems. Inoculation of the virus into the hippocampus led to the labeling of cells in various regions including the contralateral dorsal hippocampus, the ipsilateral entorhinal cortex and the mamillary bodies. Similarly, β-galactosidase expression was visible in the inferior olive following injection of the adenovirus into the cerebellum. Infection of the dorsolateral geniculate body labeled a number of cells in the ipsilateral superior colliculi and in layer 6 of the visual cortex, but retrogradely labeled cells were not observed in the ganglion cells of the retina.

These results indicate that it should be possible to use adenovirus as a tracer of neural connections. However, as a general rule, the procedure should be optimized for each individual case.

4.4.3 Titer

Efficiency of *in vivo* gene transfer of AdRSVβgal is directly related to the titer of the viral inoculum and is measured by varying the concentration of virus. However, it is not possible to indicate accurately the titer that must be used to achieve an optimal efficacy of transfection in a given structure, since this conclusion depends on several parameters. First, the specific characteristics of the virus itself, as well as the details of its preparation and expansion, can strongly influence efficacy and cytotoxicity. Second, efficacy is also dependent on other parameters, such as the volume of viral solution injected and the target structure chosen. Titers of around 10^7 p.f.u. appear appropriate. Cytopathic effects are typically observed above 10^8 p.f.u. These considerations explain why the investigator must exercise great care in preparation of the virus, must check the toxicity associated with each batch of virus for a given volume, must understand the sub-structure of the organ being injected and the intended effect: this is the only way to optimize the ratio of efficacy to cytotoxicity.

4.4.4 Diffusion from the Site of Injection

The spread of viral particles within the brain parenchyma is limited. The pattern of positively stained cells usually depends on the anatomic organization of the structure injected. In relatively homogeneous structures, e.g. striatum or inferior colliculi, transgene expression was detected in cells within a maximum of 0.3–1 mm of the injection site. To increase the total number of transgene-expressing cells it may be preferable to repeat the administration of virus at several sites a few tenths of a millimeter apart. In addition, refinements of the technique by favoring diffusion and cell penetration of the virus can be expected in the near future.

4.4.5 Volume of Virus Injected

In the brain parenchyma of the rat or mouse, volumes of about 1 μl seem appropriate. However, precautions should be taken to allow slow and regular administration of the inoculum. Slow infusion of the viral solution (0.2–0.5 μl/min) causes less damage than more rapid infusion and allows inoculation of larger volumes. To ensure a slow and regular injection rate we favor the use of a microinjection pump.

4.4.6 Target Structures

The extent of spread of viral particles within the brain parenchyma depends on the target structure. Spread tends to respect anatomical boundaries such as fiber tracts or specific cell layers. For example, the diffusion of the virus was greater in the hippocampus than in the substantia nigra and infected cells were found throughout the entire dorsal region of the hippocampus, whereas in the substantia nigra the overall pattern of infection was restricted mainly to a medial–lateral plane. The greater diffusion within the hippocampus may reflect the propensity of the virus to spread through tissues that adhere loosely, such as the hippocampal fissure. Within more compact or heterogeneous structures infected cells are more regularly distributed around the injection site.

The specificity of the infection pattern in a given structure may also depend on retrograde transport of virus following local neuronal pathways. Further variations in the distribution of transgene-expressing cells could also arise from a differential sensitivity of the virus for specific neuronal populations or from certain cells being more vulnerable to virus-induced cytotoxicity than others.

Several brain structures are difficult to infect because of their location within the central nervous system: cell groups only a few tenths of a millimeter below a ventricle are difficult, if not impossible, to infect using a dorsal stereotactic approach. For example, lowering the needle into the brain may displace the tissue, the injected solution may leak through the ventricles during or just after administration—this explains why gene transfer is difficult in the CA1 layer of the hippocampus. Similarly, if the injection needle has to traverse a ventricle or space to reach its target, the injected solution will tend to escape from the tissue into the space or ventricle and thus spread away. In such conditions the final number of particles remaining in the target structure could be greatly reduced, resulting in reduced infection of a substantial number of cells. An example of such a structure is the CA3 region of the hippocampus, which is mostly surrounded by ventricles.

These considerations explain the difficulty we have encountered during an *in vivo* survey of the susceptibility to vector transduction of all hippocampal subfields following localized adenovirus inoculations.

4.5 On Protocol #41: *In vivo* CNS Gene Transfer in Adult Rats Using Recombinant Adenovirus; Gene Transfer into the Striatum

To adapt the adenovirus-mediated gene transfer to large nuclei of the central nervous system such as the striatum, we have used the Ad-RSVβGal expressing *E. coli* β-galactosidase, varying parameters of intracerebral injection to optimize the level of expression and the diffusion of the enzyme from the site of infection. The widest distribution of infected cells was obtained after injecting into three sites at three different anteroposterolateral coordinates within the striatum. Each principal site was subdivided into three subsites by depositing the virus at three places (0.4 mm apart) while removing the cannula. We have also analysed the effect of varying the amount of virus from 3×10^5 p.f.u. to 3×10^8 p.f.u. A total dose of 1.5×10^8 per striatum provided the optimal level of transgene expression, and a rate of injection of 0.5 μl/min increased the diffusion of the virus.

4.6 On Protocol #42: Adenovirus-mediated Gene Transfer; *in vivo* Gene Transfer by Intraventricular Administration

Adenovirus vectors can effectively transfer a foreign gene to the ependymal cells lining the ventricles. A volume of 5–10 μl may be administered into the lateral or third ventricle through a microsyringe. It is critical that the inoculum is delivered solely by gravitational force, with no externally applied pressure.

4.6.1 Advantages and Limitations of Intracerebral Compared with Intraventricular Administrations

The spread of adenovirus particles in the brain appears to be limited to regions close to the site of injection. This could be very useful when targeting a foreign gene to a specific, well circumscribed area. In contrast, the poor diffusion of the virus will impede applications in which the transgene activity is aimed at a widespread population of neuronal cells. Interestingly, the ability of adenovirus to infect ependymal cells lining the ventricles following intracerebroventricular injection may offer a suitable route for delivering the transgene into the cerebroventricular fluid, provided that the gene product can cross the brain–ventricle barrier. Compared with the direct infusion of a protein that is rapidly degraded into the cerebrospinal fluid, adenovirus-mediated gene transfer into ependymal cells may provide sustained, long-lasting production of the desired protein.

REFERENCES

Akli, S., Caillaud, C., Vigne, E., Stratford-Perricaudet, L.D., Poenaru, L., Perricaudet, M., Kahn, A. and Peschanski, M.R. 1993. Transfer of a foreign gene into the brain using adenovirus vectors. *Nature Genet.* **3,** 224–228.

Bajocchi, G., Feldman, S.H., Crystal, R.G. and Mastrangeli, A. 1993. Direct *in vivo* gene transfer to ependymal cells in the central nervous system using recombinant adenovirus vectors. *Nature Genet.* **3,** 229–234.

Björklund, A. and Stenevi, U. 1979. Reconstruction of the nigrostriatal dopamine pathway by intracerebral nigral transplants. *Brain Res.* **177,** 555–560.

Davidson, B.L., Allen, E.D., Kozarsky, K.F., Wilson, J.M. and Roessler, B.J. 1993. A model system for *in vivo* gene transfer into the central nervous system using an adenoviral vector. *Nature Genet.* **3,** 219–223.

Fisher, L.J., Jinnah, H.A., Kale, LC., Higgins, G.A. and Gage, F.H. 1991. Survival and function of intrastriatally grafted primary fibroblasts genetically modified to produce L-Dopa. *Neuron* **6,** 371–380.

Freed, C., Breeze, R., Rosenberg, N., Scneck, S., Criek, E., Qi, J., Lone, T., Zhang, Y., Snyder, J., Wells, T., Ramig, L., Thomson, L., Mazziotta, J., Huang, S., Grafton, S., Brooks, D., Sawle, G., Schroter, G. and Ansari, A. 1992. Survival of implanted fetal dopamine cells and neurologic improvement 12 to 46 months after transplantation for Parkinson's disease. *N. Engl. J. Med.* **327,** 1549–1555.

Gluzman, Y. and Van Doren, K. 1983. Palindromic Adenovirus type 5-SV40 hybrid. *J. Virol.* **45,** 91–103.

Graham, F.L., Smiley, J., Russell, W.C. and Nairu, R. 1977. Characteristics of a human cell line transformed by DNA from human adenovirus type 5. *J. Gen. Virol.* **36,** 59–72.

Horellou, P., Brundin, P., Kalen, P., Mallet, J. and Björklund, A. 1990. *In vivo* release of DOPA and dopamine from genetically engineered cells grafted to the denervated rat striatum. *Neuron* **5,** 393–402.

Horellou, P., Vigne, E., Castel, M.N., Barbeoud, P., Colin, P., Perricaudet, M., Delaere, P. and Mallet, J. 1994. Direct intracerebral gene transfer of a adenoviral vector expressing tyrosine hydroxylase in a rat model of Parkinson's disease. *Neuroreport* **6,** 49–53.

Jiao, SS, Guerevich, V. and Wolff, J.A. 1993. Long-term correction of rat model of Parkinson's disease by gene therapy. *Nature* **362,** 450–453.

Kelsey, D.S. 1978. Adenovirus meningo-encephalitis. *Pediatrics* **61,** 291–293.

Le Gal La Salle, G., Robert, J.J., Berrard, S., Ridoux, V., Stratford-Perricaudet, L.D., Perricaudet, M. and Mallet, J. 1993. Adenovirus as a potent vector for gene transfer in neurons and glia in the brain. *Science* **235,** 986–988.

Lindvall, O., Brundin, P., Widner, H., Rehncrona, S., Gustavii, B., Frackowiak, R., Leeders, K., Sawle, G., Rothwell, J.C., Marsden, C. and Björklund, A. 1990. Grafts of fetal dopamine neurons survive and improve motor function in Parkinson's disease. *Science* **247,** 574–577.

Olson, L., Nordberg, A., von Holst, H., Backman, L., Ebendahl, T., Alafuzoff, I., Amberla, K., Hartvig, P., Herlitz, A., Lilja, A., Lundquist, H., Langstron, B., Meyerson, B., Persson, A., Viitanene, M., Windblad, B. and Seiger, A. 1992. Nerve growth factor affects 11C-nicotine binding, blood flow, EEG and verbal episodic memory in an Alzheimer patient. *J. Neurol. Transm.* [*P-D Sect*] **4,** 79–95.

Perlow, M.J., Freed, W.J., Hoffer, B.J., Seiger, Å., Olson, L. and Wyatt, R.J. 1979. Brain grafts reduce motor abnormalities produced by destruction of nigrostriatal dopamine system. *Science* **204,** 643–646.

Ridoux, V., Robert, J.J., Zhang, X., Perricaudet, M., Mallet, J. and Le Gal La Salle, G. 1994a. The use of adenovirus vectors for intracerebral grafting of transfected nervous cells. *Neuroreport* **5,** 801–804.

Ridoux, V., Robert, J.J., Zhang, X., Perricaudet, M., Mallet, J. and Le Gal La Salle, G. 1994b. Adenoviral vectors as functional retrograde neuronal tracers. *Brain Res.* **648,** 171–175.

Rubin, B.A. and Rorke, L.B. 1988. Adenovirus vaccines. In: Plotkin and Mortimer (Eds), *Vaccines*, W.B. Saunders, Philadelphia, pp. 492–512.

Sambrook, J., Fritsch, E.F. and Maniatis, T. 1989. *Molecular cloning. A laboratory manual.* 2nd edition. CSH Laboratory Press, pp. 16.30–16.32.

Spencer, D.D., Robbins, R.J., Naftolin, F., Marek, K.L., Vollmer, T., Leranth, C., Roth, R.H., Price, L.H., Gjedde, A., Bunney, B.S., Sass, K.J., Elsworth, J.D., Kier, E.L., Makuch, R., Hoffer, P.B. and Redmond, E. 1992 . Unilateral transplantation of human fetal mesencephalic tissue into the caudate nucleus of patients with Parkinson's disease. *N. Engl J. Med.* **327,** 1541–1548.

Thimmappaya, B., Weinberger, C., Schneider, R.J. and Shenk, T. 1982. Adenovirus VA1 RNA is required for efficient translation of viral mRNAs at late times after infection. *Cell* **31,** 543–551.

Ushida, K., Ishii, A., Kaneda, N., Toya, S., Nagatsu, T. and Kohsaka, S. 1990. Tetrahydrobiopterin-dependent production of L-Dopa in NRK fibroblasts transfected with tyrosine hydroxylase cDNA: future use for intracerebral grafting. *Neurosci. Lett.* **109,** 282–286.

Widner, H., Tetrud, J., Rehncrona, S., Snow, B., Brundin, P., Gustavii, B., Björklund, A., Lindvall, O. and Langston, J.W. 1992. Bilateral fetal mesencephalic grafting in two patients with parkinsonism induced by 1-methyl-4-phenyl-1,2,3,6-tetrahydropyridine (MPTP). *N. Engl J. Med.* **327,** 1556–1563.

CHAPTER 8

The Use of Adenovirus Vectors to Transfer Genes to Identified Target Brain Cells *in vitro*

PEDRO R. LOWENSTEIN, ANDY F. SHERING, DEREK BAIN, MARIA G. CASTRO AND GAVIN W.G. WILKINSON*

University of Manchester, School of Medicine, Department of Medicine, Molecular Medicine Unit, Room 1.302, Stopford Building, Oxford Road, Manchester M13 9PT, UK. Tel: 0161 275 5672; Fax: 0161 275 5672; Email: lowenstein@man.ac.uk.

**Department of Medicine, University of Wales College of Medicine, Tenovus Building, Heath Park, Cardiff CF4 4XX, UK. Tel: 01222 745215; Fax: 01222 745003; Email: wmdgww@cardiff.ac.uk*

1. INTRODUCTION

Classical pharmacology used to teach that cell functions could not be altered. This particular statement has now been rewritten. The capacity of novel gene transfer techniques to introduce almost any required function into any target cell has raised the prospect of gene therapy, and with it new strategies for combating the wide range of diseases that continue to afflict mankind. As this book testifies, there are many ways to introduce genes into the brain, and the one selected will depend on the investigator's or clinician's aims and expectations. *Ex vivo* techniques can be employed to deliver genes encoding soluble factors to the brain (e.g. neurotransmitters such as dopamine or growth factors such as nerve growth factor). Such an approach involves first inserting the transgene into a precursor platform cell that can then either be transplanted directly into the brain or infused into the bloodstream from where it can repopulate the CNS. Although this approach may be effective in treating some disorders, other disorders will require genes to be introduced directly into target neurons (Table 8.1) or other brain cells *in vivo*. In such cases, vectors can be used that directly target genes into resident brain cells; for example neurons of diverse sorts, astroglial cells, oligodendroglial cells and endothelial cells.

Viral vectors currently provide a number of advantages to the experimentalist, both to those working with *in vivo* paradigms, and to those working with neurons *in vitro*. As recently as 5 years ago the only way to introduce genes into post-mitotic neurons was by microinjection of DNA. Although this methodology is being perfected (SEE CHAPTER 3), it is still a difficult technique limited to studies *in vitro*. Certain viruses can accomplish the following processes with particular facility (Shenk, 1995):

- Packaging of transgenes
- Cell delivery (Curiel et al., 1991; Wickham et al., 1993, 1994)
- Endosomolysis
- Nuclear delivery (Greber et al., 1993)
- Promotion of high levels of expression

Protocols for Gene Transfer in Neuroscience: Towards Gene Therapy of Neurological Disorders
Edited by P.R. Lowenstein and L.W. Enquist

Table 8.1 Strategies for human neurological gene therapy

Strategy	*Disease*	*Gene/gene product*	*Consequence of mutation*	*Target tissue*	*Vectors*
Gene augmentation	Leash–Nyhan	HPRT	Loss of activity	Basal ganglia	HSV-1; adenovirus, AAV
	Tay–Sachs	Hexosaminidase A	Loss of activity	Forebrain neurons	Bone marrow, HSV-1, adenovirus, AAV
	Gaucher's	Glucocerebrosidase	Loss of activity	Forebrain neurons	Bone marrow, HSV-1, adenovirus, AAV
	Kennedy's	Androgen receptor	Loss of function?	Anterior horn, motor neurons	HSV-1, adenovirus, AAV
	Fragile X	FMR1	Loss of function	CNS	HSV-1, adenovirus, AAV
	Familial dysautonomia	Unidentified	Unknown	Dorsal root ganglion neurons, posterior horn neurons	HSV-1, adenovirus, AAV
Gene inhibition	Huntington's	IT15 (huntingtin)	Gain of function (unknown effect)	Basal ganglia, cerebral cortex	AAV, HSV-1, adenovirus, genetic suppressor elements
	Creutzfeld–Jakob	Prion protein gene	Accumulation of gene product	Forebrain neurons and glial cells	AAV, HSV-1, adenovirus, genetic suppressor elements
	Spinocerebellar ataxia I	Trinucleotide expanded allele (gene unidentified)	Gain of function (unknown effect)	Dorsal root ganglion neurons, cerebellum	HSV-1, adenovirus, genetic suppressor elements
	CNS infections: HSV-1, HIV	Viral genes	Gain of function (expression of viral genes)	Neurons, macrophages	AAV, retroviruses, genetic suppressor elements
Cell replacement	Parkinson's	Tyrosine hydroxylase	n/a	Basal ganglia neurons; alternatively fibroblasts, myoblasts, neuronal vell progenitors	Retroviruses and cell transplantation, direct gene transfer into neurons (e.g. HSV-1)
	Alzheimer's	Neuronal growth factors? Choline acetyltransferase?	n/a	Neuronal cell progenitors, embryonic neurons, fibroblasts etc. for transplantation, cortical neurons	Retroviruses and cell transplantation, direct gene transfer into neurons (e.g. HSV-1)
	Charcot–Marie–Tooth IA	PMP-ss	Increase of function (duplication)? Dominant negative mutation (point mutations)?	Schwann cells	Retroviruses, liposomes, adenovirus particle-mediated gene transfer and cell transplantation

	Charcot–Marie–Tooth X1	Connexin 32	Loss of function	Schwann cells	Retroviruses, liposomes, adenovirus particle-mediated gene transfer and cell transplantation
	Pelizaeus–Merzbacher	PLP	Increase of function (duplication)? Dominant negative mutation (point mutations)?	Oligodendrocytes	Retroviruses, liposomes, adenovirus particle-mediated gene transfer and cell transplantation
	Multiple sclerosis	?	?	Oligodendrocytes	Retroviruses, liposomes, adenovirus particle-mediated gene transfer and cell transplantation
Cell killing, tumors	Neurofibromatosis	HSV-1 TK, other toxic genes	NF1 (decreased amount of protein), NF2 (loss of function?)	Tumors	Retrovirus, HSV-1, adenovirus particle-mediated gene transfer, liposomes, antisense or genetic suppressor elements for growth factors etc.
	von-Hippel Lindau	HSV-1 TK, other toxic genes	Loss of function	Cerebellar tumors	Retrovirus, HSV-1, adenovirus particle-mediated gene transfer, liposomes, antisense or genetic suppressor elements for growth factors etc.
	Tuberous sclerosis	HSV-1 TK, other toxic genes	Loss of function	Brain tumors	Retrovirus, HSV-1, adenovirus particle-mediated gene transfer, liposomes, antisense or genetic suppressor elements for growth factors etc.
	Neuroblastoma	HSV-1 TK, other toxic genes		Tumors	Retrovirus, HSV-1, adenovirus particle-mediated gene transfer, liposomes, antisense or genetic suppressor elements for growth factors etc.

From Lowenstein, 1995

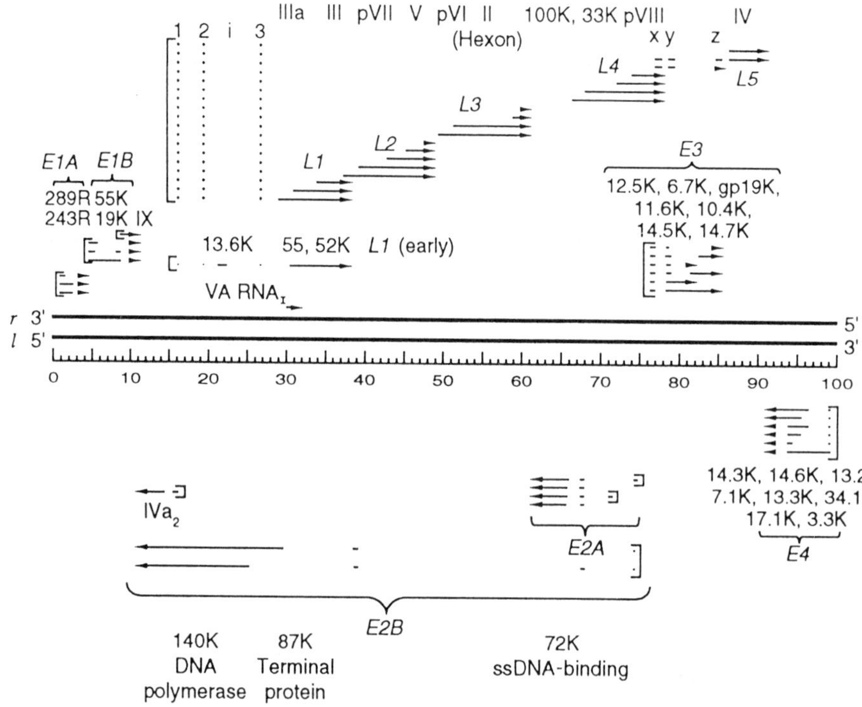

Figure 8.1 Map of the adenovirus 2 genome, which is a linear duplex DNA of 36 000 base pairs. The letters *r* and *l* refer to rightward and leftward transcription; the split arrows indicate the spliced structures of the mRNAs (exons are shown). Proteins are given as, for example, 289R, 55K, IIIa. Transcriptional units are given as *E1A*, *E1b*, *E3*. *L1*–*L5* are families of "late" mRNAs. ss, Single stranded. This figure can be compared with Fig. 8.2 to identify those regions deleted from adenoviral vectors. (Reproduced by permission from Wold et al., 1994)

This makes them attractive vehicles to the gene therapist in general, and to the experimental neurobiologist in particular. Viral vectors are now being exploited as tools to explore the molecular basis of neuronal function and developed as vehicles for human neurological gene therapy.

1.1 The Adenovirus System

The adoption of adenovirus as a model system by molecular biologists in the 1970s led to the generation of an invaluable body of information on adenovirus genetics and virus:cell interaction. There are some 47 serotypes in humans, and many more in birds and mammals, but most vectors are based on the human adenovirus serotypes 2 or 5 (Ad2 or Ad5; Fig 8.1) (Top et al., 1971a,b; Schwartz et al., 1974; Rubin and Rorke, 1988). Adenoviruses all have an intermediate-sized genome of about 36 kb, for which the complete sequence of Ad5 is available. Like the herpesviruses, adenoviruses operate a cascade system of gene expression. The first genes to be expressed following infection (the E1 gene region) are responsible for activating transcription of the early genes (E2–E4) and eventually, following viral DNA replication, late genes are expressed (Shenk, 1995). Adenoviruses compensate for the limited size of their genomes by utilizing an astonishing complex system of post-transcriptional control involving a complex pattern of RNA splicing. While most of the viral genome is essential for virus growth, replication-competent adenovirus recombinants could be constructed with transgene insertion into the E1, E3 or E4 regions (Armentano et al., 1994; Bett et al., 1994; Engelhardt et al., 1994).

Replication-deficient adenovirus vectors are normally deleted in the E1 gene region (excluding the region containing the coding sequence for protein IX, 10-11map units, an essential virion structural protein) but may carry additional deletions or mutations elsewhere in the viral genome. As the E1 genes are essential, adenovirus $E1^-$ vectors are normally propagated on a helper cell line expressing an E1 helper function (typically 293 cells) (Graham et al., 1977). In normal cells, although the $E1^-$ virus is taken up and transported to the nucleus (Greber et al., 1993), there is usually no expression from the $E1^-$ genome. The absence of background expression from the vector is the feature which makes adenovirus an ideal candidate for gene therapy. Transgenes are normally inserted into the adenovirus genome under the control of a constitutive promoter (e.g. the HCMV IE promoter or RSV LTR), which can drive efficient expression using pre-existing, unmodified cellular transcription factors. In principle the adenovirus vector simply acts as an extremely efficient DNA delivery system, permitting expression in a high proportion of target cells both *in vitro* and *in vivo*.

Thus adenovirus vectors provide a powerful technology to direct gene transfer either *in vitro* or *in vivo*. Some important features of these vectors include:

- Ability to infect neurons
- Long-term expression in brain (described in mice)
- Rarely associated with brain infections
- Transgene expression in post-mitotic neurons
- Well characterized vector systems
- High-level expression in a wide range of cell types
- Recombinants can readily be grown to high titers (up to 10^{12} p.f.u./ml)
- Exclusive expression of transgene in target cell
- Controlled expression by gene dosage and promoter selection
- Targeted and regulated expression might be achieved using an appropriate promoter
- Target cells can be infected with more than one adenovirus recombinant
- Experience has been obtained with adenoviruses in human gene therapy (cystic fibrosis clinical trials).

(See Stratford-Perricaudet et al., 1990, 1992; Graham and Prevec, 1991; Quantin et al., 1991; Rosenfeld et al., 1991, 1992, 1994; Akli et al., 1993; Bajocchi et al., 1993; Davidson et al., 1993; Engelhardt et al., 1993; Herz and Gerard, 1993; Ishibashi et al., 1993; Kass-Eisler et al., 1993, 1994; Kozarsky and Wilson, 1993; Le Gal La Salle et al., 1993; Mastrangeli et al., 1993; Simon et al., 1993; Smith et al., 1993; Zabner et al., 1993a,b, 1994; Acsadi et al., 1994a,b; Armentano et al., 1994; Boucher et al., 1994; Bout et al., 1994a,b; Boviatsis et al., 1994; Brody et al., 1994a,b; Jomary et al., 1994; Kozarsky et al., 1994; Mittereder et al., 1994; Ridoux et al., 1994a,b; Welsh et al., 1994; Wilson et al., 1994; Yei et al., 1994a,b; Schewach et al., 1994; Lowenstein et al., 1995; Shering et al., 1996).

We have exploited adenovirus vectors to target expression to brain neocortical cells in culture. In this chapter the protocols used in our laboratories to generate adenoviruses, to explore whether they infect identified brain cells in culture, and to transfer missing functions to cellular models of human diseases are described. The adenovirus vector is not limited to mammalian neural systems—therefore these protocols may be of value to researchers working in other fields as well.

2 MATERIALS AND EQUIPMENT

2.1 Plasmids for the Construction of Adenovirus Recombinant

pΔE1sp1A, pΔE1sp1B, pFG140 and pJM17 (Kit A). Shuttle vector pJM17 contains the entire genome of Ad5dl309, the recipient viral backbone. It contains an E3 deletion and the prokaryotic vector pBRX inserted into the E1 region, which hinders packaging of genomic DNA. The E1 plus pBRX regions are replaced, in the final recombinant, by a smaller promoter-transgene cassette. The pBRX sequences also allow propagation in bacteria. These plasmids can all be obtained from:

Microbix Biosystems Inc,
341 Bering Avenue,
Toronto,
Ontario
Tel: 416-234-1624; Fax: 416-234-1626

Some commercial sources of eukaryotic promoters:

Invitrogen BV
De Schelp 26, 9351 NV Leek
The Netherlands
Tel: 31 5945 15175; Fax: 31 5945 15312

Invitrogen Corporation
3985 B Sorrento Valley Blvd.
San Diego CA, 92121
Tel: 800 955 6288; Fax: 619 597 6201

Clontech Laboratories Inc
4030 Fabian Way
Palo Alto CA 94303-4607

Qiagen
Diagen Gmbh
Max-Volmer Strasse 4
40724 Hilden
Germany
Tel: 49 2103 892 230; Fax: 49 2103 892 222

Qiagen Inc.
9600 De Soto Avenue
Chatsworth CA, 91311
Tel: 800 426 8157; Fax: 800 718 2056

2.2 Cotransfection and Isolation of Recombinant Adenovirus Vectors

(1) 293 cells available from ECACC, Catalog Number 85120602 or ATCC CRL 1573 or from Microbix Biosystems (Cat No PD-02-01). These cells are available adapted for growth as adherent cells (Graham et al., 1977; Graham, 1987; Graham and Prevec, 1991) or in suspension (designated 293-N3S; ECACC Catalog number 92052131). For most purposes adherent cells are adequate.
(2) Medium: to 500 ml MEM, 8% FCS add 10 ml penicillin/streptomycin (5000 mg/ml and 5000 U/ml respectively) (Sigma, S-7647; P-0781) and 5 ml 100 mM L-glutamine (Sigma, G-7513).
(3) Transfection buffers: 2 M CaCl; Low TE buffer (100 μl 1 M Tris–HCl, pH 7.5; 10 μl 0.5 M EDTA, pH 8.0, made up to a final volume of 100 ml); 2 × HBS buffer (5.6 ml 5 M NaCl; 50 mM HEPES; 0.75 ml 0.2 M Na_2HPO_4, made up to a final volume of 100 ml, final pH 7.12. The pH is critical for efficient transfection, and the pH electrode must be well washed before use, especially if held in phosphate buffer).

2.3 Preparation of Virus Stock

Arklone P (Basic Chemical Company, High Wycombe, UK)—for cleaning up virus preparation.

2.4 Neocortical Neuronal Cultures

2.4.1 Chromic Acid for Coverslip Preparation

(1) Add 100g of potassium dichromate to 850 ml distilled water.
(2) Dissolve for a few minutes then add 50 ml of sulfuric acid. Allow the solution to cool for several minutes then add a further 50 ml of sulfuric acid.
(3) Adjust volume to 1000 ml with distilled water.

2.4.2 Poly-L-lysine

(Sigma P-2636) at 1 mg/ml in 0.1 M borate buffer, pH 8.5.

(1) Prepare borate buffer by dissolving 3.81 g sodium tetraborate (borax) in approximately 90 ml distilled water. Adjust pH to 8.5 and warm gently.

(2) Dissolve 100 mg poly-L-lysine in the borate buffer.
(3) Adjust volume to 100 ml and filter sterilize into two sterile 50 ml centrifuge tubes. Store at 4°C.

2.4.3 Cleaning the Coverslips

(1) Place 22 mm² coverslips (Carolina Biological Supply Company 63-3095) in PTFE racks and wash twice for 10 min in distilled water.
(2) Place racks in chromic acid for 18–36 h.
(3) Wash off all traces of chromic acid and leave in distilled water for 2 h. Wash again in distilled water for 2 h.
(4) Place racks in 100 ml beakers and cover with aluminum foil. Cut two small holes in the foil half way down the beaker to allow moisture to escape.
(5) Sterilize in an oven at 225°C overnight. Allow beakers to cool to room temperature.

2.4.4 Putting Wax Beads on Coverslips

(1) Sterilize paraffin wax (Fisons P/0680/90) in a 50 ml beaker in an autoclave.
(2) Move to a laminar flow hood. Clean a hot plate and thermometer with 70% ethanol and place in hood.
(3) Heat wax to 100°C ([+]2°C). (Too cool and the beads will fall off, too hot and the beads will spread too much).
(4) Place coverslips into each well of a six-well tissue culture dish with sterile forceps.
(5) Dip the tip of a sterile Pasteur pipette 1–2 cm into the molten wax. Allow a small amount of wax to enter the pipette by capillary action.
! DO NOT PULL THE WAX INTO THE PIPETTE !
(6) Place a thumb over the top of the pipette and quickly remove excess wax from the pipette on the side of the beaker.
(7) Very quickly touch the pipette tip onto the corners of the coverslip. Gently press on top of the pipette with thumb to expel a wax bead. Repeat until the wax runs out or solidifies. The beads should be approximately 2 mm high.
(8) Replace pipette into molten wax to remelt the wax in the pipette (if any). Triturate (pipette up and down 3–4 times) and repeat application procedure.

2.4.5 Coating Coverslips with Poly-L-lysine

(1) Using a sterile Pasteur pipette add 5–7 drops of poly-L-lysine to each coverslip. If the coverslips are properly cleaned, and the poly-L-lysine is dropped from a height of 2–3 cm, the solution will spread out to cover all but the corners of the coverslip.
(2) Slowly rotate the six-well dish, allowing the solution to spread into the corner of the coverslips.
(3) Tip the dish slightly to ensure the poly-L-lysine accumulates in the corners of the coverslips.
(4) Use minimum amount of poly-L-lysine that will cover the coverslips.
(5) Leave in the laminar flow hood overnight.
(6) Wash with sterile distilled water twice for 2 h each washing.
(7) Add 1 ml neuronal plating medium to each well and incubate at 37°C in an atmosphere of 5% CO_2. If the coverslips are to be stored for more than a couple of days they should be stored dry after washing in distilled water (Step 6).

2.4.6 Preparation of Mowiol for Mounting Immunolabeled Cells

(1) Dispense 6.9 g 87% glycerol in a 15 ml centrifuge tube.
(2) Add 2.4 g Mowiol (Calbiochem, Cat No. 475904) and stir.
(3) Add 6 ml distilled water, stir well, and leave for 2 h at room temperature.
(4) Transfer to a 50 ml centrifuge tube, add 12 ml 0.2 M Tris, pH 8.5, and incubate for 10 min at 50°C with occasional stirring. A shaking bath with occasional stirring may be useful, because

Mowiol is very difficult to dissolve. The solution is not light sensitive.
(5) Transfer the tube to a shaking platform and leave overnight.
(6) Spin at 5000 r.p.m. for 15 min.
(7) Remove supernatant.
(8) Aliquot and store at −20°C.
(9) Thaw just before use and do not refreeze.

2.5 Glial and Neuronal Media

(1) Glial Plating Medium (GPM): 450 ml MEM (Sigma S-7647); 50 ml horse serum (Gibco 041-04190M); Penicillin (100 U/ml)/streptomycin (100 μg/ml), 5 ml per 500 ml medium. (Sigma P-0781); 0.6% (w/v) glucose. (BDH) 3 g per 500 ml medium.
(2) Neuronal plating medium (NPM): Prepare in the same way as the glial plating medium, but with a reduced glucose concentration of 0.06% w/v.
(3) Neuronal maintenance medium (NMM): 500 ml MEM (Sigma S-7647); transferrin (Apo-human, cell culture tested), 10 mg/l (Sigma T-1147); vitamin E (DL-α-tocopherol, 10 mg/l. (Sigma T-3251); bovine serum albumin, 4 g/l (Organon Teknika 141440); vitamin A (all *trans*-retinol), 1 mg/l (Sigma R-7632); lipoic acid (DL-6,8, thiotic acid, oxidized), 250 μg/l (Sigma T-1395); bovine pancreatic insulin, 10 mg/l (Sigma I-6634); progesterone, 6.28 μg/l (Sigma P-0130); putrescine, 40 μg/l (Sigma P-7505); selenium dioxide, 3.32 μg/l (Sigma S-9379); sodium pyruvate, 1 mM (Sigma S-8636); penicillin 100 U/ml; streptomycin, 100 μg/ml (Sigma P-0781).
(4) Trypsin ×10 solution: 2.5% (1:250) (Gibco 043-05090 D).
(5) DNAse: 1% DNAse in 0.15 M NaCl (Sigma DN-25).
(6) Fixation solution: 4% Paraformaldehyde in 0.12 M sucrose, pH 7.4.
   - Dissolve 4 g sucrose (Sigma S-0389) in 50 ml 0.2 M phosphate buffer and place on ice.
   - Heat approximately 30 ml of distilled water to 55–60°C and add 4 g of paraformaldehyde (TAAB). Add a few drops of NaOH.
   - Filter the paraformaldehyde solution into the ice-cold phosphate buffer.
   - Adjust pH to 7.4.
   - Store at 4°C.

2.6 Specific Antibodies for Identifying Cell Types and Transgenes

(1) Neurons: mouse monoclonal anti-MAP-2 (Sigma, Cat. No. M-4403)1:500; rabbit polyclonal anti-MAP-2 (Fisher et al., 1987) 1:2000.
(2) Astrocytes: mouse monoclonal and rabbit polyclonal anti-GFAP (Sigma, Cat. No. G-3893/9269) 1:200.
(3) Oligodendrocytes: rabbit polyclonal anti-MBP (P.Morgan, University of Wales College of Cardiff) 1:100; mouse monoclonal anti-GC (Johnson et al., 1988) 1:1000.
(4) Schwann cells: mouse monoclonal anti-NGF-R (Rauscht et al., 1982) 1:100; rabbit polyclonal anti-S100 (Dakopatts) 1:1000.
(5) Fibroblasts: mouse monoclonal anti-Thy1.1 (Sigma) 1:1000.
(6) β-galactosidase: mouse monoclonal anti-β-galactosidase (Sigma, G-8021) 1:1000; rabbit polyclonal anti-β-galactosidase (J. Price, SmithKline Beecham, UK) 1:1000; mouse monoclonal anti-β-galactosidase (Promega) 1:5000.
(7) Chloramphenicol acetyl transferase (CAT): monoclonal anti-CAT (D. Lane, University of Dundee, UK) 1:1000.
(8) **Adenovirus proteins:** monoclonal anti-E1a (E. Harlow) 1:2; polyclonal goat anti-adenovirus hexon (Chemicon) 1:50.
(9) **Secondary antibodies:** Rhodamine-conjugated goat anti-mouse (Jackson Immunochemicals Inc., Catalog No. 115-025-146); Fluorescein-conjugated swine anti-rabbit (Dakopatts, Catalog No. F-205).

3 THE PROTOCOLS

Protocol #44: Making an Adenovirus Recombinant

(SEE EXTENSIVE NOTES IN SECTION 4.)

(1) Thinly seed 293 cells in a fresh 25 cm^2 tissue culture flask the day before transfection, aiming for about 40% confluency to obtain best transfection efficiencies.
(2) Add fresh prewarmed medium (5 ml) to cells immediately before transfection.
(3) Pipette 10 μg of DNA (5 μg transfer vector containing transgene plus 5 μg pJM17) into 6 ml (12 × 75 mm) polypropylene Falcon tubes (serial number 2063).
(4) Add low TE buffer to a final volume of 210 μl and mix.
(5) Add 30 μl $CaCl_2$ dropwise to the tube and mix by vortexing.
(6) Add the DNA–$CaCl_2$ mixture to a second tube containing 240 μl of 2× HBS, and mix by vortexing.
(7) Allow a precipitate to form for 30 min.
(8) Add solution and precipitate directly to fresh tissue culture medium, in a 25 cm^2 tissue culture flask containing the 293 cells. Check that a fine precipitate has formed on the cells by viewing at high magnification.
(9) Leave DNA precipitate on the cells for 16 h.
(10) Wash cells once with PBS.
(11) Wash cells once with medium.
(12) Add fresh medium to cells.
(13) Replenish medium every 3 days, or more often if it turns acidic.
(14) If transfection is successful plaques will be visible 6–8 days after transfection (Fig. 8.3: see Plate III).
(15) Do not attempt to pick plaques. Allow the virus to spread through the monolayer. All the progeny generated by this system invariably contain the desired insert.
(16) Retain all cultures and inspect up to 2 weeks after transfection before discarding any as negative.
(17) Plaque-purify the recombinant three times to ensure that the virus stock is derived from a single infectious unit.

Protocol #45: Titration of Adenovirus Stocks by End Point Dilution

(1) Seed a 96-well plate with 293 cells at approximately 30% confluency. Do not seed too densely, as cells will overgrow the well, rapidly deplete the media and substantially slow down virus growth.
(2) Prepare a series of 10-fold dilutions. Most adenovirus stocks will have a titer of 10^8–10^{11} p.f.u./ml so sufficient serial dilutions must be made to cover this broad range. Prepare three tubes with 4.95 ml medium. Add 50 μl of the stock to the first tube (10^{-2} dilution). Mix well and, with a fresh pipette, add 50 μl of this dilution to the next tube (10^{-4} dilution). Mix well and, with a fresh pipette, add 50 μl of this dilution to the next tube (10^{-6} dilution). Prepare five tubes with 4.5 ml medium. Add 500 μl of the 10^{-6} dilution to the first tube (10^{-7} dilution). Continue this process of 10-fold dilutions through the remaining tubes, changing pipette tips each time. The final dilution will be 10^{-11}.
(3) Remove media from the 96-well plate using a multichannel pipetting device.
(4) Add 100 μl medium to the central 10 wells at the bottom of the plate.
(5) Add 100 μl of each dilution to 10 wells in the remaining seven rows. Start with the highest dilution (10^{-11}) and work down to the 10^{-4} dilution in order. As you are progressing to higher concentrations (lower dilutions) of virus it is not necessary to change tips on the pipette.
(5) Leave virus on cells for 16 h and then change the medium.
(6) Replenish medium every 3 days, or when the medium becomes acid.
(7) Read adenovirus plaques after 8 days.
(8) Count the number of viral plaques at each dilution.

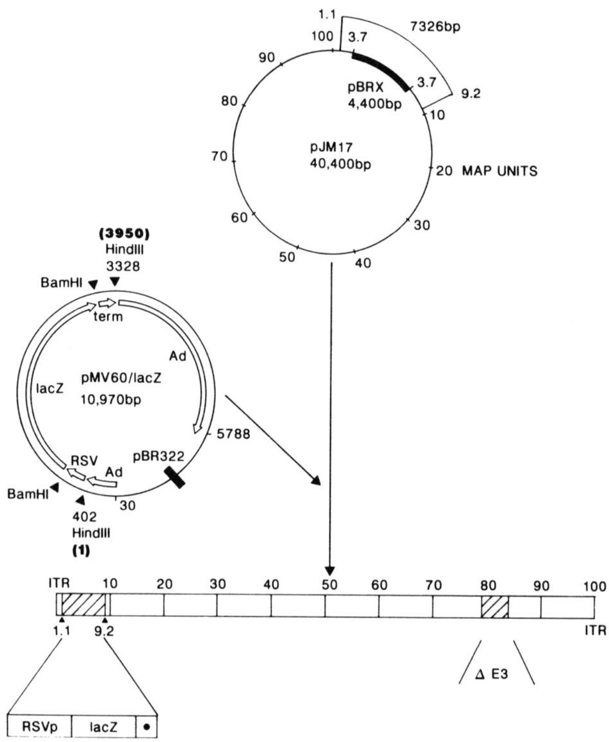

Figure 8.2 Construction of recombinant adenovirus vectors. Generation of recombinant virus RAd-RSV/*lacZ*. The transfer vector pMV60/*lacZ* was constructed from plasmid pXCX2 (Spessot et al., 1989) with the addition of a linker (containing the *Hin*dIII cloning site) at the unique *Xba*I cleavage site. *lacZ* was cloned into pMV60 under RSV promoter control and upstream of a polyadenylation signal on a *Hin*dIII expression cassette (1–3950 bp, in bold). The transfer vector provides the expression cassette with flanking homology from either side of the Ad E1a gene region, fine numbers on pMV60 refer to the Ad5 genomic sequence. *lacZ* was excised from the transfer vector by *Bam*H1 digestion. Plasmid pJM17 contains the entire Ad5dl309 genome with the prokaryotic vector pBRX (4400 bp) inserted into the E1a gene at 3.7 map units. Insertion of the prokaryotic vector makes pJM17 too large to package into Ad nucleocapsids (McGrory et al., 1988). The transfer vectors and pJM17 were cotransfected into 293 cells. Homologous recombination between the plasmids results in the *Hin*dIII expression cassettes replacing both the E1a region, 402–3328 and the intervening prokaryotic vector. This results in the removal of 7326 bp (pBRX 4400 bp and 2926 bp of the E1a gene) and insertion of the *lacZ* expression cassette 3950 bp in length. The recombinant pJM17 size is thus reduced sufficiently to be packaged into nucleocapsids, resulting in plaques in the 293 cell monolayer and generation of E1a$^-$ recombinant virus, RAd–RSV/*lacZ*. A linear expression of the RAd genome is shown at the bottom of the figure, illustrating the position of the expression cassettes, RSV/*lacZ*

(9) Use the method of Reed and Meunch to calculate $TCID_{50}$:

$$\text{proportionate distance} = \frac{(\%\text{ positive above }50\%) - 50\%}{(\%\text{ positive above }50\%) - (\%\text{ positive below }50\%)}$$

and,

$$\log ID_{50} = (\log\text{ dilution above }50\%) + (\text{proportionate distance} \times \text{dilution factor});$$

then, obtain ID_{50}.

The dilution of the virus stock thus obtained (ID_{50}) is the one required to infect 50% of the wells.

Two further calculations must be made to obtain the final titer:

- The reciprocal of this value represents the number of tissue culture infectious doses per unit volume.
- Because 100 μl of the virus dilutions was added to each well, multiply by a factor of 10 to give the final titer as $TCID_{50}$/ml.

Example of the method of Reed and Meunch to calculate virus titer

The method is best illustrated by an example. If a titration gave 9/10 positive wells (90%) at the 10^{-8} dilution and above, 3/10 (30%) at the 10^{-9} dilution and 0/10 at the 10^{-10} dilution then:

$$\text{proportionate distance} = \frac{90\% - 50\%}{90\% - 30\%} = \frac{40}{60} = 0.67$$

$$\log ID_{50} = -8 + (0.67 \times -1) = -8.67$$

$$ID_{50} = 10^{-8.67}$$

This dilution of the virus stock is required to infect 50% of wells.

Two further adjustments must be made to this figure:

- The reciprocal of this value represents the number of tissue culture infectious doses per unit volume (i.e. $10^{8.67}$ $TCID_{50}$/100 μl).
- Only 100 μl of virus was added to each well; therefore this must be multiplied by 10 to give a final value of $10^{9.67}$ $TCID_{50}$/ml.

Protocol #46: Preparation of Recombinant Adenovirus Stock

(1) Grow 15 175 cm^2 flasks of 293 cells to 80% confluence.
(2) Remove the medium by aspiration and inoculate each flask with 25 ml viral stock at a multiplicity of infection (MOI) of 0.1 or less.
(3) Incubate for 90 min, rotating the flasks every 15 min to circulate the virus.
(4) Remove the inoculum by aspiration.
(5) Add 25 ml of 293 medium to each flask.
(6) After 2 days replace the old medium with fresh. A clear cytopathic effect (CPE) will spread rapidly through the monolayer.
(7) Tap the flask to detach cells from the monolayer once the whole monolayer exhibits a gross CPE.
(8) Collect the cell suspension in 50 ml centrifuge tubes.
(9) Recover infected cells by centrifugation at 500*g* for 5 min. Perform all potentially aerosol-generating steps in an appropriate microbiological safety cabinet. Use detachable centrifuge buckets and open these inside the cabinet.
(10) Discard the supernatant into approved disinfectant and resuspend the cells in PBS at a concentration of 2×10^7 cells/ml. The cells may be stored at -70°C at this stage.
(11) Add an equal volume of Arklone P (a fluorocarbon compound) to the cell suspensions and mix vigorously.
(12) Centrifuge the emulsion at 1000*g* for 5 min, then remove the upper aqueous phase in a tissue culture laminar flow cabinet.
(13) Maximize the yield by re-extracting the interface with PBS.
(14) Discard the lower fluorocarbon phase.
(15) Aliquot virus immediately or purify further by CsCl gradient centrifugation (Precious and Russell, 1985; SEE CHAPTER 7).

Protocol #47: Neocortical Glial Cultures

(1) Immerse sacrificed 1–2-day-old rat pups (5–12 pups per neuronal culture, depending on number of cells required) in 100% ethanol (in laminar flow hood) and decapitate with a sterile scalpel.

(2) Place the head in a Petri dish containing Balanced Salts Solution (BSS) without calcium or magnesium (Gibco 041-04170), with 10 mM Hepes (Sigma H-0887).
(3) Hold the head with curved forceps inserted into the eye sockets. Insert one point of a fine pair of scissors into the spinal column at the base of the skull. Make a cut through the skull to just below the ear on both sides of the head.
(4) Open the skull to reveal the top of the brain and using fine curved forceps to remove it to a fresh Petri dish containing BSS with Hepes. Repeat with the remaining heads.
(5) Transfer the brains to a Petri dish containing BSS without calcium and magnesium only.
(6) With the aid of a dissection microscope remove the meninges with fine forceps and dissect out the cortex. Cut each into pieces approximately 1 mm^3.
(7) Transfer tissue to a 15 ml centrifuge tube and dissociate the cortex in 5 ml BSS (without Calcium/Magnesium) five times with a 5 ml pipette, then a flame polished Pasteur pipette until no clumps are visible.
(8) Adjust volume to 12 ml with BSS and add 1.5 ml DNAase and trypsin.
(9) Incubate for 15 min at 37°C, inverting every 5 min.
(10) Filter the homogenate through nylon cell strainer, pore size 70 μm (Falcon, Cat. No. 2350) into 15 ml glial plating medium in a sterile 50 ml centrifuge tube.
(11) Centrifuge for 15 min at 500 r.p.m. at 4°C with no brake.
(12) Remove supernatant carefully with a pipette. Resuspend the cell pellet in 6 ml glial plating medium.
(13) Count cells and adjust density to approximately 2×10^6 cells/ml.
(14) Add 1 ml glial plating medium to each well of a six-well tissue culture dish.
(15) Add 1 ml glial suspension to each well of the dish and place in a incubator at 37°C/5% CO_2.
(16) Next day aspirate all the media and replace with 1 ml of glial plating medium. Feed every 3–4 days with glial plating medium until the cells are confluent (1–2 weeks).
(17) One or two days before preparing a neuronal culture, replace the glial plating medium with 1 ml neuronal maintenance medium.

Protocol #48: Neocortical Neuronal Cultures

(1) Kill a pregnant rat (E17–18) using an accepted procedure and disinfect the animal's fur with 70% ethanol.
(2) Using sterile dissection tools make a large opening in the skin of the abdomen, leaving the internal abdominal wall intact.
(3) Use fresh sterile tools, open a large area of the abdominal wall to reveal the embryos in the uterus.
(4) Remove both horns of the uterus with fresh sterile forceps, move to a laminar flow hood and place each horn into a Petri dish containing a small volume of BSS without calcium or magnesium, with 10 mM Hepes.
(5) Remove the embryos from the uterus. Decapitate them, discard the bodies and place the heads in a Petri dish containing a small volume of BSS with Hepes.
(6) Remove the brains and dissect the cortex as described in Protocol #47.
(7) Using a pipette gather tissue in as little volume of BSS as possible.
(8) Transfer tissue to a 15 ml centrifuge tube. Adjust volume to 12 ml with fresh BSS without calcium or magnesium. Add 1.5 ml DNAse and trypsin.
(9) Incubate for 15 min at 37°C. Mix by inversion every 5 min.
(10) Allow the tissue to settle and remove as much medium as possible. Add 15 ml fresh BSS and leave for 5 min. Repeat three times. Resuspend the last wash in 15 ml neuronal plating medium. Invert three times and allow to settle.
(11) Remove all but 5 ml of medium. Using a 5 ml pipette triturate 5–6 times carefully.
(12) Dissociate tissue on the side of the tube using a flame-polished Pasteur pipette. Once suspension is homogeneous adjust volume to 15 ml with neuronal plating medium.
(13) Filter through a nylon cell strainer, pore size 70 μm (Falcon 2350) into a sterile 50 ml centrifuge tube.
(14) Count cells using a counting chamber.

(15) Adjust the density of cells to 2×10^5–5×10^5 per ml by diluting with neuronal plating medium.
(16) Add 1 ml neuronal plating medium to each well of a six-well tissue culture dish containing pre-prepared coverslips.
(17) Add 1 ml of the neuronal suspension to each well and place the dish in an incubator at 37°C/5% CO_2 incubator for 3 h.
(18) Using sterile forceps invert the coverslips (with the neurons facing down) over the confluent glia. Add a further 1 ml of neuronal maintenance medium.
(19) Feed cells every 3–4 days by removing half the maintenance medium (1 ml) and replacing it with fresh medium.

Protocol #49: *In vitro* Viral Infections of Neuronal Cultures

(1) Remove the viral aliquot(s) from the freezer and place in a 37°C water bath until ice just disappears then place tubes on ice.
(2) Move to a suitable laminar flow hood, with absorbent mats or aluminum foil to contain drips etc. Use a beaker containing 1% w/v Virkon (Day Impex Ltd. 330003) for disposal of contaminated plastic and liquids.
(3) Transfer the viral aliquot(s) in an ice bucket to the laminar flow hood. Dilute the virus to the appropriate concentration in neuronal maintenance medium taken from the wells of the coculture. Dilute the virus in a minimal volume of medium (e.g. 700 μl/well). Keep on ice.
(4) Using sterile forceps transfer the coverslips with the appropriate neurons to a fresh sterile six-well tissue culture dish.
(5) Add 700 μl of the viral inoculum to each well and return the cultures to the 37°C/5% CO_2 incubator.
(6) Incubate the cells at 37°C for 2 h, rocking gently every 15 min.
(7) Transfer the infected culture to the laminar flow hood, remove the viral inoculum and discard.
(8) Wash the cells three times with 2 ml neuronal maintenance medium.
(9) Using sterile forceps return the coverslips to the coculture and replace in the 37°C/5% CO_2 incubator.
(10) Sterilize all plasticware and forceps by autoclaving.

Protocol #50: Fluorescent Immunocytochemistry of Infected Cultures

(1) At the appropriate time after infection, within the laminar flow hood transfer the coverslips with infected neurons to a six-well culture dish containing 2 ml prewarmed 0.1 M PBS/well using sterile forceps.
(2) Quickly wash cells in each well with 2 ml 0.1 M PBS three times, disposing of each wash in 1% Virkon as in Protocol #49.
(3) Fix cells by adding 2 ml of 4% paraformaldehyde in 0.12 M sucrose to each well. Keep at room temperature for 20 min.
(4) Remove fixative solution by gentle aspiration, and wash each well with 5 ml of 0.1 M PBS for 5 min, taking care not to disturb the cells. Repeat wash three times.
(5) Permeabilize cells (if necessary) by adding 1 ml 0.1% Triton X-100 (BDH 30632 4N) in PBS to each well for 5 min.
(6) Wash three times in PBS.
(7) Incubate for 30 min in 10% normal blocking serum (for example, swine serum).
(8) Wash briefly with 1% blocking serum.
(9) Place drops with primary antibody dilutions (100 μl per coverslip) onto clean Parafilm in a humid chamber, and invert coverslips over antibody dilutions.
(10) Use two primary antibodies (e.g. mouse (monoclonal) and rabbit (polyclonal)), where one is directed against the transgene and the other against a cell type-specific marker.
(11) Wash off unbound primary antibody thoroughly with six washes with 1% blocking serum in PBS.

(12) Incubate in 100 μl secondary antibodies in 1% blocking serum, keeping coverslips in a dark box and perform subsequent washes under dimmed ambient light.
(13) Wash thoroughly six times for 5 min each wash in PBS to remove unbound secondary antibodies.
(14) Wash briefly in distilled water before mounting in 10% Mowiol containing 25% glycerol in 50 mM Tris–HCl, pH 8.5.
(15) Allow to harden at 4°C overnight before viewing under epifluorescence.
(16) Photograph using, for example, a Kodak TMAX 3200 (black and white) or an AGFA RS1000 (color) film (For Fig. 8.4 see Plate II.)

4 NOTES AND TROUBLESHOOTING

4.1 On Protocol #44: Making an Adenovirus Recombinant

4.1.1 The Transgene

The source of the DNA will vary. Adenovirus is a nuclear virus and can be used to express spliced genes. However, we prefer to use cDNA copies to minimize the potential for exons from the expressed transgene to splice into adenovirus sequences. In general, transgenes are expressed using their own ATG codon but may be tailored using fortuitous restriction sites or polymerase chain reaction (PCR) to avoid additional non-coding sequences which may affect expression. Levels of expression obtained using the same vector system can vary enormously; this has been observed with all eukaryotic expression systems. A large number of factors affect expression—e.g. turnover of mRNA, turnover of protein, efficiency of RNA processing, efficiency of translation, toxicity of protein, target cell type.

4.1.2 Promoter Selection

The adenovirus vector acts as a highly efficient vehicle for delivery of the genetic material to the cell. The promoter chosen to express the transgene is critical in regulating the level, kinetics and even the cell-specificity of expression (Friedman et al., 1986). In our hands the CMV major IE promoter proved to be 50 times stronger than the SV40 promoter and 20 times stronger than the RSV LTR in driving expression from a reporter gene in HeLa cells (Wilkinson and Akrigg, 1991). These three viral promoters are excellent in driving constitutive expression in a wide range of cell types. Nevertheless, our recent results indicate that the RSV promoter may be preferable to the CMV IE promoter in targeting neurons (Lowenstein et al., 1995; Shering et al., 1995). Although cellular promoters tend to be less efficient they may be desirable for some, perhaps most, gene therapy protocols as cell-specific promoters can be effective in restricting expression to the appropriate cell type (Friedman et al., 1986).

Not all promoters with the same name are identical. For example, we use an exceptionally strong, truncated version of the CMV promoter (−299 to +69), but other versions can extend further upstream or even contain the first intron of the CMV immediate early gene (which has been found to stimulate expression). The strong CMV enhancer element can also be found linked to an actin promoter. The tripartite leader sequence from the adenovirus late promoter is linked to the RSV LTR in many constructs. To ensure efficient RNA processing most mammalian expression vectors provide a polyadenylation signal downstream of the site for transgene insertion, this element can also affect the efficiency of expression.

4.1.3 Transfection Buffers

All buffers should be made from the best quality reagents available and filter-sterilized, rather than autoclaved, before use. Aliquots should be stored frozen, preferably at −70°C. Fresh buffers should be made up at regular intervals.

4.1.4 Preparation of Plasmids

Transfection-quality plasmid DNA can be readily prepared by at least two methods. Centrifugation on CsCl gradient routinely produces high-grade DNA (especially if the plasmid is subjected to two rounds of centrifugation) suitable for most purposes, but the procedure is time-consuming and requires expensive, specialized equipment (Sambrook et al., 1989). Alternatively, DNA may be prepared using Qiagen affinity columns: DNA purified by such columns has been reported to contain bacterial lipopolysaccharide (LPS), which can be removed by further processing (Cotten et al., 1994). Although, in our hands, 293 cells usually tolerate Qiagen-purified plasmid DNA and are efficiently transfected with such preparations, other cell types can be less forgiving. In order to make adenovirus recombinants we normally use the 42 kb plasmid pJM17 (kindly provided by Professor F.L. Graham and available from Microbix; SEE SECTION 2.1), which contains the entire Ad5 dl309 genome. *Escherichia coli* carrying this plasmid, not surprisingly, grows slowly and yields are characteristically low. With this particular plasmid we obtain higher yields on Qiagen columns.

4.1.5 Cloning Step 1

The first step is to insert the transgene under the control of the appropriate promoter. Typically, we use a plasmid such as pMV100 which has the HCMV major IE promoter upstream of a multiple cloning site and a polyadenylation signal. *Xba*I and *Bam*HI are particularly useful cloning sites for inserting transgenes as *Xba*I will accept *Spe*I or *Nhe*I sticky ends while *Bam*HI will accept a *Bgl*II or *Bcl*I sticky end. A wide range of vectors containing eukaryotic promoters has been produced and a number are commercially available.

4.1.6 Cloning Step 2

The expression cassette comprising the promoter/transgene/polyadenylation signal is then excised and inserted into an adenovirus transfer vector such as pΔE1sp1A or pΔE1sp1B. The resultant transfer vector supplies the expression cassette with flanking sequence homology from either side of the adenovirus E1 gene region. The orientation of insertion into this vector will control the orientation of insertion into the adenovirus genome. Orientation does not appear to significantly affect the level of expression. Although this cloning step is routine, the size of the vector and the recombinant plasmid being sought are larger than average and consequently the efficiency of *E. coli* transformation is relatively low.

4.1.7 Generation of Recombinant Virus

In order to make the recombinant virus the adenovirus transfer vector and pJM17 are cotransfected into 293 cells. There is no requirement to linearize plasmids before transfection. pJM17 contains the complete Ad5 dl309 genome including sequences from the prokaryotic vector pBRX inserted in E1; the insertion of the prokaryotic sequences make pJM17 too large to package into adenovirus particles so transfection of pJM17 alone does not generate replicating virus. However, following homologous recombination the E1 gene region and all prokaryotic sequences are replaced with the expression cassette which reduces the overall size of the viral genome to one that can be packaged into the adenovirus particles. This extremely elegant system, developed by Graham and coworkers at McMaster University (Graham et al., 1977; Graham, 1987; Graham and Prevec, 1991), has not only greatly facilitated the generation of recombinants but also ensures that all the progeny of the transfection are invariably the desired recombinant. Thus, while it is still necessary to confirm the identity of the recombinant, there is no need to screen plaques.

Although the technology for generating adenovirus recombinants is efficient, problems may still be encountered. It is crucial that the transfection be extremely efficient. 293 cells can be transfected with extraordinary efficiency: up to 80% of cells can take up plasmid DNA and express a recombinant protein. However, it is not enough simply to get DNA into the cell, it is necessary also to obtain recombination between the plasmids, which occurs at low efficiency. In order to monitor the efficiency of transfection we use a plasmid containing the HCMV IE promoter driving β-galactosidase, and Microbix supply a control plasmid (pFG140), which will generate adenovirus plaques following transfection. As a rough guide, if a transfection system enables the HCMV IE promoter/β-gal construct to express in more than 20% of cells, adenovirus recombinants may normally be generated (Fig. 8.4; See Plate II).

4.1.8 Transfection and Virus Generation

Virus plaques appear more rapidly in growing cells; thus low seeding density is recommended (approx. 40%). Transfection should not be toxic to the 293 cells.

4.1.9 Constraint on Insert Size

The size of insert attainable with current replication-deficient adenovirus vectors is limited to the region of 8.3 kb (Bett et al., 1994). Few regions of the viral genome (notably the E3 region) are dispensable for growth *in vitro* and the complexity of the adenovirus transcription is such that the deletion of essential genes (to be complemented in *trans*) is problematical. Additionally the packaging capacity of the adenovirus particle is limited to 1.5–2 kb in addition to the wild-type genome. Current vectors therefore will permit large enough insertions to accommodate most cDNAs. However, it is theoretically possible to clone much larger inserts (approx. 35 kb) between the adenovirus inverted terminal repeats (ITRs) of the adenovirus genome and to package such constructs using a replicating adenovirus helper virus. This system is analogous to the herpes simplex amplicon system (See Chapters 11–13) and shares many of its limitation; most notably it is difficult to control the ratio of helper virus to the transgene-carrying particle.

4.1.10 Safety

There are strict guidelines or legislation governing the use of recombinant viruses in many countries that require the potential hazards associated with the construction of such agents to be carefully evaluated and appropriate precautions determined and enacted for biological containment. These precautions include physical containment (in the laboratory, tissue culture cabinets, centrifugation and animal isolators), operating procedures and disinfection policy.

Wild-type Ad2 and Ad5 are common serotypes normally associated with mild upper respiratory tract infections of childhood, although they have been rarely associated with more serious disease (Kelsey, 1978; Lowenstein et al., 1996). Essentially, adenovirus is not a significant cause of neurological disease, although cases of meningoencephalitis caused by the organism (mainly Ad7 serotype) have been described in the literature (Rubin and Rorke, 1988). Certain properties of adenovirus E1$^-$ deletion mutants are positive safety features. Being replication-deficient, the virus is incapable of independent spread within or between individuals (Oualikene, 1994). Additionally, the transforming potential associated with the E1 gene region has been removed. There are, however, a number of caveats against its use: (1) the E1 deletion can potentially be rescued by coinfection with either a wild-type adenovirus or a herpesvirus (e.g. HSV-1 or CMV), thus promoting spread and enhancing expression of the transgene; (2) the adenovirus recombinants are propagated on a helper cell line carrying the E1 gene function—the potential therefore exists for the generation of a helper-independent recombinant during growth in 293 cells, although this is not routinely observed (Lochmuller et al., 1994); (3) adenovirus as a non-lytic system is capable of transducing cells, albeit at low efficiency—the expression of transforming genes carries specific hazards; (4) the expression of diffusible gene products with pharmacological properties could reach much higher levels than predicted if the recombinant virus was rescued by a helper virus. Therefore, the potential effects of combining each transgene with any viral vector must be considered individually. See also Cotten et al. (1994) for other sources of toxicity and Wold et al (1994) for effects of adenovirus proteins on host immune function.

We usually insert transgenes into the E1 locus so that (1) if homologous recombination resulted in the recombinant "recapturing" the E1 gene region then it would favor deletion of the transgene and (2) inserting the transgene under the late transcription unit (e.g. in E3 locus) is avoided. Genes in the E3 locus tend to be expressed from the adenovirus late promoter in 293 cells.

If 293 cells can be transfected, but no plaques are obtained, check that the cells are still expressing the necessary *trans*-complementing functions. An easy way to check this is to immunostain the cells with antibodies recognizing the E1a proteins. If cells are negative, they should be discarded and new stocks obtained.

4.1.11 General Notes

pJM17 is an extremely large plasmid which can undergo rearrangement following transformation. Check this by doing a restriction digest with *Hin*dIII and compare with the standard *Hin*dIII digest shown in the information provided with the Microbix catalog. Try always to go back to a glycerol culture that is known to be effective.

It is critical to mix extremely vigorously, so make sure your vortexer is up to speed.

293 cells are human embryonic kidney cells which have been immortalized/transformed using an Ad5 DNA fragment. Although this is a rapidly growing immortalized cell line that can grow back from a single cell, 293 cells should be handled with care and are sensitive to "over-trypsinization". Best results are achieved with these cells when they are subcultured regularly (so that they are kept growing), and by regularly changing the growth medium. If allowed to overgrow 293 cells become "clumpy" and they do not survive on maintenance media. They tend to grow poorly on roller bottles but are adaptable to microcarrier systems. Some groups recommend the use of low-passage (below 50) 293 cells.

Clumps of 293 cells routinely detach from monolayers to give the appearance of a plaque; researchers should be very certain that there actually is a plaque before proceeding. Adenovirus infection characteristically causes cells to form "grape-like" clusters that round up and detach. A plaque will rapidly increase in size and spread through the monolayer.

4.2 On Protocol #45: Titration of Adenovirus Stocks by End Point Dilution

In order to accurately titer an adenovirus recombinant virus or purify a recombinant, a plaque assay may be performed according to the procedure described by Revah and coworkers (SEE CHAPTER 7). However, 293 cells are relatively difficult to handle and a plaque assay may not give satisfactory results (Precious and Russell, 1985). An alternative approach is to use a "quantal" rather than a quantitative assay. End point dilution assays are relatively straightforward to perform and can be used to quantify or purify a recombinant virus stock (Burleson et al., 1992). The value obtained from such an assay is called the $TCID_{50}$ (50% tissue culture infective dose). A number of ways of performing such an assay are possible, and we give a method routinely used in our laboratories.

Pipetting the virus dilutions using a multichannel pipette may be made easier by using special presterilized medium reservoirs (Sigma R9384) to feed the multichannel pipette.

4.2.1 General Notes on Virus Titration

One $TCID_{50}$ is **roughly** equivalent to 0.7 p.f.u.

Replication-deficient adenovirus recombinants can be titered only in the presence of the helper function. As with other viruses, the infectivity of adenovirus for different cell types is variable, 293 cells being more permissive than most. The titer in an adenovirus recombinant in 293 cells provides a benchmark that allows experimental procedures to be standardized. Adenovirus recombinants expressing reporter genes (e.g. *lacZ*) can be used in preliminary experiments to establish the conditions necessary for efficient gene expression in the target cell.

At the lowest dilution in an end point assay it is probable that a well is infected with only one infectious virus particle. Selecting virus from such a well is therefore broadly equivalent to a single round of virus plaque purification.

4.3 On Protocol #46: Preparation of Recombinant Adenovirus Stock

Preparation of virus stocks requires scale-up of 293 cells. The volume of cells used will depend on the final use of the virus. We give details of the method for generating a stock of virus partially purified by extraction with the fluorocarbon Arklone P. Where highly purified virus (is needed e.g. animal inoculation) virus must be further purified by a CsCl gradient (SEE CHAPTER 7).

4.4 On Protocol #47: Neocortical Glial Cultures

This protocol should be followed for glial cultures enriched in astrocytes—with the exception that the cerebral cortex of 2–4-day-old pups are used and glial plating medium (GPM) is used instead of NPM (GPM is almost identical to NPM, except that glucose concentration is increased to 0.6% (w/v)). Low numbers of cortical oligodendrocytes do grow within the astrocyte cultures, but separate protocols exist to obtain pure oligodendrocyte cultures.

Schwann cells are isolated from the sciatic nerves of rat pups 2–4 days old. The nerves are removed and chopped into small lengths then incubated for 30 min in 0.1% collagenase in HBSS followed by incubation for 30 min in 0.1% collagenase plus 0.25% trypsin. The subsequent steps are the same as for neuronal cultures (Kleitman et al., 1991; Morgan, 1994).

4.5 On Protocol #48: Neocortical Neuronal Cultures

Low-density primary cultures of neurons are cocultured with glia for long-term maintenance. The protocols described above demonstrate the establishment of glial primary cultures for coculture with neurons, the preparation of coverslips for neuronal cultures and the establishment of a low-density primary culture of neurons. Glia are grown to confluence in six-well dishes fed with glial plating medium. One or two days before a neuronal culture, the glia are switched to the serum-free, defined medium (neuronal maintenance medium), which they "condition" for the neurons. Three hours after plating the coverslips containing the neurons are inverted over the glia. The neurons are kept in close proximity to, but separate from, the glia by the wax dots.

4.6 On Protocol #49: *In vitro* Viral Infections of Neuronal Cultures

At a low input MOI replication-deficient adenovirus recombinants can promote efficient transgene expression with no detectable cytotoxicity or breakthrough to early: late phase adenovirus gene expression. Using the powerful constitutive CMV IE promoter, extremely high-level expression can be achieved (up to 35% cell protein; Wilkinson and Akrigg, 1992). Such overexpression can itself be toxic: indeed, the expression of certain transgenes even in low amounts may be toxic. Toxicity has been associated with the *in vivo* administration of adenovirus recombinants where it is difficult to ensure an even distribution of virus to the target cell population. At extremely high MOI, toxicity can be associated with the virion penton–base protein, although a greater problem is that there may be a breakthrough to adenovirus early/late gene expression. Breakthrough can result in an inflammatory response associated with the induction of a cell-mediated response to adenovirus proteins. Research in vector development is directed to preventing this effect and mutations in the adenovirus E2a gene have been shown to be beneficial by preventing readthrough to late gene expression.

Recombinant adenoviruses are added for 3 days in 0.7–1 ml of NPM, with fixation on the third day. HSV and HCMV should be added for only 1–2 h and fixed less than 12 h later.

For short-term expression experiments with recombinant adenovirus, vectors are added for the length of the experiments (e.g. 72 h).

An advantage of using adenovirus is that multiple infections with different recombinant vectors are possible. This may be useful in evaluating interactions between transgenes, e.g. certain receptors and possible associated G proteins.

4.7 On Protocol #50: Fluorescent Immunocytochemistry of Infected Cultures

If antibodies recognize an extracellular epitope of a plasma membrane protein, permeabilization can be omitted. However, fixation with paraformaldehyde will cause some limited permeabilization of the plasma membrane (for an example, see Figure 9 in Lowenstein et al., 1994).

The serum used for the 10% blocking step should not interfere with the subsequent immunocytochemical procedure; to avoid any possible cross-reactions, the species of the blocking serum should be the same as the secondary antibody carrying the detection system (e.g. if secondary antibody is goat anti-rabbit fluorescein, the blocking serum should be normal goat serum). Depending on the experimental procedure followed this might not be possible; however, the blocking antiserum should **never** be of the same species as the primary antibody—this will generate high background levels.

If the experiments reveal a high level of background labeling, the background may be reduced by quenching the remaining reactive aldehyde groups by incubating with ammonium chloride (50 mM in PBS) for 15 min, or by adding 1% lysine or glycine to the 10% blocking serum.

Guidelines on primary dilutions of antibodies are usually provided by the supplier. However, it is usually necessary to optimize the exact dilutions of all antibodies to be used for the particular applications.

Owing to the relatively short half-life of the fluorophors of some fluorescently labeled secondary antibodies it is important to perform most of the experimental analysis and photography shortly after the experiment is finished. While some preparations may be examined over relatively long periods (days to weeks) if kept in the dark and cold, some experimental results can fade too rapidly to be photographed or even examined properly—also, much quenching of the samples will occur while photographing the samples. Other commercial or home-made coverslipping agents usually allow lower light intensity to be detected only when examined with fluorescence microscopy and compared to Mowiol, and they do not become hard enough for easy examination under oil-immersion lenses.

For further information on getting the viruses across the brain see Chapter 23; on getting the viruses into cells and then into thc brain see Chapter 7 and for information on the immune response and vector toxicity see Chapter 26.

ACKNOWLEDGMENTS

We are indebted to Professor F.L. Graham for developing the adenovirus vector system and pointing us in the right direction, and we thank Roger Everett for invaluable advice on DNA transfection. E1A antibodies were kindly provided by Ed Harlow and Keith Leppard who also provided advice on Ad5. Polyclonal rabbit anti-Map2 antibodies were a kind gift of Itzhak Fischer. P.R.L. is a Research Fellow of The Lister Institute of Preventive Medicine. The research undertaken by G.W. and discussed in this chapter was supported by The Welsh Scheme for the Development of Health and Social Science. P.R.L. and M.G.C. acknowledge the support received from The Wellcome Trust, The Royal Society, The Muscular Dystrophy Group, UK, and The Welsh Scheme for the Development of Health and Social Science.

REFERENCES

Acsadi, G., Hani, A., Massie, B., Simoneau, M., Holland, P., Blaschuk, K. and Karpati, G. 1994a. A differential efficiency of adenovirus-mediated *in vivo* gene transfer into skeletal muscle cells of different maturity. *Hum. Mol. Genet.* **3,** 579–584.

Acsadi, G., Jani, A., Huard, J., Blaschuk, K., Massie, B., Holland, P., Lochmuller, H. and Karpati, G. 1994b. Cultured human myoblasts and myotubes show markedly different transducibility by replication-defective adenovirus recombinants. *Gene Ther.* **1,** 338–340.

Akli, S., Caillaud, C., Vigne, E., Stratford-Perricaudet, L.D., Poenaru, L., Perricaudet, M., Kahn, A. and Peschanski, M.R. 1993. Transfer of a foreign gene into the brain using adenovirus vectors. *Nature Genet.* **3,** 224–228.

Armentano, D., Sookdeo, C., White, G. et al. 1994. Second generation adenovirus vectors for cystic fibrosis gene therapy. *J. Cell Biochem.* **18A (Suppl.),** abstract DZ102.

Bajocchi, G., Feldman, S.H., Crystal, R.G. and Mastrangeli, A. 1993. Direct *in vivo* gene transfer to ependymal cells in the central nervous system using recombinant adenovirus vectors. *Nature Genet.* **3,** 229–234.

Bett, A.J., Haddara, W., Prevec, L. and Graham, F.L. 1994. An efficient and flexible system for construction of adenovirus vectors with insertions or deletions in early regions 1 and 3. *Proc. Natl Acad. Sci. USA* **91,** 8802–8806.

Boucher, R.C., Knowles, M.R., Johnson, L.G., Olsen, J.C., Pickles, R., Wilson, J.M., Engelhardt, J., Yang, Y. and Grossman, M. 1994. Clinical protocol: Gene therapy of cystic fibrosis using E1-deleted adenovirus: A phase I trial in the nasal cavity. *Hum. Gene Ther.* **5,** 615–639.

Bout, A., Imler, H.L, Schultz, H., Perricaudet, M., Zurcher, C., Herbrink, P., Valerio, D. and Pavirani, A. 1994a. *In vivo* adenovirus mediated transfer of human CFTR cDNA to rhesus monkey airway epithelium: efficacy, toxicity and safety. *Gene Ther.* **1,** 385–394.

Bout, A., Perricaudet, M., Baskin, G., Imler, J.L., Scholte, B.J., Pavirani, A. and Valerio, D. 1994b. Lung gene therapy: *in vivo* adenovirus-mediated gene transfer to rhesus monkey airway epithelium. *Hum. Gene Ther.* **5,** 3–10.

Boviatsis, E.J., Chase, M., Wei, M.X., Tamiya, T., Hurford, R.K. Jr, Kowall, N.W., Tepper, R.I., Breakefield, X.O. and Chiocca, E.A. 1994. Gene transfer into experimental brain tumors mediated by adenovirus, herpes simplex virus, and retrovirus vectors. *Hum. Gene Ther.* **5**, 183–191.

Brody, S.L., Jaffe, H.A., Han, S.K., Wersto, R.P. and Crystal, R.G. 1994a. Direct *in vivo* gene transfer and expression in malignant cells using adenovirus vectors. *Hum. Gene Ther.* **5**, 437–447.

Brody, S.L., Metzger, M., Danel, C., Rosenfeld, M.A. and Crystal, R.G. 1994b. Acute responses of non-human primates to airway delivery of an adenovirus vector containing the human cystic fibrosis transmembrane conductance regulator cDNA. *Hum. Gene Ther.* **5**, 821–836.

Burleson, F.G., Chambers, T.M. and Wiedbrauk, D.L. 1992. *Virology: A Laboratory Manual.* Academic Press Inc, San Diego.

Cotten, M., Baker, A., Saltik, M., Wagner, E. and Buschle, M. 1994. Lipopolysaccharide is a frequent contaminant of plasmid DNA preparations and can be toxic to primary human cells in the presence of adenovirus. *Gene Ther.* **1**, 239–246.

Curiel, D.T., Agarwal, S., Wagner, E. and Cotten, M. 1991. Adenovirus enhancement of transferrin-polylysine-mediated gene delivery. *Proc. Natl Acad. Sci. USA* **88**, 8850–8854.

Davidson, B.L., Allen, E.D., Kozarsky, K.F., Wilson, J.M. and Roessler, B.J. 1993. A model system for *in vivo* gene transfer into the central nervous system using an adenoviral vector. *Nature Genet.* **3**, 219–223.

Davidson, B.L., Doran, S.E., Shewach, D.S., Latta, J.M., Hartman, J.W. and Roessler, B.J. 1994. Expression of *Escherichia coli* β-galactosidase and rat HPRT in the CNS of *Macaca mulatta* following adenoviral mediated gene transfer. *Exp. Neurol.* **125**, 258–267.

Engelhardt, J.F., Simon, R.H., Yang, Y., Zepeda, M., Weber Pendleton, S., Doranz, B., Grossman, M. and Wilson, J.M. 1993. Adenovirus-mediated transfer of the CFTR gene to lung of nonhuman primates: biological efficacy study. *Hum. Gene Ther.* **4**, 759–769.

Engelhardt, J.F., Ye, X., Doranz, B. and Wilson, J.M. 1994. Ablation of E2a in recombinant adenoviruses improves transgene persistence and decreases inflammatory response in mouse liver. *Proc. Natl Acad. Sci. USA* **91**, 6196–6200.

Fischer, I., Kosik, K.S. and Saphstein, V.S. 1987. Heterogeneity of microtubule-associated protein (MAP-2) in vertebrate brains. *Brain Res.* **436**, 39–48.

Friedman, J.M., Babiss, L.E., Clayton, D.F. and Darnell, J.E. 1986. Cellular promoters incorporated into the adenovirus genome: cell-specificity of albumin and immunoglobulin expression. *Mol. Cell. Biol.* **6**, 3791–3797.

Graham, F.L., Smiley, J., Russell, W.C. and Nairu, R. 1977. Characteristics of a human cell line transformed by DNA from human adenovirus type 5. *J. Gen. Virol.* **36**, 59–72.

Graham, F.L. 1987. Growth of 293 cells in suspension culture. *J. Gen. Virol.* **68**, 937–940.

Graham F.L. and Prevec, L. 1991. Manipulation of adenovirus vectors. In Murray, E.J., ed., *Methods in Molecular Biology* Vol. 7. 109–128, The Humana Press Inc, Clifton NJ.

Greber, U.F., Willetts, M., Webster, P. and Helenius, A. 1993. Stepwise dismantling of adenovirus 2 during entry into cells. *Cell* **75**, 477–486.

Herz, J. and Gerard, R.D. 1993. Adenovirus-mediated transfer of low density lipoprotein receptor gene acutely accelerates cholesterol clearance in normal mice. *Proc. Natl Acad. Sci. USA* **90**, 2812–2816.

Ishibashi, S.M., Brown, M.S., Goldstein, J.L., Gerard, R.D., Hammer, R.E. and Herz, J. 1993. Hypercholesterolemia in low density lipoprotein receptor knockout mice and its reversal by adenovirus-mediated gene delivery. *J. Clin. Invest.* **92**, 883–893.

Johnson, E., You, Q. and Hohnson, E.M. 1988. An immunohistochemical study of nerve growth factor receptors in developing rats. *J. Neurosci.* **8**, 3481–3498.

Jomary, C., Piper, T.A., Dickson, G., Couture, L.A., Smith, A.E., Weal, M.J. and Jones, S.E. 1994. Adenovirus-mediated gene transfer into murine retinal cells *in vitro* and *in vivo*. *FEBS Lett* **347**, 117–122.

Kass-Eisler, A., Falck-Pedersen, E., Alvira, M., Rivera, J., Buttrick, P.M., Wittenberg, B.A., Cipriani, L. and Lewinwand, L.A. 1993. Quantitative determination of adenovirus-mediated gene delivery to rat cardiac myocytes *in vitro* and *in vivo*. *Proc. Natl Acad. Sci. USA* **90**, 11498–11502.

Kass-Eisler, A., Falck-Pedersen, E., Elfenbein, D.H., Alvira, M., Buttrick, P.M. and Leinwand, L.A. 1994. The impact of developmental stage, route of administration and the immune system on adenovirus-mediated gene transfer. *Gene Ther.* **1**, 395–402.

Kelsey, D.S. 1978. Adenovirus meningo-encephalitis. *Pediatrics* **61**, 291–293.

Kleitman, N., Wood, P.M. and Bunge, R.P. 1991. Tissue culture methods for the study of myelination. In: Banker, G. and Goslin, K., eds., *Culturing Nerve Cells*, pp. 337–377. MIT Press, Cambridge, MA.

Kozarsky, K.F., McKinley, D.R., Austin, L.L., Raper, S.E., Stratford-Perricaudet, L.D. and Wilson, J.M. 1994. *in vivo* correction of low density lipoprotein receptor deficiency in the Watanabe heritable hyperlipidemic rabbit with recombinant adenoviruses. *J. Biol. Chem.* **269**, 13695–13702.

Kozarsky, K.F. and Wilson, J.M. 1993. Gene therapy: adenovirus vectors. *Curr. Opin. Gen. Dev.* **3**, 499–503.

Le Gal La Salle, G., Robert, J.J., Berrard, S., Ridoux, V., Stratford-Perricaudet, L.D., Perricaudet, M. and Mallet, J. 1993. Adenovirus as a potent vector for gene transfer in neurons and glia in the brain. *Science* **235**,

986–988.

Lochmuller, H., Jani, A., Huard, J., Prescott, S., Simoneau, M., Massie, B., Karpati, G. and Acsadi, G. 1994. Emergence of early region 1-containing replication-competent adenovirus in stocks of replication-defective adenovirus recombinants ([D]E1 + [D]E3) during multiple passages in 293 cells. *Hum. Gene Ther.* **5,** 1485–1491.

Lowenstein, P.R. 1994. Molecular neurosurgery: mending the broken brain. Gene therapy for neurological disease? *Bio/Technol* **12,** 1075–1079.

Lowenstein, P.R. 1995. Degenerative and inherited neurological disorders. In: Dickson, G., ed., *Molecular and Cell Biology of Human Gene Therapeutics*, pp.301–349. Chapman & Hall, London.

Lowenstein, P.R., Morrison, E.E., Bain, D., Hodge, P., Preston, C.M., Clissold, P., Stow, N.D., McKee, T.A. and Castro, M.G. 1994. Use of recombinant vectors derived from herpes simplex virus 1 mutant *ts*K for short-term expression of transgenes encoding cytoplasmic and membrane anchored proteins in post-mitotic polarized cortical neurons and glial cells *in vitro*. *Neuroscience* **60,** 1059–1077.

Lowenstein, P.R., Bain, D., Shering, A.F., Wilkinson, G.W.G. and Castro, M.G. 1995. Cell type specific expression from viral promoters within replication deficient adenovirus recombinants in primary neocortical cultures. *Restor. Neurol. Neurosci.* **8,** 37–39.

Lowenstein, P.R., Wilkinson, G.W.G., Castro, M.G., Shering, A.F., Fooks, A.R. and Bain, D. 1996. Non-neurotropic adenovirus: a vector for gene transfer to the brain and possible gene therapy of neurological disorders. In: Latchmann, D., ed., *Genetic Manipulation of the Nervous System*, pp.11–39. Academic Press, New York.

Mastrangeli, A., Danel, C., Rosenfeld, M.A., Stratford-Perricaudet, L., Perricaudet, M., Pavirani, A., Lecocq, J.P. and Crystal, R.G. 1993. Diversity of airway epithelial cell targets for *in vivo* recombinant adenovirus-mediated gene transfer. *J. Clin. Invest.* **91,** 225–234.

McGrory, W.J., Bautista, D.S. and Graham, F.L. 1988. A simple technique for the rescue of early region-1 mutations into infectious human adenovirus type-5. *Virology* **163,** 614–617.

Mittereder, N., Yei, S., Bachurski, C., Cuppoletti, J., Whitsett, J.A., Tolstoshev, P. and Trapnell, B.C. 1994. Evaluation of the efficacy and safety of *in vitro*, adenovirus-mediated transfer of the human cystic fibrosis transmembrane conductance regulator cDNA. *Hum. Gene Ther.* **5,** 717–729.

Morgan, L. 1994. Schwann cell culture. In: Cohen, J. and Wilkinson, G., eds, *Nerve Cell Culture, Volume* 1. *A practical approach.* IRL Press, Oxford.

Precious, B. and Russell, W.C. (1985) Growth, purification and titration of adenoviruses. In: Mahy, B.W.J., ed, *Virology: A Practical Approach*, pp. 193–205. IRL Press, Oxford.

Oualikene, W., Gonin, P. and Eloit, M. 1994. Short and long term dissemination of deletion mutants of adenovirus in permissive (cotton rat) and non-permissive (mouse) species. *J. Gen. Virol.* **75,** 2765–2768.

Quantin, B., Perricaudet, L.D., Tajbakhsh, S. and Mandel, J.L. (1991) Adenovirus as an expression vector in muscle cells *in vivo*. *Proc. Natl Acad. Sci. USA* **89,** 2581–2584.

Rauscht, B., Clopshaw, P.A., Price, J., Noble, M. and Seifert, W. 1982. Development of oligodendrocytes and Schwann cells studied with a monoclonal antibody against galactocerebrosidase. *Proc. Natl Acad. Sci USA* **79,** 2709–2713.

Ridoux, V., Robert, J.J., Zhang, X., Perricaudet, M., Mallet, J. and Le Gal La Salle, G. 1994a. The use of adenovirus vectors for intracerebral grafting of transfected nervous cells. *NeuroReport* **5,** 801–804.

Ridoux, V., Robert, J.J., Zhang, X., Perricaudet, M., Mallet, J. and Le Gal La Salle, G. 1994b. Adenoviral vectors as functional retrograde neuronal tracers. *Brain Res.* **648,** 171–175.

Rosenfeld, M.A., Chu, C.S., Seth, P., Danel, C., Banks, T., Yoneyama, K., Yoshimura, K. and Crystal, R.G. 1994. Gene transfer to freshly isolated human respiratory epithelial cells *in vitro* using a replication-deficient adenovirus containing the human cystic fibrosis transmembrane conductance regulator cDNA. *Hum. Gene Ther.* **5,** 331–342.

Rosenfeld, M.A., Siegfried, W., Yoshimura, K., Yoneyama, K., Fukayama, M., Stier, L.E., Paakko, P.K., Gilardi, P., Stratford-Perricaudet, L.D., Perricaudet, M., Jallat, S., Pavirani, A., Lecocq, J.P. and Crystal, R.G. 1991. Adenovirus-mediated transfer of a recombinant α_1-antitrypsin gene to the lung epithelium *in vivo*. *Science* **252,** 431–434.

Rosenfeld, M.A., Yoshimura, K., Trapnell, B.C., Yoneyama, K., Rosenthal, E.R., Dalemans, W., Fukayama, M., Bargon, J., Stier, L.E., Stratford-Perricaudet, L., Perricaudet, M., Guggino, W.B., Pavirani, A., Lecocq, J.P. and Crystal, R.G. 1992. *in vivo* transfer of the human cystic fibrosis transmembrane conductance regulator gene to the airway epithelium. *Cell* **68,** 143–155.

Rubin, B.A. and Rorke, L.B. 1988. Adenovirus vaccines. In: Plotkin, S.A. and Mortimer, E.A., eds, *Vaccines*, 2nd edn, pp. 475–502. W.B. Saunders, Philadelphia.

Sambrook, J., Fritsch, E.F. and Maniatis, T. 1989. *Molecular Cloning. A Laboratory Manual*, 2nd edition. CSH Laboratory Press, Cold Spring Harbor.

Schwartz, A.R., Togo, Y. and Hornick, R.B. 1974. Clinical evaluation of live, oral types 1, 2, and 5 adenovirus vaccines. *Am. Rev. Respir. Dis.* **109,** 233–238.

Shenk, T. 1995. Adenoviridae: the viruses and their replication. In: Fields, B.N, Knipe, D.M., Howley, P.M., eds, *Virology*, pp. 979–1016.

Shering, A.F., Bain, D., Wilkinson, G.W.G., Castro, M.G. and Lowenstein, P.R. 1995. The cytomegalovirus major immediate early promoter within a replication-deficient adenovirus recombinant drives transgene expression in astrocytes and fibroblasts, but not neurons or Schwann cells. *J. Virol.*, submitted.

Shewach, D.S., Zerve, L.K., Hughes, T.L., Roessler, B.H., Breakefield, X.O. and Davidson, B.L. 1994. Enhanced cytotoxicity of antiviral drugs mediated by adenovirus directed transfer of the herpes simplex virus thymidine kinase gene in rat glioma cells. *Cancer Gene Ther.* **1,** 107–112.

Simon, R.H., Engelhardt, J.F., Yang, Y., Zepeda, M., Weber Pendleton, S., Grossman, M. and Wilson, J.M. 1993. Adenovirus-mediated transfer of the CFTR gene to lung of nonhuman primates: toxicity study. *Hum. Gene Ther.* **4,** 771–780.

Smith, T.A.G., Mehaffey, M.G., Kayda, D.B., Saunders, J.M., Yei, S., Trapnell, B.C., McClelland, A. and Kaleko, M. 1993. Adenovirus mediated expression of therapeutic plasma levels of human factor IX in mice. *Nature Genet.* **5,** 397–402.

Spessot, R., Inchley, K., Hupel, T.M. and Bacchetti, S. 1989. Cloning of the herpes-simplex virus ICP4 gene in an adenovirus vector—effects on adenovirus gene-expression and replication. *Virology* **168,** 378–387.

Stratford-Perricaudet, L.D., Makeh, I., Perricaudet, M. and Briand, P. 1992. Widespread long-term gene transfer to mouse skeletal muscles and heart. *J. Clin. Invest.* **90,** 626–630.

Stratford-Perricaudet, L.D., Levrero, M., Chasse, J.F., Perricaudet, M. and Briand, P. 1990. Evaluation of the transfer and expression in mice of an enzyme-encoding gene using a human adenovirus vector. *Hum. Gene Ther.* **1,** 241–256.

Top, F.H. Jr., Buescher, E.L, Bancroft, W.H. and Russell, P.K. 1971a. Immunization with live types 7 and 4 adenovirus vaccines. II. antibody response and protective effect against acute respiratory disease due to adenovirus type 7. *J. Infect. Dis.* **124,** 155–160.

Top, F.H. Jr., Grossman, R.A., Bartelloni, P.J. et al. 1971b. Immunization with live types 7 and 4 adenovirus vaccines. I. Safety, infectivity, antigenicity, and potency of adenovirus type 7 vaccine in humans. *J. Infect. Dis.* **124,** 148–154.

Welsh, M.J., Smith, A.E., Zabner, J., Rich, D.P., Graham, S.M., Gregory, R.J., Pratt, B.M. and Moscicki R.A. 1994. Clinical Protocol: Cystic fibrosis gene therapy using an adenovirus vector: *in vivo* safety and efficacy in nasal epithelium. *Hum. Gene Ther.* **5,** 209–219.

Wickham, T.J., Mathias, P., Chenesh, D.A. and Nemenow, G.R. 1993. Integrins $\alpha v\beta 3$ and $\alpha v\beta 5$ promote adenovirus internalization but not virus attachment. *Cell* **73**: 309–313.

Wickham, T.J., Filardo, E.J., Cheresh, D.A. and Nemerow, G.R. 1994. Integrin $\alpha v\beta 5$ selectively promotes adenovirus mediated cell membrane permeabilization. *J. Cell Biol.* **127,** 257–264.

Wilkinson, G.W.G. and Akrigg, A. 1991. The CMV major IE promoter and it use in eukaryotic expression systems. In: Greenaway, P.J., ed., *Advances in Gene Technology*, pp.287–310. JAI Press, London.

Wilkinson, G.W.G. and Akrigg, A. 1992. Constitutive and enhanced expression from the CMV major IE promoter in a defective adenovirus vector. *Nucl. Acid Res.* **20,** 2233–2239.

Wilson, J.M., Engelhardt, J.F., Grossman, M., Simon, R.H. and Yang, Y. 1994. Clinical protocol: Gene therapy of cystic fibrosis lung disease using E1 deleted adenoviruses: a phase I trial. *Hum. Gene Ther.* **5,** 501–519.

Wold, W.S.M., Hermiston, T.W. and Tollefson, A.E. 1994. Adenovirus proteins that subvert host defenses. *Trends Microbiol.* **2,** 437–443.

Yang, Y., Nunes, F.A., Berencsi, K., Gonczol, E., Engelhardt, J.F. and Wilson, J.M. 1994. Inactivation of E2A in recombinant adenoviruses improves the prospect for gene therapy in cystic fibrosis. *Nature Genet.* **7,** 362–369.

Yei, S., Bachurski, C.J., Weaver, T.E., Wert, S.E., Trapnell, B.C. and Whitsett, J.A. 1994. Adenoviral-mediated gene transfer of human surfactant protein B to respiratory epithelial cells. *Am. J. Respir. Cell. Mol. Biol.* **11,** 329–336.

Yei, S., Mittereder, N., Wert, S., Whitsett, J.A., Wilmott, R.W. and Trapnell, B.C. 1994. *In vivo* evaluation of the safety of adenovirus-mediated transfer of the human cystic fibrosis transmembrane conductance regulator cDNA to the lung. *Hum. Gene Ther.* **5,** 731–744.

Zabner, J., Couture, L.A., Gregory, R.J., Graham, S.M., Smith, A.E. and Welsh, J.M. 1993a. Adenovirus-mediated gene transfer transiently corrects the chloride transport defect in nasal epithelia of patients with cystic fibrosis. *Cell* **75,** 207–216.

Zabner, J., Petersen, D.M., Puga, A.P., Graham, S.M., Couture, L.A., Keyes, L.D., Lukason, M.J., St-George, J.A., Gregory, R.J., Smith, A.E. and Welsh, M.J. 1993b. Safety and efficacy of repetitive adenovirus-mediated transfer of CFTR cDNA to airway epithelia of primates and cotton rats. *Nature Genet.* **6,** 75–83.

Zabner, J., Couture, L.A., Smith, A.E. and Welsh, J.M. 1994. Correction of cAMP-stimulated fluid secretion in cystic fibrosis airway epithelia: efficiency of adenovirus-mediated gene transfer *in vitro*. *Hum. Gene Ther.* **5,** 585–593.

CHAPTER 9

Adeno-associated Virus Vectors for Gene Transfer

JEFFREY S. BARTLETT, XIAO XIAO AND RICHARD J. SAMULSKI

Gene Therapy Center and Department of Pharmacology, School of Medicine, University of North Carolina at Chapel Hill, Chapel Hill, C.B. #7352, North Carolina 27599-7352, USA. Tel: 919 966 0905; Fax: 919 966 0908; Email: jbart @med.unc.edu

1 INTRODUCTION

The concept of gene therapy involves a form of molecular surgery by which a defective gene is replaced by a characterized normal counterpart. Although the concept is simple and appears straightforward, researchers have been presented with the daunting task of achieving effective gene delivery to the affected cells in an individual. This has hampered advances in the exciting potential of performing gene therapy. When perfected, gene therapy will have far-reaching impact on the estimated 4000 genetic disorders now characterized. Of these disorders 2000 genes have been identified and are readily available for gene replacement therapy. As our capability of identifying candidate genes increases, through efforts such as the Human Genome Project, we can predict that these candidate genes will quickly move from the laboratory bench to a clinical setting. This is best illustrated by cystic fibrosis (CF). The gene for CF was identified in 1989 (Riordan et al., 1989; Rommens et al., 1989), which led to the understanding that this disease involved a defective chloride transport channel (Anderson et al., 1991; Bear et al., 1991; Kartner et al., 1991). Access to the CF gene enabled generation of the first animal model with this disease in 1992 (Snouwaert et al., 1992), and to approved clinical gene therapy protocols for humans, which first started in April 1993—a blistering pace considering how long this genetic disorder has been observed in the medical profession. The recent advances in gene replacement have provided the means to tackle such life threatening disorders as sickle-cell anemia, diabetes and CF. Successful gene therapy approaches will not only be applicable to genetic disorders but will also have a tremendous impact on cancer and infectious diseases (e.g. HIV, herpes, and hepatitis). In search of efficient delivery systems, many workers hope that the molecular surgery required for gene replacement can be efficiently performed by viral vectors.

Viral vectors, capable of infecting almost every cell in a target population, are the most efficient way of delivering nucleic acids into mammalian cells. Viral expression vectors, reviewed by Rigby (1983) have been developed using DNA viruses, such as papova (i.e. SV40), adeno, herpes, and pox viruses, and RNA viruses, such as retrovirus. The most commonly used model vectors are derived from murine and avian retroviruses (Cone and Mulligan, 1984; Mann et al., 1983; Sorge et al., 1984; Watanabe and Temin, 1983). All steps required for use of these replication-defective vectors (infection, replication, integration, and gene expression) have been thoroughly studied and

Protocols for Gene Transfer in Neuroscience: Towards Gene Therapy of Neurological Disorders
Edited by P.R. Lowenstein and L.W. Enquist

characterized, providing a well developed vector system which can randomly deposit genes into the host genome. However, drawbacks restrict the usefulness of this system for gene therapy:

- At present, recombinant retrovirus stocks can only be made to low titers
- Although the retrovirus vectors can infect a broad class of cell types, cell replication and DNA synthesis are required for provirus integration, restricting their efficient use to replicating cells
- The recognition of human retroviruses as the etiologic agents of acquired immune deficiency syndrome (AIDS), some cases of T-cell and hairy cell leukemia and numerous examples of oncogenic animal retroviruses, has created an awareness of the potential health risks associated with the use of retrovirus vectors, which is particularly relevant to their use in human gene therapy.

Although further study may overcome these problems, they have fueled the search for alternative vectors. Ideally, a virus vector should lead to efficient infection and stable gene expression, through the use of high-titer stocks free of wild-type recombinants. It should also systematically target a specific site(s) in the genome, and the appropriate cells and organs.

Many of the viral vectors currently available either do not integrate into host cells at high frequency (such as adenovirus), are limited in their host range, or include other viral genes. For this reason 10 years ago we began to focus on the human DNA virus, adeno-associated virus (AAV), a promising alternative to the vectors currently used. This virus is a defective member of the parvovirus family. It can be propagated as a lytic virus or maintained as a provirus integrated into the host cell genome (Cukor et al., 1984). In a lytic infection, replication requires the presence of either adenovirus (Atchison et al., 1965; Parks et al., 1967), or herpes simplex virus (Buller et al., 1981); hence the classification of AAV as a "defective" virus. The requirement of a helper virus for productive infection has made it difficult to understand the AAV life cycle. However, from a vector point of view, it has added a level of control when generating non-replicative vectors in that they can be propagated under controlled conditions. One of the most interesting aspects of the organism's life cycle is its ability to integrate into the host genome in the absence of helper virus. When AAV infects cells in the absence of helper virus, it becomes latent by persisting in the host cell genome as an integrated provirus (Berns et al., 1975; Cheung et al., 1980; Samulski, 1993). If these cells are subsequently infected with wild-type helper virus the latent AAV can be rescued from the chromosome, and enters its lytic cycle.

The present method for producing stocks of recombinant AAV (rAAV) utilizes a two-component plasmid system: (1) AAV plasmid vector, containing the viral inverted terminal repeats; (2) AAV helper plasmid, which provides the necessary AAV capsid and replication proteins in *trans* (Fig. 9.1). The vector and helper plasmid DNAs should be sufficiently non-homologous to preclude homologous recombination events between the two which could generate wild-type AAV. Although there are many variations on this theme, this chapter will focus on the AAV plasmid vector *psub201* (Samulski et al., 1987) and helper plasmid *pAAV/Ad*, which contains adenovirus type 5 terminal sequences in place of the normal AAV termini. This helper plasmid has no homology to the *psub201*, and can not be packaged into AAV virions because it lacks the terminal *cis*-acting domains required for this function. In addition, *pAAV/Ad* contains no adenovirus packaging sequences, therefore there is no chance of obtaining unwanted adenovirus recombinants.

By cotransfecting *pAAV/Ad* and *psub201* containing a foreign gene inserted between the two AAV terminal repeats in the presence of adenovirus, rescue, replication and packaging of the foreign gene into AAV particles occurs as depicted in Fig. 9.1. The results of such a packaging scheme are an adenovirus helper and an AAV particle carrying the recombinant DNA. This recombinant adeno-associated virus (rAAV) may then be used to transfer the recombinant DNA into an appropriate target cell. The adenovirus helper may be removed by a number of physical and genetic techniques. Heating the virus lysate to 56°C for 30 min is one such strategy. Using this packaging system unconcentrated helper-free stocks of AAV vectors can be generated at titers of 10^4–10^5 particles/ml.

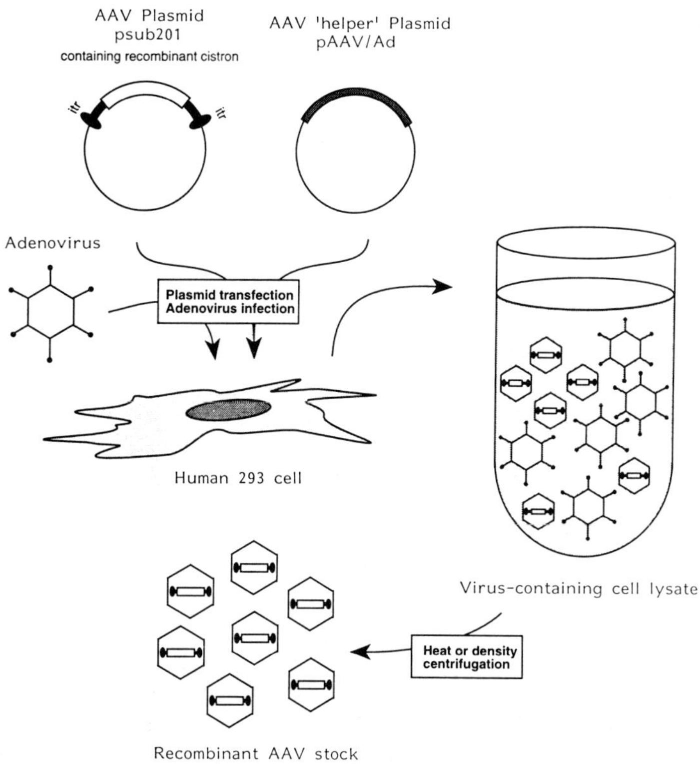

Figure 9.1 Production of recombinant AAV. Cells are transfected with an AAV recombinant plasmid based on the *psub201* vector, containing foreign DNA inserted between the two AAV inverted terminal repeats (itr), and a "helper" plasmid, *pAAV/Ad*, which supplies the necessary AAV gene products in *trans*. The cells are also infected with adenovirus (Ad) to supply helper function. The virus stock produced contains both adenovirus and the recombinant AAV. Adenovirus can be inactivated by heat treatment or removed by density gradient centrifugation

2 MATERIALS AND EQUIPMENT

2.1 Cell Culture: General

(1) Human 293 cells should be split 1/5 every 3–4 days or at about 70% confluence. They should not be allowed to overgrow and should be of low passage (less than passage 50). These cells may be obtained from the American Type Culture Collection, Rockville, MD (ATCC cat. no. CRL 1573) or the European Collection of Animal Cell Cultures, Centre for Applied Microbiology and Research, Porton Down, Salisbury, SP4 OJG, UK (ECACC cat. no. 85120602).
(2) Phosphate-buffered saline (PBS): 1.0% NaCl, 0.025% KCl, 0.14% Na_2HPO_4, 0.025% KH_2PO_4 (all w/v), pH 7.2. Sterile.
(3) Dulbecco's Modified Eagle's Medium (DMEM) with glutamine containing 100 U/ml penicillin G and 100 μg/ml streptomycin.
(4) Tissue culture dishes (100 mm diameter).
(5) Fetal bovine serum (FBS).
(6) Trypsin–EDTA solution (0.05% Trypsin, 0.53 mM EDTA–4Na in Hank's balanced salt solution) for the routine passage of 293 cells.
(7) Humidified incubator, 37°C, 5% CO_2.

2.2 Production of Recombinant AAV Plasmid

(1) AAV plasmid vector *psub201*.
(2) DNA insert containing the desired transgene, appropriate promoter, enhancer and RNA processing elements flanked by *Xba*I restriction enzyme recognition sites (as discussed in Protocol #51). The use of *psub201* requires that the foreign gene cassette is excised with a restriction enzyme that produces *Xba*I sticky ends. Alternatively, the insert and digested vector may be treated with a suitable enzyme to produce flush ends for blunt-end ligation.
(3) Restriction enzyme *Xba*I and appropriate buffer.
(4) Shrimp alkaline phosphatase (SAP) and buffer.
(5) T4 DNA ligase and buffer containing ATP.
(6) Electrocompetent *E. coli* SURE® cells (See Section 4, Page 121).
(7) GlassMAX® (Gibco/BRL) DNA extraction cartridges and vendor supplied reagents.
(8) Additional reagents and equipment for electroporation of *E. coli* cells, DNA minipreps, large-scale plasmid isolation and purification of plasmid DNA by CsCl gradient centrifugation, and agarose gel electrophoresis.

2.3 Generation of Recombinant Virus

(1) Monolayers of 293 cells at approximately 80% confluence.
(2) Lipofectin[t] reagent (Gibco/BRL).
(3) Polystyrene tubes (Falcon): 17 × 100 mm (#2059) or 12 × 175 mm (#2058).
(4) AAV "helper" plasmid *pAAV/Ad*, as described in Section 1. Very pure DNA should be used for transfection; therefore plasmid should be purified by double CsCl gradient centrifugation (See Chapter 10 for CsCl purification).
(5) Recombinant AAV plasmid constructed as described in Section 2.2 and purified by double CsCl gradient centrifugation.
(6) Tissue culture dishes as described in Section 2.1.
(7) Opti-MEM® medium (Gibco).
(8) DMEM, as described above, containing 10% FBS.
(9) PBS as described in Section 2.1.
(10) Adenovirus stock (type dl309 or equivalent). Methods for the propagation and purification of adenovirus have been described by Graham and Prevec, 1991.

2.4 Purification of Recombinant Virus

(1) PBS as prepared in Section 2.1.
(2) Clinical centrifuge for low-speed centrifugation.
(3) Sonicator (for example, Branson Model 2000, fitted with 0.5 cm microtip).
(4) Saturated solution of NH_4SO_4.
(5) Chloroform.
(6) Ultracentrifuge tubes, 13 × 51 mm.
(7) CsCl solution for density gradient centrifugation (1.37 g/ml CsCl in 0.01 M Tris–HCl, pH 8.0; 0.001 M EDTA).
(8) Ultra centrifuge capable of reaching 150 000*g*.
(9) Disposable syringe fitted with a 21 gauge needle.
(10) Dialysis tubing.

3 THE PROTOCOLS

Protocol #51: Production of Recombinant AAV Plasmid

(1) In a 20.0 μl reaction, digest 2.0–10.0 μg of *psub201* DNA with *Xba*I restriction enzyme in the appropriate buffer for 1 h at 37°C. *Xba*I digestion of *psub201* should generate two DNA

fragments (4.5 and 3.8 kb). The larger (4.5 kb) fragment containing the plasmid backbone and AAV terminal repeats are used to generate the rAAV plasmid vector (SEE SECTION 4, PAGE 121).

(2) In a second restriction endonuclease reaction, digest a similar amount of plasmid containing the desired transgene with *Xba*I or other appropriate restriction enzyme.

(3) Once the reactions are complete, inactivate the enzymes by heating for 15 min. at 75°C.

(4) Add 2.0 μl 10 × SAP buffer and 1 U shrimp alkaline phosphatase to the DNA fragments; incubate for 1 h at 37°C.

(5) Inactivate the SAP reaction by heating for 15 min. at 75°C. If no further enzymic treatments are necessary, proceed to Step 7.

(6) If the ends generated by the *Xba*I restriction endonuclease must be converted to blunt ends (SEE DISCUSSION IN SECTION 4, PAGE 121), add 1.0 μl of a solution containing all four dNTPs (0.5 mM each) and an appropriate amount of Klenow fragment of *E. coli* DNA polymerase. Incubate at 30°C for 15 min. When the reaction is complete, inactivate the enzymes by heating to 75°C for 15 min.

(7) Isolate the desired DNA segments by gel electrophoresis, or by other methods if appropriate. Electrophoresis in agarose gels is the most common method. Purification is not essential, but is very helpful.

(8) Visualize the DNA fragments by placing the gel on a long wavelength transilluminator. Protect yourself from UV exposure. Cut out the desired DNA band(s) from the gel with a scalpel or single-edge razor blade and purify the DNA from the gel slices using GlassMAX® DNA extraction cartridges and the procedures described by the manufacturer. Quantitate the purified DNA fragments by absorbance at 260 nm.

(9) Set up the following ligation reaction (20.0 μl total volume): 100 ng purified *psub201* DNA fragment; 4.0 μl 5 × T4 DNA ligase buffer containing ATP; 20–200 U T4 DNA ligase (blunt-end ligations require more ligase); 300 ng of the DNA segment containing the transgene cassette.

(10) Allow the ligation reaction to proceed overnight at 15°C.

(11) Electroporate 1.0 μl of a 1/10 dilution of the ligation reaction mixture into *E. coli* cells and select for transformants using the ampicillin resistance marker present on the *psub201* vector.

(12) Analyse individual *E. coli* transformants by miniprep analysis for those that contain the desired insert.

(13) Prepare a large-scale preparation of the recombinant AAV plasmid and purify by banding twice on CsCl gradients and extensive dialysis against 10 mM Tris–HCl, 1 mM EDTA, pH 8.0.

(14) Quantitate the final DNA preparation by absorbance at 260 nm.

Protocol #52: Generation of Recombinant AAV

(1) Grow 293 cells on 100 mm tissue culture dishes in DMEM containing 10% fetal bovine serum until they are 60–80% confluent. The number of dishes used will depend of the amount of rAAV needed for a particular application. We routinely transfect 10–20 plates at a time for the production of recombinant virus. Large *in vivo* experiments may require significantly more plates.

(2) Suspend the DNAs in a 15 ml polystyrene tube containing 1.0 ml Opti-MEM medium per 100 mm tissue culture dish. The amount of DNA used for each transfection is related to the amount of Lipofectin reagent and the number of cells (SEE SECTION 4, PAGE 121). We routinely use between 5 and 25 μg of total DNA *pAAV/Ad* helper plasmid, and rAAV vector plasmid at a 3:1 ratio per 100 mm tissue culture dish.

(3) Suspend Lipofectin reagent in 1.0 ml of Opti-MEM medium in a second polystyrene tube. The DNA/Lipofectin ratio should be 1:4 (SEE SECTION 4).

(4) Mix the DNA and Lipofectin by inverting the tube several times or vortexing gently.

(5) Incubate the DNA/Lipofectin mixture at room temperature for 5 min.

(6) Remove the medium by aspiration and wash the monolayer twice with Opti-MEM medium or PBS.

(7) Add 2 ml DNA/Lipofectin/Opti-MEM mixture to the cells.

(8) Incubate at 37°C, 5% CO_2 for 3–6 h.
(9) Remove medium by aspiration and replace with DMEM containing 2% FBS and adenovirus (1–10 p.f.u./cell). The exact amount of adenovirus may need to be empirically determined. It is important that each cell in the monolayer is infected. However, the infection must proceed slowly and only a moderate cytopathic effect (CPE) should be evident on the second day after infection.
(10) Continue incubation for 48 h.

Protocol #53: Isolation and Purification of Recombinant AAV

(1) 48 h after infection, scrape the cells into the medium and collect in appropriate 50 or 250 ml conical centrifuge bottles. Keep the samples on ice.
(2) Sonicate the material to disrupt the cells and shear the cellular DNA. The conditions will need to be empirically determined for each sonicator and will depend on the sample volume and kind of vessel the sample is in. The procedure we use consists of 20 intermittent pulses, 1 s on, 1 s off. The 20 pulses are repeated two or three times.
(3) Centrifuge the bottles at low speed to pellet the cellular debris. Remove the supernatant to a new bottle.
(4) Extract the supernatant three times with an equal volume of chloroform to remove lipid from the preparation, which often interferes with subsequent purification steps (See Section 4, Page 121).
(5) Add saturated ammonium sulfate solution to a final 25% saturation, and incubate on ice for 15–30 min. Collect the precipitate by low-speed centrifugation. Remove the supernatant to a new bottle and add saturated ammonium sulfate to a final 50% saturation. Incubate on ice for 15–30 min. Collect the precipitate by low speed centrifugation, discarding the supernatant.
(6) Resuspend the pellet in 12.0 ml CsCl solution (1.37 g/ml), mix well to dissolve, and divide the sample between two 13 × 51 mm ultracentrifuge tubes. Spin at 35 000 r.p.m. in a Beckman SW-50.1 rotor (or equivalent) for 20–36 h.
(7) The recombinant viral band may be visible after centrifugation but it should not be confused with the slightly less dense adenovirus helper band. If it is visible, collect the banded virus with a syringe through the side of the tube. If there is no discrete rAAV band, the gradient should be fractionated into 10 fractions of 0.5 ml. The recombinant AAV should band at a density of 1.42–1.45. Determine the density of CsCl in each fraction either by weighing a small amount of each fraction or by using a refractometer. Pool those fractions with densities in the appropriate range. If the rAAV being produced is easily assayed biologically, the assay may also be used to determine which fractions contain recombinant virus.
(8) Reband the recombinant virus on a second CsCl gradient: adjust the volume of the collected fractions to 6.0 ml with CsCl solution (1.37 g/ml), spin down and collect as described in Steps 6 and 7.
(9) Dialyse the banded virus in boiled dialysis tubing for about 2 h against two changes of 100 volumes of PBS to remove the cesium from the preparation. If virus aggregation is a problem, the CsCl may be removed by gel filtration on Sephadex G-50 spin columns (Boehringer Mannheim).
(10) Freeze aliquots at −70°C. These virus stocks are stable for many years at this temperature.

Protocol #54: Titration of Recombinant AAV by Replication Center Assay

(1) Plate 293 cells into 96-well tissue culture dishes the day before performing the assay at a density of approximately 2–3 × 10^4 cells/well (about 50% of confluence). Set up one row of the plate for determining the recombinant titer (row A) and a second row for wild-type AAV contamination (row H). Up to 11 different preparations of AAV can be titered on a single plate (Fig. 9.2).
(2) The next day, remove the media from the cells, leaving behind just enough to cover the cells. Add 1 μl of the rAAV-containing lysate or purified rAAV preparation to a well in the first row

on the plate (row A), and the same amount to a well in the last row (row H). Other wells can be used to monitor rAAV purification or concentration. Leave the last well in the row A for an "Ad only" control. Rock the plate gently to mix.

(3) Add a predetermined amount (see Step 4) of adenovirus to 2.4 ml of DMEM/2% FBS in a 15 ml polystyrene tube. Mix well, and dispense 100 μl into each well in row H and the "Ad only" control well at the end of row A.

(4) Add a calculated amount of wild-type AAV to the remaining, approximately 1.2 ml, medium/Ad mixture, and dispense 100 μl into each well in row A. The final multiplicity of infection (MOI) of adenovirus and AAV should be 20 and 2, respectively.

(5) Incubate for 30 h.

(6) Remove the medium and rinse the cells with a small volume of PBS.

(7) Add 250 μl of PE solution to each well and place the dish on ice.

(8) Mark each nylon hybridization membrane with pen, prewet with PBS, and mount in the filter holder.

(9) Apply 5.0 ml PBS to each filter.

(10) Resuspend the cells from a well of the plate by moving up and down gently in a pipette. Apply 50 μl of the cell suspension into the PBS buffer on the top nylon filter mounted in the filter holder and mix gently. Apply suction.

(11) Carefully remove the nylon filter disk from the manifold with flat-tipped forceps. Place the disk with the cell side up onto a pool of 0.5 M NaOH on plastic wrap. Stretch the plastic wrap to insure that all disks wet evenly. After 2 min, remove disks and place on blotting paper, cell side up.

(12) Repeat Step 11 with a new sheet of plastic wrap and fresh 0.5 N NaOH.

(13) On a new sheet of plastic wrap place a small amount of 1.0 M Tris–HCl, pH 7.5. Place the nylon filter disks, cell side up, onto this pool. Stretch the plastic wrap to insure that all of the disks wet evenly. After 2 min, remove the disk and place on blotting paper (cell side up).

(14) Repeat Step 13 with a new sheet of plastic wrap and fresh Tris–HCl.

(15) Allow the disks to dry at room temperature. Fix the DNA to the disks by microwaving for 5 min at full power.

(16) Hybridize the filters from row H with a radioactively labeled wild-type AAV probe and those from row A with a radioactively labeled foreign gene DNA probe. Hybridization using probes with a specific activity of 10^7 c.p.m./μg DNA gives a strong signal on overnight exposure of the filter to X-ray film.

(17) The titer of the original rAAV preparation is equal to the number of positive cells per filter multiplied by 5×10^3, expressed as infectious units (i.u.) per milliliter.

4 NOTES AND TROUBLESHOOTING

4.1 On Protocol #51: Production of Recombinant AAV Plasmid

This section describes the DNA manipulations necessary to obtain a recombinant plasmid vector containing the gene of interest flanked by the AAV terminal repeats. This plasmid will then be transfected into tissue culture cells in conjunction with AAV helper plasmid and adenovirus infection to generate rAAV. For the purposes of this chapter, it is assumed that an appropriate transgene, containing the necessary transcriptional and translational control elements, is already at hand. These will inevitably include enhancer as well as promoter elements, and may be either virally derived or cellular in origin.

Commonly used viral elements include the human cytomegalovirus (HCMV) immediate early gene enhancer–promoter and the Rous sarcoma virus long terminal repeat (RSV LTR) promoter. These viral sequences provide a very high-level of transgene expression and are commercially available as part of eukaryotic expression plasmids.

Tissue-specific expression can be obtained by including cellular control elements in the recombinant cistron. Previously described CNS-specific elements include the mouse myelin basic protein gene promoter for selective expression in glioma cells (Miyao et al., 1993), the human dopamine β-hydroxylase gene promoter for selective expression in the neurons of the locus

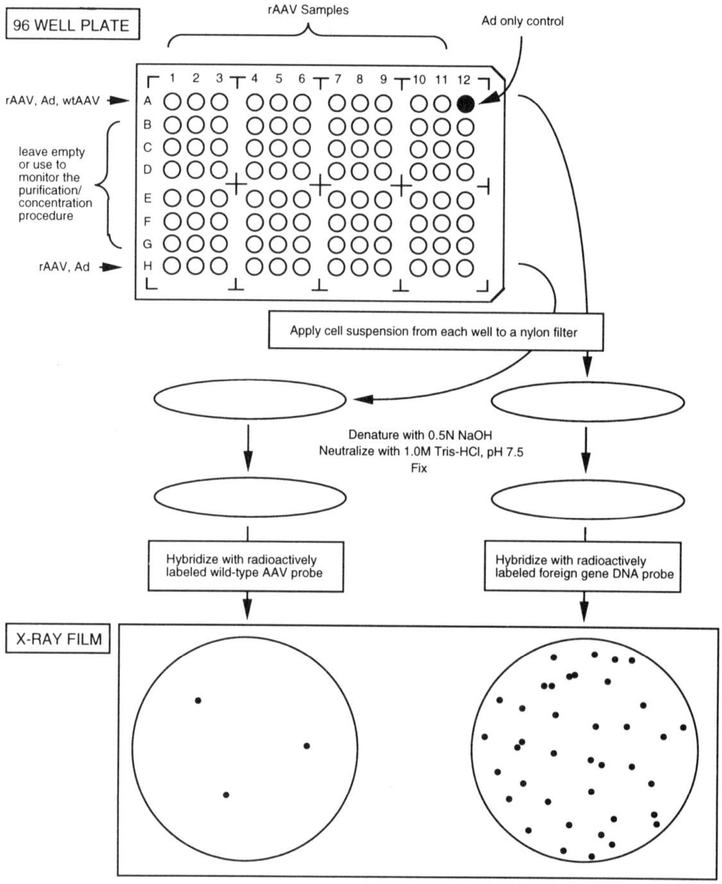

Figure 9.2 Infectious center assay. Cells are grown in a 96 well plate, as described in Protocol #54, resuspended in PBS and applied to nylon filter membranes. After denaturation and binding of the replicated AAV DNA to the filters, the filters are probed with radioactively labeled wild-type or foreign DNA probes to determine the titer of the recombinant AAV preparation

ceruleus and other noradrenergic brain stem neurons, sympathetic ganglion neurons and adrenal chromaffin cells (Mercer et al., 1991), and the rat preproenkephalin promoter for specific expression in the caudate nucleus, amygdala, piriform cortex, olfactory tubercle and ventromedial hypothalamus (Kaplitt et al., 1994a).

Promoters, enhancers, splice signals, and other *cis*-acting elements do not function as fully independent elements. In some instances there may be preferred and non-functional combinations. In many cases, appropriate tissue-specific expression depends on the assembly of an appropriate expression cassette; ideally matching enhancer with promoter and promoter with splice signal and polyadenylation signal. The selection and arrangement of *cis*-acting elements in a recombinant cistron is thus critical in achieving the desired expression upon gene transfer. Therefore, before attempting to construct recombinant virus, take your time in engineering your recombinant plasmid. Additionally, if possible, the plasmid should be tested by transfection into the target cell type and assayed for expression before assembly of the virus vector.

The transgene and appropriate control elements will probably be constructed and contained within a separate plasmid vector. The transgene cassette should be no larger than 4.5 kb. When cloned into the AAV plasmid *psub201*, this reflects the maximum size that can be efficiently rescued and packaged into viral particles (an insert size of 4.27 kb is ideal). The method described in Protocol #51 assumes that the entire gene cassette can be excised by digestion with *Xba*I and subsequently ligated to *Xba*I digested *psub201*. If this approach is not practical, *Xba*I digested *psub201* can be blunt-ended by treatment with the Klenow fragment of *E. coli* DNA polymerase and NTPs, and then ligated to a similarly treated transgene insert fragment.

All DNA preparations should be pure; double banding through CsCl gradients (Maniatis et al., 1982) or a preparation of equivalent high quality is essential.

The AAV terminal repeats may be unstable in plasmids propagated in several commonly used laboratory strains of *E. coli*. Host strains carrying *rec*A, *rec*J and *rec*B mutations, such as the SURE® strain of cells, are recommended.

It may be desirable to sequence the final recombinant AAV plasmid to ensure the sequence is correct before investing the time and reagents necessary to produce recombinant virus. Likewise, gene expression can be determined before virus production by transfecting the recombinant plasmid into the anticipated target cell type and performing an appropriate expression assay. Protein expression may be detected by fluorescence microscopy, flow cytometry or radiolabeling followed by immunoprecipitation. RNA analysis and immunohistochemistry may also be carried out.

4.2 On Protocol #52: Generation of Recombinant AAV

This protocol outlines methods for cotransfecting 293 cells with recombinant AAV and helper plasmids, for rescue of the recombinant AAV genome and packaging into viral particles. The cell line of choice is always 293, because these cells are good recipients of DNA in DNA-mediated gene transfer procedures, and allow the use of replication-deficient adenovirus as helper virus.

We routinely use the transfection procedure outlined to obtain recombinant virus from the recombinant plasmid clones. Although we have investigated a number of other methods (calcium-phosphate precipitation, DEAE–dextran, electroporation, etc.) the method of choice is most often the one the investigator has the most experience with and is most comfortable with. The reader is encouraged to evaluate other transfection techniques.

The small cationic lipid vesicles in the Lipofectin reagents can fuse to form large multilamellar structures in the presence of polyvalent anions, such as EDTA, citrate or phosphate (Felgner and Ringold, 1989). Preparations of these large fused vesicles are less effective than the small vesicles. Therefore, tissue culture media containing high concentrations of polyanionic buffers should be avoided.

Serum contains components that may inhibit Lipofectin-mediated transfection. Although a wide variety of serum-free media give good results with lipofection, in a number of cell lines Opti-MEM 1 gives the best results with respect to both viability in the presence of Lipofectin and the level of expression obtained.

The toxicity of the transfection reagent varies with cell type, and elimination of serum from the transfection media further reduces viability. Screening has identified Opti-MEM as an acceptable serum-free medium, which results in improved viability, relative to DMEM, for human 293 cells.

Large non-functional DNA/lipid aggregates may form if the DNA concentration during formation of the lipid/DNA complexes is too high (100 μg/ml or above). Formation of these large aggregates is exacerbated by increased ionic strength; if a concentrated stock solution of premixed Lipofectin/DNA complexes is needed, it should be prepared at low ionic strength. In an effort to maintain concentrations of both DNA and transfection reagent as low as possible, the DNA and transfection reagent should be separately diluted into equal volumes of media and then mixed before complex formation.

The concentration-dependent ionic species and ionic strength-dependent aggregates that can form under different transfection conditions are sticky, and adhere to glassware and plastic. Polypropylene and glass attract these aggregates more than polystyrene: polystyrene mixing containers are preferred for transfection.

Optimum transfection activity occurs under conditions in which the net negative charge on the DNA is substantially reduced. Complexes with an excess of positive charge are taken up by cells more effectively than neutral or negatively charged complexes. The optimum transfection activity for DNA seems to occur when the ratio of positively charged molar equivalents (contributed by

DOTMA in Lipofectin exceeds by 1.1–2.5 the number of molar equivalents of negative charge contributed by the DNA. The molarity of DOTMA (molecular weight 669.5) in a 1 mg/ml Lipofectin solution containing 50/50 (w/w) of DOPE (neutral lipid) is 0.75 mM, and the molar equivalents of negative charge in a 1 mg/ml DNA solution (average molecular weight of the nucleotide monomer 330) 3 mM. Based on this estimate, the optimum activity occurs when the total mass of lipid (DOTMA + DOPE) exceeds the mass of DNA by four- to tenfold.

4.3 On Protocol #53: Isolation and Purification of Recombinant AAV

This protocol is for production of large, high titer viral stocks. However, concentrated crude virus stocks may be prepared rapidly from infected 293 cells by scraping the cells into the culture medium and recovering them by pelleting at low speed in a benchtop centrifuge. The cells are then resuspended in a hypotonic buffer (e.g. PBS) and the virus released by three cycles of freeze-thawing or brief sonication. The cell debris may be removed by a second low-speed centrifugation if desired, and the lysate stored at −70°C until needed.

Before using this crude cell lysate to infect cells, it may be desirable to inactivate the adenovirus by heating the cell lysate at 56°C for 1 h. This treatment will effectively remove the heat-labile adenovirus from the preparation without significantly decreasing the titer of recombinant AAV.

Although these rapid crude viral stocks are often all that is needed to transduce cells in tissue culture, *in vivo* gene transfer necessitates the production of larger, higher titer, viral stocks as described in the protocol. These crude viral preparations are often toxic to primary neuronal cell cultures at high MOI. As the titer of recombinant AAV from the two-component plasmid system described here is relatively low, the procedure may need to be scaled up. The volumes described are for 100 mm tissue culture plates but plates of 150 mm or larger may also be used. For larger tissue culture dishes, the amounts may need to be adjusted to take into account the change in culture surface area. The protocol should facilitate recovery and concentration of rAAV from large volumes of culture medium.

Ether may be used instead of chloroform in the purification of recombinant virus, although care must be taken to remove all of the ether before ammonium sulfate precipitation and centrifugation.

Virus yields will depend on plasmid transfection efficiency, titer of adenovirus helper, level of AAV gene product expression, the length of time between infection and harvesting, and the ability to remove and concentrate virus from the culture medium. As many variables as possible should be optimized.

When making virus stocks, growing the virus in multiple passages will generate defective particles that will decrease the efficiency of expression of inserted genes. This should be avoided.

4.4 On Protocol #54: Titration of Recombinant AAV by Replication Center Assay

It is often important to determine the titer of recombinant AAV. This is a "defective" virus and direct titration of infectious units by their ability to form plaques on permissive cells is not possible. Therefore rAAV must be indirectly titered by a replication center assay, or by its ability to transduce an assayable marker gene. The replication center assay is more applicable to a broader range of rAAV vectors. A detailed description of this method is provided by Bartlett and Samulski (1995).

4.5 On Recombinant AAV Transduction of Neuronal Cells

Recombinant AAV-mediated transduction of neuronal cells and tissues has many applications. The infection protocol will vary slightly among applications, and should be optimized for each application. Recombinant AAV is only beginning to be used to deliver genes to the CNS and detailed procedures have yet to be developed—and only general guidelines for infection of cells in some typical experiments are presented here. Fortunately, the published literature contains several protocols that have been used successfully to transduce neuronal cells with other viral vectors; many of these may provide good starting points for protocols involving transduction by rAAV.

4.5.1 *Transduction* in vitro

Infection of target cells *in vitro* is accomplished by simply incubating the virus with the cells. When incubating some neuronal cells with virus *in vitro*, problems may occur if undiluted crude viral preparations are used. This may be due to the presence of toxic cellular metabolites in the crude viral preparations. To avoid this problem, the recombinant virus should be banded in CsCl gradients as described in Protocol #53. However, any CsCl remaining in the virus preparation may also lead to cytotoxicity or reduced transduction frequency, so it should be completely removed before use.

It is difficult to generalize about the efficiency of infection, although it can approach 100%. The variables that influence infectability of a given cell are mostly unknown. The vector genomes appear to be able to persist in non-dividing cells, but transduction seems to preferentially occur in cells after they have entered S phase (Russell et al., 1994). Although proliferating cells may be better transduced by AAV vectors, proliferation is not absolutely required for transduction. In fact, experiments *in vivo* have shown that recombinant AAV vectors are able to transduce at remarkably high efficiencies cell populations thought to be largely quiescent. These include human bone marrow progenitors in culture (Zhou et al., 1993; Goodman et al., 1994; Miller et al., 1994), and rat brain *in vivo* (Kaplitt et al., 1994b) (Fig. 9.3: SEE PLATE III). Histological analysis of rat brains injected with recombinant virus encoding β-galactosidase has demonstrated long-term expression in many regions of the rat brain, including striatum, hippocampus and substantia nigra (Kaplitt et al., 1994b). In addition to demonstrating the potential for gene therapy approaches targeting neuronal cells using rAAV, this finding represents the most conclusive demonstration that recombinant AAV vectors can transduce non-dividing cells.

Usually, gene activity is assayed 2–7 days after transduction. However, no systematic determination of gene expression and persistence of expression in neuronal tissue has been carried out for the recombinant AAV vectors. Also unresolved is the way in which the low mitotic activity of this tissue effects viral integration and persistence of the transgene.

Tissue explants may be infected essentially as described for transduction of cells grown in culture. A tissue explant can be bathed in as much virus stock as desired for several hours before moving it to fresh culture medium.

4.5.2 *Transduction* in vivo

Genes may also be transduced *in vivo* using recombinant AAV vectors. Detailed protocols for the handling of laboratory animals are beyond the scope of this chapter. The reader should refer to other sources for instructions on the techniques essential to the infection methods described.

The volume of recombinant virus that can be delivered to the CNS *in vivo* is generally quite small (0.1–5.0 μl). It is therefore important to prepare virus stock of high titer. In general, the virus titer should range from 10^6 to 10^8 infectious units/ml. It is also important to deliver the virus directly to the desired target area. It not clear whether factors in tissue fluids (e.g. cerebrospinal fluid) may inhibit viral infectivity; therefore the virus should be injected directly into the target tissue. Viral delivery is fairly straightforward. For stereotactic injection into rat brain, we suggest exposing the skull and lowering a 33-gauge stainless steel injector through a hole drilled over the hippocampus. However, when performing infections of brain tissue for the first time, or when transduction and expression of the transferred gene in the brain is unknown, preliminary experiments should be performed using an AAV vector carrying a histochemical marker gene such as *lac*Z. The injected animal should be examined a few days after infection to determine if the target cells have been infected and are capable of expressing the transduced gene.

In our hands, transduction frequencies with recombinant AAV containing the bacterial β-galactosidase gene have been very high. The ability of rAAV to transduce and express the *lac*Z gene in brain tissue is demonstrated in Fig. 9.3 (Plate III). The ability of recombinant AAV to deliver other genes, including therapeutic genes, to rat brain is currently being examined. Kaplitt et al. (1994b) have showed that an AAV vector could deliver a tyrosine hydroxylase gene to cells in the CNS. They also showed that the functional defects in tyrosine hydroxylase activity could be partially reversed following gene transfer. Based on the ability of recombinant AAV to carry genes expressed from exogenous tissue-specific control elements (Miller et al., 1993, 1994; Zhou et al., 1993), and the efficiency of recombinant AAV transduction in the CNS (Kaplitt et al., 1994b) we believe that this vector system may prove invaluable for the treatment of neurological disorders and malignancies.

REFERENCES

Anderson, M.P., D.P. Rich, et al. (1991). Generation of cAMP-activated chloride currents by expression of CFTR. *Science* **251:** 679–682.

Atchison, R.W., B.C. Casto, et al. (1965). Adenovirus-associated defective virus particles. *Science* **149:** 754–756.

Bartlett, J.S. and R.J. Samulski (1996). Methods for the Construction and Propagation of Recombinant Adeno-Associated Virus Vectors. *Methods in Molecular Biology: Gene Therapy Protocols* Ed. P. Robbins. New York, Humana Press.

Bear, C.E., F. Duguay, et al. (1991). Cl^- channel activity in *Xenopus* oocytes expressing the cystic fibrosis gene. *J Biol Chem* **266:** 19142–19145.

Berns, K.I., T.C. Pinkerton, et al. (1975). Detection of adeno-associated virus (AAV)-specific nucleotide sequences in DNA isolated from latently infected Detroit 6 cells. *Virology* **68:** 556–560.

Buller, R.M., J.E. Janik, et al. (1981). Herpes simplex virus types 1 and 2 completely help adenovirus-associated virus replication. *J Virol* **40:** 241–247.

Cheung, A.K., M.D. Hoggan, et al. (1980). Integration of the adenoassociated virus genome into cellular DNA in latently infected human Detroit 6 cells. *J Virol* **33:** 739–748.

Cone, R.D. and R.C. Mulligan (1984). High-efficiency gene transfer into mammalian cells: Generation of helper-free recombinant retrovirus with broad mammalian host range. *Proc Natl Acad Sci USA* **81:** 6349–6353.

Cukor, G., N.R. Blacklow, et al. (1984). Biology of Adeno-Associated Virus In: *The Parvoviruses* Ed. K.I. Berns. New York, Plenum Press, pp.33–66.

Felgner, P.L. and G.M. Ringold (1989). Cationic liposome-mediated transfection. *Nature* **337:** 387–388.

Goodman, S., X. Xiao, et al. (1994). Recombinant adeno-associated virus-mediated gene transfer into hematopoietic progenitor cells. *Blood* **84:** 1492–1500.

Graham, F.L. and L. Prevec (1991). In *Methods in Molecular Biology*, vol 7. Clifton, New Jersey, Humana, pp.109–127.

Kaplitt, M.G., A.D. Kwong, et al. (1994a). Preproenkephalin promoter yields region-specific and long-term expression in adult brain after direct *in vivo* gene transfer via a defective herpes simplex viral vector. *Proc Natl Acad Sci USA* **91:** 8979–8983.

Kaplitt, M.G., P. Leone, et al. (1994b). Adeno-associated virus vectors yield safe delivery and long term expression of potentially therapeutic genes into the mammalian brain. *Nature Genet* **8:** 148–154.

Kartner, N., J.W. Hanrahan, et al. (1991). Expression of the cystic fibrosis gene in non-epithelial invertebrate cells produces a regular anion conductance. *Cell* **64:** 681–691.

Maniatis, T., E.F. Fritsch, et al. (1982). *Molecular Cloning* (*A Laboratory Manual*). New York, Cold Spring Harbor Prcss.

Mann, R., R.C. Mulligan, et al. (1983). Construction of a retrovirus packaging mutant and its use to produce helper-free defective retrovirus. *Cell* **33:** 153–159.

Mercer, E.H., G.W. Hoyle, et al. (1991). The dopamine β-hydroxylase gene promoter directs expression of *E. coli lacZ* to sympathetic and other neurons in adult transgenic mice. *Neuron* **7:** 703–716.

Miller, J.L., C.E. Walsh, P.A. Ney, R.J. Samulski and A.W. Nienhuis (1993). Single-copy transduction and expression of human gamma-globulin in K562 erythroleukemia cells using recombinant adeno-associated virus vectors: The effect of mutations in NF-E2 and GATA-1 binding motifs within the hypersensitivity site 2 enhancer. *Blood* **82:** 1900–1906.

Miller, J.L., R.E. Donahue, et al. (1994). Recombinant adeno-associated virus (rAAV) mediated expression of a human β-globin gene in human progenitor derived erythroid cells. *Proc Natl Acad Sci USA* **91:** 10183–10187.

Miyao, Y., K. Shimizu, et al. (1993). Selective expression of foreign genes in glioma cells: use of the mouse myelin basic protein gene promoter to direct toxic gene expression. *J Neurosci Res* **36:** 472–479.

Parks, W.P., J.L. Melnick, et al. (1967). Physical assay and growth cycle studies of a defective adeno-satellite virus. *J Virol* **1:** 171–180.

Rigby, P.W. (1983). Cloning vectors derived from animal viruses. *J Gen Virol* **64:** 255–266.

Riordan, J.R., J.R. Rommens, et al. (1989). Identification of the cystic fibrosis gene: cloning and characterization of complementary DNA. *Science* **245:** 1066–1073.

Rommens, J.M., M.C. Iannuzzi, et al. (1989). Identification of the cystic fibrosis gene: chromosome walking and jumping. *Science* **245:** 1059–1065.

Russell, D.W., A.D. Miller, et al. (1994). Adeno-associated virus vectors preferentially transduce cells in S phase. *Proc Natl Acad Sci USA* **91:** 8915–8919.

Samulski, R.J. (1993). Adeno-associated virus: Integration at a specific chromosomal locus. *Curr Opin Gen Dev* **3:** 74–80.

Samulski, R.J., L.-S. Chang, et al. (1987). A recombinant plasmid from which an infectious adeno-associated virus genome can be excised *in vitro* and its use to study viral replication. *J Virol* **61:** 3096–3101.

Snouwaert, J.N., K.K. Brigman, et al. (1992). An animal model for cystic fibrosis made by gene targeting. *Science* **257:** 1083–1088.

Sorge, J., A.E. Cutting, et al. (1984). Integration-specific retrovirus expression in embryonal carcinoma cells. *Proc Natl Acad Sci USA* **81:** 6627–6631.

Watanabe, S. and H.M. Temin (1983). Construction of a helper cell line for avian reticuloendotheliosis virus cloning vectors. *Mol Cell Biol* **3:** 2241–2249.

Zhou, S.Z., H.E. Broxmeyer, et al. (1993). Adeno-associated virus 2-mediated gene transfer in murine hematopoietic progenitor cells. *Exp Hematol* **21:** 928–33.

SECTION 4

Protocols for Gene Delivery Using Herpes Simplex Virus-1 Vectors

CHAPTER 10

Transcriptional Regulation of Herpes Simplex Virus Gene Expression: Implications for our Understanding of Latency

DAVID S. LATCHMAN

Department of Molecular Pathology, University College London Medical School, The Windeyer Building, Cleveland Street, London W1P 6DB, UK. Tel: 0171 380 9343; Fax: 0171 387 3310

1 INTRODUCTION

During lytic infection with herpes simplex virus (HSV), the viral genome is expressed in a precise temporally regulated cascade (Honess and Roizman, 1974). Immediately after initial infection, the five genes encoding the immediate–early (IE) proteins ICP0, ICP4, ICP22, ICP27 and ICP47 are transcribed, in a process that does not require viral protein synthesis in the infected cell (Anderson et al., 1980; Watson et al., 1980). These regulatory proteins subsequently play a critical role in inducing the expression of the early genes, whose protein products are primarily involved in replication of the viral genome, and the late genes, which encode structural components of the viral particle (O'Hare and Hayward, 1985). For this reason the IE proteins ICP4 and ICP27 play an essential role in the lytic cycle, and their deletion or inactivation by mutation prevents the virus from undergoing lytic replication (Preston, 1979; Watson and Clements, 1980; Sacks et al., 1985).

Although the lytic cycle follows initial infection of most cell types, it is aborted in sensory neurons; in these cells the virus can establish long-lived latent infections which contain no replicating viral DNA (for reviews see Roizman and Sears, 1987; Latchman, 1990). Although entirely asymptomatic, these latent infections serve as a reservoir for lytic infection elsewhere in the body because the latent virus can reactivate in response to specific stimuli such as stress or fever and migrate to the periphery, where it can carry out the lytic cycle in susceptible epithelial cells.

A major step forward in the understanding of latency was provided by the finding that, with the exception of one region encoding the latency-associated transcripts (LAT), the viral genome is completely silent in latently infected neuronal cells of humans (Croen et al., 1987) and mice (Stevens et al., 1987). In particular, the viral genes encoding the IE proteins are not transcribed in latently infected cells. Much data has emerged to suggest that the initial establishment of latency itself depends on failure of viral IE gene expression after infection of neuronal cells. Thus, mutants lacking the genes for viral proteins such as the virion transactivator Vmw65 (Valyi-Nagi et al., 1991), which is essential for IE gene transcription (SEE SECTION 1.1), or the IE protein ICP4 (Katz et al., 1990) readily establish latency in neuronal cells despite the lack of significant viral gene expression following infection. Similarly, latent infection with wild-type HSV can be established in

Protocols for Gene Transfer in Neuroscience: Towards Gene Therapy of Neurological Disorders
Edited by P.R. Lowenstein and L.W. Enquist

ganglionic neurons in which no previous viral IE gene expression or DNA replication has taken place (Margolis et al., 1992; Speck and Simmons, 1992).

Hence both the establishment and maintenance of latent infections in neuronal cells are likely to be critically dependent upon a failure of viral IE gene expression, focusing attention on the manner in which IE gene expression is regulated. This chapter will consider the mechanisms regulating IE gene expression, focusing particularly on the mechanisms that inhibit expression in latent infections, but also considering the implications of such regulatory processes for the design of safer HSV vectors that could be used in gene therapy.

1.1 Regulation of the IE Promoters in the HSV Lytic Cycle

The IE promoters contain numerous binding sites for cellular transcription factors, such as the Sp1 factor (Jones and Tjian, 1985), which produce a significant basal activity of these promoters in different cell types (Gelman and Silverstein, 1987a,b). In lytic infection the activity of the IE promoters critically depends on their *trans*-activation by a multiprotein complex formed between the HSV virion protein Vmw65, the cellular transcription factor Oct-1 (O'Hare and Goding, 1988; Preston et al., 1988) and several other cellular cofactors (Kristie and Sharp, 1993; Werstuck and Capone, 1993). The Oct-1 protein usually binds to the octamer motif present in a number of cellular genes, such as those encoding histone H2B and the snRNAs (for a review, see Falkner et al., 1986). However, in the presence of Vmw65 and the various cofactors, the complex containing Oct-1 binds with high affinity to the octamer-related TAATGARAT (R = purine) motif in the viral IE gene promoters and transactivates their expression (for a review see Goding and O'Hare, 1989). This transactivation is very important for the success of the viral lytic cycle because viruses in which the Vmw65 protein has been altered so that it is unable to transactivate the IE promoters are capable of lytic growth only at high multiplicities of infection (Ace et al., 1989).

The promoters of the IE1, IE2 and IE3 genes (which encode the ICP0, ICP27 and ICP4 proteins respectively) also contain binding sites for the ICP4 protein itself. Binding of ICP4 to these sites results in an inhibition of promoter activity and serves to autoregulate the production of these proteins during the lytic cycle (Faber and Wilcox, 1986; Resnick et al., 1989).

1.2 Regulation of the HSV IE Promoters in Neuronal Cells

The evidence that latent infection involves a failure of IE gene expression has focused attention on the processes regulating IE gene expression after infection of neuronal cells. Initial investigations of these regulatory processes focused on the regulation of HSV gene expression in neuronal cell lines, which provided a large-scale source of material. The non-permissivity of the C1300 neuroblastoma cell line for HSV infection (Vahlne and Lycke, 1977, 1978) was shown to be due to a failure of viral IE protein synthesis following infection (Ash, 1986), as occurs in latently infected neurons *in vivo*. This failure of IE protein synthesis is caused by the lack of transcription of the IE genes in HSV-infected C1300 cells (Kemp and Latchman, 1989).

The gene encoding the viral latency-associated transcript (LAT) is not transcribed following infection of C1300 cells (Kemp and Latchman, 1989), although this does occur in latently infected cells *in vivo* (Croen et al., 1987), suggesting that C1300 cells may not entirely mimic the processes occurring following initial infection of neuronal cells *in vivo*.

We therefore studied the effect of HSV on a range of ND cell lines derived by the fusion of rat primary sensory neurons (the natural site of HSV latency *in vivo*) with C1300 cells (for information on these cell lines see Wood et al., 1990). The ND cell lines exhibited a range of permissivities for the viral lytic cycle, ranging from highly non-permissive to a level of permissivity similar to that observed in fibroblast cells readily supporting the viral lytic cycle *in vitro* (Wheatley et al., 1990). This range of permissivities parallels that observed by others for populations of primary sensory neurons both *in vitro* and *in vivo* (Kennedy et al., 1983; Sacks et al., 1985). One cell line, ND3, was identified as highly non-permissive and, as in C1300 cells, this non-permissivity was caused by the lack of IE gene transcription following infection. However, unlike C1300 cells, these cells **did** transcribe the LAT gene following infection (Wheatley et al., 1990), suggesting that they may represent a better model system. The ND3 cell line and another non-permissive ND cell line, ND7, were therefore used, together with C1300 cells, in subsequent experiments.

Transfection of these cells with constructs in which the HSV IE promoters drive expression of the readily assayable chloramphenicol acetyltransferase gene revealed a very low level of IE promoter activity compared with that observed in permissive fibroblasts (Kemp et al., 1990; Wheatley et al., 1991). Hence the failure of IE gene transcription following infection is dependent on the weak activity of the IE promoters in ND3, ND7 and C1300 cells. The lack of IE promoter activity could be due to the absence in neuronal cells of a positively acting cellular transcription factor required for IE gene transcription or to the presence in neuronal cells of a negatively acting cellular factor which inhibits IE gene transcription. In initial studies, both C1300 and ND cells contained high levels of the positively acting Oct-1 factor, which was capable of forming a functional complex with the viral Vmw65 protein.

The presence of the Oct-1/Vmw65 complex in neuronal cell lines is paralleled by evidence from sensory neurons *in vivo*. It was suggested that the failure of IE gene expression in neuronal cells may arise from the loss of Vmw65 as the virus moves up the nerve process from the periphery, resulting in a lack of *trans*-activation within the sensory neuron nucleus (Roizman and Sears, 1987). This is, however, unlikely because latency can be established in transgenic mice in which Vmw65 has been artificially expressed in all cell types, including sensory neurons (Sears et al., 1991). It seems more likely that the block to IE gene expression in sensory neurons is due to differences in the complement of cellular octamer-binding proteins between these cells and permissive cells.

One possibility in this regard is that neuronal cells contain an inhibitory protein capable of binding to the TAATGARAT motif and preventing binding of the Oct-1/Vmw65 complex, thereby inhibiting *trans*-activation. Both IE promoter activity and viral permissivity can be increased by cotransfecting ND cells with a plasmid containing binding sites for octamer-binding proteins (Kemp et al., 1990; Wheatley et al., 1991). Thus, this plasmid would titrate out an inhibitory octamer-binding protein, removing it from the IE promoter and hence increasing its activity and viral permissivity.

1.3 The Oct-2 Protein

Having shown using functional assays that neuronal cells contain an inhibitory octamer-binding protein, we used DNA mobility shift assays to identify it. These experiments showed that although permissive cells contained only the ubiquitously expressed octamer-binding protein Oct-1, neuronal cells expressed both Oct-1 and another protein that bound specifically to the octamer motif to form a DNA–protein complex of higher mobility than that formed by Oct-1 (Kemp et al., 1990; Wheatley et al., 1991).

Several different octamer-binding proteins have been identified in neuronal cells by DNA mobility shift assays (Scholer et al., 1989) or by hybridization analysis (He et al., 1989). In particular, the Oct-2 protein (originally thought to be specific to B cells (Singh et al., 1986; Staudt et al., 1988)) has been detected in neuronal cells in the brain (He et al., 1989; Scholer et al., 1989). The additional octamer-binding protein detectable using DNA mobility shift assays in our neuronal cell lines showed a mobility similar to that of B cell Oct-2 and reacted with a polyclonal antibody to Oct-2 (Lillycrop et al., 1991). Moreover, the Oct-2 mRNA was the only mRNA (apart from the Oct-1 mRNA) encoding an octamer-binding protein detectable in ND cells using the polymerase chain reaction (PCR), and cDNA cloning of the PCR product revealed that the ND cell Oct-2 protein was identical to that of B cells in the central POU domain (which mediates DNA binding (Lillycrop et al., 1991, 1992)). Hence the octamer-binding repressor protein identified in our earlier experiments is a neuronally expressed form of the Oct-2 protein.

Identification of the repressor as Oct-2 raises a paradox: B cell Oct-2 was originally identified as a strong **activator** of immunoglobulin gene transcription acting via the octamer motif in the gene promoter or enhancer (Muller et al., 1988; Scheidereit et al., 1988) but in our experiments neuronal Oct-2 **inhibited** the IE promoter. In additional experiments Oct-2 stimulated the IE promoter in B cells and repressed it in neuronal cells (Dent et al., 1991). This paradox is explained by the finding that Oct-2 mRNA exists in at least eight different alternatively spliced forms (Wirth et al., 1991;

Stoykova et al., 1992). Two of these forms, Oct-2.4 and Oct-2.5, lack a gene activation domain at the C-terminus of the molecule (Wirth et al., 1991) and are overexpressed in neuronal cells. B cells contain predominantly the Oct-2.1 form, which contains a functional C-terminal activation domain (Lillycrop and Latchman, 1992). In experiments in which various forms are transiently transfected into cells lacking any endogenous Oct-2, both Oct-2.4 and Oct-2.5 repress the IE promoter but Oct-2.1 stimulates it (Lillycrop and Latchman, 1992). Similarly, both Oct-2.4 and Oct-2.5 can prevent *trans*-activation of the IE promoters by Vmw65 (Lillycrop et al., 1993). Moreover, BHK cells that are usually permissive can be rendered non-permissive for the HSV lytic cycle when stably transfected with Oct-2.4 or Oct-2.5 expression vectors, whereas transfection of an Oct-2.1 expression vector enhances their permissivity (Lillycrop et al., 1994a). These experiments demonstrate that Oct-2 can repress the IE promoter in neuronal cells and when artificially expressed in other cell types, resulting in a failure of the HSV lytic cycle. Its ability to do so depends on alternative splicing which produces predominantly inhibitory forms in neuronal cells.

The ability of Oct-2.4 and Oct-2.5 to inhibit the IE promoter in neuronal cells probably depends on their lack of a strong C-terminal activation domain and their inability to form a complex with the viral Vmw65 protein. This inability is mediated by differences between Oct-1 and Oct-2 in the POU domains (Gerster and Roeder, 1988; Stern et al., 1989) and should therefore be observed for all the alternatively spliced forms of Oct-2, which are identical in the POU domain region (Wirth et al., 1991; Lillycrop and Latchman, 1992). Hence Oct-2.4 and Oct-2.5 cannot activate IE gene transcription following binding to the TAATGARAT motif because they lack an activation domain and cannot recruit the strong activation domain of Vmw65 to the promoter. The binding of these proteins thus blocks activation of the promoter by the Oct-1/Vmw65 complex and therefore prevents transactivation of the IE promoter by Vmw65. In agreement with this idea, transactivation by Vmw65 can also be blocked by the isolated DNA binding POU domain of Oct-2, indicating that no regions of Oct-2 other than the DNA binding domain are required for this effect (Lillycrop et al., 1993).

Interestingly, Oct-2.4 and Oct-2.5 also strongly inhibit the basal activity of the IE promoters in the absence of Vmw65, an effect that does not appear to depend on their ability to inhibit the binding of other factors. Thus, as Oct-1 alone transactivates the IE promoter only weakly, inhibition of its binding could not explain the strong inhibitory effect of Oct-2.4 and Oct-2.5 on basal activity. Moreover, the basal activity of the IE promoter is not significantly inhibited by the isolated POU domain of Oct-2, indicating that other regions of the protein are required for this effect (Lillycrop et al., 1994b).

We have recently defined a 40 amino acid region near the N-terminus of Oct-2 which is responsible for this effect. This region acts as an independent inhibitory domain to directly repress promoter activity when linked to a heterologous DNA binding domain (Lillycrop et al., 1994b). This region is present not only in the inhibitory Oct-2.4 and Oct-2.5 forms of Oct-2 but also in the stimulatory (Oct-2.1) form. Deletion of the C-terminal activation domain from Oct-2.1 results in a strong repressor whereas deletion of the N-terminal inhibitory region results in an increase in the activating ability of Oct-2.1. Hence the presence of a functional C-terminal activation domain, as in Oct-2.1, overcomes the effect of the inhibitory domain, allowing activation of transcription. Where the activation domain is deleted, either naturally by alternative splicing (as in Oct-2.4 and Oct-2.5) or artificially (as in the C-terminal deletion mutant of Oct-2.1), the inhibitory domain will repress transcription following DNA binding. Oct-2.4 and 2.5 are thus able to inhibit IE promoter activity by two mechanisms involving passive blocking of binding of the transactivating Oct-1/Vmw65 complex to DNA and active inhibition of transcription following DNA binding.

1.4 Oct-2 is Expressed in Primary Sensory Neurons

The experiments described above show that the neuronal Oct-2 protein is responsible for the failure of IE gene expression and hence of the lytic cycle following infection of neuronal cell lines. Having demonstrated the role of Oct-2 using material available from the cell lines studied, it is necessary to confirm that Oct-2 is present in normal unimmortalized sensory neurons and so able to play a similar role in the failure of the HSV lytic cycle and consequent latent infection in sensory neurons *in vivo*. The Oct-2 mRNA is readily detectable in neuronal cells in intact dorsal root ganglia dissected directly from the animal or in primary culture, using both PCR and *in situ* hybridization (Lillycrop et al., 1991). The Oct-2 protein itself is detectable in dorsal root ganglia by DNA mobility shift assay (Wood et al., 1992).

1.5 Oct-2 and Latency

The demonstration of a role for Oct-2 in the initial establishment of latency raises the question of whether changes in its levels play a part in the reactivation of latent virus in response to specific stimuli. Does a fall in Oct-2 levels result in the release of the inhibitory effect and lead to the activation of IE gene expression and consequent reactivation of the virus?

This mechanism does appear to operate, in the case of reactivation of the virus by withdrawal of nerve growth factor (NGF). In the original demonstration of HSV latency by Cushing (1905), cutting of the trigeminal nerve in patients with neuralgia resulted in the appearance of herpetic lesions caused by reactivated virus. This reactivation is now known to be due to blockage of retrograde transport of NGF from the innervated tissue to the neuronal cell body, the presence of NGF being essential for the maintenance of viral latency (Wilcox and Johnson, 1987). We have shown that withdrawal of NGF from cultures of sensory neurons decreases the Oct-2 mRNA and protein levels with no alteration in the level of Oct-1 (Wood et al., 1992). In the absence of NGF, Oct-2 is no longer bound to the TAATGARAT motif in the promoter. The Oct-2 protein may therefore play a critical role in the maintenance as well as establishment of latency.

1.6 Implications for the Design of Gene Therapy Vectors

The ability of HSV to latently infect neuronal cells has led to the suggestion that it could be used as a vector to express genes of therapeutic benefit in neuronal cells. Although HSV has many advantages as a gene therapy vector, such as its large genome size and ability to infect non-dividing neuronal cells, its use has a major disadvantage because it can replicate lytically under certain circumstances in neuronal cells. Thus, for example, when high multiplicities of virus are used to infect either primary sensory neurons (Kennedy et al., 1983) or ND7 cells (Wheatley et al., 1990), the Oct-2 inhibitor is titrated out by the excess of TAATGARAT sequences, exactly as in the experiments where permissivity was increased by transfecting plasmids carrying TAATGARAT sequences (see above). This results in increased IE gene expression and consequent lytic infection. This lytic replication in cells of neuronal origin parallels the effect of direct HSV injection into the brain leading to lytic replication and a potentially lethal encephalitis.

The virus must be disabled to prevent it carrying out a lytic infection in either neuronal or non-neuronal cells before its use as a vector can be contemplated. Similarly, even in the case of herpes amplicon vectors which contain only a viral origin of replication and packaging signal, the helper virus that provides the viral proteins required for DNA replication and packaging must be disabled to prevent it from replicating lytically after injection (Geller et al., 1990).

Initial approaches to this problem have involved deletion of the IE gene encoding ICP4, either from the viral vector itself (Dobson et al., 1990) or from the helper virus used in conjunction with the amplicon vectors (Geller et al., 1990). As ICP4 is essential for the activation of the early and late genes (see above), this causes the lytic cycle to fail at an early stage. However, this method suffers from two disadvantages. Firstly, a stock of the resulting virus must be grown on a cell line that artificially expresses ICP4. Although this complements the defect and allows lytic growth, it also allows the possibility of recombination between the virus and the ICP4 gene in the cell line recreating a wild type virus (Geller et al., 1990). Secondly, as ICP4 is involved in the autoregulation of the other IE genes (see above), the amounts of the other IE proteins synthesized will increase following infection with virus lacking in ICP4. This may damage the infected cell, as synthesis of the IE proteins has a significant cytotoxic effect even when other viral proteins are not synthesized and the full lytic cycle does not occur (Johnson et al., 1992).

It would be preferable therefore to prevent the synthesis of all the IE proteins in parallel. One way of doing this would be to exploit the mechanism leading to the virus becoming latent in neuronal cells. It would be possible to incorporate the gene for Oct-2 under the control of a constitutive promoter into the viral vector, so inhibiting expression of the IE genes and leading to latent rather than lytic infection. Some means of eliminating the inhibitory effect of Oct-2 would be necessary when the viral vector is grown in tissue culture: this could be achieved by using cell lines expressing high amounts of Oct-1 and Vmw65 or by using plasmids containing cloned TAATGARAT sequences. Alternatively, it might be possible to express Oct-2 in the virus under the control of a promoter which could be inhibited under specific circumstances—for example, by including *lac* operator sites in the promoter and expressing the *lac* repressor in the cell line used to grow the virus.

Even if this could be achieved, it is possible that the expression of Oct-2 in the virus would have undesirable effects on Oct-2-dependent cellular genes in the cells infected by the viral vector *in vivo*. To avoid this problem, linking the 40 amino acid domain responsible for the inhibitory effect of Oct-2 (see above) to the DNA binding domain of ICP4 would result in delivery of the inhibitory domain to all the viral genes that contain ICP4 binding sites, including the other IE genes (which it normally autoregulates (Resnick et al., 1989)) and the early genes that it normally transactivates (Tedder et al., 1989). This would result in widespread inhibition of viral gene expression without affecting cellular gene expression.

Although these ideas are evidently speculative and need to be tested both *in vitro* and subsequently *in vivo*, they do indicate the manner in which an elucidation of the mechanisms mediating HSV latency may ultimately lead to the improved design of HSV vectors for gene therapy.

CONCLUSION

The work described in this chapter has involved the use of cell lines to identify a neuronal form of the Oct-2 protein as responsible for the failure of viral IE gene expression following initial infection of neuronal cells. The insights obtained using the large amounts of material available have been confirmed using the more limited amounts of material available from primary sensory neurons. Thus Oct-2 has been shown to be expressed in these cells both *in vivo* and *in vitro* and to be modulated by nerve growth factor, which is known to play a role in the maintenance of HSV latency. Without the use of neuronal cell lines, it is unlikely that a factor first identified as an activator of immunoglobulin gene expression in B lymphocytes would have been shown to act as a repressor of HSV IE gene expression in neuronal cells and to thereby play a critical role in the initiation and maintenance of latent infection with HSV. The insights thus obtained may result in improved therapy of the clinically important problem of HSV latency as well as improvements in the design of gene therapy vectors.

REFERENCES

Ace, C.I., McKee, T.A., Ryan, M., Cameron, J.M. and Preston, C.M. (1989). Construction and characterization of a herpes simplex virus type 1 mutant unable to transduce immediate-early gene expression. *J. Virol.* **63,** 2260–2269.

Anderson, K.P., Costa, R.H., Holland, L.E. and Wagner, E.K. (1980). Characterization of herpes simplex virus type 1 RNA present in the absence of de novo protein synthesis. *J. Virol.* **34,** 9–27.

Ash, R.J. (1986). Butyrate-induced reversal of herpes simplex virus restriction in neuroblastoma cells. *Virology* **155,** 584–592.

Croen, K.D., Ostrove, J.M., Dragovic, L.J., Smialek, J.E. and Straus, S.E. (1987). Latent herpes simplex virus in human trigeminal ganglia. Detection of an immediate-early gene anti-sense transcript by *in situ* hybridization. *N. Engl. J. Med.* **317,** 1422–1432.

Cushing, J. (1905). Surgical aspects of major neuralgia of trigeminal nerve. *J. Am. Med. Assoc.* **44,** 1002–1008.

Dent, C.L., Lillycrop, K.A., Estridge, J., Thomas, N.S.B. and Latchman, D.S. (1991). The B cell and neuronal forms of the octamer binding protein Oct-2 differ in DNA binding specificity and functional activity. *Mol. Cell. Biol.* **11,** 3925–3930.

Dobson, A.T., Margolis, T.P., Sedarati, F., Stevens, J.G. and Feldman, L.T. (1990). A latent nonpathogenic HSV-1-derived vector stably expresses β-galactosidase in mouse neurons. *Neuron* **5,** 353–360.

Faber, S.W. and Wilcox, K.W. (1986). Association of the herpes simplex virus regulatory protein ICP4 with specific nucleotide sequences in DNA. *Nucl. Acids Res.* **14,** 6067–6083.

Falkner, F.G., Moickat, R. and Zachau, H.G. (1986). Sequences closely related to an immunoglobulin promoter/enhancer element occur also upstream of other eukaryotic and of prokaryotic genes. *Nucl. Acids Res.* **13,** 7847–7863.

Geller, A.I., Keyomarsi, K., Bryan, J. and Pardee, A.B. (1990). An efficient deletion mutant packaging system for defective herpes simplex virus vectors: Potential applications to human gene therapy and neuronal physiology. *Proc. Natl Acad. Sci. USA.* **87,** 8950–8954.

Gelman, I.H. and Silverstein, S. (1987a). Herpes simplex virus immediate–early promoters are responsive to virus and cell *trans* acting factors. *J. Virol.* **61,** 2286–2296.

Gelman, I.H. and Silverstein, S. (1987b). Dissection of immediate–early gene promoters from herpes simplex virus: sequences that respond to virus transcriptional activation. *J. Virol.* **61,** 3167–3172.

Gerster, T. and Roeder, R.G. (1988). A herpes virus trans-activating protein interacts with transcription factor OTF-1 and other cellular proteins. *Proc. Natl Acad. Sci. USA* **85,** 6347–6351.

Goding, C.R. and O'Hare, P. (1989). Herpes simplex virus Vmw65-octamer binding protein interaction: a paradigm for combinatorial control of transcription. *Virology* **173,** 363–367.

He, X., Treacy, M.N., Simmons, D.M., Ingraham, H.A., Swanson, L.S. and Rosenfeld, M.G. (1989). Expression of a large family of POU-domain regulatory genes in mammalian brain development. *Nature* **340,** 35–42.

Honess, R.W. and Roizman, B. (1974). Regulation of herpes virus macromolecular synthesis. I. Cascade regulation of the synthesis of three groups of viral proteins. *J. Virol.* **14,** 8–19.

Johnson, P.A., Miyanohara, A., Levine, F., Cahill, T. and Friedmann, T. (1992). Cytotoxicity of a replication-defective mutant of herpes simplex virus type 1. *J. Virol.* **66,** 2952–2965.

Jones, K.A. and Tjian, R. (1985). Sp1 binds to promoter sequences and activates herpes simplex virus immediate-early gene transcription *in vitro*. *Nature* **317,** 179–182.

Katz, J., Bodin, T. and Coen, D.M. (1990). Quantitative polymerase chain reaction analysis of herpes simplex virus DNA in ganglia of mice infected with replication incompetent mutants. *J. Virol.* **64,** 4288–4295.

Kemp, L.M., Dent, C.L. and Latchman, D.S. (1990). Transcriptional repression of herpes simplex virus immediate–early genes and of octamer containing cellular promoters in neuronal cells is mediated by the octamer DNA element. *Neuron* **4,** 215–222.

Kemp, L.M. and Latchman, D.S. (1989). Regulated expression of herpes simplex virus immediate–early genes in neuroblastoma cells. *Virology* **171,** 607–610.

Kennedy, P.G.E., Clements, G.E. and Brown, S.M. (1983). Differential susceptibility of human neural cell types in culture to infection with herpes simplex virus. *Brain* **106,** 101–119.

Kristie, T.M. and Sharp, P.A. (1993). Purification of the cellular C1 factor required for the stable recognition of the Oct-1 homeodomain by the herpes simplex virus a-*trans*-induction factor (VP16). *J. Biol. Chem.* **268,** 6525–6534.

Latchman, D.S. (1990). Molecular Biology of herpes simplex virus latency. *J. Exp. Pathol.* **71,** 133–141.

Lillycrop, K.A. and Latchman, D.S. (1992). Alternative splicing of the Oct-2 transcription factor is differentially regulated in B cells and neuronal cells and results in protein isoforms with opposite effects on the activity of octamer/TAATGARAT-containing promoters. *J. Biol. Chem.* **267,** 24960–24966.

Lillycrop, K.A., Estridge, J.K. and Latchman, D.S. (1993). The octamer binding protein Oct-2 inhibits transactivation of the herpes simplex virus immediate–early genes by the virion protein Vmw65. *Virology* **196,** 888–891.

Lillycrop, K.A., Dent, C.L., Wheatley, S.C., Beech, M.N., Ninkina, N.N., Wood, J.N. and Latchman, D.S. (1991). The octamer binding protein Oct-2 represses HSV immediate–early genes in cell lines derived from latently infectable sensory neurons. *Neuron* **7,** 381–390.

Lillycrop, K.A., Budhram, V.S., Lakin, N.D., Terrenghi, G., Wood, J.N., Polak, J.M. and Latchman, D.S. (1992). A novel POU family transcription factor is closely related to Brn-3 but has a distinct expression pattern in neuronal cells. *Nucl. Acids Res.* **20,** 5093–5096.

Lillycrop, K.A., Howard, M.K., Estridge, J.K. and Latchman, D.S. (1994a). Inhibition of herpes simplex virus infection by ectopic expression of neuronal splice variants of the Oct-2 transcription factor. *Nucl. Acids Res.* **22,** 815–820.

Lillycrop, K.A., Dawson, S.J., Estridge, J.K., Gerster, T., Matthias, P. and Latchman, D.S. (1994b). Repression of a herpes simplex virus immediate-early promoter by the Oct-2 transcription factor is dependent upon an inhibitory region at the N-terminus of the protein. *Mol. Cell. Biol.* **14,** 7633–7642.

Margolis, T.P., Sedarati, F., Dobson, A.T., Feldman, L.T. and Stevens, J.G. (1992). Pathways of viral gene expression during acute neuronal infection with HSV-1. *Virology* **189,** 150–160.

Muller, M.M., Rupert, S., Schaffner, W. and Matthias, P. (1988). A cloned octamer transcription factor stimulates transcription from lymphoid-specific promoters in non-B cells. *Nature* **336,** 544–551.

O'Hare, P. and Goding, C.R. (1988). Herpes simplex virus regulatory elements and the immunoglobulin octamer domain bind a common factor and are both targets for virion transactivation. *Cell* **52,** 435–445.

O'Hare, P. and Hayward, G.S. (1985). Evidence for a direct role for both the 175,000 and 110,000 molecular weight immediate-early proteins of herpes simplex virus in the transactivation of delayed early promoters. *J. Virol.* **53,** 751–760.

Preston, C.M. (1979). Control of herpes simplex virus type 1 mRNA synthesis in cells infected with wild-type virus or the temperature sensitive mutant tsK. *J. Virol.* **29,** 275–284.

Preston, C.M., Frame, M.C. and Campbell, M.E.M. (1988). A complex formed between cell components and a herpes simplex virus structural polypeptide binds to a viral immediate–early gene regulatory DNA sequence. *Cell* **52,** 425–434.

Resnick, J., Boyd, B.A. and Haffey, M.L. (1989). DNA binding by the herpes simplex virus type 1 ICP4 protein is necessary for efficient down regulation of the ICP0 promoter. *J. Virol.* **63,** 2497–2503.

Roizman, B. and Sears, A.E. (1987). An inquiry into the mechanisms of herpes simplex virus latency. *Annu. Rev. Microbiol.* **41,** 543–571.

Sacks, W.R., Greene, C.C., Aschman, D.P. and Schaffer, P.A. (1985). Herpes simplex virus Type 1 ICP27 is an essential regulatory protein. *J. Virol.* **55,** 796–805.

Scheidereit, C., Cromlish, J.A., Gerster, T., Kawakami, K., Balmaceda, G-C., Currie, R.A. and Roeder, R.G. (1988). A human lymphoid-specific transcription factor that activates immunoglobulin genes is a homeobox protein. *Nature* **336,** 551–557.

Scholer, J.R., Hatzopoulos, A.K., Balling, R., Suzuki, N. and Gruss, P. (1989). A family of octamer-specific proteins present during mouse embryogenesis: evidence for germline-specific expression of an Oct factor. *EMBO J.* **8,** 2543–2550.

Sears, A.E., Hukkanen, V., Labow, M.A., Levine, A.J. and Roizman, B. (1991). Expression of the herpes simplex virus 1 a transinducing factor (VP16) does not induce reactivation of latent virus or prevent the establishment of latency in mice. *J. Virol.* **65,** 2929–2935.

Singh, H., Sen, R., Baltimore, D. and Sharp, P.A. (1986). A nuclear factor that binds to a conserved sequence motif in transcriptional control elements of immunoglobulin genes. *Nature* **319,** 154–158.

Speck, P.G. and Simmons, A. (1992). Synchronous appearance of antigen positive and latently infected neurons in spinal ganglia of mice infected with a virulent strain of herpes simplex virus. *J. Gen. Virol.* **73,** 1281–1285.

Staudt, L.M., Clerc, R.G., Singh, H., Le Bowitz, J.H., Sharp, P.A. and Baltimore, D. (1988). Cloning of a lymphoid-specific cDNA encoding a protein binding the regulatory octamer DNA motif. *Science* **241,** 577–580.

Stern, S., Tanaka, M. and Herr, W. (1989). The Oct-1 homeodomain directs formation of a multi-protein complex with the HSV trans-activator VP16. *Nature* **341,** 624–630.

Stevens, J.G., Wagner, E.K., Devi-Rao, G.B., Cook, M.L. and Feldman, L.T. (1987). RNA complementary to a herpes virus alpha gene mRNA is prominent in latently infected neurons. *Science* **235,** 1056–1059.

Stoykova, A.S., Steiner, S., Erselius, J.R., Hatzopoulos, A.K. and Gruss, P. (1992). Mini-Oct and Oct-2c: Two novel functionally diverse murine Oct-2 gene products are differentially expressed in the CNS. *Neuron* **8,** 541–558.

Tedder, D.G., Everett, R.D., Wilcox, K.W., Beard, P. and Pizer, L.I. (1989). ICP4-binding sites in the promoter and coding regions of the herpes simplex virus gD gene contribute to activation of *in vitro* transcription by ICP4. *J. Virol.* **63,** 2510–2520.

Vahlne, A. and Lycke, E. (1977). Herpes simplex virus infection of mouse neuroblastoma cells. *Proc. Soc. Exp. Biol. Med.* **156,** 82–87.

Vahlne, A. and Lycke, E. (1978). Herpes simplex virus infection of *in vitro* cultured neuronal cells (mouse neuroblastoma C 1300 cells). *J. Gen. Virol.* **39,** 321–332.

Valyi-Nagi, T., Deshmane, S.L., Spivack, J.G., Steiner, I., Ace, C.I., Preston, C.M. and Fraser, N.W. (1991). Investigation of herpes simplex virus type 1 (HSV-1) gene expression and DNA synthesis during the establishment of latent infection by an HSV-1 mutant in 1814 that does not replicate in mouse trigeminal ganglia. *J. Gen. Virol.* **72,** 641–649.

Watson, R.J. and Clements, J.B. (1980). A herpes simplex virus type 1 function continuously required for early and late viral RNA synthesis. *Nature* **285,** 329–330.

Watson, R.J., Preston, C.M. and Clements, J.B. (1980). Separation and characterization of herpes simplex virus type 1 immediate–early mRNAs. *J. Virol.* **31,** 42–52.

Werstuck, G.H. and Capone, J.P. (1993). An unusual cellular factor potentiates protein-DNA complex assembly between Oct-1 and Vmw65. *J. Biol. Chem.* **268,** 1272–1278.

Wheatley, S.C., Kemp, L.M., Wood, J.N. and Latchman, D.S. (1990). Cell lines derived from dorsal root ganglion neurons are non-permissive for HSV and express only the latency associated transcript following infection. *Exp. Cell. Res.* **190,** 243–246.

Wheatley, S.C., Dent, C.L., Wood, J.N. and Latchman, D.S. (1991). A cellular factor binding to the

TAATGARAT DNA sequence prevents the expression of the HSV immediate–early genes following infection of non permissive cell lines derived from dorsal root ganglion neurons. *Exp. Cell. Res.* **194,** 78–82.

Wilcox, C.L. and Johnson, E.M. (1987). Nerve growth factor deprivation results in the reactivation of latent herpes simplex virus *in vitro*. *J. Virol.* **61,** 2311–2315.

Wirth, T., Priess, A., Annweiler, A., Zwilling, S. and Oeler, B. (1991). Multiple Oct-2 isoforms are generated by alternative splicing. *Nucl. Acids Res.* **19,** 43–51.

Wood, J.N., Bevan, S.J., Coote, P., Darn, P.M., Hogan, P., Latchman, D.S., Morrison, C., Rougon, G., Theveniau, M. and Wheatley, S.C. (1990). Novel cell lines display the properties of nociceptive sensory neurons. *Proc. Roy. Soc. Ser. B* **241,** 187–194.

Wood, J.N., Lillycrop, K.A., Dent, C.L., Ninkina, N.N., Beech, M.N., Willoughby, J.J., Winter, J. and Latchman, D.S. (1992). Regulation of expression of the neuronal POU protein Oct-2 by nerve growth factor. *J. Biol. Chem.* **267,** 17787–17791.

SECTION 4

Part A: Protocols for Gene Delivery Using Helper-dependent Herpes Simplex Virus-1 Vectors

CHAPTER 11

Herpes Simplex Virus-1 Amplicons

NIZA FRENKEL AND RONIT SARID

Department of Cell Research and Immunology, Tel Aviv University, Tel Aviv 69978, Israel. Tel: 972 3 6407166; Fax: 972 3 6422046; Email: frenkeln@ccsg.tau.ac.il

1 INTRODUCTION

The HSV amplicons are defective virus vectors capable of introducing amplified foreign genes into various types of eukaryotic cells (Spaete and Frenkel, 1982; Frenkel et al., 1994). The defective viruses follow their non-defective counterparts in the ability to infect mitotic and post-mitotic cells. This makes them potentially useful vectors for use in non-dividing cells, such as nerve cells. Retrovirus vectors employed to date for gene therapy require cell division and therefore cannot be used to target neurons.

Like other herpesviruses, HSV resides latently in the host until it is reactivated to produce recurrent infections (Stevens et al., 1987; Roizman and Sears, 1990; Whitley, 1990). Latency takes place in ganglia, with the virus traveling through nerve cells from the sites of replication to the site of latency. During latency, the virus enters a benign stable state that does not alter electrophysiological properties of the cells (Stevens et al., 1975; Fukuda et al., 1983). Farkas and colleagues (1994) found no alterations in the electrophysiological properties of cholinergic and dopaminergic neurons after infection for several days with vectors derived from HSV-1. These properties of the virus have made it an attractive vector for experimentation in nerve cells *in vivo*. HSV-1 amplicon vectors were shown to be expressed in neuronal cells *in vitro* (Geller and Breakefield, 1988; Geller, 1993) and in non-dividing neurons in the adult animal *in vivo* (Kaplitt et al., 1991; Federoff et al., 1992; Ho et al., 1993).

The amplicon contains three kinds of genetic elements:

(1) Sequences that allow its propagation in bacteria, including an *E. coli* plasmid origin of replication and the ampicillin resistance gene.
(2) Sequences from HSV that support propagation of the amplicon in virus stocks. These include an HSV origin of replication—oriS or oriL (Frenkel et al., 1982; McGeoch et al., 1986) and the two HSV packaging signals—pac-1 and pac-2 located within the "a" sequence of the HSV-1 genome. The pac-1 and pac-2 signals are consensus sequences of all herpesviruses which define distance and structure of the corresponding genomic termini (Deiss and Frenkel, 1986; Deiss et al., 1986).
(3) Transcription unit. It includes a promoter element (e.g. HSV-1 IE4/5 promoter (Kwong and Frenkel, 1985) or CMV promoter (Kaplitt et al., 1991)), an expressed foreign gene and the SV40 polyadenylation site.

Such vectors have been used to demonstrate the expression of cDNAs such as the chicken

Protocols for Gene Transfer in Neuroscience: Towards Gene Therapy of Neurological Disorders
Edited by P.R. Lowenstein and L.W. Enquist

ovalbumin gene, which was efficiently expressed in rodent, monkey and human cells under the control of IE4/5 promoter (Kwong and Frenkel, 1985; reviewed by Frenkel et al., 1994). More recently, Geller and Breakefield (1988) have shown expression of β-galactosidase from an amplicon.

For their propagation, defective viruses require a helper virus encoding *trans*-acting functions, such as DNA replication genes and enzymes, virion proteins and packaging functions (Frenkel et al., 1980). The helper virus must also contain specialized functions, essential for gene expression within the target cells and tissues. Cotransfection of cells with the seed amplicon and helper virus DNA or transfection of cells with amplicon DNA and then superinfection of the cells with the helper virus results in virus stocks typically consisting of two components: (1) defective genomes containing multiple identical head-to-tail repeats of the HSV seed amplicon, probably arising by rolling circle replication; (2) helper viruses. The concatemeric defective genomes are cleaved to unit-length genomes at their cleavage/packaging signals (pac-1-pac-2 signals). Packaged defective virus particles are about 150 kb, the size of the HSV-1 genome (Vlazny et al., 1982; Deiss and Frenkel, 1986; Deiss et al., 1986); therefore defective genomes and standard genomes cannot be separated by DNA size. The virus stocks can be routinely propagated at high MOI for several passages to amplify defective to helper virus ratios. Finally, the state of the input amplicons in defective virus stocks is analysed, by restriction enzyme analyses of viral DNAs, by using marker genes to quantify the ratios of helper and defective viruses in Southern blots, or by employing β-galactosidase as an expressed marker gene (Hall et al., 1983; Sanes et al., 1983).

Stocks containing defined ratios of helper virus and amplicon can be reproduced repeatedly and may be used in experiments aimed at development of gene therapy.

The defective viruses cannot propagate and spread in the recipient cells without their helper counterparts, as documented *in vitro* using wild-type (Frenkel et al., 1980, 1982), and mutant helper viruses (Locker et al., 1982; Geller et al., 1988, 1990).

There is a limit to the repeat unit sizes that can be constructed. Amplicons with repeat units below 15 kb are stably propagated, but larger seed repeats cause random deletions and generate deleted repeats smaller than 15 kb, which are then stable (Kwong and Frenkel, 1984).

The amplicon-derived genomes replicate efficiently, having advantages over the helper virus DNA. This is because the 152 kb of HSV-1 DNA contains three origins of replication but the amplicon vectors contain one origin of replication in each repeat unit that is smaller than 15 kb (Frenkel et al., 1980; Roizman and Sears, 1990).

2 MATERIALS AND EQUIPMENT

(1) Rabbit skin cells for DNA transfection (American Type Culture Collection, Rockville, MD, USA).
(2) Vero (African Green Monkey kidney) or Hep-2 (epidermoid carcinoma) cells for virus propagation (American Type Culture Collection).
(3) DMEM (Dulbecco's Modified Minimum Eagle's Medium).
(4) Maintenance medium: DMEM supplemented with 10% inactivated fetal calf serum (IFCS inactivated by incubation for 30 min at 56°C).
(5) Versene (0.02% EDTA solution).
(6) Sterile plastic roller bottles.
(7) 199-V medium: M199 (Hank's) medium containing 1% inactivated calf serum (ICS), inactivated by heating at 56°C for 30 min, 100 U/ml penicillin and 100 mg/ml streptomycin.
(8) 199-O medium: 199-V medium plus 0.1% screened pooled human gamma globulin.
(9) Phosphate-buffered saline (PBS): 15 mM sodium phosphate, pH 7.3, 150 mM NaCl.
(10) Methanol.
(11) Giemsa stain, filtered to remove large granules present in the stain.
(12) 2× HeBS: 8.2 g NaCl, 5.95 g HEPES and 0.105 g Na_2HPO_4 in double-distilled water to a final volume of 500 ml, brought to pH 7.05 with 5 N NaOH. Sterilize by filtering through 22 μm filter. Store at −20°C.
(13) 2 M $CaCl_2$, sterilized through 22 μm filter and stored at −20°C.

(14) Stock solutions of 1 M Na_2HPO_4, 1 M NaH_2PO_4 and 1 M $MgCl_2$: prepare in double-distilled water and store at room temperature.
(15) Stock solutions of 50 mM potassium ferricyanide ($K_3Fe(CN)_6$) and 50 mM potassium ferrocyanide ($K_4Fe(CN)_6$), prepared in double-distilled water and stored in foil-wrapped glassware (in the dark) at 4°C. Solutions are stable for at least 3 months in these conditions.
(16) X-gal stock: dissolve in *N*,*N*-dimethyl formamide at 20 mg/ml and store in a glass container (not polycarbonate or polystyrene) in the dark at −20°C.
(17) 4% paraformaldehyde: in a fume hood, dissolve 8 g paraformaldehyde powder in 150 ml 0.1 M sodium phosphate, pH 7.3 (80 mM Na_2HPO_4, 20 mM NaH_2PO_4) while stirring and heating to 60°C. Add 10 N NaOH at a rate of 1 drop per minute until the solution clears. Bring the volume to 200 ml with 0.1 M sodium phosphate, pH 7.3. Store at 4°C for up to 1 month.

! WEAR A MASK AND GLOVES WHEN HANDLING PARAFORMALDEHYDE !

(18) Working fixative (2% paraformaldehyde; 0.2% glutaraldehyde in 0.1 M sodium phosphate): combine 50 ml 4% paraformaldehyde with 49.2 ml 0.1 M sodium phosphate, pH 7.3, and 0.8 ml 25% glutaraldehyde. This may be stored at 4°C for up to 1 week.
(19) X-gal stain: 100 mM sodium phosphate, pH 7.3 (80 mM Na_2HPO_4, 20 mM NaH_2PO_4), 1.3 mM $MgCl_2$, 3 mM $K_3Fe(CN)_6$, 3 mM $K_4Fe(CN)_6$ and 1 mg/ml X-gal. Filter through a 0.45 μm disposable filtration unit before use.

3 THE PROTOCOLS

Protocol #55: HSV-1 Propagation and Titration

(1) Grow Hep-2 cells to confluence (as assessed by microscopy) in 10 roller bottles using DMEM with 10% IFCS. Each roller bottle should contain about 2×10^8 cells.
(2) Remove the medium. Add the virus inoculum at 0.01 p.f.u./cell in 10 ml 199-V medium. Determine the amount of plaque-purified "mother pool" virus required for the inoculum as follows:

Total p.f.u. to be used for each roller bottle = 2×10^8 cells/bottle × 0.01 p.f.u./cell
Volume of "mother pool" required to give MOI of 0.01 = total p.f.u./stock titer (p.f.u./ml)

(3) Incubate infected bottles at 37°C for 2 h to allow adsorption of the virus.
(4) Remove inoculum and replace with 50–100 ml 199-V medium.
(5) Incubate 3–5 days at 37°C, or until the cells are easily removed from the culture substrate by vigorous shaking and scraping.
(6) Scrape the infected cells into the medium and decant into conical centrifuge tubes.
(7) Centrifuge at 1500 r.p.m. for 10 min at 5°C.
(8) The supernatant contains virus that has been released from the cells. The pellet contains large amounts of infectious virus. Decant the medium into sterile containers.
(9) Resuspend each pellet in 2.5 ml the decanted spent medium.
(10) Freeze and thaw the suspended pellet three times by transferring between freezer at −80°C and water bath at 37°C to break down the remaining intact cells and facilitate release of virus.
(11) Freeze aliquots of the suspension at −80°C.

Protocol #56: Titration of Infectious HSV-1

(1) Thaw the virus to be titrated in a 37°C water bath until the ice just melts. Keep in ice.
(2) Serially dilute virus stocks by diluting 10 μl in 1 ml 199-V (10^{-2} dilution) and then by consecutive 10-fold dilution steps (200 μl plus 1800 μl 199-V). Dilutions in the range 10^{-6}–10^{-8} are appropriate for most virus stocks.
(3) Decant the medium and apply 1 ml of diluted virus to the Vero cells. Ensure that the flasks are level surface to allow the inoculum to spread evenly.
(4) Allow the virus to adsorb for 2 h at 37°C. Adsorption of *ts* mutants should also be at the appropriate temperature.
(5) Remove the inoculum, rinse the cells with 1–2 ml 199-O medium and overlay the plates with 5 ml 199-O medium.

(6) Incubate at 37°C for 2–3 days.
(7) After 2–3 days incubation stain with Giemsa thus. Remove medium from flask. Rinse the cells with 10 ml PBS, taking care not to disrupt the monolayer of infected cells. Carefully fix the monolayer by adding 5 ml methanol, letting it stand for 5 min then discarding the methanol. Add 5 ml Giemsa stain and leave on monolayer for 10–20 min, making sure that the stain is not too intense. Rinse monolayer twice in water.
(8) When the monolayer is dry, count plaques using a stereomicroscope. Count the dilutions giving separate and distinct plaques. Between 10 and 300 plaques per 25 cm^3 flask are appropriate for good statistics (counting error is related to the square root of the number of plaques).

Protocol #57: DNA Transfection of Rabbit Skin Cells

(1) Prepare rabbit skin cell cultures in 25 cm^2 flasks.
(2) Decant medium and overlay with fresh maintenance medium.
(3) Prepare the transfection mixture (DNA/calcium precipitate). Specifically, for each transfection prepare two sterile Eppendorf tubes, one containing 250 μl 2 × HeBS, the second (which is kept cold in ice) containing 30 μl 2 M $CaCl_2$, DNA and double-distilled water to a final volume of 250 μl. Combine the contents of the two tubes, mix gently (do not vortex) and allow precipitate to form at room temperature for 20 min.
(4) Apply transfection mixture directly to the middle of the rabbit skin cells monolayer and ensure that it is uniformly distributed.
(5) Incubate at 37°C for 4–6 h.
(6) Remove the medium and add 2 ml DMEM containing 10% glycerol.
(7) Incubate 1 min and quickly remove the medium (prolonged exposure to glycerol is toxic to cells).
(8) Rinse twice with DMEM.
(9) Overlay with maintenance medium.
(10) Incubate 4–5 days, or until the viral infection has spread throughout the culture.

Protocol #58: X-Gal Histochemical Reaction to Detect Defective Amplicon HSV-1 Viruses Expressing the *E. coli lac* Gene

(1) Remove medium from monolayers infected with virus stock.
(2) Rinse monolayer twice with PBS.
(3) Overlay with the working fixative solution. Incubate at 4°C for 5 min.
(4) Remove fixative and rinse twice with PBS at room temperature.
(5) Remove PBS and overlay the fixed cells with the X-gal stain. Incubate at 37°C until blue color develops (between 30 min and overnight).

4 NOTES AND TROUBLESHOOTING

4.1 On Protocol #55: HSV-1 Propagation and Titration

Virus stocks are produced by infection of Hep-2 cells at low MOI (0.01 p.f.u/cell) to avoid generation of defective viruses and viral variants. "First passage viral pools" are set aside and are not multiply passaged. Instead, they are used to generate multiple stocks of "mother pools" from which the virus for infection experiments is generated.

To enhance adsorption of virus to the cells, the inoculum volume is kept low (10 ml per roller bottle).

It is important to keep a record of what has been done, including name of infecting virus, name of virus generated, number of bottles infected, cell type used, dates of infection and harvest, volume used, plaque titer and temperature used.

4.2 On Protocol #56: Titration of Infectious HSV-1

The titration assay uses Vero cells grown to confluence in 25 cm^3 flasks. For each virus assayed six flasks are required (if a *ts* mutant is being titrated, 12 flasks are necessary—six for incubation at the permissive temperature and six for incubation at the non-permissive temperature). The virus under investigation is serially diluted. Duplicate tubes and plates at dilutions of 10^{-6}, 10^{-7}, 10^{-8} are used in the infectious virus plaque assay.

It is critical to change pipettes or tips at each dilution to prevent carryover of virus and anomalous high titers. Briefly vortex each tube before using the virus and after each dilution and pipette up and down in the tube to remove viruses adhering to the plastic.

4.3 On Protocol #57: DNA Transfection of Rabbit Skin Cells

Mixtures of plasmid DNA and HSV-1 helper virus DNA are used to transfect rabbit skin cells in 25 cm^2 flasks by the calcium-phosphate coprecipitation technique (Graham and van der Eb, 1973; Gorman et al., 1982). Transfection efficiencies should be determined by estimating the proportion of blue cells/total cells after transfecting with plasmid containing β-galactosidase driven by adequate promoter (alternatively, amplicon DNA can be transfected followed by superinfection with the helper virus). The derived virus stocks are harvested by three cycles of freeze–thawing (−80°C/37°C). The virus stocks derived from the cotransfection or transfection–superinfection (passage 0) are serially passaged, taking a fixed ratio for each passage (e.g. 1 : 4 dilution) in Vero or Hep-2 cells to generate virus stock passages. Propagation continues while determining the ratio of defective to helper virus in each passage. The number of passages needed depends on the amplicon and helper virus employed. The choice of passage to be used as constructed amplicon stock depends on the amount of foreign gene expression aimed. Concentration of helper virus is determined by titration plaque assay. Defective virus may be assayed in culture using histochemical detection of bacterial β-galactosidase—each blue cell is considered to represent one infectious defective virion.

Amplicon propagation could begin with cotransfection of the cells with amplicon and helper virus DNA, or could involve transfection of the cells with amplicon DNA followed by superinfection with the helper virus. For transfection–superinfection begin by transfecting the cells with amplicon DNA and follow by infection with the helper virus at a MOI of 1 p.f.u./cell. Incubate in 199-V medium.

ACKNOWLEDGMENTS

We thank The Israel Science Foundation, administered by the Israel Academy of Sciences and Humanities, Israel Health Ministry and the Wolfson Foundation for support.

REFERENCES

Deiss, L.P. and N. Frenkel. 1986. The herpes simplex amplicon: cleavage of concatemeric DNA is linked to packaging and involves the amplification of the terminally reiterated a sequence. *J. Virol.* **57:** 933–941.

Deiss, L.P., Chou, J. and N. Frenkel. 1986. Functional domains within the sequence involved in the cleavage-packaging of herpes simplex virus DNA. *J. Virol.* **59:** 605–618.

Farkas, R.H., S. Nakajima and Y. Nakajima. 1994. Cultured neurons infected with an HSV-1-derived vector remain electrically excitable and responsive to neurotransmitter. *Neurosci. Lett.* **165:** 153–156.

Federoff, H.J., M.D. Geschwind, A.I. Geller and J.A. Kessler. 1992. Expression of nerve growth factor *in vivo* from a defective herpes simplex virus 1 vector prevents effects of axotomy on sympathetic ganglia. *Proc. Natl Acad. Sci. USA* **89:** 1636–1640.

Frenkel, N., H. Locker and D.A. Vlazny. 1980. Studies of defective herpes simplex viruses. *Ann. N Y Acad. Sci.* **354:** 347–370.

Frenkel, N., R.R. Spaete, D.A. Vlazny, L. Deiss and H. Locker. 1982. The herpes simplex virus amplicon—A novel animal virus cloning vector. In: Gluzman, Y. (ed): *Eukaryotic viral vectors.* Cold Spring Harbor: Cold Spring Harbor Laboratory, p.205.

Frenkel, N., O. Singer and A.D. Kwong. 1994. Minireview: The Herpes simplex virus amplicon—a versatile defective virus vector. *Gene Ther.*, **1:** 537–546.

Fukuda, J., I. Kurata, A. Yamamoto and K. Yamaguchi. 1983. Morphological and physiological studies on cultured nerve cells from guinea pigs infected with herpes simplex virus in vivo. *Brain Res.* **262:** 79–89.

Geller, A.I. and X.O. Breakefield. 1988. A defective HSV-1 vector expresses *Escherichia coli* β-galactosidase in cultured peripheral neurons. *Science* **241:** 1667–1669.

Geller, A.I., K. Keyomarsi, J. Bryan and A.B. Pardee. 1990. An efficient deletion mutant packaging system for defective herpes simplex virus vectors: Potential applications to human gene therapy and neuronal physiology. *Proc. Natl Acad. Sci. USA* **87:** 8950–8954.

Geller, A.I. 1993. Herpesviruses: expression of genes in postmitotic brain cells. *Curr. Opin. Genet. Dev.* **3:** 81–85.

Gorman, C.M., G.T. Merlino, M.C. Willingham, I. Pastan and B.H. Howard. 1982. The Rous sarcoma virus long terminal repeat is a strong promoter when introduced into a variety of eukaryotic cells by DNA mediate transfection. *Proc. Natl Acad. Sci. USA* **79:** 6777–6781.

Graham, F.L. and A.J. van der Eb. 1973. A new technique for the assay of infectivity of human adenovirus 5 DNA. *Virology* **52:** 456–467.

Hall, C.V., P.E. Jacob, G.M. Ringold, and F. Lee. 1983. Expression and regulation of *Escherichia coli lacZ* gene fusions in mammalian cells. *J. Mol. Appl. Genet.* **2:** 101–109.

Ho, D.Y., E.S. Mocarski and R.M. Sapolsky. 1993. Altering central nervous system physiology with a defective herpes simplex virus vector expressing the glucose transporter gene. *Proc. Natl Acad. Sci. USA* **90:** 3655–3659.

Kaplitt, M.G., J.G. Pfaus, S.P. Kleopoulos, B.A. Hanlon, S.D. Rabkin and D.W. Pfaff. 1991. Expression of a functional foreign gene in adult mammalian brain following in vivo transfer via a herpes simplex virus type 1 defective viral vector. *Mol. Cell. Neurosci.* **2:** 320–330.

Kwong, A.D. and Frenkel, N. 1984. Herpes simplex virus amplicon: Effect of size on replication of constructed defective genomes containing eukaryotic DNA sequences. *J. Virol.* **51:** 595–603.

Kwong, A.D. and N. Frenkel. 1985. The herpes simplex virus amplicon IV. Efficient expression of a chimeric chicken ovalbumin gene amplified within defective virus genomes. *Virology* **142:** 421–425.

Locker, H., N. Frenkel and I. Halliburton. 1982. Structure and expression of class II defective herpes simplex virus genomes encoding infected cell polypeptide number 8. *J. Virol.* **43:** 574–593.

McGeoch, D.J., A. Dolan, S. Donald and D.H.K. Brauer. 1986. Complete nucleotide sequence of the short repeat region in the genome of herpes simplex virus type 1. *J. Gen. Virol.* **71:** 125–132.

Roizman, B. and Sears, A.E. 1990. Herpes simplex viruses and their replication. In: Fields, B.N., D.M. Knipe, R.M. Chanock et al. (eds.) *Virology*, 2nd edn. New York: Raven Press, pp.1795–1841.

Sanes, J.R., J.L.R. Rubenstein and J.F. Nicolas. 1983. Use of a recombinant retrovirus to study post-implantation cell lineage in mouse embryos. *EMBO J.* **5:** 3133–3142.

Spaete, R.R. and N. Frenkel. 1982. The herpes simplex virus amplicon: A new eukaryotic defective-virus cloning–amplifying vector. *Cell* **30:** 295–304.

Stevens, J.G., M.L. Cook and M.C. Jordan. 1975. Reactivation of latent herpes simplex virus after pneumococcal pneumonia in mice. *Infect Immun.* **11:** 635–639.

Stevens, J.G., E. Wagner, O. Devi-Rao, M. Codi and L. Feldman. 1987. RNA complementary to a herpesvirus alpha mRNA is prominent in latently infected neurons. *Science* **235:** 1056–1059.

Vlazny, D.A., A.D. Kwong, and N. Frenkel. 1982. Site specific cleavage/packaging of herpes simplex virus DNA and the selective maturation of nucleocapsids containing full length viral DNA. *Proc. Natl Acad. Sci. USA* **79:** 1423–1427.

Whitley, R.J. 1990. Herpes simplex viruses. In: Fields, B.N., D.M. Knipe, R.M. Chanock et al. (eds.) *Virology*. 2nd edn. New York: Raven Press, pp.1843–1887.

CHAPTER 12

The Use of Herpes Simplex Virus 1 for Gene Transfer into *in vitro* Maintained Brain Slices

HOWARD J. FEDEROFF, BHASKAR MUKHERJEE* AND PETER BERGOLD†

Department of Neurology, University of Rochester Medical Center, Box 673, 601 Elmwood Avenue, Rochester, NY 14642, USA. Tel: 716 273 4851; Fax: 716 442 6646; Email: hfed@medinfo.rochester.edu.

**Department of Medicine, Albert Einstein College of Medicine, 1300 Morris Park Avenue, Bronx, NY 14061, USA.*

†Department of Pharmacology, SUNY Downstate, NY, USA

1 INTRODUCTION

The wild-type herpes simplex virus type-1 (HSV-1) genome is approximately 150 kb and two strategies have been developed to utilize the virus as a vehicle for gene transfer. The first, the recombinant virus vector, incorporates a heterologous transcription unit into a full-length genome (Shih et al., 1984; Palella et al., 1988; Dobson et al., 1990; Fink et al., 1992; see also Chapters 14, 15, 16, this book). The second, the amplicon virus vector, is a eukaryotic expression plasmid that has been modified by the addition of an HSV origin of DNA replication (Fig. 12.1, *ori*) and an HSV DNA cleavage/packaging site (Fig. 12.1, *pac*). The cloning of the *ori* and *pac* sequences in *cis* allows the amplicon vector to be replicated and packaged into virions when supplied with these enzymatic functions by a copropagated helper virus (Frenkel et al., 1981, 1982; Stow and McMonagle, 1982; Geller and Breakefield, 1988). This chapter will present methods for the growth and use of HSV amplicon vectors, with particular emphasis on use for infecting hippocampal brain slices.

Amplicon vectors can be constructed to contain different types of transcription units. The promoter may be of viral or cellular origin and the expressed sequence a cDNA or gene (Federoff et al., 1992; Bergold et al., 1993). Multiple transcription units (Greenlund et al., 1993), as well as bicistronic transcription units driven by a single promoter (Hartnick et al., 1994), can be accommodated. Owing to the requirement for a nearly full-length genome size (approx. 150 kb) to be cleaved and incorporated into a virion the amplicon vector is packaged in a concatenated form. For example, approximately 15 unit lengths of a 10 kb amplicon will be packaged into a single viral particle.

Replication-defective amplicon virus stocks are best produced by use of a complementing cell line and helper virus (DeLuca et al., 1985; DeLuca and Schaffer, 1987; Geller and Breakefield, 1988; Geller et al., 1990; Kaplitt et al., 1991, 1994). The HSV-1 helper virus has been made replication defective by deletion of the essential immediate–early 3 gene (IE3; also called ICP4 or

Protocols for Gene Transfer in Neuroscience: Towards Gene Therapy of Neurological Disorders
Edited by P.R. Lowenstein and L.W. Enquist

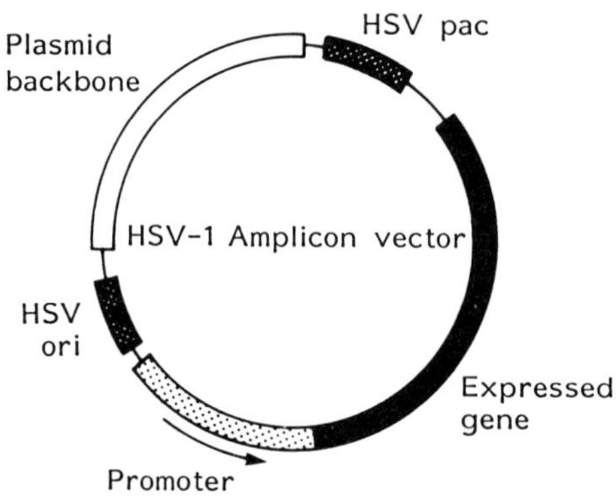

Figure 12.1 Structure of an HSV amplicon vector. The amplicon vector consists of a plasmid backbone composed of a β-lactamase gene and *Col*E1 origin of replication, HSV origin of replication (HSV *ori*), a promoter, expressed gene and an HSV cleavage and packaging site (HSV *pac*)

Table 12.1 HSV-1 Helper viruses and complementing cell lines

Virus/Cells	*Reference*
Helper virus	
*D30 EBA	Paterson and Everett, 1990
dl 120	DeLuca et al., 1985
Cell lines	
M64A (BHK)	Paterson and Everett, 1990
*RR1 (BHK)	Johnson et al., 1992
E5 (Vero)	DeLuca et al., 1985

*Helper virus and cell line described in this chapter

Vmw175). It will grow only on stably transfected cell lines that express the complementing IE3 gene. Several IE3Δ HSV-1 viruses and complementing cell lines have been described (Table 12.1). More extensive deletion of IE3 gene sequences within the helper virus is preferred as it reduces the frequency of recombination with the integrated IE3 gene that results in wild-type virus generation.

Amplicon vectors can be used to produce focal infections in the brain and in organotypic slice cultures prepared from brain (Bergold et al., 1993; Casaccia-Bonnefil et al., 1993a). In our studies organotypic cultures were prepared from the neonatal rat hippocampus. These cultures continue to develop *in vitro* (Gahwiler, 1984; Zimmer and Gahwiler, 1984, 1987; Frotscher and Gahwiler, 1988) and can be maintained for up to 6 weeks (Gahwiler, 1981; Stoppini et el., 1991). Synaptic neurotransmission in slice cultures is similar to that observed in acute slices. Slices placed in culture are deafferented and the loss of these connections, and the relative immaturity of the slice at time of culture, results in a variable degree of aberrant synaptogenesis (Gahwiler, 1984; Zimmer and Gahwiler, 1984, 1987; Frotscher and Gahwiler, 1988), depending on how the slice cultures are prepared. The methods described here tend to reduce variability and have facilitated studies with HSV amplicons that transduce ionotropic glutamate receptor genes.

In the HSV microapplication technique localized gene transfer is accomplished by extracellular application of nanoliter volumes of HSV vector stocks to slice cultures. Localized gene transduction is the direct result of the high virus titer and efficient infectivity of HSV vectors. Amplicon HSV vector stocks contain 10^{6}–10^{7} recombinant virions so even nanoliter amounts of virus stocks contain hundreds of virions. As HSV vectors transduce and express genes with high efficiency, small numbers of virions can be applied successfully. Over 80% of HSV virions applied to slice cultures successfully transduce and express genes. Microapplication of 10 nl of virus stock containing 10–12 HSVlac virions resulted in 8–10 transduced cells. Similar efficiencies were observed with 10–250 recombinant HSV virions.

HSV vectors avidly attach to cells at the site of microapplication, causing tight clustering of transduced cells. The amount of clustering depends on the volume applied, smaller volumes resulting in more clustering. Hippocampal slice cultures retain the characteristic laminar structure of the hippocampus and clustering of transduced cells results in gene transduction to specific hippocampal regions. Multiple applications to the same culture may be performed if extra transduced cells are required. Expression of transduced genes can be extremely rapid using HSV vectors: using vectors containing HSV IE promoters transcripts of the transduced gene accumulate within 2 h of application (Bergold et al., 1993; Casaccia-Bonnefil et al., 1993a). Other promoters can be used to achieve slower accumulation of gene product and to target specific cell types.

Using methods similar to those described below for hippocampus, organotypic slice cultures have been prepared from other brain regions (Stoppini et al., 1991; Yammato et al., 1992; Rothstein et al., 1994). Such cultures have been used to study synaptic plasticity (Thomson and Gahwiler, 1989; Stoppini et al., 1991; Muller et al., 1993), epileptogenesis (Shin et al., 1992), modulation of ion channels (Thomson and Gahwiler, 1989), process outgrowth (Yammato et al., 1992) and neurotoxicity (Benedikz et al., 1993; Casaccia-Bonnefil et al., 1993b; Rothstein et al., 1994). Many genes have been successfully expressed using HSV vectors, suggesting that microapplication of HSV vectors to organotypic slice cultures will be useful for a variety of neurobiological studies.

2 MATERIALS AND EQUIPMENT

(1) Helper virus: D30 EBA (Paterson and Everett, 1990) and dl120 (DeLuca et al., 1985) are all HSV-1 mutants defective for expression of the IE gene ICP4.
(2) Helper cell lines: M64A (BHK) cells (Paterson and Everett, 1990); RR1 (BHK) cells (Johnson et al., 1992) and E5 (Vero) cells (DeLuca et al., 1985). These cell lines contain the HSV-1 ICP4 gene and express it on HSV-1 infection.
(3) Culture media: Dulbecco's minimal essential medium (DMEM) supplemented as described in the protocols. Medium for helper cell line propagation is 1 × DMEM containing high glucose (4.5 g/l), 10% fetal calf serum, 1% penicillin/streptomycin and 400 μg/ml of bioactive geneticin (G418, Gibco, Grand Island, NY, USA).
(4) Cup sonicator (Heat Systems, Inc., Farmingdale, NY, USA).
(5) Low melting agarose (#A9414, Sigma, St Louis, MO, USA)
(6) Lipofectin (Gibco–BRL)
(7) Neutral Red solution (Sigma N2889)
(8) McIlwain tissue chopper (Brinkman, Westbury, NY).
(9) Gey's balanced salt solution (Gibco) supplemented with 25 mM HEPES (pH 7.2) and glucose (6.5 mg/ml).
(10) Millicell CM filters (Millipore, Bedford, MA).
(11) Six-well culture dishes (Falcon #3046).
(12) Slice culture medium: 50% Eagle's basal medium, 25% horse serum, 25% Earle's balanced salt solution, 1 mM glutamine, glucose 6.5 mg/ml, 25 mM HEPES, pH 7.2).
(13) Mitotic cells elimination medium: slice culture medium containing 100 nM 5′-fluorodeoxyuridine, 100 nM cytosine arabinoside, 100 nM uridine (Sigma).
(14) Glass capillaries, 0.8 mm (Kimble Glass Inc., Vineland, NJ).
(15) Mineral oil (Squibb)
(16) Standard inverted microscope (model TMS, Nikon)
(17) Vibrationless table (Kinetic Systems) Alternatively, the microapplication apparatus can be placed on a marble slab 60 × 90 × 7 cm positioned on 18 equally spaced squash balls (Casaccia-Bonnefil et al., 1993a).
(18) Manual micromanipulator (Narishige, Tokyo, Japan).

3 THE PROTOCOLS

Protocol #59: Cell Growth and Preparation of Helper HSV-1 Virus

(1) Maintain RR1 cells in DMEM with all supplements including G418 at 37°C in an atmosphere containing 5% carbon dioxide and 95% air.
(2) Passage cells before reaching confluence, typically at 1:4. For all steps involving virus production, grow cells as above but in the absence of G418.
(3) Prepare D30 EBA helper virus by infecting nearly confluent RR1 cells at an MOI of 0.1.
(4) Add virus in approximately 100 μl to a 60 mm plate and rock the plate to obtain adequate coverage of virus over the monolayer.
(5) After 1 h add 5 ml DMEM (with 5% FCS, 1% penicillin/streptomycin) and incubate at 34°C for 2–3 days until more than 95% of cells display a rounded-up appearance (cytopathic effect, CPE).
(6) Place the cells at 37°C for 1–2 h to increase release of virus.
(7) Scrape the cells into the medium, rotating the plate three or four times to insure all areas are removed from the plate.
(8) Collect the cell suspension in a 15 ml polypropylene conical tube and quick-freeze in a dry ice/ethanol bath (virus can be left at −70°C at this stage).
(9) Thaw virus at 34°C and sonicate five times in 30 s bursts using a cup sonicator (Heat Systems, setting 6–8) cooled with circulating ice-cold water.
(10) Spin down cellular debris at 1200 r.p.m. for 10 min.
(11) Aliquot supernatant (25–100 μl) and freeze in dry ice/ethanol.
(12) Titer helper virus on RR1 cells as described in Protocol #62.

Protocol #60: Production of HSV-1 Amplicon Viral Stocks

Transfection of RR1 Cells with Amplicon DNA: Day 1

(1) Plate 3 × 10^6 RR1 cells in medium containing 10% FCS.
(2) Ethanol precipitate DNA. In a sterile tube add 30 μg amplicon DNA, 0.1 volume 3 M sodium acetate and 2 volumes of ethanol. Place at −70°C for 15 min.
(3) Spin at maximum speed in a microfuge at 4°C to collect precipitate.
(4) Wash pellet with 70% ethanol to remove salt and invert in a tissue culture hood for 15 min to remove trace ethanol.
(5) Resuspend pellet in 30 μl of sterile water.
(6) Four hours after plating the cells, remove medium and wash twice with 2 ml serum-free medium (SFM).
(7) After washing, add 2 ml SFM to each plate.
(8) To each plate add 40 μl lipofectin and rotate plate to disperse.
(9) Place plate in tissue culture hood for 5 min.
(10) Add amplicon DNA solution from Step 5 dropwise to each plate.
(11) Rotate gently and return to incubator at 34°C.
(12) After 6 h in the incubator add 2 ml medium containing 10% FCS to each plate and return to incubator.

Superinfection of Transfected Cells: Day 2

(1) Approximately 20 h after starting the transfection, remove all but about 1 ml of medium from each plate.
(2) Add D30 EBA virus in 50–100 μl to achieve a MOI of 0.2. Rotate plate to distribute virus four times over the next hour.
(3) Add 5 ml complete medium with 5% FCS to each plate and incubate at 34°C.

Harvest Virus Stock: Days 3 and 4

(1) Monitor the superinfected cells for CPE. Within 2 days of adding the helper virus more than 95% of cells should be rounded up.
(2) When CPE is about 95%, incubate plates at 37°C for 2 h.
(3) Remove medium from each plate and save in a sterile polypropylene tube.
(4) Scrape the remaining cells from each plate and pool with the medium collected in Step 3.
(5) Freeze tube containing cell suspension and medium in a dry ice/ethanol bath for 5 min.
(6) Store at −70°C overnight.
(7) Plate fresh RR1 cells in 60 mm plates at a density of 4×10^6 cells/plate.

Sonication and Repassaging: Day 5

(1) Thaw virus stocks at 34°C.
(2) Sonicate five times using 30 s bursts in a cup sonicator (Heat Systems, setting 6–8) cooled with circulating ice-cold water.
(3) Spin down cellular debris at 1200 r.p.m. for 10 min. Save the supernatant.
(4) Remove all but about 1 ml of media from the RR1 cells plated the previous day.
(5) Warm the viral supernatants to 34°C and add to the RR1 plates,
(6) Return plates to incubator at 34°C.

Harvesting the Final Virus Stock: Days 6 and 7

(1) Monitor the infected cells and harvest when more than 95% of cells show CPE.
(2) Sonicate as described in Step 2 for Day 5.
(3) Spin down cellular debris at 1200 r.p.m. for 10 min.
(4) Save the supernatant and freeze in dry-ice/ethanol bath.
(5) Store stocks at −70°C.

Protocol #61: Titering an HSV-1 Amplicon that Expresses β-Galactosidase

(1) Plate Vero cells or NIH 3T3 cells at 1×10^6 cells per 35 mm dish in their usual growth medium.
(2) Apply (in duplicate) increasing volumes of HSV amplicon containing the *lacZ* reporter gene. Typically this will range from 1 μl to 150 μl.
(3) Twenty-four hours after infection, fix cells and stain with X-gal using standard methods.
(4) Count the number of X-gal$^+$ (blue) cells. The titer is expressed as the number of blue units forming per ml.

Protocol #62: Titering the HSV-1 Helper Virus Component

Titer the D30 EBA helper virus or similar helper virus by plaque assay on RR1 cells.

(1) RR1 are plated at 1×10^6 cells per 35 mm dish in DMEM containing 10% FCS.
(2) Make dilutions of the amplicon stocks to cover a range of 10^{-3} to 10^{-8}. Prepare dilutions in medium (5% FCS) in a volume of 500 μl.
(3) Approximately 12–20 h after plating the RR1 cells, remove the medium and add virus to each plate. Rotate to spread virus inoculum evenly over the monolayer.
(4) Return plates to incubator at 37°C.
(5) Prepare 100 ml of 2% low-melting agarose in sterile water and heat until molten.
(6) Place melted agarose in a 42°C water bath for 15 min.
(7) Approximately 45 min after returning the plates to the incubator, prepare in the hood 100 ml 2× DMEM with 20% FCS and 2% penicillin/streptomycin.
(8) Warm prepared media in a 42°C water bath for 10 min.
(9) Mix 2× DMEM with 2% low-melting agarose solution in hood. Place a sterile thermometer in the mixture.

(10) After 1 h, remove plates from incubator and remove medium (this contains the virus).
(11) Wash monolayers with fresh medium and add 2 ml of the DMEM–agarose mixture by pipetting down the side of the dish. Gently swirl to cover the entire surface. Let the agarose solidify in tissue culture hood before returning plates to the incubator at 37°C.
(12) The next day, add 2 ml Neutral Red solution (Sigma N2889, diluted 1:100 in DMEM) to each plate. Cover plates in aluminum foil and return to the incubator.
(13) Count plaques (clear areas in a lawn of red cells). To obtain statistically relevant titers, count plates that have 10–100 plaques (counting error is related to the square root of the number of plaques).
(14) Titer the wild-type recombinant viruses in each stock by repeating this protocol using non-complementing Vero cells or BHK cells.

Protocol #63: Purification and Concentration of HSV-1 Amplicon Stocks

(1) In a sterile chilled swing-bucket centrifuge tubes (SW41), pipette 2 ml 25% sucrose in PBS (containing calcium and magnesium, filter sterilized).
(2) Overlay viral stock. Use medium to achieve optimal volume and balance.
(3) Centrifuge at 25 000 r.p.m., 4°C, for 16–18 h.
(4) Open centrifuge buckets in hood. Mark location of the viral pellet.
(5) Remove medium and sucrose with a sterile pipette. Remove residual liquid with sterile Pasteur pipette, taking care not to disturb the virus pellet.
(6) Resuspend the virus pellet by first overlaying it with ice-cold PBS (containing calcium and magnesium): 0.01 volumes for *in vivo* use or 0.5 volumes for tissue culture experiments.
(7) Let tubes sit on ice for 2 h in hood and then resuspend pellet by gently pipetting for 2 min, every 30 min, for a further 2 h.
(8) Aliquot pellet suspension in sterile tubes appropriate for the experiment planned. Freeze aliquots in a dry-ice/ethanol bath. For example, we freeze concentrated virus for *in vivo* use in 7–10 μl aliquots.
(9) Store aliquots at -70°C.

Protocol #64: Preparation of Organotypic Hippocampal Slice Cultures

This protocol is modified from the method of Stoppini et al. (1991).

(1) Anesthetize 9–11-day-old Sprague-Dawley rats by intraperitoneal injection of ketamine (0.1 mg/animal) and decapitate the animals.
(2) Remove the brains and dissect in ice-cold Gey's balanced salt solution supplemented with 25 mM HEPES (pH 7.2) and glucose (6.5 mg/ml).
(3) Cut the hippocampi into 400 μm transverse slices using a McIlwain tissue chopper.
(4) Incubate the slices at 4°C for 1 h in Gey's balanced salt solution. Plate only those slices having smooth edges and well defined neuronal layers.
(5) Plate two slices at least 3 mm apart on Millicell CM filters.
(6) Place the insert into six-well culture dishes containing 1 ml slice culture medium.
(7) Maintain the slices at 35°C in a 95% air, 5% CO_2 atmosphere.
(8) After 4–5 days in culture, eliminate mitotic cells by transferring slices for 24 h to mitotic cells elimination medium.
(9) After antimitotic treatment feed the cultures with slice culture medium every 3–5 days. About 70–80% of slice cultures containing a continuous stratum pyramidale will be used for HSV infection.

Protocol #65: Gene Transfer into Hippocampal Slice Cultures with HSV-1 Amplicon Stocks

Slice cultures can be transduced with HSV vectors at any time after culture preparation. Microliter quantities of HSV viral stock will be applied to slice cultures, using a manually driven microapplication apparatus.

(1) Fill 0.8 mm glass capillaries with mineral oil and back-fill the capillary with 1–2 μl HSV virus stocks by aspiration.
(2) Attach the micropipettes using oil-filled rigid plastic tubing to an airtight oil-filled 50 μl Hamilton syringe. Attach a micrometer to the plunger of the syringe to enable regulation of the volume to be delivered.
(3) To avoid vibration, place the microinjection apparatus and a standard inverted microscope on a vibrationless table or on a marble slab (60 × 90 × 7 cm) positioned on 18 equally spaced squash balls (Casaccia-Bonnefil et al., 1993a).
(4) Calibrate the microapplication apparatus by measuring the number of micrometer increments necessary to deliver a known volume of solution.
(5) In a laminar flow hood, transfer a Millicell insert containing two slice cultures to a 10 × 35 mm culture dish containing 1 ml of slice culture medium.
(6) Transfer the dish to the vibrationless table. Wash the surface of the microscope stage with 70% ethanol to ensure sterility of the cultures during the procedure.
(7) Using a manual micromanipulator position a micropipette at a 20° angle directly over the site of microapplication.
(8) Insert the micropipette tip directly into stratum pyramidale or stratum granulosum.
(9) Apply 25–500 nl of viral stock at a flow rate of 100 nl/min.
(10) After completion of the microapplication, remove the micropipette and return the cultures to the incubator.

4 NOTES AND TROUBLESHOOTING

4.1 On Protocol #60: Production of HSV-1 Amplicon Viral Stocks

4.1.1 Transfection Efficiency Control for Amplicon Production

One extra plate should be transfected with an amplicon vector that expresses *lacZ* from a strong promoter. This plate should be processed for X-gal histochemistry the next day in order to assess the transfection efficiency. The percentage of blue cells should be about 5%.

4.1.2 Amplicon Stocks

Each virus stock will contain both an amplicon component and a helper component. The helper virus contains a lethal mutation in an essential IE gene (e.g. IE3) and can be propagated only on helper cells containing the wild-type IE3 gene. Wild-type recombinant virus will arise at a frequency of approximately 1×10^{-6} by recombination of helper virus with the viral DNA carried by the helper cells. It is important to titer this wild-type virus in your stocks.

4.1.3 Rearrangement of Amplicons

Amplicon rearrangement can occur in a number of ways, including recombination with helper virus. To ensure that the amplicon vector has not been rearranged during packaging, perform a Southern blot analysis on DNA extracted from stocks of virus. This is easily done by extracting 0.5 ml of amplicon virus stock with phenol and concentrating the DNA by ethanol precipitation. The DNA is digested with a restriction enzyme that will excise the entire transcription unit and these digests fractionated with a similar digest of the initial amplicon plasmid. Standard methods for Southern blot analysis should be followed, using a probe derived from the transcription unit. Rearrangement is observed by an alteration in the predicted size of the hybridizing band.

4.2 On Protocol #61: Titering an HSV-1 Amplicon that Expresses β-Galactosidase

Amplicons can be titered by an expression assay if the transcription unit cloned into the vector will be expressed in tissue culture cells. For example, vectors expressing the *E. coli lacZ* gene from a viral promoter can be readily titered by infecting cells, allowing for expression and performing

X-gal histochemistry. Expression of gene products can also be detected if suitable antibodies are available.

Amplicon stocks can be used without purification. The cellular debris within the stock may produce some cytotoxicity for some cell types. The stock should be purified before use in cell culture; this is strongly recommended for *in vivo* use.

4.3 On Protocol #62: Titering the HSV-1 Helper Virus Component

4.3.1 Virus Titer Problems

If your viral titers are lower than expected, consider the following and make changes as appropriate.

HSV-1 viruses are sensitive to environmental conditions. Virus should be frozen in a dry-ice/ethanol bath and stored at $-70°C$. Repeated freeze/thaw cycles may inactivate the virus so, when the final packaging step is complete, store virus in volumes slightly larger than will be used for experiments.

Do not let stock RR1 cells grow to very high density. Cells plated at 5×10^5/100 mm dish can be left for 3–4 days without splitting.

Several HSV genes have been shown to cause cellular toxicity and/or damage in infected cells. The expression of HSV IE genes has been correlated with cytotoxicity (Johnson et al., 1992) and may reflect their interaction with cellular transcription factors. The transcription of the IE gene set strongly depends on the HSV transcription factor VP16, a product of an HSV late gene. Thus, efforts to make packaging cell systems or recombinant viruses that are mutated in VP16 may reduce cytotoxicity. Cytotoxicity appears to be less severe using amplicon than with recombinant vectors. This may reflect the fact that amplicon vectors do not contain IE genes, although the copropagated helper virus does. Thus amplicon stocks may contain fewer virions with IE genes than recombinant vector stocks with comparable amounts of transducing particles. Other HSV genes, such as UL41 which encodes the virus host shutoff function (vhs), may also produce toxicity (Johnson et al., 1992). The development and systematic testing of new helper viruses with mutations in these genes will probably lead to reductions in cellular toxicity.

4.4 On Protocol #65: Gene Transfer into Hippocampal Slice Cultures with HSV-1 Amplicon Stocks

4.4.1 Microdelivery of Amplicons to Hippocampal Slices

It is critical to calibrate the microapplication apparatus by measuring the number of micrometer increments necessary to deliver a known volume of solution. Because the virus can aggregate, it is important to confirm that microapplication of additional virus stock results in application of additional HSV virions. This can be done by microapplication of HSV vector stocks (25–500 nl) to microcentrifuge tubes and direct assay by PCR amplification using primers specific for thc recombinant HSV vector (Bergold et al., 1993). In this analysis, additional amplification product should be observed when larger volumes are microapplied. Alternatively, HSV vectors expressing *E. coli lacZ* can be microapplied to slice cultures and the number of transduced cells assayed with X-gal histochemistry (Casaccia-Bonnefil et al., 1993a).

REFERENCES

Benedikz, E., P. Casaccia-Bonnefil, A. Stelzer and P.J. Bergold. Hyperexcitability and cell loss in kainate-treated hippocampal slice cultures. 1993. *NeuroReport* **5:** 90–92.

Bergold, P., P. Casaccia-Bonnefil, H. Federoff and A. Stelzer. Transduction of CA3 neurons by a herpes virus vector containing a GluR6 subunit of the kainate receptor induces epileptiform discharge. 1993. *Soc. Neurol. Abstr.* **19:** 21.

Bergold, P., P. Casaccia-Bonnefil, Z. Xiu-Liu and H. Federoff. Transsynaptic neuronal loss induced in hippocampal slice cultures by a herpes simplex virus vector expressing the GluR6 subunit of the kainate receptor. 1993. *Proc. Natl Acad. Sci. USA* **90:** 6165–6169.

Casaccia-Bonnefil, P., E. Benedikz, H. Shen, A. Stelzer, D. Edelstein, M. Geschwind, M. Brownlee, H. Federoff and P. Bergold. Localized gene transfer into hippocampal slice cultures and acute hippocampal slices. 1993a. *J. Neurosci. Meth.* **50:** 341–351.

Casaccia-Bonnefil, P., E. Benedikz, R. Rai and P.J. Bergold. Excitatory and inhibitory pathways modulate kainate excitotoxicity in hippocampal slice cultures. 1993b. *Neurosci. Lett.* **154:** 5–8.

DeLuca, N. and P. Schaffer. Activities of herpes simplex virus type 1 (HSV-1) ICP4 genes specifying nonsense peptides. 1987. *Nucl. Acids Res.* **15:** 4491–4511.

DeLuca, N., A. McCarthy and P. Schaffer. Isolation and characterization of deletion mutants of Herpes Simplex Virus Type 1 in the gene encoding immediate–early regulatory protein ICP4. 1985. *J. Virol.* **56(2):** 558–570.

Dobson, A., T.P. Margolis, F. Sedarati, J. Stevens and L.T. Feldman. A latent, nonpathogenic HSV-1 derived vector stably expresses beta-galactosidase in mouse neurons. 1990. *Neuron* **5:** 353–360.

Federoff, H.J., M.D. Geschwind, A.I. Geller and J.A. Kessler. Expression of nerve growth factor *in vivo*, from a defective HSV-1 vector, prevents effects of axotomy on sympathetic ganglia. 1992. *Proc. Natl Acad. Sci. USA* **89:** 1636–1640.

Fink, D., L. Sternberg, P. Weber, M. Mata, W. Goins and J. Glorioso. *In Vivo* Exprcssion of beta-galactosidase in hippocampal neurons by HSV-1 mediated transfer. 1992. *Hum. Gene. Ther.* **3:** 11–19.

Frenkel, N. Defective interfering herpesviruses. In *The human herpesviruses—an interdisciplinary prospective.* Nahmias, A.J., Dowdle, W.R. and Scchinazy, R.F., eds. 1981. Elsevier–North Holland, Inc. New York.

Frenkel, N., R. Spaete, D. Vlazny, L. Deiss and H. Locker. The herpes simplex virus amplicon—a novel animal–virus cloning vector. In *Eukaryotic viral vectors*, pp.205–209. Gluzman, Y., ed. 1982. Cold Spring Harbor Laboratory, New York.

Frotscher, M. and B. Gahwiler. Synaptic organization of the intracellularly stained CA3 pyramid neurons in slice cultures of hippocampus. 1988. *Neuroscience* **24:** 541–551.

Gahwiler, B. Development of the hippocampus *in vitro*: Synapses and receptors. 1984. *Neuroscience* **11:** 751–760.

Gahwiler, B. Organotypic monolayer cultures of nervous tissue. 1981. *J. Neurosci. Meth.* **4:** 329–342.

Geller, A.I. and X.O. Breakefield. A defective HSV-1 vector expresses *Escherichia coli* beta-galactosidase in cultured peripheral neurons. 1988. *Science* **241:** 1667–1669.

Geller, A.I., K. Keyomarsi, J. Bryan and A.B. Pardee. An efficient deletion mutant packaging system for defective herpes simplex vectors: potential applications to human gene therapy and neuronal physiology. 1990. *Proc. Natl Acad. Sci. USA* **87:** 8950–8954.

Greenlund, L., J. Chang, P. Olivo and J. Johnson. Trk oncogene and Bcl-2 oncogene introduced via HSV-1 vectors prevents neuronal programmed cell death. 1993. *Soc. Neurosci. Abstr.* **19:** 886.

Hartnick, C., M. Geschwind, H. Federoff and T. Van De Water. Use of a defective herpes simplex virus to deliver BDNF to auditory neurons promotes neurite outgrowth. 1994. *Soc. Neurosci. Abstr.* **20:** 680.

Ho, D., E. Mocarski and R. Sapolosky. Altering central nervous system physiology with a defective herpes simplex virus vector expressing the glucose transporter gene. 1993. *Proc. Natl Acad. Sci. USA* **90:** 3655–3659.

Johnson, P., A. Miyanohara, F. Levine, T. Cahill and T. Friedman. Cytotoxicity of replication-defective mutant of herpes simplex virus type 1. 1992. *J. Virol.* **66:** 2952–2965.

Kaplitt, M., P. Leone, R. Samulski, X. Xiao, D. Pfaff, K. O'Malley and M. During. Long-term gene expression and phenotypic correction using adeno-associated virus vectors in the mammalian brain. 1994. *Nature Genet.* **8:** 148–154.

Kaplitt, M.G., J.G. Pfauss, S.P. Kleopoulous, B.A. Hanlon, S.D. Rabkin and D.W. Pfaff. Expression of a functional foreign gene in adult mammalian brain following *in vivo* transfer via a herpes simplex virus type 1 defective viral vector. 1991. *Mol. Cell. Neurosci.* **2:** 320–330.

Muller, M., B. Gahwiler, E. Peterhans and S. Thompson. Reversible loss of dendritic spines and altered excitability after chronic epilepsy in hippocampal slice cultures. 1993. *Proc. Natl Acad. Sci. USA* **90:** 257–261.

Palella, T., L. Silverman, C. Schroll, F. Homa, M. Levine and W. Kelley. Herpes simplex virus-mediated human hypoxanthine-guanine phosphoribosyltransferase gene transfer into neuronal cells. 1988. *Mol. Cell. Biol.* **8:** 457–460.

Paterson, T. and R. Everett. A prominent serine-rich region in Vmw175, the major transcriptional regulator protein of herpes simplex virus type 1, is not essential for virus growth in tissue culture. 1990. *J. Gen. Virol.* **71:** 1775–1783.

Rothstein, J., L. Bristol, B. Hosler, R. Brown Jr and R. Kuncl. Chronic inhibition of superoxide dismutase produces apoptotic death of spinal neurons. 1994. *Proc. Natl Acad. Sci. USA* **91:** 4155–4159.

Shih, M., M. Arsenakis, P. Tiollais and B. Roizman. Expression of hepatitis B S gene by a herpes simplex type 1 vectors carrying α- and β-regulated gene chimeras. 1984. *Proc. Natl Acad. Sci. USA* **81:** 5867– 5870.

Shin, C., Y. Tamaki, J. Wilson, L. Butler and T. Sakaguchi. NMDA-receptor mediated electrical epileptogenesis in the organotypic culture of rat hippocampus. 1992. *Brain Res.* **589:** 129–134.

Stoppini, L., P.-A. Buchs and D. Muller. A simple method for organotypic culture of nervous tissue. 1991. *J. Neurosci. Meth.* **37:** 173–182.

Stow, N. and E. McMonagle. Propagation of foreign DNA sequences linked to a herpes simplex virus origin of replication. In *Eukaryotic Viral Vectors*, pp.199–204. Gluzman, Y., ed. 1982 Cold Spring Harbor Laboratory, New York.

Thomson, S. and B. Gahwiler. Activity dependent disinhibition. I. Repetitive stimulation reduces IPSP driving force and conductance in the hippocampus *in vitro.* 1989. *J. Neurophys.* **61:** 501–511.

Yammato, N., K. Yamada, T. Kurotani and K. Toyama. Linear specificity of extrinsic cortical connections studied in co-culture preparations. 1992. *Neuron* **9:** 217–228.

Zimmer, J. and B. Gahwiler. Cellular and connective organization of slice cultures of the rat hippocampus and the fascia dentata. 1984. *J. Comp. Neurol.* **228:** 432–436.

Zimmer, J. and B. Gahwiler. Growth of hippocampal mossy fibers: A lesion and co-culture study of organotypic slice cultures. 1987. *J. Comp. Neurol.* **264:** 1–13.

CHAPTER 13

Amplicon Vectors: Mind the Helper!

ALBERTO L. EPSTEIN AND P.R. LOWENSTEIN*

Centre de Génétique Moléculaire et Cellulaire, CNRS – UMR 106 – Université Claude Bernard Lyon, 143, boulevard du 11 Novembre 1918, 69622 Villeurbanne Cedex, France. Tel: 33 72 43 13 25; Fax: 33 72 44 05 55; Email: epstein@biomserv.univ-lyon1.fr

**University of Manchester, School of Medicine, Department of Medicine, Molecular Medicine Unit, Room 1.302, Stopford Building, Oxford Road, Manchester M13 9PT, UK. Tel: 0161 275 5672; Fax: 0161 275 5672; Email: lowenstein@man.ac.uk*

1 INTRODUCTION

Two types of vector can be derived from herpes simplex type 1 virus (HSV-1): recombinant vectors and amplicons (Denniston et al., 1981; Spaete and Frankel, 1982; Barnett et al., 1983; Bear et al., 1984; Breakefield and DeLuca, 1991; Epstein, 1992; Leib and Olivo, 1994; Frenkel et al., 1994). In recombinant vectors the exogenous DNA sequences (the transgene) and the whole set of virus genes are located in the same DNA molecule and hence are carried by the same virus particle. In amplicons the transgene is on one DNA molecule (the vector genome) and the virus genes are in a different one (the helper genome). As HSV-1 capsids appear to package a single continuous DNA molecule it follows that the transgene and the virus genes are packaged into different virus particles. Thus, although recombinant vectors form (theoretically) homogeneous populations of particles, amplicon vector populations are genetically heterogeneous. The binary character of amplicon populations is the basis of the advantages and disadvantages of amplicons when compared with recombinant vectors.

One of the most interesting properties of amplicons is that only with these vectors is it possible to study transgene expression in cells that have not received the whole complement of lytic cycle genes. Because amplicon vector populations are composed of two different types of particle (Spaete and Frenkel, 1982) some target cells are infected only by the vector, some simultaneously by both vector and helper particles and others only with the helper virus (Lowenstein et al., 1994a, 1995).

Although both the vector and the helper virions contain structural proteins that are imported into the cells during infection, *de novo* expression of virus genes can be induced only in helper-infected cells, even if the helper virus used to prepare the amplicon is defective for replication (for a review on HSV-1 see Roizman and Sears, 1995). As a consequence, most of the cytopathic effects and toxicity associated with amplicon infection will be produced by the helper particles, not by the amplicon vector. For this reason, the phenotypic modifications induced by transgenic expression differ in cells infected with vector and those infected simultaneously with vector and helper particles. Furthermore, when studying the behavior of tissue-specific regulatory

Protocols for Gene Transfer in Neuroscience: Towards Gene Therapy of Neurological Disorders
Edited by P.R. Lowenstein and L.W. Enquist

promoters it is crucial to be sure that transgenic expression is not being influenced by immediate–early transcriptional activators encoded by the helper virus.

Thus, only by monitoring the infected cultures to distinguish cells that have been infected by vector particles alone from cells that have been infected with both vector and helper particles could results be reasonably ascribed exclusively to the transgenic transcription unit. The aim of this chapter is to illustrate how to use immunocytochemical procedures to fully exploit this unique advantage of amplicons.

1.1 Simultaneous Detection of Amplicon and Helper-encoded Proteins

In our experiments primary cultures of neocortical glial cells and neurons and an astrocytoma cell line were independently infected with different amplicon vectors. To distinguish cells infected by the amplicon particles alone from those infected by both types of particle, double-labeling immunofluorescence experiments were performed using antibodies specific for the transgenic protein encoded by the amplicon and for antigens encoded by the helper virus.

1.1.1 Plasmids and Helper Viruses

The plasmids used to prepare the amplicon vectors, pA-SF1 and pA-TT1, are shown in Fig. 13.1. Both contain an amplicon cassette composed of one virus origin of replication (Ori-S) and one packaging "a" sequence (Spaete and Frenkel, 1982). Plasmid pA-SF1 carries a phleomycin resistance/*lacZ* fusion gene under the control of IE-HCMV regulatory sequences and also contains SV40 splicing and polyadenylation signals (Baron et al., 1992). The β-galactosidase protein expressed from the fusion gene contains no apparent nucleophilic signal so is expected to remain essentially in the cytoplasm of infected cells. Plasmid pA-TT1 contains the TT1 transcription unit under HSV-1 IE3 gene regulatory sequences and an HSV-1 thymidine kinase (TK) polyadenylation signal (Lowenstein et al., 1994b). The TT1 gene encodes a chimeric construct consisting of a non-neuronal protein tissue inhibitor of metalloproteinases (TIMP), linked to the last exon of the protein Thy1, which contains a GPI anchor and was shown previously to target proteins to the external leaflet of the plasma membrane (Lowenstein et al., 1994b).

Two helper viruses were employed: the wild-type HSV-1 strain F (HSV-1 wt) and HSV-1 CgalΔ42 (Johnson et al., 1991). HSV-1wt was grown and assayed on Vero cells, the second on V9 cells (Johnson et al., 1991), as described previously (Machuca et al., 1986)–HSV-1 CgalΔ42 lacks the essential UL42 gene and can only be grown and assayed on *trans*-complementing cell lines such as V9 cells (Johnson et al., 1991). It expresses β-galactosidase from a bacterial *lacZ* gene inserted into an intergenic region located within the unique short sequence of HSV-1 under the control of the IE-HCMV promoter/regulatory element (Johnson et al., 1991). Thus, using this virus as the helper β-galactosidase can be considered as a virus antigen.

1.1.2 Construction and Assay of Vectors

Three different amplicon populations were prepared, as shown in Table 13.1. The pA-SF1/wt amplicon vectors were constructed by transfecting Vero cells with pA-SF1 using the calcium phosphate method (Graham and van der Eb, 1973) followed 4 h after transfection by a 15% glycerol shock. Transfected cells were superinfected the following day with HSV-1 wild-type at 1 p.f.u./cell. Two pA-TT1 amplicon vectors were produced, either by transfecting Vero cells with pA-TT1 and superinfecting with HSV-1 wt (pA-TT1/wt) or by transfecting pA-TT1 into V9 cells and superinfecting with HSV-1CgalΔ42 (pA-TT1/CgalΔ42). Helper virus titers were obtained on Vero or V9 cells. Titers of pA-SF1 were estimated by counting blue cells after X-Gal staining. Titers of pA-TT1 were estimated by counting the number of cells expressing TT1 in immunofluorescence experiments. Alternatively, amounts of pA-SF1 and pA-TT1 DNA are compared, after extraction and cleavage of total DNA from each virus population by blot hybridization of electrophoretically separated DNA fragments using a radiolabeled pSKII probe. As the titers of

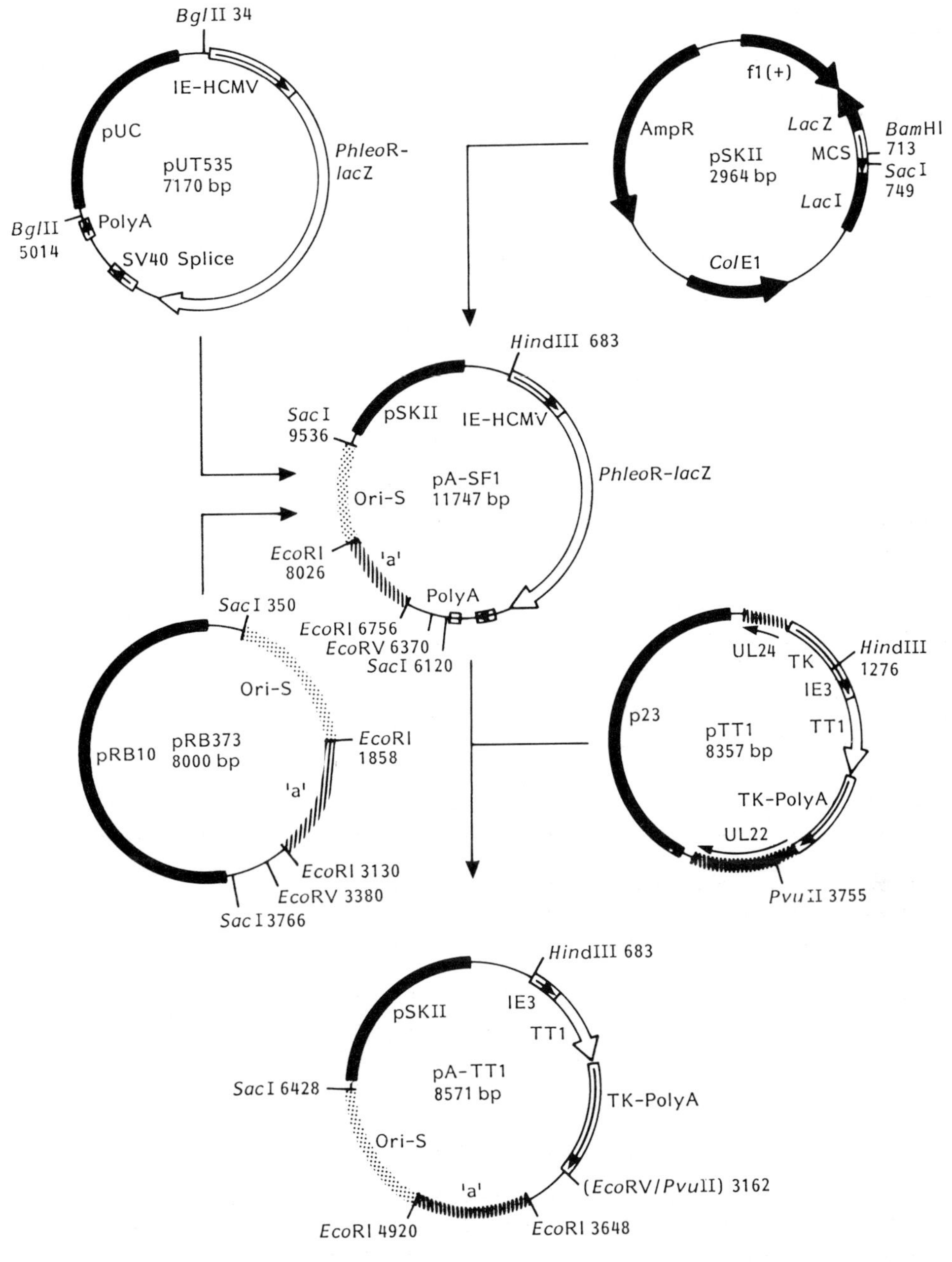

Figure 13.1 Plasmids used to generate the amplicon vectors. pA-SF1 is a pSKII-derived plasmid carrying a 3.4 kbp *Sac*I fragment, which contains the "amplicon cassette" (from pRB373) and a 4.9 kbp *Bgl*II fragment containing the β-galactosidase transcription unit (from pUT535), both inserted into the multiple cloning site (MCS) of pSKII. In pA-TT1 the β-galactosidase transcription unit (*Hin*dIII–*Eco*RV fragment) has been replaced by the TIMP–Thy 1 unit (*Hin*dIII–*Pvu*II fragment) from pTT1. Other abbreviations not described in the text are: PhleoR/*lacZ* = phleomycin resistance/*lacZ* fusion open reading frame; SV40 splice and polyA = SV40 sequences allowing splicing and polyadenylation of corresponding transcripts; "a" = HSV-1 sequences containing the virus packaging (cleavage/encapsidation) signal; TK = thymidine kinase; TK-polyA = polyadenylation signal from HSV-1 thymidine kinase gene; UL22 and UL24 = two HSV-1 genes surrounding HSV-1 TK (UL23); AmpR = ampicillin resistance gene. Restriction enzyme sites used for cloning are presented in the figure. Reproduced by permission

Table 13.1 Amplicon populations used in this work

		Helper virus	
		HSV-1 (wt)	*HSV-1CgalΔ42*
Plasmids	pA-SF1	pA-SF1/wt	—
	pA-TT1	pA-TT1/wt	pA-TT1/CgalΔ42

Each amplicon population was passaged three times (pA-SF1/wt and pA-TT1/wt in Vero cells and pA-TT1/CgalΔ42 in UL42 expressing V9 cells). Southern blots of DNA from all virus populations gave no evidence for recombination between helper and vector DNA (data not shown)

Table 13.2 Primary and secondary antibody combinations used to detect vector and helper expression

Amplicon population	*Ab anti-vector*[a]	*Ab anti-helper*[b]
pA-SF1/wt	1° β-galactosidase (RPC) 2° Rhodamine	1° UL42 (MMC) 2° Fluorescein
pA-TT1/wt	1° TIMP (MMC) 2° Fluorescein	1° ICP27 (RPC) 2° Rhodamine
pA-TT1/CgalΔ42	1° TIMP (MMC) 2° Fluorescein	1° β-galactosidase (RPC) 2° Rhodamine

[a]Antibodies specifically recognizing the protein encoded by the amplicon vector; [b]antibodies specifically recognizing a protein encoded by the helper virus (either viral or transgenic); RPC: rabbit polyclonal antibodies; MMC: mouse monoclonal antibodies; 1°: primary antibodies; 2° secondary antibodies

pA-SF1 vector particles were known and the original plasmids were very similar in size, the relative amounts of pA-TT1 vector could be estimated. Both methods consistently indicated that at corresponding passages the titers of both vector particles were similar. Southern blots of DNA from all populations, independently probed with virus and plasmid radiolabeled DNA, showed no recombination between helper and amplicon DNA (not shown here).

Primary cultures of rat neocortical neurons, glial cells and 1321NI human astrocytoma cells, prepared as described elsewhere (Lowenstein et al., 1994b; SEE ALSO CHAPTER 8), were independently infected with pA-SF1/wt, pA-TT1/wt or pA-TT1/CgalΔ42 at an MOI of about 1 p.f.u./cell of helper, corresponding to about 0.3 particles/cell of vector. In all experiments we used the P_2 passages because they gave the best amplicon to helper ratios. The infectivity of the virus depends in part on the susceptibility of the cell type being infected, so 1 p.f.u./cell in Vero cells does not necessarily mean 1 p.f.u./cell in nerve cells: we observed fewer infected nerve cells than we expected from the titers. Infected cells were fixed 12–15 h later with paraformaldehyde and immunoreacted with antibodies specific for anti-β-galactosidase, anti-TIMP, anti-ICP27 and anti-UL42 antibodies in double immunofluorescence experiments, as shown in Table 13.2.

Analysis of the results obtained with the pA-SF1/wt population revealed that neurons, glia and astrocytoma cells infected with the vector did express β-galactosidase, as assessed by immunolabeling of infected cells with antibodies to β-galactosidase, in both the absence (β-gal$^+$/UL42$^-$ cells) and presence (β-gal$^+$/UL42$^+$ cells) of helper coinfection. This experiment revealed that in cells infected only with vector pA-SF1 β-galactosidase diffused throughout the cytoplasm but did not enter the nuclei. In contrast, cells that were infected by pA-SF1 and the wild-type helper virus also displayed nuclear β-galactosidase immunoreactivity (Figs 13.2, Plate IV and 13.3, Plates IV/V). That the pA-SF1 vector expressed β-galactosidase in infected neurons was further confirmed by double labeling of infected cells with antibodies against β-galactosidase and neuronal specific Map2 antibodies. Infected cells appeared healthy at the time of the immunofluorescence experiments.

Similar studies were carried out in cells infected with pA-TT1/CgalΔ42. As before, neurons, glia and astrocytoma cells infected with the vector particles expressed TIMP protein with and without helper coinfection. Expression from the helper genome was assessed in this case using antibodies to β-galactosidase. The intracellular distribution of TIMP was identical in cells singly infected with vector and doubly infected (vector + helper). TIMP immunoreactivity was found mainly as a punctuate staining over the plasma membrane. Intracellular immunoreactivity could also be detected in a juxtanuclear area usually occupied by Golgi cisternae, as TIMP traverses the ER and Golgi before entering plasma membrane-bound transport vesicles. Double labeling of infected cells using anti-TIMP and anti-Map2 antibodies confirmed that neurons expressed TT1 protein. Similar studies conducted with the pA-TT1/wt population gave identical results.

2 MATERIALS AND EQUIPMENT

(1) Media, solutions and equipment for producing amplicons and helper viruses, as described in Chapter 11.
(2) Olympus Vanox AHBS photomicroscope with brightfield illumination or with the fluorescent attachment AH2-RFL.
(3) AGFA RS1000, or Fuji-color 1600D color transparency film.
(4) Sterile standard phosphate-buffered saline (PBS): 1.0% NaCl, 0.025% KCl, 0.14% Na_2HPO_4, 0.025% KH_2PO_4 (all w/v), pH 7.2.
(5) 4% paraformaldehyde, 0.12 M sucrose in PBS, pH 7.4.
(7) 0.3% Triton X-100 in PBS.
(8) Blocking solution (10% normal goat serum (NGS, Vector Labs, Peterborough, UK) in PBS).
(9) 1% v/v NGS in PBS (Vector Labs).
(10) Secondary antibodies: rabbit anti-mouse and/or swine anti-rabbit (Dakopatts, UK).
(11) Mowiol (Calbiochem).
(12) Primary antibodies (final dilution): mouse monoclonal anti-Map2 (1 : 250), rabbit polyclonal anti-Map2 (1 : 100), mouse monoclonal anti-human TIMP (1 : 100), rabbit polyclonal anti-β-galactosidase (1 : 100), mouse monoclonal anti-UL42 (1 : 200), rabbit polyclonal anti-ICP27 (1 : 500), all in 1% (v/v) NGS in PBS. UL42 is an early HSV-1 gene encoding a protein essential for virus replication. ICP27 is an essential immediate–early virus protein.

3 THE PROTOCOLS

See Protocols #58, #60 and #61 for preparation and titration of amplicons.

Protocol #66: Infection of Cultured Nerve Cells with Amplicon Preparations

(1) Grow neuronal cultures on slides for immunofluorescence, as described in Chapter 8.
(2) Infect cells with a small volume of diluted virus (in PBS or in virus medium), adjusted to give a MOI of 0.1–0.5 p.f.u./cell.
(3) After 90 min contact remove non-adsorbed virus.
(4) Wash cells twice with fresh virus medium and add fresh virus medium to re-feed cells.
(5) Fix infected cells after infection for 10–15 h.

Protocol #67: Labeling HSV-1 Amplicon Infected Cells Simultaneously with Two Different Antibodies; Detection of Single and Double Infected Cells

(1) For immunocytochemical experiments, rinse cultures in prewarmed PBS (37°C) and fix for 20 min in 4% paraformaldehyde, 0.12 M sucrose in PBS, pH 7.4.
(2) Wash cultures four times with PBS and permeabilize cells in 0.3% Triton X-100 in PBS for 5 min.
(3) Rinse and incubate in blocking solution for 1 h.
(4) Wash once in 1% v/v NGS in PBS, and then incubate in primary antibodies for 1–2 h at 4°C.
(5) Wash cultures four times in 1% NGS in PBS, and incubate in fluorescently labeled secondary antibodies (rabbit anti-mouse and/or swine anti-rabbit diluted 1 : 100 in 1% NGS in PBS) for 1 h.
(6) Wash cultures four times in PBS, quickly dip in distilled water and mount on glass slides with Mowiol.

4 NOTES AND TROUBLESHOOTING

Vero, HEp-2, HeLa, CV1, rabbit skin and BHK21 cells are fully permissive for HSV-1 virus production. Viruses that have been deleted for an essential function can only be grown and assayed in specially constructed permissive cell lines expressing that function (helper cells or complementing cells). Several such lines and corresponding defective viruses are available (SEE CHAPTER 12). When choosing the helper virus for constructing the amplicon vector population, remember that the earlier the virus cycle is blocked, the lower the cytotoxic effects.

Always prepare, in parallel, the amplicon vector expressing the transgenic protein of interest and a β-galactosidase expressing vector, both as a control for the transfection step and for each of the infections (passages).

Vector particles can be estimated in cells that are non-permissive for helper particles. The advantage of this is that quantitative estimations of vector particles will be aided by the absence of helper-induced plaques. However, distinct cell lines may differ in susceptibility to virus infection, so assaying both components of the population in different cell lines will give only an approximation to actual amplicon/helper ratios.

For most experiments it is important to be sure that recombinants between the helper and the vector genomes have not been generated. Recombination is very frequent during the HSV replication cycle. The only equipment required to ascertain the genetic purity of the helper and the vector genomes is that currently used for Southern blotting and hybridization. A sample of total DNA extracted from cells infected by the helper virus (but not transfected with the amplicon plasmid) and, in a separate well, a sample of amplicon plasmid DNA, both digested by the same enzyme, should be used as control. The lanes containing the amplicon vectors should display the fragments observed in the HSV-1 control plus the fragment(s) observed in the plasmid control (the plasmid and the HSV-1 DNA will cross-react with either probe because they share Ori-S and "a" HSV-1 sequences) but the controls should lack two minor fragments that represent the termini of the concatemeric amplicon vector. The appearance of any other fragment in the vector lanes, or a difference in mobility of any of the fragments, could indicate recombination or rearrangement. The molarity of vector and helper-derived fragments will probably be different (this depends on the relative concentrations of both genomes and is caused by the vector genome containing several tandem copies of the original plasmid).

By monitoring expression from the two elements comprising the amplicon population we have confirmed double infection of a significant number of cells, while other cells were singly infected with the amplicon vector or the helper virus (Lowenstein et al., 1994a, 1995). The relative proportion of singly and doubly infected cells is thought to depend on the internal structure of the amplicon population (the amplicon/helper ratio) and on the MOI used (infectious particles/cell ratio).

Targeting to the plasma membrane of TIMP protein expressed from pA-TT1/wt or pA-TT1/CgalΔ42 was unaffected by coinfection with helper virus. This suggests that HSV-1 does not significantly alter protein targeting to the plasma membrane of nerve cells and that HSV-1 encoded proteins are not necessary for correct targeting of TIMP-Thy1 to the plasma membrane (Lowenstein et al., 1994a). The distribution of TIMP in cells infected with pA-TT1 was, however, indistinguishable from that achieved by infecting similar cells with the recombinant HSV-1 tsK vector TIMP/Thy1 (TT21), which encodes the same transcription unit as amplicon pA-TT1 (Lowenstein et al., 1994b).

In the case of cytoplasmic β-galactosidase, coinfection with helper and vector particles did affect the expression or distribution of the transgene product encoded by the vector, as shown with pA-SF1/wt amplicons (Lowenstein et al., 1994a). Entry of β-galactosidase into the nuclei of coinfected cells could be related to changes in the permeability of the nuclear membranes in HSV-1 infected cells, overall changes in the expression of β-galactosidase in doubly infected cells, or association of the transgenic protein with nuclear targeted HSV-1 proteins.

These experiments suggest that transgenes under the control of HSV-1 IE3 or IE-HCMV regulatory sequences can be expressed from amplicon vectors in neurons, glia and astrocytoma cells that have not been coinfected with the helper virus, and hence in the absence of synthesis of HSV-1 proteins (Lowenstein et al., 1995).

REFERENCES

Barnett JW, Eppstein DA and Chan HW. 1983. Class I defective herpes simplex virus DNA as a molecular cloning vehicle in eukaryotic cells. *Journal of Virology* **48**:384–395.

Baron M, Reynes JP, Stassi D and Tiraby G. 1992. A selectable bifunctional β-galactosidase: phleomycin resistance fusion protein as a potential marker for eukaryotic cells. *Gene* **114**:239–243.

Bear SE, Colberg-Poley AM, Court DL, Carter BJ and Enquist LW. 1984. Analysis of two potential shuttle vectors containing herpes simplex virus defective DNA. *Journal of Molecular and Applied Genetics* **2**:471–484.

Breakefield XO and DeLuca. NA. 1991. Herpes Simplex Virus for gene delivery to neurons. *New Biologist* **3**:203–218.

Denniston KJ, Madden MJ, Enquist LW and Vandewoude G. 1981. Characterization of coliphage lambda hybrids carrying DNA fragments from herpes simplex virus type 1 defective interfering particles. *Gene* **15**:365–378.

Epstein AL. 1992. Les vecteurs herpetiques pour le transfer de genes. *Medicine/sciences* **8**:902–911.

Frenkel N, Singer O and Kwong AD. 1994. The herpes simplex virus amplicon—a versatile defective virus vector. *Gene Therapy* **1**:(Suppl.1) S40–S46.

Graham FL. and van der Eb AJ. 1973. A new technique for the assay of infectivity of human Adenovirus 5 DNA. *Virology* **52**:456–467.

Johnson P, Best M, Friedmann T and Parris DS. 1991. Isolation of a herpes simplex virus type 1 mutant deleted for the essential UL42 gene and characterisation of its null phenotype. *Journal of Virology* **65**:700–710.

Leib DA and Olivo PD. 1994. Gene delivery to neurons: is herpes simplex virus the right tool for the job? *Bioessays* 1994 **15**:547–554.

Lowenstein PR, Fournel S, Bain D, Tomasec P, Clissold P, Castro MG and Epstein AL. 1994a. Herpes simplex virus 1 (HSV-1) helper co-infection affects the distribution of an amplicon encoded protein in glia. *Neuroreport* **5**:1625–1630.

Lowenstein PR, Fournel S, Bain D, Tomasec P, Clissold P, Castro MG and Epstein AL. 1995. Simultaneous detection of amplicon and HSV-1 helper encoded proteins reveals that neurons and astrocytoma cells do express amplicon-borne transgenes in the absence of synthesis of virus immediate early proteins. *Molecular Brain Research* **30**:169-175.

Lowenstein PR, Morrison EE, Bain D, Hodge P, Preston CM, Clissold P, Stow ND, McKee TA and Castro MG. 1994b. Use of recombinant vectors derived from herpes simplex 1 mutant tsK for short-term expression of transgenes encoding cytoplasmic and membrane anchored proteins in post mitotic polarised cortical neurons and glial cells. *Neuroscience* **60**:1059–1077.

Machuca I, Jacquemont B and Epstein AL. 1986. Multiple adjacent or overlapping loci affecting the level of gC and cell fusion mapped by intratypic recombinants of HSV-1. *Virology* **150**:117–125.

Roizman B and Sears A. 1995. Herpes simplex viruses and their replication. In: *Virology*, Third edition, eds BN Fields, DM Knipe et al. Raven Press, New York, pp. 1043–1107.

Spaete RR and Frenkel N. 1982. The herpes simplex virus amplicon: a new eukaryotic defective-virus cloning-amplifying vector. *Cell* **30**:295–304.

SECTION 4

Part B: Protocols for Gene Delivery Using Helper-independent Herpes Simplex Virus-1 Vectors

CHAPTER 14

Herpes Simplex Virus Temperature-sensitive Mutant *ts*K as a Vector for Neuronal Gene Transfer

PETER TOMASEC, DEREK BAIN, MARIA G. CASTRO, CHRIS M. PRESTON* AND PEDRO R. LOWENSTEIN

University of Manchester, School of Medicine, Department of Medicine, Molecular Medicine Unit, Room 1.302, Stopford Building, Oxford Road, Manchester M13 9PT, UK. Tel: 0161 275 5672; Fax: 0161 275 5672; Email: lowenstein@man.ac.uk

**MRC Virology Unit, Institute of Virology, Glasgow G11 5JR, UK. Tel: 0141 339 8855, ext. 4635/4630; Fax: 0141 337 2236; Email: cpreston@vir.gla.ac.uk*

1 INTRODUCTION

Vectors derived from Herpes simplex virus-1 are powerful tools for transfer of foreign genes into post-mitotic mature neurons both *in vivo* and *in vitro*. Main advantages are their neurotropism, their large capacity for cloning foreign sequences, the large number of defective or mutant viruses that can be adapted as gene transfer vectors, the possibility of using a single gene transfer vector system *in vivo* and *in vitro* and the ease with which recombinant vectors can be generated. An in-depth treatment of the virology of HSV-1 can be found in the detailed chapters by Roizman (1995).

We have used HSV-1 vectors derived from the temperature-sensitive mutant *ts*K by cloning transgenes into the thymidine kinase (TK) locus under the control of an active HSV-1 immediate–early (IE) promoter. *ts*K contains a lesion in the IE gene 3 (IE3) encoding the protein ICP4 (also called Vmw175). The permissive temperature for growth when ICP4 is functional is 31°C and the non-permissive temperature (when ICP4 is non-functional) is 38.5°C; however, this vector is still non-permissive at 37°C (Lowenstein et al., 1994).

Using *ts*K as a vector has several advantages: (1) a complete cloning system is available (vector plus necessary plasmids; see Figs 14.1 and 14.2); (2) recombinant vectors can be used *in vitro* as wild-type vectors (at 31°C), as ICP4$^-$ mutants at 37–38.5°C or *in vivo* as ICP4$^-$ mutants, given that its growth is non-permissive at 37°C; (3) no *cis*-complementing cell lines are needed to grow it; (4) because selection methods are available when cloning into the TK locus screening for recombinant virus vectors containing the genes of interest is greatly facilitated; (5) high levels of expression can be obtained by inserting the transgenes under HSV-1 IE promoter control after relatively short post-infection times (e.g. 8 h).

Unfortunately this system also has disadvantages: (1) the vectors are toxic after 48–72 h, due to a HSV-1 function (e.g. host shutoff functions or viral IE protein expression) or the very high levels of

Protocols for Gene Transfer in Neuroscience: Towards Gene Therapy of Neurological Disorders
Edited by P.R. Lowenstein and L.W. Enquist

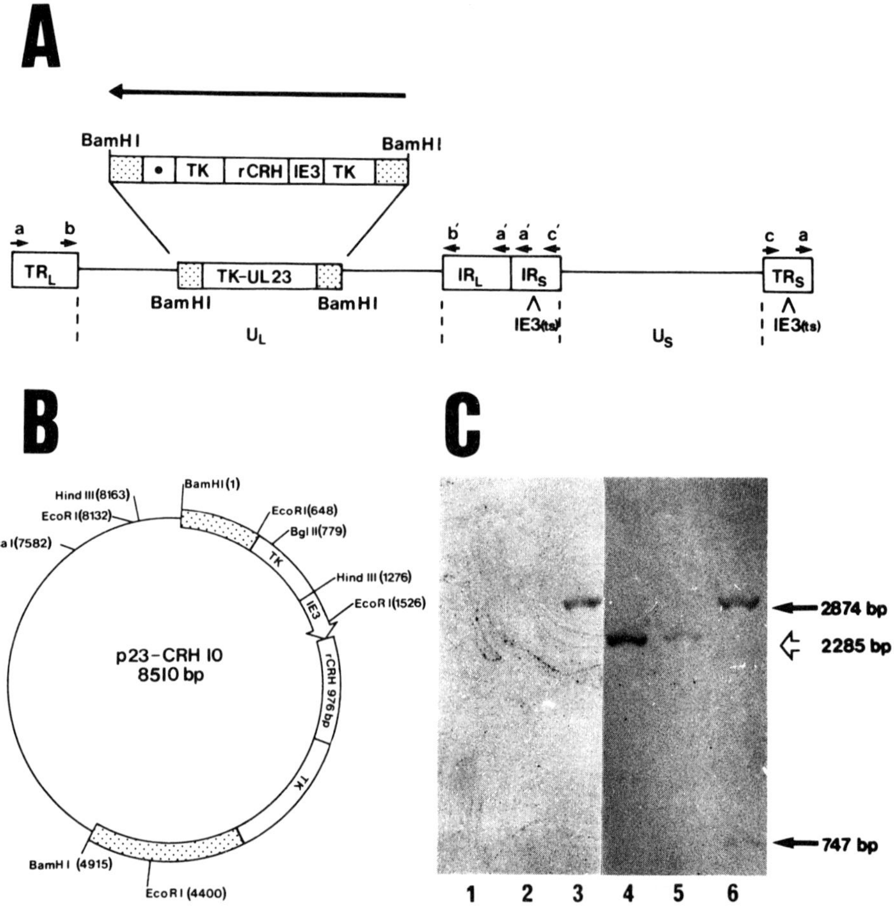

Figure 14.1 Construction of a recombinant HSV-1 *ts*K derived vector expressing the cDNA encoding the neuropeptide pre-pro rat corticotropin releasing hormone (rCRH) under the transcriptional control of the HSV-1 IE3 promoter. The overall recombinant production strategy is depicted in (A). The rCRH cDNA was inserted into plasmid p23 and the resulting plasmid (B) cotransfected with *ts*K DNA into BHK cells as described in the text. Recombination occurs between the flanking homologous sequences in the plasmid and *ts*K DNA (stippled regions), leading to the production of the recombinant *ts*K with a TK locus containing an insertion of the IE3 promoter followed by rCRH. The arrow (A) indicates the direction of transcription and the black dot (A) indicates the presence of a polyadenylation signal. Individual plaques obtained from the cotransfection were purified once, DNA isolated, cut with *Eco*RI and *Bgl*II and then probed with DIG labelled rCRH ((C): lanes 1–3) or with DIG labelled *Eco*RI "n" fragment of HSV-1 ((C): lanes 4–6) in a Southern blot analysis. The presence of a 2874 bp band in lane 3 and 2874 and 747 bp bands in lane 6 indicate that DNA from the plaque in lanes 3 and 6 contains the rCRH insert within the TK locus. The 2285 bp band in lane 4 indicates that only the parent *ts*K virus was present in this plaque. The absence of the 2285 bp band from lane 6 demonstrates that the plaque consists of pure recombinant virus, and contains no parent *ts*K

transgene expression; (2) length of expression is usually therefore limited to 48–72 hours; (3) temperature-independent revertants can appear with a frequency of 10^{-6}.

To generate these vectors for gene transfer, host cells must be grown, stocks of virus and viral DNA prepared, foreign genes introduced into the virus, the virus vectors plaque purified and grown, and the recombinant virus vectors identified. In this chapter we describe the procedures used in our laboratory for preparation of HSV-1 *ts*K recombinants using the permissive temperature of incubation of 31°C. Please note that this temperature will not apply if viruses which are not temperature sensitive are used.

2 MATERIALS AND EQUIPMENT

2.1 Cell Culture and Virus Production Media

(1) Culture medium: Glasgow MEM (BHK-21) medium supplemented with 10% or 5% (v/v) newborn calf serum, 5% (v/v) tryptose phosphate broth, 100 U/ml penicillin, 100 μg/ml streptomycin (from Life Technologies), sterile. MEM is Glasgow modified Eagle's medium.
(2) Freezing medium: 40% (v/v) Glasgow MEM, 40% (v/v) newborn calf serum, 20% (v/v) glycerol, sterile.
(3) 199 medium: 199 medium with Earle's balanced salt solution (EBSS) supplemented with 1% (v/v) inactivated newborn calf serum, 100 U/ml penicillin, 100 μg/ml streptomycin, sterile. Serum in 199 medium is inactivated by heating at 56°C for 30 min.
(4) Titration medium: 199 medium with EBSS supplemented with 5% (v/v) pooled human serum, 100 U/ml penicillin, 100 μg/ml streptomycin, sterile.
(5) 199/acycloguanosine medium: 199 medium with EBSS supplemented with 1% (v/v) inactivated newborn calf serum, 100 U/ml penicillin, 100 μg/ml streptomycin, 5 μM acycloguanosine (Sigma, UK), sterile.
(6) 1 × Trypsin/EDTA, sterile.

2.2 Cell and Virus Growth/Titration Reagents

(1) Phosphate-buffered saline (PBS) (without Ca^{2+}, Mg^{2+}) (Life Technologies), sterile.
(2) Giemsa stain solution (Sigma), prepared by mixing 0.65 g crystalline Giemsa stain (Sigma), 22 ml glycerol, 100 ml methanol.
(3) Ficoll 400.
(4) 1% agar in tissue culture grade water, autoclaved. The grade of agar used is important for cell viability. Agar normally used for bacterial plates is no good; we recommend Noble agar. Solidified agar can be melted in microwave oven or hot water before putting into 45°C water bath.
(5) Methanol.

2.3 Viral DNA Preparation and Transfection Reagents

(1) 10 × HEPES-buffered saline (HBS): 8.18% (w/v) NaCl, 5.94% (w/v) HEPES, 0.2% (w/v) Na_2HPO_4, filter sterilized and kept at 4°C.
(2) 2 × HBS: prepare before transfection by diluting 10 × HBS and adjust pH to exactly 7.12 with 1 M NaOH before adjusting to final volume. Filter sterilize and keep at 4°C.
(3) 2 M $CaCl_2$, filter sterilized and kept at 4°C.
(4) Glycerol solution: 15% glycerol in 1 × HBS pH 7.12, filter sterilized and kept at 4°C.
(5) Dimethylsulfoxide (DMSO) solution: 20–25% DMSO in 1 × HBS pH 7.12, filter sterilized. Some observations suggest that DMSO shock works better for BHK cells than glycerol shock.

! DO NOT USE CELLULOSE ACETATE FILTERS FOR DMSO !

(6) Lysis buffer 1: 1 : 10 mM NaCl, 10 mM Tris, 1.5 mM $MgCl_2$, 2% N P-40, 1% SDS, 1 mg/ml pronase (added fresh before use), pH 7.5.
(7) Lysis buffer 2: 10 mM Tris pH 8, 10 mM EDTA, 0.5% sodium dodecyl sulfate (SDS), 1 mg/ml pronase (add fresh before use).
(8) 100% and 70% ethanol.
(9) 10 M LiCl.
(10) TE: 10 mM Tris–HCl pH 8, 1 mM EDTA, sterile filtered.
(11) 10% SDS.
(12) EDTA, 0.5 M, pH 8.
(13) Chloroform, molecular biology grade.
(14) NP-40 buffer: 10 mM NaCl, 10 mM Tris pH 7.5, 1.5 mM $MgCl_2$, 1% NP-40.
(15) Tris buffer: 10 mM NaCl, 10 mM Tris, 1.5 mM $MgCl_2$, pH 7.5.

2.4 Reagents for Growth and Analysis of Bacterial Plasmids

(1) Nutrient broth (NB) and nutrient agar (NA) (Oxoid).
(2) Ampicillin: prepare a 25 mg/ml solution of the sodium salt of ampicillin in distilled water. Filter sterilize and store in aliquots at −20°C. Use final concentration of 25 μg/ml of NB and 50 μg/ml of NA. Allow autoclaved media to cool to 48°C before adding ampicillin. Ampicillin/NA plates must not be stored longer than 1–2 weeks at 4°C.
(3) Tris-borate buffer (TBE) for agarose gels: 0.089 Tris-borate pH 8.3, 0.002 M EDTA. Prepare 5× stock by mixing 54 g Tris base, 27.5 g boric acid, 20 ml 0.5 M EDTA pH 8 and distilled water to 1 liter.
(4) Tris-acetate buffer (TAE) for low melting point agarose gels: 0.04 M Tris-acetate pH 7.6, 0.001 M EDTA. Prepare 50× stock by mixing 242 g Tris base, 57.1 ml glacial acetic acid, 100 ml 0.5 M EDTA pH 8 and distilled water to 1 liter.
(5) DNA gel loading buffer (6× concentrated): 0.25% bromophenol blue, 30% glycerol in water. Store at 4°C.
(6) Ethidium bromide (EtBr) for DNA staining: Prepare 10 mg/ml stock of EtBr in water, store in a dark bottle at 4°C. Add EtBr to a final concentration of 0.5 μg/ml of gel. Gel could be run without EtBr and after electrophoresis stained in a 0.5 μg/ml EtBr solution at room temperature for 45 min. Gel may be destained in 1 mM $MgSO_4$ at room temperature. It is preferable to stain supercoiled DNA after agarose gel electrophoresis is complete rather than during electrophoresis, because EtBr introduces positive supercoils into the negatively supercoiled plasmid molecule.

! EtBr is a Powerful Mutagen and a Carcinogen.
It Must be Handled and Disposed of Carefully !

(7) Low melting point agarose, electrophoresis grade.
(8) Tris buffer: 10 mM NaCl, 10 mM Tris pH 7.5, 1.5 mM $MgCl_2$.
(9) Lysis buffer 2: 10 mM NaCl, 10 mM Tris pH 7.5, 1.5 mM $MgCl_2$, 2% NP-40, 1% SDS.
(10) Phenol/chloroform reagent. Use molecular biology grade of phenol (pink or yellow batches must be redistilled). Melt frozen stock at 68°C. Add 8-hydroxyquinoline to a final concentration of 0.1% (8-hydroxyquinoline serves as antioxidant and its yellow color also serves as indicator to identify phenolic phase). Extract melted phenol several times with an equal volume of 1 M Tris-HCl pH 8, then with 0.1 M Tris-HCl pH 8, 0.2% β-mercaptoethanol. The pH of the aqueous phase after last extraction must be above 7.6—if not, it must be extracted further. Make a 25 : 24 : 1 mixture of phenol : chloroform : isoamylalcohol; this is finally used to remove proteins from DNA preparations. Store at 4°C.
(11) 1% agar in tissue culture grade water, autoclaved. Do not use agar normally used for bacterial plates. We recommend Noble agar. Solidified agar can be melted in microwave oven or hot water before putting into 45°C water bath (for details see Protocol #73).

3 THE PROTOCOLS

All protocols in this chapter are described for use with temperature-sensitive HSV-1 *ts*K, permissive temperature 31°C, non-permissive temperature 38.5°C.

Protocol #68: Passage of BHK Cells (Syrian Hamster Kidney Cell Line)

(1) Grow BHK cells to confluence in an atmosphere of 5% CO_2 at 37°C.
(2) Remove medium and wash cell monolayer with warm PBS (without Ca^{2+}, Mg^{2+}) by rocking the dish. Remove PBS.
(3) Add warm trypsin/EDTA solution (1.5 ml per 175 cm² dish), cover the cell monolayer and incubate at 37°C for approximately 3 min. The cells should detach readily.
(4) Resuspend cells in warm culture medium by pipetting and ensure that they are evenly dispersed. To passage cells, split 1 : 3–1 : 6 (seeding at 2×10^4–4×10^4 cells/cm²). Incubate at 37°C to confluence. Cells become confluent in 2–4 days.

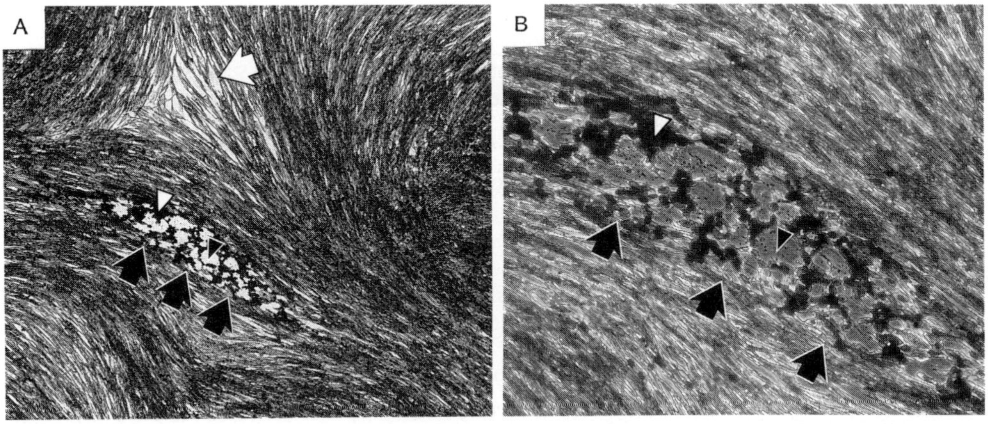

Figure 14.2 A confluent monolayer of BHK cells was infected with *ts*K virus and overlaid with medium supplemented with human HSV-1 hyperimmune serum. Three days after incubation at 31°C the cells were stained with Giemsa. (A) (low magnification, 850 ×) and (B) (high magnification, 2100 ×) show the morphology of a single plaque in the BHK monolayer. Black arrows indicate the viral plaque. The white arrowhead indicates an area of dead cells within the plaque, and the black arrowhead indicates a hole left after dead cells have lifted off the plastic dish surface. The white arrow in (A) points to an area of reduced cell density, without displaying any cytopathology. Such areas can be seen in monolayers of BHK cells. It is important to differentiate these morphologies

Protocol #69: Storage of BHK Cells

(1) Grow cells to confluence and trypsinize as described in Protocol #68, Steps 1–3. Wait until cells detach.
(2) Resuspend cells in 10 ml warm culture medium by pipetting. Ensure cells are evenly dispersed.
(3) Transfer suspension into a 15 ml centrifuge tube and spin at 1500 r.p.m. for 5 min.
(4) Discard the supernatant and disperse the cells by tapping the tube. Resuspend the cells by pipetting in freezing medium to give a final concentration of approximately 5 × 10^6 cells/ml (cells from one 175 cm^2 flask in 8–10 ml medium).
(5) Disperse 1 ml aliquots of the cell suspension into sterile cryotubes. Place the tubes upright in an expanded polystyrene container. Allow cells to freeze slowly by placing the container overnight at −70°C, then transfer to liquid nitrogen for long-term storage.

Protocol #70: Recovery of BHK Cells

(1) Thaw frozen cells rapidly while agitating in a 37°C water bath until the last little bit of ice is seen floating on the top.
(2) Transfer cell suspension into a 15 ml centrifuge tube and slowly add 5 ml of cold (4°C) culture medium.
(3) Pellet the cells at 1500 r.p.m. for 5 min, discard supernatant and disperse the pellet by tapping the tube.
(4) Resuspend the cells in cold culture medium and transfer to a tissue culture dish. Incubate at 37°C, 5% CO_2 until cells are confluent.

Protocol #71: Growth of HSV-1 and Preparation of Virus Stocks

(1) Grow several 175 cm^2 tissue culture flasks or roller bottles of BHK cells to confluence.
(2) Remove medium and add virus inoculum at a multiplicity of infection (MOI) of 0.001–0.1 plaque forming units (p.f.u.) per cell (3 × 10^6 p.f.u./175 cm^2 flask (approximately 3 × 10^7 cells)) in warm 199 medium sufficient to just cover the cell monolayer. Always prepare virus inoculum just before use.

(3) Incubate at 31°C for 90 min, gently agitating every 15 min.
(4) Remove inoculum, briefly wash cells with warm 199 medium, add warm 199 medium and incubate at 31°C for 3–5 days, until the complete cytopathic effect is seen in cultured cells (the cells become rounded and detach from the plastic when the flask is shaken; Fig.14.3).
(5) Scrape the infected cells into the medium using a sterile scraper and transfer into sterile centrifuge tubes. Spin at 3000 r.p.m., 4°C for 20 min.
(6) If a virus strain that releases significant amounts of virus particles into the medium is grown, transfer supernatant to fresh sterile tubes and centrifuge at 23 000*g* for 2 h at 4°C to pellet the virus released by the cells. Resuspend the pellet in cold 199 medium. Store small aliquots in sterile cryotubes at −70°C.
(7) If a strain that does not release significant amounts of virus into the medium is grown, safely dispose of the supernatant obtained in Step 5 and go to Step 8. The cell pellet contains most of the infectious virus.
(8) Resuspend the cell pellet in 5 ml cold 199 medium and freeze/thaw three times in liquid nitrogen. Disrupt the cells further by homogenizing on ice. This crude preparation could be used for infections i.e. for *in vitro* but not for *in vivo* experiments (Ficoll gradient purified virus should be used for these).
(9) Spin homogenate at 10 000 r.p.m. for 5 min at 4°C to remove cell debris. Retain the supernatant as a virus stock. Store small aliquots in sterile cryotubes at −70°C.
(10) To further purify the virus stock, take supernatant from step 9 and centrifuge at 23 000*g* for 2 hours at 4°C. This pellets the virus. Resuspend the pellet in cold 199 medium. Dispense small aliquots into sterile cryotubes and store at −70°C.
(11) For *in vivo* experiments, gradient-purified virus preparation should be used (Szilagyi and Cunningham, 1991). Pour linear 5–15% (w/v) Ficoll gradient in PBS (use clear tubes) and layer the virus preparation from Steps 6 or 10 (in approximately 1 ml medium) on the top of the gradient (all at 4°C).
(12) Spin at 19 000*g* for 2 h at 4°C. Under top illumination with dark background the virion appears as the heaviest band in the middle of the gradient.
(13) Collect the intense virion band by puncturing the side of the tube.
(14) Dilute virion band from the Ficoll gradient in the virion preparation with cold PBS (e.g. virions from one gradient to a final volume of 30 ml) and spin at 65 000*g* for 2 h at 4°C to pellet the virus.
(15) Resuspend the pellet in cold PBS. Store small aliquots in sterile cryotubes at −70°C.

Protocol #72: HSV-1 Titration

(1) Grow BHK cells on four six-well plates to confluence.
(2) Remove medium from the plates and add 0.5 ml warm 199 medium to each well.
(3) Make serial dilutions of virus stock by first diluting 50 μl in 450 μl 199 medium (10^{-1} dilution) and then by consecutive tenfold dilutions (50 μl added to 450 μl medium). Use a fresh pipette tip for each dilution to prevent carryover of virus. Work on ice.
(4) Apply 100 μl diluted virus (10^{-5}–10^{-8} for permissive temperature and 10^{-2}–10^{-8} for non-permissive temperature) to duplicate wells for each temperature. Gently rock the plates to ensure virus is evenly spread. Adsorb virus at the appropriate temperature for 90 min, rocking plates occasionally.
(5) Remove inoculum, wash plates with warm 199 medium and add 2.5 ml warm titration medium to each well. Incubate at the appropriate temperature for 3–4 days without disturbing the plates to allow plaques to develop.
(6) Remove medium and fix cells for 20 min in methanol. Remove the methanol and add Giemsa stain, leave for 30 min, then wash with tap water.
(7) Count the plaques using a stereo microscope or inverted microscope. On the basis of the number of plaques formed at various dilutions calculate the titer of the virus stock as p.f.u./ml.

Example Titer Calculation

At 10^{-6} dilution 60 and 55 p.f.u. were found per well; at the 10^{-7} dilution 5 and 6 p.f.u./well.

Transform all counts to the same order and calculate the mean; for example 60, 55, 50 and 60 p.f.u./well at 10^{-6} dilution, giving a 56 p.f.u./well at 10^{-6} dilution. Enter this count in the following formula:

$$\text{Titer} = \frac{\text{p.f.u./well}}{\text{dilution}} \times 10$$

$$\text{Titer} = \frac{56}{10^{-6}} \times 10$$

$$= 5.6 \times 10^{8} \text{ p.f.u./ml}$$

Protocol #73: Plaque Purification of HSV-1

(1) Grow BHK cells on six-well plates to confluence.
(2) Prepare agar overlay medium by mixing one volume of 2 × 199 medium with one volume of 1% molten agar, both equilibrated to 45°C. Keep the overlay medium at 45°C in a water bath until use.
(3) Remove medium and add 0.5 ml warm 199 medium to each well.
(4) Make serial tenfold dilutions of virus stock to be plaque purified as described in Protocol #72, Step 3.
(5) Apply 100 μl of diluted virus (10^{-3}–10^{-8}) to each well. Gently rock the plates to ensure virus is evenly spread. Incubate at 31°C for 90 min, rocking plates occasionally.
(6) Remove all medium (leftover liquid between cells and agar renders the monolayer very susceptible to damage during manipulation). Work quickly so that the cell monolayer does not dry out.
(7) Pipette 2 ml overlay medium into each well. Allow plaques to grow at 31°C to a reasonable size (about 3 days).
(8) Select wells containing a low number of well separated plaques. Mark plaques by viewing plates under inverted microscope. Then, viewing plates under a stereo microscope (dark field can help in plaque identification), using a yellow tip (Eppendorf) to avoid cross-contamination, withdraw cells from individual plaques and transfer them to a tube containing 200 μl cold 199 medium (Fig. 14.2).
(9) Freeze/thaw cells three times in liquid nitrogen to release the virus. Store plaques at −70°C.
(10) At this stage the plaques may be titrated further (dilution range 10–10^{-4}) and Steps 1–9 repeated until the plaque isolate is homogeneous.
(11) Grow up the plaque isolate by inoculating 5 cm plates of confluent BHK cells with 50 μl aliquots of plaque isolate. Incubate at 31°C for 90 min, rocking occasionally. Remove the medium by aspiration and add fresh warm 199 medium. Grow at 31°C.
(12) Harvest cells when complete cytopathic effect is visible (the cells become rounded and detach from the flask when shaken). Scrape infected cells into the medium with a sterile scraper and transfer into a 15 ml centrifuge tube. Spin at 1500 r.p.m. for 10 min.
(13) If a virus strain is grown that releases significant amount of virus particles into the medium follow Step 6 of Protocol #71. If a strain that does not release significant amount of virus into the medium is being grown, dispose of the supernatant from Step 12 and go to Step 14. The cell pellet contains most of the infectious virus.
(14) To release cell associated virus, resuspend the cell pellet from Step 12 in 1 ml cold 199 medium and freeze/thaw three times in liquid nitrogen. Disrupt the cells further by homogenizing. This crude preparation of virus could be used for infection and stored as plate harvest at −70°C.
(15) Spin down the cell debris at 10 000 r.p.m. for 5 min at 4°C. Retain the supernatant as a plate harvest. Store aliquots in sterile cryotubes at −70°C.

Protocol #74: Preparation of HSV-1 DNA from Virions

(1) Prepare HSV-1 virus as described in Protocol #71 Steps 1–10, but infect cells with a MOI of up to 5 p.f.u./cell. Cell-released virions from Step 7 are cleaner and better than cell-associated virions from Step 10.

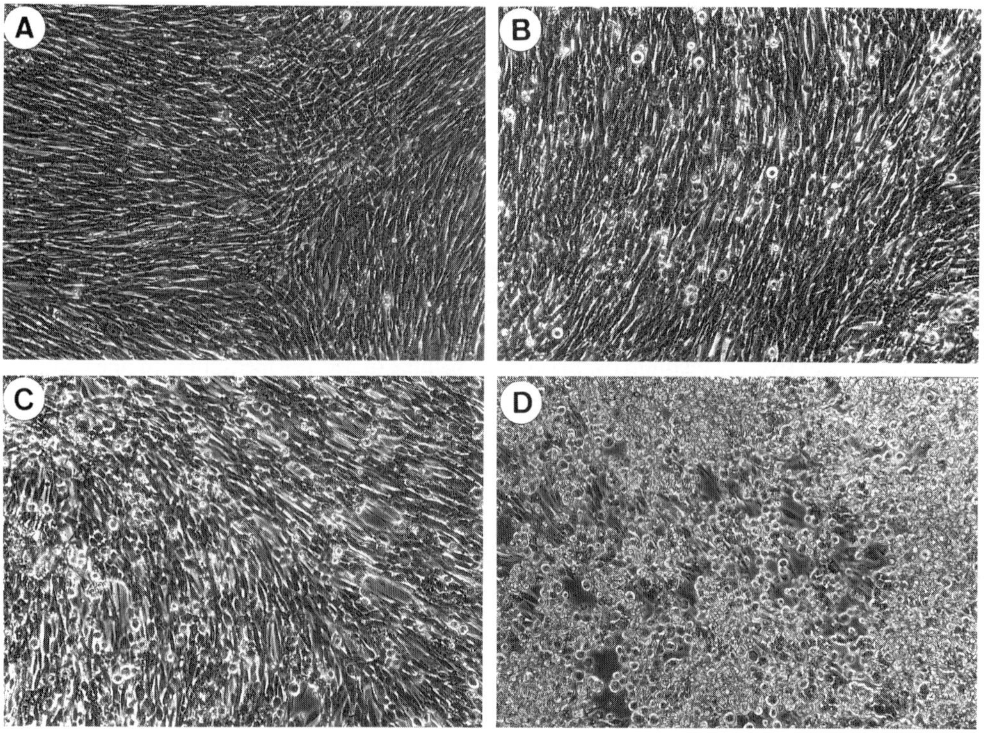

Figure 14.3 Morphological sequence of cell infection. Confluent BHK cells (A) were infected with *ts*K at a MOI of 0.01 and incubated at 31°C. It takes approximately 4 days for cells to show the complete cytopathic effect (D). The uninfected monolayer is shown in (A). (B) Shows the monolayer after 1–2 days, and some infected cells are visible, already showing a different morphology from the uninfected cell layer. (C) The monolayer near the stage of complete cytopathic effect. At the time of complete cytopathic effect (D) virus should be harvested

(2) Resuspend the virion pellet in 300 μl of cold Tris buffer. Transfer the suspension to a 1.5 ml polypropylene tube and add 300 μl cold lysis buffer 1. Invert the tube gently several times to mix and incubate at 37°C overnight.
(3) Very gently (important) extract the lysate with phenol/chloroform. Centrifuge at 12 000 r.p.m. for 5 min and transfer upper aqueous phase to a fresh tube.
(4) Repeat the extraction with phenol/chloroform and then extract the aqueous phase with chloroform. Keep the top aqueous phase.
(5) Ethanol precipitate the DNA in the presence of 0.5 M LiCl by adding 10 M LiCl to 0.5 M final concentration, then add two volumes of cold absolute ethanol, gently inverting the tube several times.
(6) Harvest the DNA by centrifugation at 12 000*g* for 20 min at 4°C. Discard the supernatant and rinse the pellet with 70% (v/v) ethanol. After removing all the ethanol, let the pellet air dry briefly and allow to dissolve gently in an appropriate volume of sterile water or TE overnight at 37°C.
(7) Store at −20°C.

Protocol #75: Preparation of Cytoplasmic HSV-1 DNA

(1) Grow eight 175 cm^3 flasks of BHK cells to confluence.
(2) Remove the medium and infect cells by adding virus inoculum at a MOI of 5 p.f.u/cell (1.7×10^8p.f.u/flask) in sufficient warm 199 medium to just cover the cell monolayer.

(3) Incubate at 31°C for 90 min, agitating gently every 15 min.
(4) Remove the inoculum, briefly wash with warm 199 medium, add more 199 medium and incubate at 31°C for days, until a cytopathic effect is seen in the cultured cells (the cells become rounded but do not detach from the sides of the flask) (Fig 14.3).
(5) Scrape the infected cells into the medium with a sterile scraper into 50 ml centrifuge tubes. Spin at 1500 r.p.m. for 20 min at 4°C.
(6) Dispose of the medium. Resuspend cells by pipetting in 6 ml of ice-cold NP-40 buffer and spin at 1500 r.p.m. for 10 min at 4°C. Keep the supernatant on ice. Resuspend the pellet in 2 ml cold NP-40 buffer and homogenize (10–20 strokes). The level of cell disruption may be observed under the microscope and homogenization stopped as soon as the cells are evenly disrupted.
(7) Spin the homogenate at 6000 r.p.m. for 5 min at 4°C. Discard the pellet and pool the supernatant with supernatant from Step 6.
(8) Add EDTA to 100 mM, SDS to 0.5% and gently agitate by inverting the tube several times. Add pronase to 1 mg/ml, gently mix by inverting several times and incubate overnight at 37°C.
(9) Very gently extract the lysate with an equal volume of phenol/chloroform. Centrifuge at 12 000 r.p.m. for 10 min and transfer top aqueous phase to a fresh tube.
(10) Repeat the phenol/chloroform extraction and then extract the aqueous phase with chloroform. Keep the top aqueous phase from chloroform extraction.
(11) Ethanol precipitate, harvest and store the DNA as described in Protocol #74.

Protocol #76: Calcium Phosphate Transfection of HSV-1 DNA

(1) Grow BHK cells to confluence at 37°C in 5% CO_2.
(2) Remove medium and wash the cell monolayer with warm PBS (without Ca^{2+}, Mg^{2+}) by tilting the dish. Remove PBS.
(3) Add warm trypsin/EDTA solution to cover the cell monolayer (1.5 ml per 175 cm^2 dish) and incubate at 37°C for approximately 3 min. The cells should detach readily.
(4) Resuspend the cells in culture medium by pipetting and ensure that they are evenly dispersed. Divide cells onto two 10 cm plates at about 50% confluence.
(5) 12–16 h after plating and 1 h before transfection replace medium with 5 ml fresh warm culture medium.
(6) Prepare DNA solution by mixing 62 μl $CaCl_2$ solution, calf thymus DNA and 0.5–4 μg HSV-1 *ts*K DNA in sterile deionized water (total volume 500 μl). Adjust the amount of calf thymus DNA to make up total DNA in solution to 5 μg. Mix very gently by inverting the tube a few times. When pipetting HSV-1 DNA, use a sterile tip with the end cut off.
(7) Pipette 500 μl of 2 × HBS buffer into a cryovial. Using 2 ml pipette, add DNA solution dropwise, very slowly, while rotating the vial. Close and invert the vial very gently. The DNA will precipitate. Immediately bring BHK plates from the incubator and using a 2 ml pipette spread 0.5 ml of precipitate dropwise on each plate.
(8) Leave the precipitate to settle for 3.5 h at 37°C.
(9) Remove the medium and add 5 ml warm glycerol or DMSO solution to the side of the plate and tilt gently once or twice to cause hypertonic shock to the cells. Incubate one plate for 1 min and one for 2 min at room temperature. Remove the glycerol (or DMSO) solution by aspiration and gently wash cells with 199 medium. Aspirate medium add 10 ml warm 199 medium and incubate at 31°C. Plaques should appear after 3–5 days. Grow the virus until the cells are showing complete cytopathic effect.
(10) Scrape the infected cells into the medium with a sterile scraper and transfer into a 15 ml centrifuge tube. Spin at 1500 r.p.m. for 10 min at 4°C.
(11) If you grow a strain which releases significant amounts of virus into the medium, follow Protocol #71 Step 6. If you grow a strain that does not release significant amount of virus into the medium, dispose of the supernatant from Step 10 and go to Step 12. The cell pellet then contains most of the infectious virus.

(12) Release cell-associated virus, purify and store as in Protocol #73, Steps 14 and 15, with the exception that the supernatant is stored as virus stock.

Protocol #77: Production of tk⁻ HSV-1 Recombinants by Homologous Recombination

(1) Transfect a mixture of 1 μg of digested plasmid DNA containing the gene of interest and 1 μg HSV-1 *ts*K DNA into BHK cells and prepare progeny of transfection using the method described in Protocol #76.
(2) Grow BHK cells on four six-well plates to confluence.
(3) Remove medium and add 0.5 ml warm 199 medium to each well.
(4) Make serial tenfold dilutions of virus stock from Step 1 as described in Protocol #72.
(5) Label two plates as Duplicate 1 and two plates as Duplicate 2. Apply 100 μl diluted virus (dilution range 10–10^{-5}) to each of two duplicates. Gently rock the plates to ensure virus is evenly spread over the surface. Incubate at 31°C for 90 min, rocking occasionally.
(6) Remove the inoculum, wash plates with warm 199 medium. Add 2 ml warm titration medium to each well in Duplicate 1 and 2 ml of warm 199/acycloguanosine medium to each well of Duplicate 2. Incubate at 31°C for 3–4 days. During this time do not disturb the plates containing titration medium.
(7) After 3–4 days remove the medium from Duplicate 1 and fix the cells in methanol for 20 min. Remove the methanol and add Giemsa stain for 30 min, then wash under tap water.
(8) Count the plaques in Duplicate 1 using a stereo microscope or inverted microscope. On the basis of the number of plaques formed in various dilutions calculate the titer of virus as described in Protocol #72. Identify the well which received approximately 10^4 p.f.u.
(9) Harvest the corresponding well from Duplicate 2 when cells are showing complete cytopathic effect by scraping into the medium and transfer to a sterile tube. Freeze/thaw three times in liquid nitrogen. Store this virus preparation at −70°C.
(10) Retitrate the stock obtained in Step 9 and prepare new stock as described in Steps 2–9. The resultant virus stock should be sufficiently enriched for tk⁻ virus to allow individual plaques to be picked.
(11) Plaque purify the virus stock from Step 10 by titration (dilution range 10^{-4}–10^{-7}). Incubate cells with virus for 90 min. Prepare agar overlay medium by mixing one volume of 2 × 199 medium with one volume of 1% molten agar, both equilibrated to 45°C. Keep the overlay medium in a 45°C water bath until use.
(12) Carefully remove all medium; liquid between cells and agar renders the monolayer very susceptible to damage during manipulation. However, work quickly and do not let the cell monolayer dry out.
(13) Pipette 2 ml of overlay medium into each well. Allow plaques to grow at 31°C to a reasonable size (about 3 days).
(14) Select plaques and process as described in Protocol #73, Steps 8–15. This stock, plate harvest, serves to grow large-scale preparations of virus.
(15) As tk⁺ viruses can also be generated spontaneously, individual plaque isolates should be checked by Southern blot analysis before growing up stocks. Choose probes which will hybridize to inserted sequences and to tk sequences to distinguish between pure recombinant virus, wild-type virus and mixtures.

Protocol #78: Preparation of Total DNA for Southern Blotting

(1) Harvest infected BHK cells showing complete cytopathic effect. Approximately 1×10^5–2×10^5 infected cells should be sufficient for one analysis.
(2) Add 0.5 ml lysis buffer 2 to the cell pellet, mix by vortexing and incubate at 37°C overnight.
(3) Extract lysates with an equal volume of phenol/chloroform. Add an equal volume of phenol/chloroform and vortex the tube for 1 min, or rotate on the wheel for 10 min. Centrifuge at 12 000 r.p.m. for 1 min and transfer upper aqueous phase to a fresh tube.
(4) Repeat the extraction with phenol/chloroform and then extract the aqueous phase with chloroform. Keep the top aqueous phase from chloroform extraction.

Table 14.1 Conversion of molar ratios to mass ratios for p23 plasmid and 0.5, 1 and 2 kbp DNA fragments to be inserted

Molar ratio	*Vector p23 7.5 kbp (ng)*	*Insert 0.5 kbp (ng)*	*Insert 1 kbp (ng)*	*Insert 2 kbp (ng)*
1:1	200	14	29	54
1:3	200	40	80	160
3:1	200	5	9	18

(5) Harvest the DNA as described in Protocol #74, Steps 5–7. It is now ready for Southern blot analysis.

Protocol #79: Preparation of DNA for Cloning

(1) Prepare sufficient DNA for cloning using any suitable technique. (SEE SECTION 4.10 for details.)

(2) Prepare vector p23 DNA by *Xho*I digestion. This 50 μl reaction is provided as an example. Mix p23 DNA, 5 μg, *Xho*I 10× buffer, 5 μl, *Xho*I, 10 U, deionized sterile water to a final volume of 50 μl in a sterile Eppendorf tube, mix by gentle tapping spin for 5 s and incubate at 37°C for 1 h. Check that the reaction has gone to completion by quick electrophoresis of a sample (0.3 μg DNA) on a 1% agarose minigel. If the reaction is complete add 10 μl calf intestinal alkaline phosphatase (CIP) 10× buffer, 0.01 U of ends and sterile deionized water to 100 μl. Incubate 60 min at 37°C. Add same amount of CIP as before and incubate for 30 min at 37°C (SEE SECTION 4.10). Purify the DNA by any suitable method. Cut out the insert cDNA by *Xho*I digestion as described above and purify the correct restriction fragment using electrophoresis on low melting agarose gel.

(3) To obtain the optimal ratio of vector to insert DNA, 1:1, 1:3 and 3:1 molar ratios should be used when cloning the fragment into a plasmid vector (see Table 14.1).

(4) Set up a ligation reaction by mixing vector and insert DNAs in a sterile Eppendorf tube as described in Table 14.1, add 2 μl 10× ligation buffer, 0.1 U T4 DNA ligase and deionized sterile water to a final volume of 20 μl. Mix all components by tapping the tube and spin for 5 s (Marsden et al., 1976; Lowenstein et al., 1994).

(5) Allow to ligate overnight at 4°C. Following the reaction, transform competent cells with DNA.

(6) Colonies will appear overnight. Each colony is a progeny of a single bacterial cell and thus a genetically pure culture. To grow up pure cultures, transfer each colony with a sterile loop to a liquid culture supplemented with ampicillin and grow at 37°C overnight with vigorous shaking.

(7) Prepare plasmid DNA from these cultures for restriction analysis. Several commercial kits are available which allow rapid isolation of small amounts of plasmid DNA for restriction analysis.

(8) Cut the DNA with one or more suitable restriction enzyme/s to check for the presence and orientation of the required insert, then select and grow up suitable recombinants.

(9) If the ends of the insert are incompatible, having 5′ overhangs or blunt ends, perform blunt end ligation as follows in Steps 10–16.

(10) Digest p23 vector as in Step 2 and cut out the insert cDNA fragment with suitable enzyme/s (or use a purified insert).

(11) Add to each mixture 10 μl of 10× T4 DNA polymerase buffer, 25 U T4 DNA polymerase, dNTPs to 100 μM each and sterile deionized water to 100 μl. Mix by tapping the tube.

(12) Incubate at 37°C for 10 min. Stop reaction by heating to 75°C for 10 min. To purify the DNA use any suitable method. To obtain the optimal ratio of vector to insert DNA, a 1:3 molar ratio should be used when cloning the blunt-ended fragment into a blunt-ended plasmid vector. The conversion of molar ratios to mass ratios for p23 plasmid and 0.5, 1 and 2 kbp DNA fragment to be inserted is given in Table 14.2.

(13) Set up ligation reaction by mixing DNAs as described in Table 14.2, add 2 μl 10× ligation buffer, 3 U T4 DNA ligase, Ficoll 400 to 15% w/v and deionized sterile water to a final

Table 14.2

Size of insert (kbp)	0.5	1	2
Plasmid p23 (ng)	1650	1400	1100
Insert (ng)	350	600	900

volume of 20 μl. Mix by tapping the tube and spin in a microfuge for 5 s.

(14) Ligate for 16 h at 15°C. Following the reaction, transform competent cells with the DNA.

(15) Colonies will appear overnight, each colony being a progeny of a single bacterial cell and thus genetically pure. To grow up pure cultures transfer each colony to a liquid culture supplemented with ampicillin and grow at 37°C overnight with vigorous shaking.

(16) Prepare plasmid DNA, check insert and grow up suitable recombinants as described in Steps 7 and 8.

4 NOTES AND TROUBLESHOOTING

4.1 Safety

HSV is a human pathogen of modest to low pathogenicity under normal circumstances. Nevertheless, all work with HSV should be undertaken in accordance with relevant local and national safety procedures. Appropriate approval from local and national genetic manipulation regulatory bodies must be obtained if a foreign protein is to be expressed using a HSV-derived vector.

When handling HSV, always wear protective clothing. Never touch mouth, eyes or genitals with fingers or articles that could be contaminated. Always work in a tissue culture hood to avoid inhalation of aerosols or splashes. If it is necessary to work outside the tissue culture hood face mask and eye protection should be worn.

For virus wastes use robust, leak-proof containers that can be handled easily. Always decontaminate or seal in an autoclave bag all articles that could have been exposed to virus (including gloves) before removing them from the hood, decontaminate work surfaces (using, for example, Virkon, 70% ethanol or bleach). An autoclave in the tissue culture room will avoid transferring virus contaminants out of the laboratory.

Avoid any activities that may produce aerosols or splashes, such as violent pipetting, blowing out of last drop, violent homogenization or sonication with exposed probes, use of unplugged pipette tips or leaking centrifuge tubes.

If small-scale spillage occurs, notify other workers in the area, cover the area with paper towels to soak up the fluid, gently pour disinfectant over these towels, leave for a while and transfer towels together with solid fragments into a bag for autoclaving. Mop area with more disinfectant. If large-scale spillage occurs, evacuate the room immediately, close the doors and contact safety staff.

Be cautious when handling animal sera and human serum.

Phenol is corrosive and can burn. Gloves should be worn when handling it. Only polypropylene or high-density polyethylene tubes should be used when extracting with phenol and chloroform.

Ethidium bromide is a mutagen and must be handled carefully. Avoid direct contact with skin. Also avoid direct exposure to ultraviolet light when examining agarose gels stained with ethidium bromide—wear a face mask.

4.2 On Protocol #68: Passage of BHK Cells

Because HSV-1 has a wide host range in tissue culture a number of host cell lines can be used for virus growth. However, the yield of virus varies widely between cell types. Hep-2 and Syrian Hamster Kidney BHK-21 (clone 13) cells, ECACC No. 85011433, have been widely used to make HSV stocks. Both grow to a high cell density in dishes or roller bottles.

The cell line to be used for virus stock preparation should be tested for mycoplasma contamination before use. We routinely use BHK cells, which are not immortal and can typically be passaged up to 15 times before becoming senescent. Consequently, frozen stocks, which can be recovered at regular intervals, must be stored as described in Protocol [#69]. Stored cells should be of a low passage number and high viability.

4.3 On Protocol #71: Growth of HSV-1 and Preparation of Virus Stocks

We use the HSV-1 mutant *ts*K of strain 17 for producing recombinant viruses (Marsden et al., 1976; Preston, 1979). When growing the temperature-sensitive mutant the cells must be incubated at the permissive temperature (31°C.) It is a useful feature of HSV-1 *ts*K that the virus behaves as an essential immediate early mutant at 37°C, allowing experiments to be performed at the physiological temperature of most primary cell lines, without the vector entering a lytic replicative cycle. However, results obtained at 37°C and 38.5°C should be compared in any system. For example a typical titer at 31°C may be 10^8 p.f.u./ml. At 37°C and above, the proportion of replicating wild-type revertants will be 10^{-5} or less, and so the titer will be 10^3 p.f.u./ml or lower.

HSV can generate populations of defective interfering (DI) particles containing incomplete genomes if consistently passaged at high MOI, so host cells should be infected at MOI of 0.001–0.1 p.f.u/cell to prevent accumulation of defective viruses. A high MOI (1 p.f.u./cell or above) should be used only for preparations that will not serve as working stocks (e.g. preparation of virus DNA, since high MOI infections will increase DNA yield). However, note that passages at high MOI are required to prepare amplicon type vectors, because amplicons are essentially DI particles.

Repeated passages of virus could cause accumulation of defective virus. To avoid this, prepare a master stock (or a plate harvest) from a single viral plaque, after infecting a 5 cm plate, as described in Protocol #73 and stored at −70°C in 199 medium. This stock is used to prepare first passage. Working stocks are routinely grown from this first passage, avoiding the risk of creating stocks so far apart in passage number as to make direct comparison between experiments invalid, as well as to avoid accumulation of non-lethal mutations in the large HSV-1 genome.

For long-term storage, freeze HSV-1 stocks at −70°C. **Never** store HSV-1 at −20°C because damage to the virus envelope results in a considerable drop in titer. The virus is stable for short-term storage (a few days) at 4°C, but stability varies between strains. Virus should be stored frozen in small enough volumes to avoid thawing and refreezing.

The time needed to develop complete cytopathic effect varies with the strain and mutant of the virus and the cell lines used, and must be determined empirically. Cells should be harvested when they look right, not when the clock indicates they are ready.

The amount of virus released into the medium and remaining cell associated is dependent on the strains of virus and cell type used. If significant lysis of cells occurs during infection, the culture supernatant is a better source of clean virus stock than the cell-associated virus. In most cases most virus remains cell associated and can be harvested from cells. Strain 17 releases well, about 50% of the total virus being present in the medium. It can be recovered by centrifugation at 23 000*g*, resuspended well or dispersed by sonication.

Once infected cells have been harvested the virus must be separated from cell debris. However, many laboratories successfully use preparations that are not completely cell-free. In our laboratory the virus is released by quick freeze/thaw cycles using liquid nitrogen and a 37°C water bath with vigorous agitation, followed by homogenization. Another method used routinely involves sonication.

If the sterility of your virus preparation is in doubt the stock should be filtered carefully through a 0.45 μm Nalgene filter with great care since a blocked filter could explode under pressure, risking exposure to the virus.

4.4 On Protocol #72: HSV-1 Titration

It is important to prevent released virus forming secondary plaques and inflating the titer. A variety of media can be used to prevent virus spreading other than through direct cell-to-cell contact. The most practical of these is to use titration medium containing pooled human serum (which contains neutralizing antibodies against HSV) or overlaying with agar (as in Protocol #73).

Viral titers may vary considerably between different cell types and it might be necessary to titrate the virus in the cell type in which it will be used. For routine applications BHK, Hep-2 or Vero cells are commonly used. Whatever cell line is chosen, cells must be able to maintain a confluent monolayer until the plaques appear, a minimum of 3 days. It is possible to maintain confluent monolayers for longer periods by reducing the serum level in the titration medium.

4.5 On Protocol #74: Preparation of HSV-1 DNA from Virions

To check the purity of the DNA preparation measure the absorbance ratio at 260 and 280 nm. Pure DNA has a ratio of 1.8; preparations usually are in the range 1.6–1.8. Ratios below 1.8 indicate protein or phenol contamination, above 1.8 indicate RNA contamination. By digesting 3 μg of HSV-1 DNA with 10 units of *Bam*HI for 2 h at 37°C and running the DNA on 0.7% agarose gel any contaminating DNA or RNA will be visible. HSV-I digests show the typical restriction pattern, if the preparation is impure smears of cellular DNA or RNA will be seen. To establish the infective quality of the DNA BHK cells should be transfected with 0.5–2μg HSV-1 DNA by calcium phosphate transfection (Protocol #76).

The DNA of HSV is large, almost 150 000 base pairs, so is sensitive to shear. After addition of lysis buffer (as in Step 2), the DNA is no longer protected within virions and will shear easily. The DNA solution should not be shaken or vortexed and yellow plastic tips with the ends cut off used.

Methods for preparation of viral DNA differ according to the degree of purity required. For each application the minimal purity required should be determined. For example, the crude viral DNA prepared in Protocol #78 is usually heavily contaminated with cellular DNA. It may be used successfully for transfection and recombinants generated but DNA from Protocol #77 will give higher success rates. For strain 17 viruses better results will be obtained by extracting DNA from cell-released virions and purifying it by spinning at 23 000*g* for 2 h: this will be cleaner than DNA obtained from cell-associated virus.

HSV-1 DNA precipitates rapidly and should be visible after mixing in ethanol. Centrifugation after thorough mixing should pellet the viral DNA. Leaving it at −70°C or −20°C will not increase recovery but could cause more contamination with RNA. Alcohol-dehydrated HSV DNA often takes longer to rehydrate than expected because of its size.

Preparations of pronase could be contaminated with DNAase and RNAase. These enzymes can be inactivated by incubating the pronase stock solution for 2 h at 37°C. As an alternative proteinase K 100 μg/ml may be used. It is purer but more expensive than pronase.

4.6 On Protocol #75: Preparation of Cytoplasmic HSV-1 DNA

Viral DNA minimally contaminated with cellular DNA can be obtained if homogenization is kept to a minimum sufficient to just lyse the cells without breaking nuclei and infected cells are harvested when they are rounded but still in good shape, quite firmly attached to the plastic.

4.7 On Protocol #76: Calcium Phosphate Transfection of HSV-1 DNA

Calf thymus DNA should be deproteinized by treating with proteinase K or pronase, followed by extraction with phenol and chloroform before use. The extent of residual protein in the DNA can be measured as optical density ratio at 260 and 280 nm. Pure DNA has a ratio about 1.8 and a ratio below 1.8 is a sign of protein contamination. Low-quality DNA should not be used for transfection.

4.8 On Protocol #77: Production of tk⁻ HSV-1 Recombinants by Homologous Recombination

Recombination is more efficient using a linearized plasmid. The plasmid should be digested with a restriction enzyme which cuts outside the inserted DNA more than 500 base pairs from the site of insertion.

When selecting recombinant viruses with acycloguanosine, cells are infected at low MOI,

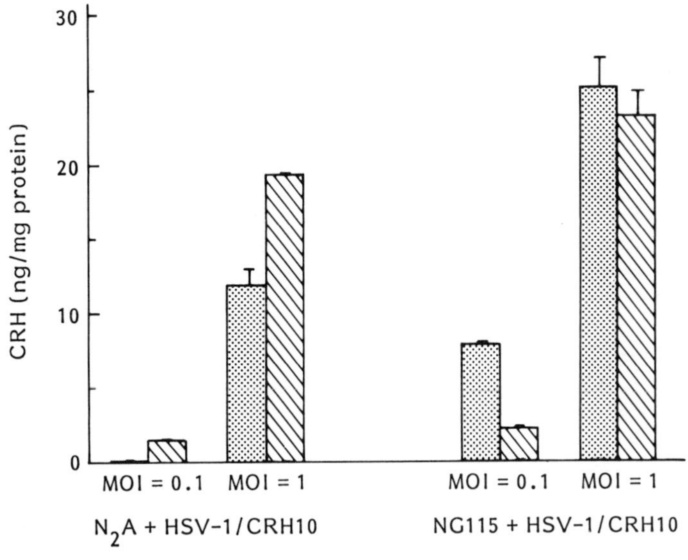

Figure 14.4 The result of infecting two neuronal cell lines with a *ts*K derived recombinant encoding the neuropeptide rCRH. Cells were infected at the MOI shown and medium or cells were collected 12 h after infection. rCRH was measured using a specific radioimmunoassay. Stippled bars: CRH stored; striped bars: CRH released

approximately 0.01 p.f.u/cell, to reduce the possibility of complementing TK^+ virus masking the effects of selection.

Homologous recombination relies on the introduction of full-length deproteinized HSV-1 *ts*K DNA into cells together with excess of a plasmid molecule containing the foreign DNA linked to a TK region of the viral genome. Because deproteinized viral DNA is infectious, a lytic cycle will take place in the infected cell and homologous recombination will occur between the region of viral TK sequences linked to foreign DNA and the corresponding TK region of the virus, causing the foreign DNA to be inserted into a recombinant virus (Figs 14.4–14.6; for Fig 14.5 see Plate VI). The TK gene is not essential in HSV-1; its inactivation in recombinant viruses can be detected and used for selecting recombinants by growing in the presence of deoxynucleotide analogs (such as acycloguanosine) that are phosphorylated by HSV-1 wild-type TK and are hence incorporated into its DNA, blocking DNA replication. For examples of *ts*K derived recombinants see Figs 14.4–14.6. For Fig. 14.5 see Plate VI.

4.9 On Protocol #78: Preparation of Total DNA for Southern Blotting

This method is suitable for applications involving large numbers of samples, such as checking the structure of a recombinant virus, for which crude DNA containing cellular as well as viral DNA (broken or intact) is sufficient. If this DNA is digested with the appropriate restriction enzymes viral DNA bands could be seen within the cellular DNA smear on gel electrophoresis. The size of regions of interest is easily determined by Southern blotting using appropriate probes. The yield of viral DNA for Southern blotting can be increased by using high MOI.

4.10 On Protocol #79: Preparation of DNA for Cloning

The structures of vector DNA and plasmid containing cDNA should be confirmed before use by digesting preparations with restriction enzymes and comparing with restriction maps.

Construction of p23 plasmid is described by Lowenstein et al. (1994). Briefly, vector p23 contains sequences of the HSV-1 *Bam*HI p fragment coding for viral thymidine kinase. It has a

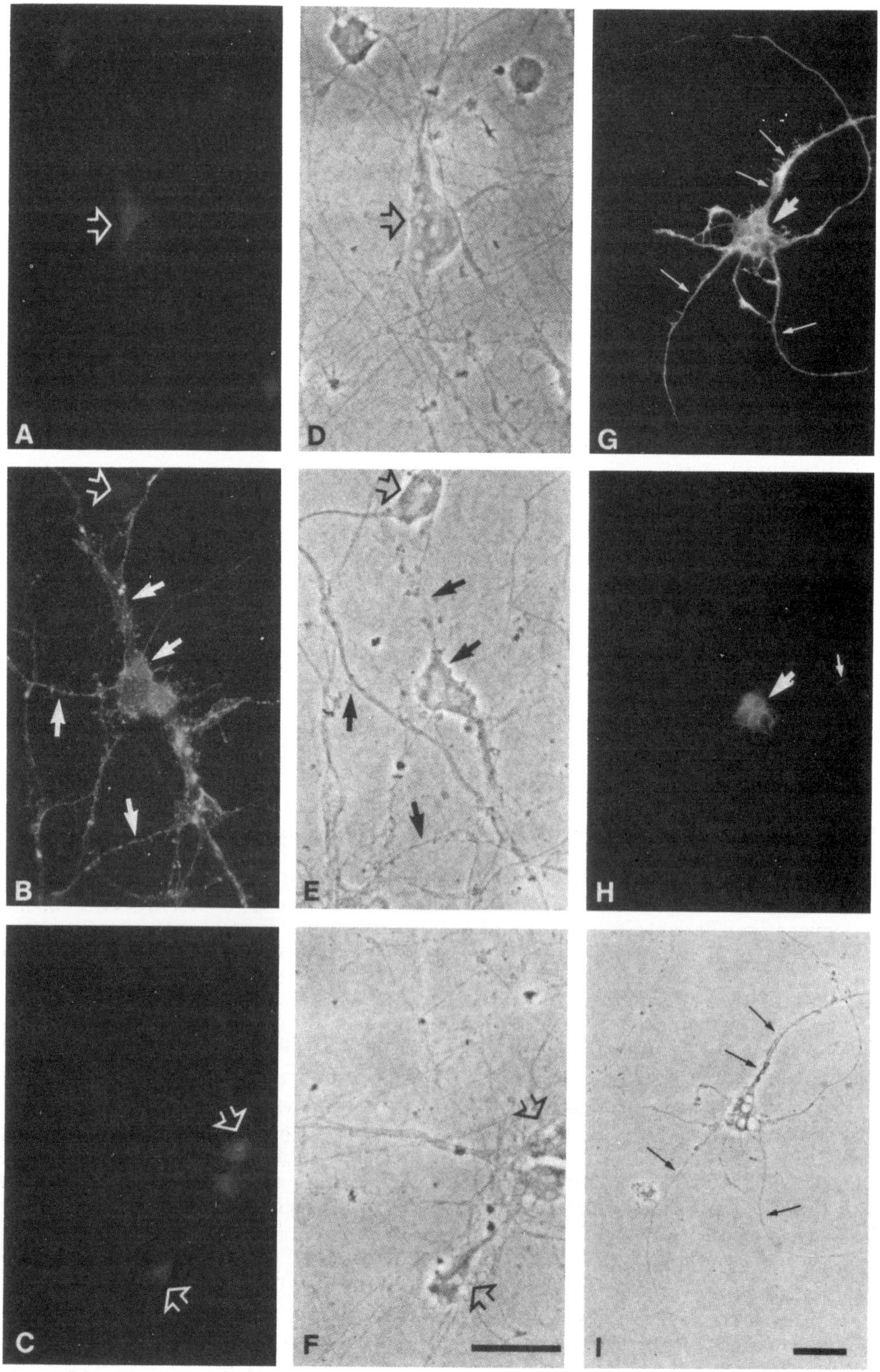
A
D
G
B
E
H
C
F
I

unique *Xho*I site within the HSV-1 TK coding sequences, flanked upstream by the IE3 promoter and cap site and downstream by TK coding sequences and, ultimately, the TK gene transcription termination signals. It carries an ampicillin resistance gene.

Each restriction enzyme should be used following the optimal conditions given by the supplier. One unit of restriction enzyme is defined as the amount required to completely digest 1 μg of DNA in 1 h at recommended conditions in 50 μl. Enzyme should be added last to a reaction mixture. When removing the enzyme from the freezer (**not** a frost-free freezer) the tube containing it should be placed immediately on ice. A new sterile tip should be used every time enzyme (and any other components of reaction mixture) is dispensed and once used it should be returned immediately to the freezer. The restriction enzyme should not contribute more than 10% of the volume of the final reaction mixture, because its activity may be inhibited by glycerol in the storage buffer. Multiple freeze/thaw cycles of the 10× ligation buffer should be avoided because the ATP it contains is unstable.

Alcohol precipitation of DNA in the presence of ammonium acetate enhances subsequent digestibility or ligation. The following method for preparing DNA fragments before ligation, end-filling or restriction enzyme digests is suggested.

(1) Add half volume of 7.5 M NH_4OAc to a DNA solution, mix, add two volumes of ethanol, mix.
(2) Incubate mixture at −20°C overnight.
(3) Spin out the DNA at 13 000 r.p.m. for 20 min.
(4) Wash the pellet with 70% ethanol and spin again.
(5) Briefly dry the pellet and dissolve in an appropriate volume of sterile deionized water or sterile TE.

Treating DNA with CIP removes 5′ phosphorylated groups and thus prevents recircularization of the vector during ligation. To assess the efficiency of the dephosphorylation, competent cells should be transformed with cut and religated vector DNA and cut, dephosphorylated and religated vector DNA.

The amount of ends (in moles) generated by restriction endonuclease cleavage of circular dsDNA is calculated thus:

2 × (moles of DNA) × (number of cuts) = 2 × (moles of DNA) × (number of cuts) + 2 × (moles of DNA)

Moles of dsDNA = weight of DNA base pairs (g) × 650 Da (molecular weight of a base pair).

If the insert DNA cannot be cut out with *Xho*I and does not have compatible sticky ends, suitable enzyme(s) should be used to purify the cDNA fragment and a method chosen to modify the vector and/or insert DNA for ligation.

For transformations we usually use *Escherichia coli* HB101 and the method described by

Figure 14.6 Effect of the enzyme PI-PLC on the immunoreactivity of neocortical neurons infected 24 h earlier with TT21, and effects of lack of membrane permeabilization of cells on the accessibility of intracellular and membrane bound antigens. (A–C): neurons immunoreacted with antibodies against TIMP; (D–F) the corresponding phase-contrast images. (A) and (D) represent non-infected cells, (B) and (E) infected cells, (C) and (F) infected cells after treatment with protease-free bacterial PI-PLC. No TIMP immunoreactivity can be detected in uninfected cells (open arrows in A and D), but can be localized in infected cells on cell bodies and neurites (straight arrows in B and E). Notice also an uninfected cell present in B and E (open arrow). Following PI-PLC treatment no TIMP immunoreactivity was detectable (C); open arrows indicate the presence of two cell bodies in both TIMP immunoreacted (C) and phase-contrast (F) images. Notice in (F) that the morphological appearance of cells is not affected by the PI-PLC treatment. This demonstrates that TIMP is linked to the external leaflet of the plasma membrane via a GPI anchor as predicted. G–I show that intracellular antigens are not accessible to antibodies in non-permeabilized cells. Infected non-permeabilized cells were double immunostained with TIMP (G) and MAP2 (H) antibodies. Notice that TIMP immunoreactivity is not affected by lack of cell permeabilization (G), while MAP2 antibodies can only stain the nucleus (straight thick arrow in H) and a short portion of a neurite (straight fine arrow in H). (I) shows a phase-contrast image of the cell shown in (G–H). Scale bars (shown in F and I) = 20 μm. Reproduced by permission from Lowenstein et al. (1994)

Maniatis (1982). Host cells may be transformed with uncut p23 and cut, religated p23 to monitor the efficiency of the transformation and ligation steps and mock-transformed cells could be plated onto nutrient agar and nutrient agar/ampicillin plates to check for cross-contamination. The microbial procedures for molecular cloning are straightforward, but require basic sterile techniques and common sense. All colony isolates should be purified at least twice by single-colony purification.

Colonies on agar plates may be stored wrapped in Parafilm and inverted at 4°C for a few weeks. No water of condensation should be allowed to fall onto the plate because it will quickly cause cross-contamination of colonies. For long-term storage, sterile overnight culture should be thoroughly mixed with sterile glycerol (15% v/v final) or DMSO (10% v/v final), frozen in liquid nitrogen and stored at −70°C. To recover bacteria, the surface of the frozen stock should be scratched with a sterile loop and transferred to nutrient broth, or the vial thawed quickly and cells grown in 100 ml nutrient broth.

Cleavage with two restriction enzymes may be carried out simultaneously if both enzymes work in the same buffer. If this is not the case, the enzyme that works in a buffer of lower ionic strength should be used first. The appropriate amount of the salt and the second enzyme can then be added and the incubation continued. *Eco*RI is a frequently used enzyme with star activity. To avoid star activity such an enzyme should be inactivated at 70°C for 10 min before changing salt concentration.

To check for occasional tandem insertions or isolation of multimer plasmids, uncleaved or supercoiled mobilities of recombinants should be compared with vector alone at the time minipreps are checked.

ACKNOWLEDGMENTS

This work was supported by a grant from the Wellcome Trust (03773529321.5/WRE/GM/JAT) to M.G.C. and P.R.L., and by the Medical Research Council (C.M.P.). P.R.L. is a Research Fellow of the Lister Institute of Preventive Medicine.

REFERENCES

Lowenstein, P. R., Morrison, E. E., Bain, D., Hodge, H., Preston, C. M., Clissold, P., Stow, N. D., McKee, T. A. and Castro, M. G. 1994. Use of recombinant vectors derived from Herpes simplex virus 1 mutant *ts*K for short term expression of transgenes encoding cytoplasmic and membrane anchored proteins in postmitotic polarized cortical neurons and glial cells *in vitro*. *Neuroscience* **60**:1059–1077.

Maniatis, T. 1982. *Molecular cloning*. (*A laboratory manual*). Cold Spring Harbor Laboratory. 249–250.

Marsden, H. S., Crombie, I. K. and Subak-Sharpe, J. H. 1976. Control of protein synthesis in herpes-virus-infected cells: analysis of the polypeptides induced by wild type and sixteen temperature-sensitive mutants of strain 17. *J. Gen. Virol.* **31**:347–371.

Preston, C. M. 1979. Control of herpes simplex virus type 1 mRNA synthesis in cells infected with wild type virus or the temperature-sensitive mutant *ts*K. *J. Virol.* **29**:275–284.

Roizman, B. 1995. Herpes simplex viruses and their replication. In *Fundamental Virology*. B.N. Fields, D.M. Knipe and P.M. Howley, chief editors. Raven Press, New York. 1043–1107.

Szilagyi, J. F. and Cunningham, C. 1991. Identification and characterization of a novel non-infectious herpes simplex virus related particle. *J. Gen. Virol.* **72**: 661–668.

CHAPTER 15

Manipulation of the Herpes Simplex Virus Genome for the Construction of Viral Vectors

NEAL A. DELUCA AND JOSEPH C. GLORIOSO

Department of Molecular Genetics and Biochemistry, University of Pittsburgh School of Medicine, Pittsburgh, PA 15261–2072, USA. Tel: 412 648 8105; Fax: 412 624 8997; Email: joe@server1.mgen.pitt.edu

1 INTRODUCTION

Viruses efficiently enter their hosts, usurping the cellular macromolecular machinery to varying degrees to express their own gene products and replicate their genomes. This often produces large numbers of viral progeny and ultimate death of the host cell. The potential for using viruses to introduce and express genes in mammalian cells has long been recognized. This potential is realized by delivering a viral genome to the cell nucleus in a form that is functional but unable to produce progeny virions or adversely affect host cell metabolism. To do this requires a detailed understanding of the life cycle of the virus and genetic tools to manipulate the virus.

Viruses being developed and used as gene transfer vehicles include retrovirus, adeno-associated virus (AAV), adenovirus and herpes simplex virus type 1 (HSV-1). Of these, retroviruses and AAV are naturally non-pathogenic and as part of their natural life cycle integrate into the genome of cells they infect. Retroviruses in particular have been most useful for gene transfer studies, both as a research tool and for clinical gene therapy protocols. However, the inability of retroviral and AAV vectors to obtain high titers of infectious virus and/or to infect non-dividing cells limits their use to mainly *ex vivo* approaches where cells in culture are infected, expanded and then selected for transduction events. The transduced cells are then transplanted into the organism at their intended site of action.

Adenovirus and HSV are both large DNA viruses that can be propagated to relatively high titers in culture. Both can easily be used to uniformly infect cells in culture and for *in vivo* or direct gene transfer in organisms. In addition, both are capable of infecting non-dividing cells, do not integrate in the cellular genome and can carry more foreign DNA than either retroviruses or AAV. HSV in particular can potentially package tens of kilobases of foreign DNA, making it possible to transduce large or multiple genes. It also has the capacity to establish latency in nerve cells, the viral genome persisting in an episomal form for prolonged periods. This feature makes HSV a promising gene transfer vector for the nervous system and a potential vehicle for treatment of neurological disorders (Chiocca et al., 1990; Dobson et al., 1990). Wild-type HSV is extremely pathogenic and cytolytic but it is possible to block its life cycle at a very early stage and to limit its pathogenic and cytotoxic potential.

Protocols for Gene Transfer in Neuroscience: Towards Gene Therapy of Neurological Disorders
Edited by P.R. Lowenstein and L.W. Enquist

1.1 Genetics and Viral Vectors of HSV

When nerve cells are infected by wild-type HSV the virus progresses through the lytic cycle, resulting in the production of infectious progeny, or (owing to events as yet to be elucidated) virus gene expression is severely restricted, resulting in latency (Wildy et al., 1982). During latency no lytic expression is observed (Spivack and Fraser, 1987; Stevens et al., 1987) and the genome persists in cells for prolonged periods without affecting host cell metabolism. The main approach used to design HSV vectors is to block virus gene expression at an early stage, abrogating the lytic cycle and mimicking the situation observed in latency. The natural silencing of the HSV genome and the establishment of latency are thought to involve mechanisms predominantly functioning in nerve cells. Mutating the virus so that lytic gene expression is attenuated in all cells might allow the virus to persist in any cells regardless of their tissue of origin. As mutant viruses blocked at a very early stage in the lytic regulatory cascade can establish latency, silencing the viral genome by mutation holds promise for development of HSV as a general gene transfer vehicle.

The HSV genome consists of 152 kbp of linear dsDNA encoding approximately 75 genes (McGeoch et al., 1988). The protein products of these genes augment and change the host cell transcriptional machinery, RNA processing, nucleotide pools and glycoprotein processing. HSV also specifies its own DNA replication machinery and proteins that affect homologous recombination. The virion is made up of approximately 30 structural proteins. It is important to understand how HSV affects host cell metabolism so that any deleterious effects on the host cell can be ameliorated. This is briefly discussed below with respect to the genetic manipulation of HSV for use as a vector.

Immediately after the HSV genome enters the nucleus of the infected cell, five viral genes are transcribed: infected cell polypeptides (ICPs) 4, 0, 27, 22, and 47 (Honess and Roizman, 1974). The promoters for these genes are activated by cellular factors and VP16 in the virion (Post et al., 1981; Batterson and Roizman, 1983; Campbell et al., 1984), and hence do not require viral protein synthesis for their expression. This operational definition is the basis on which they are referred to as immediate–early (IE) genes. The remaining HSV genes require one or more of the protein products of the IE genes for efficient expression (Honess and Roizman, 1975). Therefore the expression of HSV genes is determined mostly by components of the virion and IE proteins.

The functions of individual IE proteins and their contribution to the regulatory cascade in viral infection have been studied by constructing mutant viruses lacking individual IE genes. ICP22 and ICP47 are not essential for viral growth and have relatively little effect on the growth of HSV in culture systems but ICP22 mutants are slightly impaired for growth in certain cell types (Sears et al., 1985). ICP22 is also involved in the phosphorylation of the carboxy terminal domain of the large subunit of RNA *pol*II (Rice et al., 1994). ICP47 reduces MHC class I molecules on the cell surface (York et al., 1994). ICP0 mutants are impaired for growth in culture, producing yields 20–50 times lower per infected cell than wild-type virus (Stow and Stow, 1986; Sacks and Schaffer, 1987; Everett, 1989). However, this difference is apparently sufficient to dramatically reduce the ability of ICP0 mutants to reactivate from latency in murine trigeminal ganglia (Leib et al., 1989; Cai et al., 1993). ICP0 is a potent transactivator of test genes in transient assays (Everett, 1994) and this activity is thought to correlate with the role of ICP0 in reactivation from latency. It has recently been shown to alter the distribution of intranuclear structures referred to as pods (Everett and Maul, 1994). The significance of this observation with respect to cell metabolism and the viral life cycle is unknown, as is the mechanism by which ICP0 activates gene expression.

ICP4 and ICP27 are absolutely essential for viral growth (Dixon and Schaffer, 1980; Preston, 1981; Sacks et al., 1985). Mutants must be propagated on transformed cell lines that supply complementing levels of the corresponding protein in *trans* (DeLuca et al., 1985; DeLuca and Schaffer, 1987; McCarthy et al., 1989). The use of such cell lines to grow viruses deleted in these genes is central to the development of HSV "vector" strains. ICP4 transcriptionally activates most of the HSV genome (Preston, 1979; Dixon and Schaffer, 1980) and many heterologous RNA polymerase II promoters. ICP4 is a large nuclear phosphoprotein (Courtney and Benyesh-Melnick, 1974) that activates and represses transcription through interactions with the host basal transcriptional machinery (Gu et al., 1993; Smith et al., 1993; Gu and DeLuca, 1994). Viruses deleted for ICP4 efficiently express only the four other IE genes and ICP6 (DeLuca et al., 1985);

enzymes involved in viral DNA replication (Challberg, 1986) and virion structural proteins are not synthesized. ICP27 is required for efficient late gene expression (McCarthy et al., 1989). It is thought to affect the processing and activity of ICP4 and ICP0 (Hardwicke et al., 1989; Su and Knipe, 1989; McMahan and Schaffer, 1990) and mRNA processing (McLauchlan et al., 1992; Sandri-Goldin and Mendoza, 1992; Hardy and Sandri-Goldin, 1994).

Together, ICP4 and ICP27 constitute activities that have the greatest influence on the expression of the HSV genome. Their effect on viral gene expression and growth is ultimately tied to how they affect the gene expression apparatus of the host cell. We are just beginning to understand the particulars of these mechanisms. Relevant to the development of HSV as a gene transfer vector is the fact that ICP4 and ICP27 are the only two essential IE genes. By isolating and propagating viruses simultaneously deleted for these genes their direct and indirect effects on host cell metabolism will be eliminated. In addition, it may also allow deletion of the genes encoding the remainder of the proteins expressed in the simultaneous absence of ICP4 and ICP27 and of certain genes encoding non-essential virion proteins that also affect host cell metabolism. These genetic manipulations have been undertaken in an effort to obtain HSV vectors that simply and solely deliver their genome to the nucleus of infected cells. This chapter outlines the procedures for the genetic manipulation of HSV relevant to its use as a gene transfer vector.

2 MATERIALS AND EQUIPMENT

(1) Plasmid pSV2neo (Southern and Berg, 1982), which encodes the neomycin resistance gene from *E. coli* under the control of the SV40 early promoter and confers resistance to the antibiotic G418.
(2) Vero cells (American Type Culture Collection (ATCC), Rockville, MD USA).
(3) See Chapters 14 and 16 for detailed lists of materials and equipment required.

3 THE PROTOCOLS

Protocol #80: Constructing Cell Lines Complementing Essential HSV-1 Functions

(1) Distribute approximately 4×10^6 Vero cells on two 85 mm Petri dishes 24 h before transfection.
(2) 3 h before transfection, remove the medium by aspiration and add 10 ml of fresh medium containing 10% FBS.
(3) For transfection, prepare calcium phosphate precipitates essentially as described by Graham and van der Eb (1973). Suspend 1 μg pSVneo, 5 μg plasmid containing the HSV gene of interest and 30 μg salmon testes DNA (SSD) in 1.0 ml of 2 × transfection buffer. The use of 5 μg of HSV plasmid is assuming that the plasmid is approximately the same size as pSV2neo. This and the concentration of SSD should be adjusted to give a fivefold molar excess of HSV plasmid over selectable marker and a total DNA concentration of 40–50 μg/ml.
(4) Add 1 ml 250 mM $CaCl_2$ dropwise and allow precipitate to form at room temperature for 20 min.
(5) Dispense 1 ml of suspension to each of the two Petri dishes of Vero cells, and incubate at 37°C for 4 h.
(6) Remove the medium and add 3 ml 15% glycerol in 1 × transfection buffer (Graham and van der Eb, 1973) to each plate.
(7) Incubate the plates at 37°C for 2 min and then remove the glycerol.
(8) Wash the cells with isotonic saline, then add medium containing 10% FBS.
(9) Incubate the cultures for 40 h at 37°C and then trypsinize the cells.
(10) Suspend the cells in medium containing 700 μg/ml of the antibiotic G418.
(11) Plate the single cell suspension into new 85 mm Petri dishes at a density of 5×10^3 cells/cm^2, and at 37°C.

(12) After 3–5 days, lower the G418 concentration to 250 mg/ml, depending on the extent of cell death, judged by when >50% of cells have rounded up.
(13) Continue incubation to allow development of G418-resistant colonies. These can be isolated 10–20 days after applying the G418 selection.
(14) Isolate individual G418-resistant colonies and grow up in the presence of 250 μg/ml G418 using standard cell culture procedures.

Protocol #81: Preparation of HSV-1 DNA

(1) Infect 10^8 Vero cells at a MOI of 0.01 p.f.u./cell and incubate at 37°C.
(2) Harvest the infected cells by scraping them into the medium. Optimum time for harvest is when generalized cytopathic effect is evident (2–3 days after infection).
(3) Pellet the infected cells by low-speed centrifugation, wash with isotonic saline and pellet again. Do **not** throw away the supernatants.
(4) Combine the supernatants from each centrifugation step and collect the extracellular virus by high-speed centrifugation (10 000 r.p.m.) for 1 h.
(5) Combine the virus and cell pellets and resuspend in a total of 9.2 ml 10 mM Tris–HCl, 1 mM EDTA, pH 8.0 (TE buffer).
(6) Add 0.6 ml 10% SDS and 0.2 ml 20 mg/ml proteinase K. Gently mix and incubate at 37°C for 4 h.
(7) In the digested suspension obtained dissolve 13.26 g CsCl slowly, to avoid shearing the HSV DNA.
(8) Remove any SDS that precipitates by low-speed centrifugation. The SDS will float to the top and the clarified viral DNA/CsCl solution may be removed with a wide-bore pipette and transferred to a 13 ml ultracentrifuge tube.
(9) Spin the DNA/CsCl solution at 35 000 r.p.m., 20°C for 65 h. The shallow CsCl gradient that develops is sufficient to separate the cellular DNA and the more dense HSV DNA, which bands at a CsCl density of 1.726 g/ml. The position of the required band in the tube is determined by measuring the refractive indices of fractions collected from the gradient.
(10) Dialyse peak fractions containing HSV DNA against a large volume of TE.

It is possible to obtain about 100 μg of HSV DNA per 10^8 cells using this procedure. This DNA is infectious and suitable for restriction enzyme analysis.

Protocol #82: Insertion of Genes into HSV-1 by Homologous Recombination

(1) Transfect approximately 10^6 complementing cells with 0.5 ml of transfection precipitate (see Protocol #80) containing 1.5 μg viral DNA and 1.5 μg of a DNA fragment containing the gene of interest with the desired mutation using the transfection protocol described above. An excess of 1 kb of flanking homology on either side of the mutation is desirable to ensure efficient marker transfer by homologous recombination.
(2) Harvest the transfected monolayers 2–3 days after transfection by scraping them into the medium.
(3) Release virus from debris by freeze/thaw then sonication. Remove the cell debris by low-speed centrifugation and save the supernatant.
(4) Titrate the clarified viral lysate for plaques on complementing cells overlaid with 2% methylcellulose in culture medium.
(5) Plaques are easily visible after 3 days and can be picked with a micropipette and put into 0.5 ml of medium. Approximately 100 plaques are sufficient to ensure the isolation of the desired mutant. The frequency of marker transfer is 1–20%.

Protocol #83: Screening Plaque Isolates for Marker Transfer from Plasmids

(1) Take the 0.5 ml single-plaque suspensions obtained in Step 5 of Protocol #82 and freeze-thaw them three times to release virus from cells and debris.
(2) Use 20–50 μl of each plaque suspension to infect 10^5 complementing cells in 24-well trays and

non-complementing cells. Incubate for 2 days.
(3) After two days of incubation, virus mutants with the marker transferred to their genomes will show numerous plaques on the complementing cells but none on the non-complementing cells.
(4) The requirement for growth on the complementing line must be verified by a quantitative plaque assay on both cell types.

As an alternative, mutants may be isolated by engineering an expressed β-galactosidase gene into the gene to be inactivated in the marker transfer. Mutants are then screened initially for β-galactosidase expression by plaque color assay of the transfection progeny on transformed cells using 0.2 mg/ml X-gal (as described by Goldstein and Weller, 1988). Plaque isolates staining blue are then analysed.

Protocol #84: Analysis of Isolated HSV-1 Genomes

(1) To verify the genotype of a suspected mutant, centrifuge 10^5 infected cells for 10 min in a standard 1.5 ml microcentrifuge tube.
(2) Remove the medium and resuspend the pellet in 190 ml TE buffer.
(3) Add 12 μl 10% SDS and 4 μl 20 mg/ml proteinase K.
(4) Incubate at 37°C for at least 4 h.
(5) Extract each digested sample twice with phenol : chloroform : isoamyl alcohol (25 : 24 : 1), once with chloroform : isoamyl alcohol (24 : 1) and then precipitate the DNA with ethanol.
(6) Resuspend the pellet in 30 ml TE.
(7) Between 5 and 10 μl is usually sufficient to see a clear restriction enzyme digest in ethidium bromide stained agarose gels; however, a Southern blot is often necessary, probing for the region corresponding to the altered gene.
(8) Plaque purify the virus isolates with the required phenotype and genotype at least twice more and prepare a stock following standard methods.

Protocol #85: Overlay Procedure for Detection of the Blue Plaque Phenotype

(1) After the appearance of plaques (48–72 h after infection), overlay the monolayers with 1 ml of 1 × MEM/Bluo-gal (300 mg/ml)/dimethylfluoride (DMF) (15%) and incubate at 37°C.
(2) Blue plaques appear 1–6 h after adding the overlay solution. The blue color can be enhanced by incubating the plates at 4°C.
(3) Pick individual, well isolated blue plaques.
(4) Resuspend the agarose plug/plaque in 0.5 ml 1 × MEM/10% FCS.
(5) Release the virus by three cycles of freeze/thaw followed by 1 min sonication.
(6) This virus preparation may then be titered by standard methods or used to prepare a higher-titer virus stock for further purification steps.

Protocol #86: Limiting Dilution Method for Isolation of Blue Plaques

(1) Add about 30 p.f.u. of virus isolated from the agarose plug (Step 2, Protocol # 85) to a 15 ml conical tube containing 3 × 10^6 Vero cells in 5 ml medium and rock the mixture slowly at 37°C for 1 h to allow the virus to adsorb.
(2) Plate aliquots of the infected cells uniformly in the wells of a 96-well plate and incubate at 37°C in a CO_2 incubator until plaques appear (2–3 days). This should give approximately 30 wells containing single plaques and the progeny in each of these wells should be derived from that single plaque.
(3) Transfer the medium from each of these wells to a new 96-well plate and store at −80°C for use as a virus stock.
(4) Test the blue plaque phenotype of these isolates by testing the cells remaining in the wells. Overlay with 0.1 ml 1 × MEM/Bluo-gal/agarose and allow the agarose to solidify at room temperature.

(5) Transfer the plate to a 37°C CO_2 incubator to facilitate the blue color reaction. Wells possessing single blue plaques are readily detectable.

4 NOTES AND TROUBLESHOOTING

4.1 On Protocol #80: Constructing Cell Lines Complementing Essential HSV-1 Functions

One of the most important prerequisites for the use of defective HSV mutants as gene transfer vehicles is the ability to isolate and efficiently propagate virus genomes deleted for one or more essential viral genes. Complementation groups, established through genetic analysis of temperature-sensitive (ts) mutants of HSV, initially defined most of the essential viral genes (Schaffer et al., 1973, 1978). The study of these mutants provided a wealth of information concerning the functions of essential genes. For example, the role of ICP4 in the expression of the HSV genome was initially defined through phenotypic analysis of ts mutants in the 1–2 complementation group (Schaffer et al., 1973; Preston, 1979, 1981; Dixon and Schaffer, 1980). Despite the central role ts mutants played in elucidating the functions of specific HSV gene products in the viral life cycle, their uses for gene transfer applications are limited. The non-permissive temperature for ts mutants is often non-physiological, they "leak" and revert back to the wild-type phenotype to varying degrees and the non-functional protein produced at the non-permissive temperature is often not biochemically and biologically inert.

Essential viral genes are inactivated using the marker transfer techniques described below. Inactivation is preceded by construction of transformed cell lines expressing complementing levels of the viral gene to be deleted to allow efficient isolation and propagation of these strains (DeLuca et al., 1985).

4.1.1 General Outline for Construction of Complementing Cell Lines

A copy of the HSV gene to be deleted is cloned, complete with its native promoter, into a standard bacterial vector. In general, each HSV gene has its own promoter and lacks intervening sequences so that the source of the HSV gene/promoter fragment is the HSV genome. A cell line that readily forms colonies and is a good host for HSV is then cotransfected with a plasmid encoding the HSV gene and one encoding a gene that confers resistance to a drug normally toxic to them. Drug resistant colonies are then isolated, expanded and subsequently screened for function. Between 10 and 50% of the cell lines that incorporate the drug resistance marker also incorporate the unlinked HSV gene. This is essentially the procedure developed by Southern and Berg (1982). The most appropriate and effective way to screen for function is to determine the ability of individual clonal isolates to complement the growth of a pre-existing deletion mutant or a ts mutant at the non-permissive temperature.

4.1.2 Testing Complementing Cell Lines

To test the cell lines for expression of the complementing viral gene, a known number of expanded cells are used to perform a plaque assay with the appropriate mutant virus under appropriate incubation conditions. A good complementing cell line will propagate mutant viruses to nearly the level seen with wild-type virus (approximately 1000 p.f.u./cell at 37°C and 20–50% of this at 39°C). This procedure was first used to generate cell lines that complement mutants in ICP4 (DeLuca et al., 1985; DeLuca and Schaffer, 1987), but has since been applied to many of the essential genes of HSV. One interesting feature of cell lines generated and screened in this way is that the viral gene resident in the cell is relatively silent. It is transcriptionally activated and the protein product synthesized only on infection with virus, because the infecting virus provides the transcriptional activators required for efficient utilization of HSV promoters. As a consequence the complementing cell lines are often phenotypically indistinguishable from their untransformed parents and are very stable upon passage with respect to the ability to complement mutant viruses. An exception to this may be cell lines providing ICP0 (Sacks and Schaffer, 1987), which are efficient hosts for ICP0 mutants for about 20 passages. The instability may be due to the toxic effects of low levels of ICP0 but this remains to be determined.

4.2 On Protocol #82: Insertion of Genes into HSV-1 by Homologous Recombination

4.2.1 Generation of HSV-1 Mutants with Deletions in Essential Genes

Engineered HSV mutants are generated by a process known as marker transfer. Infectious HSV DNA is cotransfected into complementing cells with a cloned fragment of the sequence, or gene, of interest that has been mutated in the desired way by recombinant techniques. Some homologous recombination between the cloned fragment and the HSV genome results in transfer of the mutation to the HSV genome, replacing the wild-type gene.

4.2.2 Plating Efficiency on Complementing and Non-complementing Cells

Plaques on non-complementing cells often indicate the presence of wild-type virus arising through homologous recombination between the mutant viral genome and the HSV sequences in the complementing cell line when the virus is being amplified. Typically, the frequency of this should be less than 10^{-6} per mutant virus. This problem can be eliminated by careful consideration of the HSV fragment used and design of the intended deletion in the mutant virus: if homologous recombination cannot occur, the frequency of wild-type recombinants will be extremely low. This has been achieved for deletion mutants of ICP27 and ICP4 (DeLuca et al., 1985; DeLuca and Schaffer, 1987; McCarthy et al., 1989). It is possible to obtain 10^{10}–10^{11} infectious virus deleted for ICP4 or ICP27 on transformed cell lines without detectable wild-type recombinants.

4.3 Notes on Transfer of Foreign Genes to the HSV genome using the *cre/lox* Site-specific Recombination System as an Alternative to Homologous Recombination

To introduce foreign sequences that lack homology with the virus into the viral genome they must be flanked by viral sequences so that the foreign material can be combined into the genome. We have developed strategies for introducing altered or foreign genetic information into the genome using an efficient P1 phage *cre/lox* recombination system that overcomes some of the difficulties inherent in marker transfer methods.

This system consists of:

- a *cis*-acting 34 bp DNA element, designated *lox*P, at which recombination occurs and
- a recombinase, *cre*, which mediates intra- or intermolecular site-specific recombination events within a single DNA molecule or between two DNA molecules each possessing *lox*P sites (Sternberg and Hamilton, 1981; Abremski et al., 1983; Abremski and Hoess, 1984, Hoess and Abremski, 1985).

For use in generating recombinant HSV-1 genomes, this simple cell-free system requires only a shuttle plasmid with a *lox*P site, a recipient HSV-1 vector genome containing a *lox*P site, and purified *cre* recombinase. Furthermore, we have introduced a *lac*Z reporter gene expression cassette into the *lox*P shuttle plasmid to enable rapid identification of recombinant plaques (Gage et al., 1992). We have employed this system to analyse the effect of specific amino acid substitutions in the cytoplasmic domain of HSV-1 glycoprotein B (gB) on the formation of syncytial plaques in cell culture (Gage et al., 1992, 1993).

This method was first reported by Enquist and colleagues (Sauer et al., 1987), who introduced plasmid sequences into the pseudorabies virus genome and improved efficiency of marker transfer procedures to 8% (the number of recombinants rarely exceeds 1% without selection). The method has the advantage that the plasmid may be recovered from the viral genome by treating the purified recombinant virus DNA with *cre*, in a circular form which could be directly transfected into bacteria for recovery and maintenance. This system thus involves the use of shuttle plasmids which can be repeatedly modified using random or site-directed mutagenesis and retested in the viral genome after plasmid insertion using *cre*-mediated recombination. When testing for the effects of random mutations on the behavior of promoters or other genetic elements or on protein structure and function, a population of shuttle plasmids can be randomly introduced into the viral genome. Only those mutants with interesting phenotypes are removed from the purified mutant viral genome by the reverse *cre* reaction and sequenced. The *cre/lox* system has potential for a variety of applications including rapid introduction of multiple gene cassettes contained within a single *lox* plasmid into a single viral locus. Recent efforts have optimized this system so that 20–90% of the virus plaques recovered after introduction of the *lox* plasmid into the recipient viral genome result from recombinant viral infections. These conditions can be routinely used to insert a plasmid containing novel genetic material into any locus in the viral genome where a *lox* site has been introduced, and can be applied to other herpesviruses for which recombinants are difficult to produce by marker transfer.

When considering construction of HSV vectors, the *cre/lox* system may be used to create recombinant viruses, taking care to construct a recipient viral genome and a shuttle plasmid each containing a *lox*P cis-acting recombination site. It is also important to determine the best molar ratio of plasmid DNA to target viral genomic DNA so that the highest number of recombinants possible may be obtained.

4.3.1 Construction of a lox*P-containing Recipient*

A recipient viral genome may be constructed by placing a *lox* recombination site into a suitable location in the genome using marker transfer procedures (Kucherlapati et al., 1984; Thomas et al., 1986; Wong and Capecchi, 1987). We have designed a *lox* site containing translational stop codons in all three reading frames in order to disrupt synthesis of the gene product into which the *lox* site has been inserted. The *lox* element was inserted into the thymidine kinase (*tk*) gene, creating a TK-defective virus and providing the opportunity for phenotypic selection of TK^-::lox HSV recombinants using media containing acyclovir/araT (Fig. 15.1). The *lox* site marker can also be transferred by rescuing a conditional lethal (e.g. ts) mutant or deletion mutant in an essential gene, in which case the *lox* site would be introduced into an adjacent gene non-essential for viral replication; only those viruses which form plaques are recombinants. In either approach selection methods should be used to ensure that the recombinants can be easily identified.

The Ktk::lox recombinant may be used as a target site for mutant HSV genes or foreign gene cassettes carried on *lox* plasmids. By disrupting the *tk* gene, it also provides the opportunity to introduce the tk gene into the shuttle vector in order to use HAT medium in the selection of TK^+ recombinants. The TK^- virus recombinants were identified by TK^- selection using araT (see Figure 15.1 legend for details), purified by limiting dilution and confirmed to possess the *lox*P site by dot blot hybridization using a radiolabeled *lox* sequence-specific probe.

4.3.2 Construction of a Shuttle Plasmid Containing a lox*P Site*

A shuttle plasmid containing a *lox*P element must also be constructed to enable insertion of the entire plasmid into the recipient viral genome. To aid the identification of positive recombinants following insertion of the shuttle plasmid, a *lac*Z reporter gene expression cassette was included in the shuttle plasmid (Fig. 15.2). *Cre/lox*-mediated recombination of this plasmid into the recipient viral genome yields a virus which can produce blue plaques on Bluo-gal agarose overlay.

The shuttle plasmid was created to contain a functional *lox*P site for *cre*-mediated recombination as well as the *lac*Z reporter gene cassette for rapid identification of recombinants possessing the shuttle plasmid. The strong HCMV IE promoter results in the production of high levels of β-galactosidase early in HSV infection which enables the easy identification of blue plaque recombinants. Several potential cloning sites exist within pJG116 for insertion of foreign gene cassettes. Unique *Hin*dIII and *Bam*H1 sites are present upstream from the HCMV IE promoter and two sites exist for both *Sal*I and *Pst*I within pJG116. Although the presence of the reporter gene cassette within the shuttle plasmid eases the identification of positive recombinants, we have used shuttle plasmids containing only a *lox*P site and the gene of interest in which case recombinants can be readily detected by dot-blot hybridization.

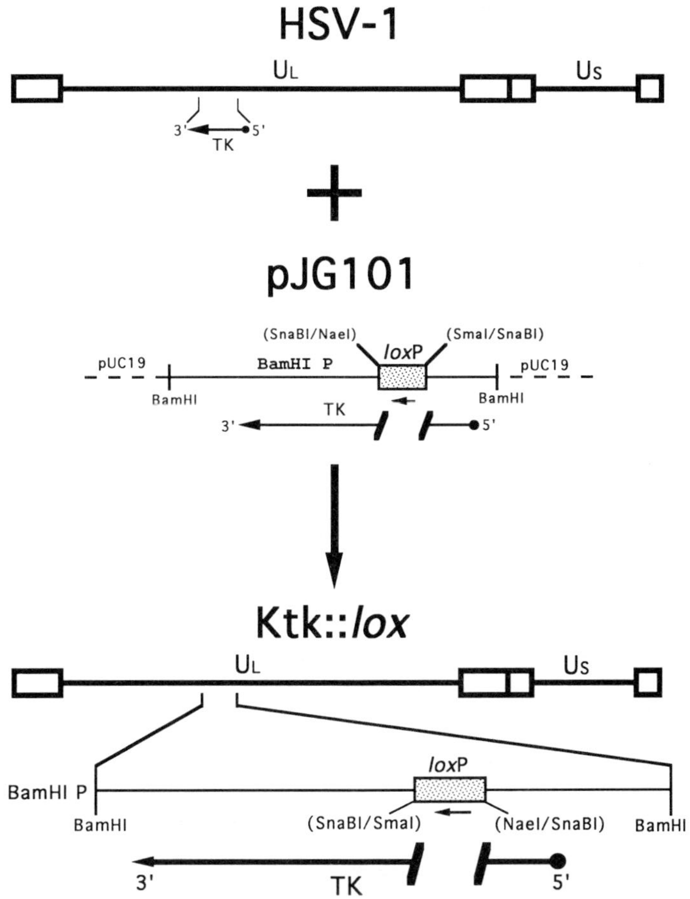

Figure 15.1 Introduction of a *lox*P site into the thymidine kinase locus. Marker rescue procedures were employed to transfer a *lox* site into the *tk* gene locus of wild-type HSV-1. A 354 bp fragment from pBS64 (Chiocca et al., 1990) containing the 34 bp *lox*P site was inserted into the unique *Sna*BI site of the plasmid pUCX1, which contains the 3.5 kb HSV-1 *Bam*H1 P fragment inserted into the *Bam*H1 site of pUC19, producing the plasmid pJG101. The *lox* site insert in pJG101 is in the same orientation as the *tk* gene and interrupts the TK coding sequence. The plasmid pJG101 (5 μg) was linearized by restriction enzyme digest, and cotransfected with the infectious wild-type strain KOS viral DNA (2 μg) into 60 mm plates containing subconfluent monolayers of Vero (African green monkey kidney) cells using the calcium phosphate transfection procedure (Graham and Van der Eb, 1973; Homa et al., 1986). TK^-::lox recombinants were identified from the mixture of progeny virus particles arising from the transfections using three rounds of limiting dilution in 96-well microtiter plates (White and Bancroft, 1982; Gage et al., 1992). TK^- recombinants were selected in 1 × MEM/10% FCS containing 100 μg/ml thymidine 1-β-arabinofuranoside (araT, Sigma, St Louis, MO) because insertion of the *lox*P site in *tk* blocks its expression. Dot-blot assays using a [^{32}P]-labeled *lox*P specific probe were performed on cell lysates from the microtiter plate wells displaying single plaques (Gage et al., 1992) in order to identify all TK^- viral recombinants which contained a *lox*P site insertion. This process was necessary because TK^- viral mutants can arise by spontaneous point mutations within the gene. Following three rounds of limiting dilution analysis in the presence of araT and dot-blot hybridization with a *lox*P specific probe, a high titer stock of the purified TK^-::*lox*P virus can be prepared for further analysis and future experiments.

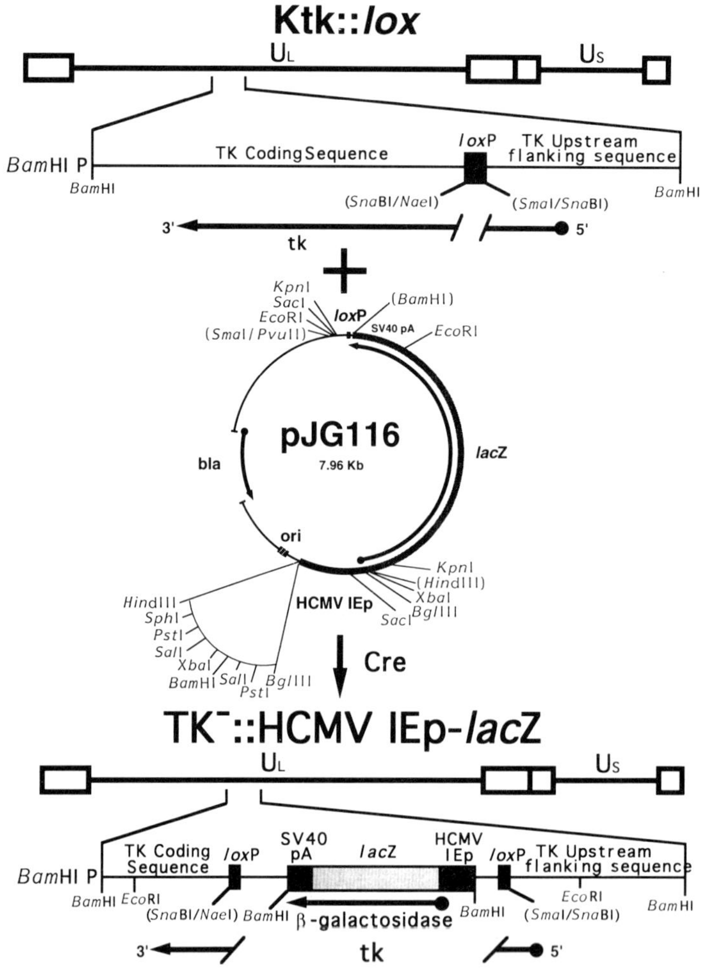

Figure 15.2 *Cre/lox*-mediated recombination for insertion of a shuttle plasmid into the HSV-1 recipient viral genome. The *lox*P- and *lac*Z-containing shuttle plasmid pJG116 was constructed by several cloning steps. First, a 252 bp *Bam*H1/*Pvu*II *lox*P containing fragment from pBS64 (Gage et al., 1992) was inserted into the *Bam*H1/*Sma*I sites of pBS-(Stratagene, La Jolla, CA) to produce the clone pBSloxP. Second, the human cytomegalovirus major IE promoter–*lac*Z reporter gene cassette (HCMV IE–*lac*Z), present on a 4.5 kb *Bam*H1 fragment from pipe-*lac*Z (Thomsen et al., 1984; Stinski and Roehr, 1985), was introduced into the *Bam*H1 site of pBSloxP producing. Since few single-cutting cloning sites were available within the newly generated plasmid, the *Hin*dIII site present at the junction of the HCMV promoter with *lac*Z, as well as the *Bam*H1 site at the 3′ end, as destroyed to produce pJG116. The plasmid of pJG116 was constructed to contain a *lox*P element for site-specific recombination and a reporter gene cassette with the HCMV major IE gene driving expression of the gene encoding *β*-galactosidase (*lac*Z) for rapid identification of recombinant viruses. When pJG116 DNA is mixed with KtK::lox viral DNA in conjunction with the *cre* recombinase, the plasmid DNA molecule is incorporated into the tk locus of the Ktk::lox target virus genome, generating the TK⁻::HCMV IEp-*lac*Z recombinant. Treatment of recombinant viral genomic DNA containing the inserted plasmid with *cre* will lead to excision of the sequences between the two *lox*P sites within the viral genome and regeneration of the original plasmid and recipient genome.

4.3.3 Ratio of Insert Plasmid DNA to Target Viral DNA in the Reaction Mixture is an Important Variable in cre/lox *Recombination*

When the insert plasmid DNA/target viral DNA ratio is too low the number of molecular interactions between the plasmid to be inserted and the target viral genome is limited and recombination frequency drops. When the ratio is too high the number of recombinants also diminishes, but this is due to the higher prevalence of plasmid molecules interacting with one another instead of the large viral DNA molecule. Using Ktk::lox viral DNA and pJG116 plasmid DNA (Fig. 15.2) we determined that the most effective molar ratio of pJG116 to Ktk::lox DNA was 50 molar equivalents of plasmid DNA to one molar equivalent of 1.0 mg of viral DNA.

The reactions were incubated at 30°C for 30 min, heat-inactivated at 70°C for 5 min, and brought up to 25.0 mg total DNA by adding salmon sperm DNA as carrier. This mixture was then used for transfection onto subconfluent monolayers of Vero cells in 60 mm Petri dishes (Homa et al., 1986; Gage et al., 1993). Virus should be isolated from each plate after all cells have rounded up. Dilutions of 10^{-4} and 10^{-6} may be used for each virus stock. To infect the cells medium was carefully removed from the cell monolayer and 0.2 ml of the appropriate dilution of virus (prepared in 1 × MEM/10% FCS) added to the cells. The plates were then incubated at 37°C for 1 h, rocking gently every 15 min to distribute the inoculum over the surface of the monolayer. Recombinant viruses were identified by their blue plaque phenotype in the presence of Bluo-Gal, as described below. A 50:1 molar ratio yields the highest yield (routinely 20–50).

4.4 On Protocol #86: Limiting Dilution Method for Isolation of Blue Plaques

This system does not require a well-isolated single blue plaque to be picked from the agarose overlay; an advantage because the blue plaque is often contaminated with a neighboring white plaque, particularly if they are numerous. Using this method wells containing single blue plaques can be used to prepare frozen stocks for subsequent rounds of limiting dilution. It is possible to use this approach to identify recombinants even if the virus recombinant lacks a *lacZ* expression cassette by extracting DNA from lysates of individual wells for use in dot-blot hybridization with *lox*-specific radiolabeled probes.

4.5 Perspectives and State-of-the-art Developments

The procedures outlined in this chapter will enable construction and isolation of HSV mutants that do not replicate in infected cells and are void of replication competent virus, and introduction of foreign genes into the mutant viral backbone.

4.5.1 Examples of Application of these Approaches

For generating viruses for use as vectors and limiting the cytotoxicity inherent to most HSV mutants (Johnson et al., 1992) we deleted the two essential IE genes, ICP4 and ICP27. It then becomes possible to delete the other genes expressed in an ICP4/ICP27 deficient background. This may allow construction of a herpesvirus that expresses none of its genes, greatly reducing its cytotoxic potential and improving on the utility of HSV vectors.

Plasmids encoding the genes for ICP27 and ICP4 were cotransfected with pSV2neo into Vero cells and selected with the antibiotic G418 as described in Protocol #80. G418-resistant colonies were amplified and tested for the ability to host KOS (wild-type virus), an ICP4⁻ virus, d120 (DeLuca et al., 1985), and an ICP27⁻ virus, 5dl1.2 (McCarthy et al., 1989). All possibilities were obtained: cells that host only KOS, only d120, cells only host 5dl1.2, and both d120 and 5dl1.2. One cell line, designated 26 cells, yielded 900 p.f.u. per cell of d120, and 350 p.f.u. per cell of 5dl1.2. These were chosen for further study. Another cell line, designated 8 cells, was retained because it was the only one that efficiently hosted 5dl1.2 and not d120.

The 26 cell line was used to generate a recombinant virus deficient for both ICP4 and ICP27 by coinfecting with d120 and 5dl1.2, plating the progeny on 26 cells, picking plaques and identifying isolates that plaque on 26 cells but not on 8 cells (ICP27 complementing), E5 cells (ICP4 complementing; DeLuca and Schaffer, 1987) and Vero cells. These corresponded to 8% of the total progeny, consistent with the distance between ICP4 and ICP27. Individual plaque isolates that grew only on 26 cells were examined by Southern blot hybridization to ascertain the presence of both mutations in *cis*. One such isolate, designated d92, was chosen for further study.

The deletions in d92 extend beyond the sequence of the DNA fragments used to incorporate the ICP27 and ICP4 genes in the complementing cell line. Therefore the copies of these genes resident in the transformed cell line lack the flanking homology necessary to rescue either of the mutations in the double mutant viral genome by homologous recombination. This puts a theoretical upper limit of 10^{-12} on the frequency of appearance of wild-type virus. The efficiency of these cell lines enabled us to obtain stock titers of this virus in excess of 10^9 p.f.u./ml (Samaniego et al., 1995).

Using d92 as a backbone we have also been able to simultaneously delete the non-essential genes encoding the virion component responsible for shutting off host cell protein synthesis (Read and Frenkel, 1983; Kwong and Frenkel, 1987) and that for the large subunit of ribonucleotide reductase. This virus does not shut off host cell protein synthesis and the only viral protein discernible on SDS gels of metabolically labeled cells is ICP0. Moreover, this virus has lower vector toxicity than ICP4 mutants and should be safe for use as an *in vivo* gene therapy vector. It remains to be seen how effective such mutants will be for gene transfer. More work is needed to perfect HSV as a gene transfer vector because toxicity remains associated with the mutants described above, most probably due to ICP0. This protein has been implicated in the reactivation of latent virus (Leib et al., 1989) and in altering the distribution of intranuclear cellular structures (Everett and Maul, 1994). Efforts are under way to generate viruses lacking this function.

For introducing genes into the mutant HSV backbones the modified *cre/lox* recombination procedure appears better than standard marker transfer procedures (Homa et al., 1986). Marker transfer procedures require considerable effort in engineering the gene cassette with homologous viral flanking sequences to provide a suitable substrate for homologous recombination. They also require the plasmid DNA molecule to be linearized by digestion at a unique restriction enzyme site before homologous recombination. This can be difficult due to the lack of single restriction sites within a large DNA fragment. Once a modified or novel gene has been placed into the viral genome by marker transfer it is not easily removed or modified.

These difficulties are largely circumvented using the *cre/lox* system. The same *lox* plasmid can be used to carry many different genetic constructs. This method is useful for testing a large number of genes which may affect a particular biological process under study or mutant genes to study their behavior. The plasmid integrates in linear form within the viral genome as part of the recombinational mechanism and is targeted to the same site each time without the need for flanking sequence homology or linearization. Importantly, the method employs a shuttle plasmid which can be introduced and removed from the viral genome for analysis either in the virus or in a bacterial system. Because it is a cell-free system there is less risk of introducing additional mutations into the HSV genome. The mutant gene may be removed and the recipient virus tested to confirm that the element removed was responsible for the particular phenotype being measured.

REFERENCES

Abremski, K. and R. Hoess. 1984. Bacteriophage P1 site-specific recombination: purification and properties of the Cre recombinase. *J. Biol. Chem.* **259:** 1509–1514.

Abremski K., R. Hoess and N. Sternberg. 1983. Studies on the properties of P1 site-specific recombination: evidence for topologically unlinked products following recombination. *Cell* **32:** 1301–1311.

Batterson, W. and B. Roizman. 1983. Characterization of the HSV-associated factor responsible for the induction of a genes. *J. Virol.* **46:** 371–377.

Cai, W., T.L. Astor, L.M. Liptak, C. Cho, D.M. Coen and P.A. Schaffer. 1993. The herpes simplex virus type 1 regulatory protein ICP0 enhances virus replication during acute infection and reactivation from latency. *J. Virol.* **67:** 7501–7512.

Campbell, M.E.M., J.W. Palfreyman and C.M. Preston. 1984. Identification of herpes simplex virus DNA sequences which encode a trans-acting polypeptide responsible for the stimulation of immediate early transcription. *J. Mol. Biol.* **180:** 1–19.

Challberg, M.D. 1986. A method for identifying the viral genes required for herpesvirus DNA replication.

Proc. Natl Acad. Sci. USA **83:** 9092–9098.

Chiocca, E.A., B.B. Choi, W. Cai, N.D. DeLuca, P.A. Schaffer, M. DiFiglia, X.O. Breakfield and R.I. Martuza. 1990. Transfer and expression of the LacZ gene in rat brain mediated by herpes simplex virus mutants. *New Biologist* **2:** 739–746.

Courtney, R.J. and M. Benyesh-Melnick. 1974. Isolation and characterization of a large molecular weight polypeptide of herpes simplex virus type 1. *Virology* **62:** 539–551.

DeLuca, N.A., A. McCarthy and P.A. Schaffer. 1985. Isolation and characterization of deletion mutants of herpes simplex virus type 1 in the gene encoding immediate-early regulatory protein ICP4. *J. Virol.* **56:** 558–570.

DeLuca, N.A. and P.A. Schaffer. 1987. Activities of herpes simplex virus type 1 (HSV-1) ICP4 genes specifying non-sense peptides. *Nucl. Acids Res.* **15:** 4491–4511.

Dixon, R.A.F. and P.A. Schaffer. 1980. Fine-structure mapping and functional analysis of temperature-sensitive mutants in the gene encoding the herpes simplex virus type 1 immediate early protein VP175. *J. Virol.* **36:** 189–203.

Dobson, A.T., T.P. Margolis, F. Sederati, J.G. Stevens and L.T. Feldman. 1990. A latent non-pathogenic HSV-1 derived vector stably expresses β-galactosidase in mouse neurons. *Neuron* **5:** 353–360.

Everett, R.D. 1984. Transactivation of transcription by herpes virus products: requirements for two HSV-1 immediate-early polypeptides for maximum activity. *EMBO J.* **3:** 3135–3141.

Everett, R.D. 1989. Construction and characterisation of herpes simplex virus type 1 mutants with defined lesions in immediate early gene 1. *J. Gen. Virol.* **70:** 2507–2513.

Everett, R.D. and G.G. Maul. 1994. HSV-1 IE protein Vmw110 causes redistribution of PML. *EMBO J* **13:** 5062–5069.

Gage, P.J., B. Sauer, M. Levine and J.C. Glorioso. 1992. A cell-free recombination system for site-specific integration of multigenic shuttle plasmids within the cytoplasmic domain of herpes simplex virus type 1 glycoprotein B. *J. Virol.* **67:** 2191–2201.

Gage, P.J., M. Levine and J.C. Glorioso. 1993. Syncytial-inducing mutations localize to two discrete regions within the cytoplasmic domain of herpes simplex virus type 1 glycoprotein B. *J. Virol.* **67:** 2191–2201.

Goldstein, D.J. and S.K. Weller. 1988. Herpes simplex virus type 1-induced ribonucleotide reductase activity is dispensable for growth and DNA synthesis: isolation and characterization and of an ICP6 *lac*Z insertion mutant. *J. Virol.* **62:** 196–205.

Graham, F.L. and A.J. Van der Eb. 1973. A new technique for the assay of infectivity of human adenovirus 5 DNA. *Virology* **52:** 456–467.

Gu, B., R. Rivera-Gonzalez., C.A. Smith and N.A. DeLuca. 1993. Herpes simplex virus infected cell polypeptide 4 preferentially represses Sp1-activated over basal transcription from its own promoter. *Proc. Natl Acad. Sci. USA* **90:** 9528–9532.

Gu, B. and N.A. DeLuca. 1994. Requirements for activation of the herpes simplex virus glycoprotein C promoter *in vitro* by the viral regulatory protein, ICP4. *J. Virol.* **68:** 7953–7965.

Hardy, W.R. and R.M. Sandri-Goldin. 1994. Herpes simplex virus inhibits host cell splicing, and regulatory protein ICP27 is required for this effect. *J. Virol.* **68:** 7790–7799.

Hardwicke, M.A., P.J. Vaughan, R.E. Sekulovich, R. O'Conner and R.M. Sandri-Goldin. 1989. The regions important for the activator and repressor functions of the HSV-1 alpha protein ICP27 map to the C-terminal half of the molecule. *J. Virol.* **63:** 4590–4602.

Hoess, R. and K. Abremski. 1985. Mechanism of strand cleavage and exchange in the Cre-*lox* site-specific recombination system. *J. Mol. Biol.* **181:** 351–362.

Homa, F.L., T.M. Otal, J.C. Glorioso and M. Levine. 1986. Transcriptional control signals of a herpes virus late (g2) gene lie within bases −34 to +124 relative to the 5′ terminus of the mRNA. *Mol. Cell. Biol.* **6:** 3652–3666.

Honess, R.W. and B. Roizman. 1974. Regulation of herpes virus macromolecular synthesis. I. Cascade regulation of the synthesis of three groups of viral proteins. *J. Virol.* **14:** 8–19.

Honess, R.W. and B. Roizman. 1975. Regulation of herpes virus macromolecular synthesis: sequential transition of polypeptide synthesis requires functional viral polypeptides. *Proc. Natl Acad. Sci. USA* **72:** 1276–1280.

Johnson, P.A., A. Miyanohara, F. Levine, T. Cahill and T. Friedmann. 1992. Cytotoxicity of a replication defective mutant of herpes simplex virus type 1. *J. Virol.* **66:** 2952–2965.

Kucherlapati, R.S., E.M. Eves, K.-Y. Song, B.S. Morse and O. Smithies. 1984. Homologous recombination between plasmids in mammalian cells can be enhanced by treatment of input DNA. *Proc. Natl Acad. Sci. USA* **81:** 3143–3157.

Kwong, A.D. and N. Frenkel. 1987. Herpes simplex virus-infected cells contain a function(s) that destabilizes both host and viral mRNAs. *Proc. Natl Acad. Sci.* USA **84:** 1926–1930.

Leib, D.A., D.M. Coen, C.L. Bogard, K.A. Hicks, D.R. Yager, D.M. Knipe, K.L. Tyler and P.A. Schaffer. 1989.

Immediate early regulatory mutants define stages in the establishment and reactivation of herpes simplex virus latency. *J. Virol.* **63:** 759–768.

McCarthy, A.M., L. McMahan and P.A. Schaffer. 1989. Herpes simplex virus type 1 ICP27 deletion mutants exhibit altered patterns of transcription and are DNA deficient. *J. Virol.* **63:** 18–27.

McGeoch, D.J., M.A. Dalrymple, A.J. Davison, A. Dolan, M.C. Frame, D. McNab, L.J. Perry, J.E. Scott and P. Taylor. 1988. The complete DNA sequence of the long unique region in the genome of herpes simplex virus type 1. *J. Gen. Virol.* **69:** 1531–1574.

McLauchlan, J., A. Phelan, C. Loney, R.M. Sandri-Goldin and J.B. Clements. 1992. Herpes simplex virus IE63 acts at the posttranscriptional level to stimulate viral mRNA 3′ processing. *J. Virol.* **66:** 6939–6945.

McMahan, L. and P.A. Schaffer. 1990. The repressing and enhancing functions of the herpes simplex virus regulatory protein ICP27 map to the C-terminal regions and are required to modulate viral gene expression very early in infection. *J. Virol.* **64:** 3471–3485.

Post, L.E., S. Mackem and B. Roizman. 1981. Regulation of alpha genes of HSV: Expression of chimeric genes produced by fusion of thymidine kinase with alpha gene promoters. *Cell* **24:** 555–565.

Preston, C.M. 1979. Control of herpes simplex virus type 1 mRNA synthesis in cells infected with wild-type virus or the temperature-sensitive mutant tsK. *J. Virol.* **29:** 275–284.

Preston, V.G. 1981. Fine-structure mapping of herpes simplex virus type 1 temperature-sensitive mutations within the short repeat region of the genome. *J. Virol.* **39:** 150–161.

Read, G.S. and N. Frenkel. 1983. Herpes simplex virus mutants defective in the virion associated shut-off of host polypeptide synthesis and exhibiting abnormal synthesis of a (immediate–early) viral polypeptides. *J. Virol.* **46:** 498–512.

Rice, S.A., M.C. Long, V. Lam and C.A. Spencer. 1994. RNA polymerase is aberrantly phosphorylated and localized to viral replication compartments following herpes simplex virus infection. *J. Virol.* **68:** 988–1001.

Sacks, W.R., C.C. Greene, D.A. Aschman and P.A. Schaffer. 1985. Herpes simplex virus type 1 ICP27 is an essential regulatory protein. *J. Virol.* **55:** 796–805.

Sacks, W.R. and P.A. Schaffer. 1987. Deletion mutants in the gene encoding the herpes simplex virus type 1 immediate–early protein ICP0 exhibit impaired growth in cell culture. *J. Virol.* **61:** 829–839.

Samaniego, L.A., A.L. Webb and N.A. DeLuca. 1995. Functional interaction between herpes simplex virus immediate early proteins during infection: gene expression as a consequence of ICP27 and different domains of ICP4. *J. Virol.* **69:** 5705–5715.

Sandri-Goldin, R.M. and G.E. Mendoza. 1992. A herpesvirus regulatory protein appears to act post-transcriptionally by affecting mRNA processing. *Gene Dev.* **6:** 848–863.

Sauer B., M. Whealy, A. Robbins and L. Enquist. 1987. Site-specific insertion of DNA in a pseudovirus virus vector. *Proc. Natl Acad. Sci. USA* **84:** 9108–9112.

Schaffer, P.A., G.M. Aron, N. Biswal and M. Benyesh-Melnick. 1973. Temperature sensitive mutants of herpes simplex virus type 1: isolation, complementation and partial characterization. *J. Virol.* **36:** 189–203.

Schaffer, P.A., V.C. Carter and M.C. Timbury. 1978. Collaborative complementation study of temperature sensitive mutants of herpes simplex virus types 1 and 2. *J. Virol.* **27:** 490–504.

Sears, A.E., I.W. Halliburton, B. Meignier, S. Silver and B. Roizman. 1985. Herpes simplex virus mutant deleted in the a22 gene: growth and gene expression in permissive and restrictive cells, and establishment of latency in mice. *J. Virol.* **55:** 338–346.

Smith, C.A., P. Bates, R. Rivera-Gonzalez, B. Gu. and N. A. DeLuca. 1993. ICP4, the major regulatory protein of herpes simplex virus type 1, forms a tripartite complex with TATA-binding protein and TFIIB. *J. Virol.* **67:** 4676–4687.

Southern, P.J. and P. Berg. 1982. Transformation of mammalian cells to antibiotic resistance with a bacterial gene under control of the SV40 early region promoter. *J. Mol. Appl. Genet.* **1:** 327–341.

Spivack, J.G. and N.W. Fraser. 1987. Detection of herpes simplex virus type 1 transcripts during latent infection in mice. *J. Virol.* **61:** 3841–3847.

Sternberg, N. and D. Hamilton. 1981. Bacteriophage P1 site-specific recombination. 1. Recombination between *lox*P site. *J. Mol. Biol.* **150:** 467–486.

Stevens, J.G., E.K. Wagner, G.B. Devi-Rao, M.L. Cook and L.T. Feldman. 1987. RNA complementary to a herpesvirus a gene mRNA is prominent in latently infected neurons. *Science* **235:** 1056–1059.

Stinski, M.F. and T.J. Roehr. 1985. Activation of the major immediate early gene of human cytomegalovirus by cis-acting elements in the promoter-regulatory sequence and by virus-specific trans-acting components. *J. Virol.* **55:** 431–441.

Stow, N.D. and E.C. Stow. 1986. Isolation and characterization of a herpes simplex virus type 1 mutant containing a deletion within the gene encoding the immediate early polypeptide Vmw110. *J. Gen. Virol.* **67:** 2571–2585.

Su, L. and D.M. Knipe. 1989. Herpes simplex virus a protein ICP27 can inhibit or augment viral gene transactivation. *Virology* **170:** 496–504.

Thomas, K.R., K.R. Folger and M.R. Capecchi. 1986. High-frequency targeting of genes to specific sites in the mammalian genome. *Cell* **44:** 419–428.

Thomsen, D.R., R.M. Stenberg, W.F. Goins and M.F. Stinski. 1984. Promoter-regulatory region of the major immediate early gene of human cytomegalovirus. *Proc. Natl Acad. Sci. USA* **81:** 6529–6533.

White, B.A. and F.C. Brancroft. 1982. Cytoplasmic dot hybridization. *J. Biol. Chem.* **257:** 8569–8572.

Wildy, P., H.J. Field and A.A. Nash. 1982. Classical herpes virus latency revisited. In: B.W.J. Mahy, A.C. Minson and G.K. Darby (eds), *Virus persistence.* Cambridge, Cambridge University Press.

Wong, E.A. and M.R. Capecchi. 1987. Homologous recombination between coinjected DNA sequences peaks in early to mid-S phase. *Mol. Cell. Biol.* **7:** 2294–2295.

York, I.A., C. Roop, D.W. Andrews, S.R. Riddell, F.L. Graham and D.C. Johnson. 1994. A cytosolic herpes simplex virus protein inhibits antigen presentation to CD8+ T lymphocytes. *Cell* **77:** 525–535.

CHAPTER 16

In vivo Expression of Reporter Genes from Herpes Simplex Virus Type 1 Recombinant Vectors

LAWRENCE FELDMAN

Department of Microbiology and Immunology, UCLA School of Medicine, Center for the Health Sciences, 10833 Le Conte Avenue, Los Angeles, CA 90024-1747, USA.
Tel: 310 206 1014; Fax: 310 206 3865; Email: lfeldman@microimmun.medsch.ucla.edu

1 INTRODUCTION

Herpes simplex virus (HSV-1) can establish latent infections in post-mitotic neurons of the peripheral and central nervous system. It is possible that a gene inserted into the viral DNA in the proper configuration may be expressed for the life of the infected host. Together with the capacity to package a large amount of foreign DNA, this makes HSV-1 a reasonable candidate for delivery and expression of foreign genes in such neurons.

The use of HSV-1 as a vector has been pursued in two ways: (1) the recombinant virus is made and plaque purified so that all progeny viruses are essentially identical; (2) the foreign DNA is packaged as an amplicon of multiple copies and the progeny viruses are a mixture of helper viruses and the defective interfering particles containing the amplicons. We favor the first approach, primarily because it delivers a known quantity of DNA in a reliable manner with each infection. By contrast, each passage of the virus in an amplicon system is subject to wide variations in the ratio of helper virus to amplicon, over which the investigator has little control.

Acute HSV-1 infection is lethal in cell culture and most animal models. To generate an effective vector system, the lethal functions of the virus must be inactivated. We routinely do this by deleting the ICP4 gene. Expression of this gene is essential for the viral growth because it activates transcription of all the early and late viral genes. ICP4 null mutants can be grown in culture by utilizing the ICP4-expressing cell line E5, developed by DeLuca et al. (1985). In this system ICP4 null mutants can be grown to titers of 1×10^9 p.f.u./ml. In infections of non-complementing cells, such as Vero cells, an ICP4 null mutant is incapable of forming plaques, although some cells in the monolayer may die, depending on the multiplicity of infection (MOI) used. Thus, a recombinant virus deleted for ICP4 is defective in low-multiplicity infections of a non-host cell. This chapter provides simple protocols for construction of HSV-1 vectors.

There are two general uses of HSV as a vector: (1) to deliver and express genes to cells in culture, such as primary neurons; (2) to deliver and express genes *in vivo*, preferably for a long time. In both cases it is of interest to remove the ICP4 gene, which is the primary transcriptional activator of the virus. The problems of infecting cells in culture are discussed briefly below; the second use of HSV is the main subject of this chapter.

Protocols for Gene Transfer in Neuroscience: Towards Gene Therapy of Neurological Disorders
Edited by P.R. Lowenstein and L.W. Enquist

1.1 Use of HSV-1 in Cell Culture

It is important to delete the ICP27 gene and the vhs gene, both of which are toxic to the cell, as well as the ICP4 gene. The ICP27 protein affects cellular mRNA processing (Sandri-Goldin and Mends, 1992), and both ICP4 and ICP27 are required for viral growth, so they are most easily removed by making a cell line expressing both genes following the protocols of DeLuca and colleagues (1985). The vhs gene shuts off host cell protein synthesis and has been mutated in HSV without causing appreciable harm to its growth properties (Read et al., 1993). Once the three genes are altered, and the gene of interest expressed from an appropriate promoter, cells in culture may be infected and the gene expressed. The chief problem is to express the gene but not the toxicity of the virus, and the investigator must keep these two variables in mind when choosing the MOI.

An important aspect of the use of vectors is the activity of the promoter element during the latent state. In HSV-1 latency a single promoter remains active to direct the synthesis of the latency-associated transcripts (LAT). However, attachment of the LAT promoter to reporter genes, or the use of promoters such as the CMV enhancer, routinely results in promoter activity for only a few days, and the promoters are not active when the virus is latent in infected neurons. In analysing this problem, we have determined that the LAT promoter contains two separate functional parts. One of these functions is the "normal" function of a promoter—the LAT promoter, from −800 to −25 relative to the start of transcription, contains DNA binding sites for common as well as neuronal specific transcription factors. Binding of specific transcription factors to the promoter determines the promoter strength, and the LAT promoter binds transcription factors which appear to be specific for dorsal root and trigeminal ganglion neurons. However, this part of the LAT promoter is functional in neurons of the peripheral nervous system for only a few days, and a second function is required to keep this promoter active. This second function maps 3′ of the start of transcription and allows promoters that are already active to continue transcription throughout the latent period but does not contribute significant transcription itself. This element might be necessary to prevent nucleosomal repression, although this is not proven.

Both the region downstream of the LAT promoter and the LTR of Maloney Murine Leukemia virus appear to keep the LAT promoter active during latency. The downstream LAT region is over 1 kb in size, contains a number of ATG sequences which disrupt the appropriate translation of the reporter gene, and is not yet well described, so we have focused attention on the LTR, which is much more clearly defined and does not contain a long leader RNA. We have paired the LTR, which also contains the site for initiation of transcription, with the upstream region of the LAT promoter, which, in this construction, contains the transcription factor binding sites upstream of the TATA box. Viruses containing this construction show high promoter activity in neurons of the peripheral nervous system and express reporter genes for many months at a level which is easily detectable by *in situ* hybridization. In the central nervous system an ICP4 null mutant with this configuration also expresses RNA for long periods, although at a much lower level (Bloom et al., 1994). These data are in accord with the model that the LTR part of the promoter provides the long term expression function and the upstream part of the LAT promoter specifies the strength of the promoter in a given neuron. It is thus not surprising that the LAT promoter shows greater activity in neurons of the peripheral nervous system than in neurons of the central nervous system.

2 MATERIALS AND EQUIPMENT

2.1 Solutions for DNA Analysis

(1) TE: 10 mM Tris pH 8.0, 1 mM EDTA.
(2) TNE: 10 mM Tris pH 7.4, 1 mM EDTA, 0.1 M NaCl, filter sterilized and stored at room temperature.
(3) 5 M NaCl.
(4) 100 mM β-mercaptoethanol (ME).
(5) 2% sodium dodecyl sulfate (SDS).
(6) TES: 50 mM Tris pH 7.8, 1 mM EDTA, 30% sucrose.
(7) Proteinase K: 20 mg/ml proteinase K in 10 mM $CaCl_2$.

(8) 7.5 M NH_4OAc in water, stored at −20°C.
(9) A 24:1 solution of chloroform:isoamyl alcohol.
(10) 95% ethanol, stored at −20°C.
(11) Phenol: saturate a bottle of phenol with water so that it separates into two phases. The phenol phase is on the bottom. Store at 4°C. Always wear gloves when handling phenol. Phenol will blister the skin by forming esters. These are reversible with alcohol; do **not** wash phenol burns with water.

2.2 Reagents for DNA Transfections

(1) Minimal essential medium containing 5% calf serum (5% CS MEM).
(2) Hypotonic lysis buffer: 10 mM Tris 8.0, 10 mM EDTA, 1% NP40, 0.5% deoxycholate.
(3) 2× HEPES buffer: Mix 16.0 g NaCl, 0.74 g KCl, 0.376 g $Na_2HPO_4{:}7H_2O$, (or 0.199 g anhydrous Na_2HPO_4), 2.0 g dextrose, 10.0 g HEPES acid (or 10.92 g of sodium salt). Bring to 800 ml and pH 7.05 with NaOH then bring to 1 liter with double-distilled water. Filter sterilize and store 25 ml aliquots in 50 ml polypropylene at −20°C.
(4) 40% Solution of dextrose in double-distilled water. Filter sterilize, store at 4°C.
(5) Minimal essential medium containing 1.5% fetal calf serum (1.5% FCS MEM).
(6) Shock buffer: 0.5 g HEPES pH 7.05, 20 g dextrose solution in 100 ml water.
(7) 2.6 M $CaCl_2$ (low sulfate, approx. 75% $CaCl_2$), filter sterilized and stored at room temperature.
(8) HSV transfection DNA (SEE PROTOCOL #87).

3 THE PROTOCOLS

Protocol #87: Rapid HSV-1 DNA for Transfection

(1) Infect one 16 oz bottle of confluent rabbit skin cells (MOI 1 p.f.u./cell) with 1–2 ml virus. Add 12 ml 5% CS MEM after adsorption.
(2) When cells are fully infected (about 48 h), harvest in a 15 ml polypropylene centrifuge tube and pellet at 1500 r.p.m. for 20 min in a low-speed centrifuge at 4°C.
(3) Save 3 ml of the supernatant as virus stock and discard the rest. Label and date this virus stock accordingly. Remove remaining medium with a Pasteur pipette.
(4) Add 5 ml hypotonic lysis buffer to cell pellet and shake gently three times over 10 min. This will lyse cells without breaking the nuclei and releasing cellular DNA.
(5) Pellet nuclei at 6000 r.p.m. for 5 min at 4°C. Place the supernatant in another 15 ml polypropylene centrifuge tube. Discard pellet.
(6) Phenol extract supernatant once: add 5 ml water-saturated phenol to the supernatant, shake vigorously (1–2 min), spin at 10 000 r.p.m. at room temperature for at least 15 min. Using a wide-mouthed plastic 5 ml pipette remove the upper aqueous phase and place into another 15 ml polypropylene centrifuge tube.
! ABSOLUTELY DO NOT TAKE ANY OF THE INTERFACE DURING THIS EXTRACTION **!**
(7) Chloroform extract the resulting aqueous phase once: add 5 ml 24:1 chloroform/isoamyl alcohol with a glass pipette. Shake vigorously (1 min). Spin for about 3 min at full speed as described in Step 6. Using a wide-mouthed plastic 5 ml pipette remove upper aqueous phase. Note volume when transferring to another 15 ml polypropylene centrifuge tube.
! ABSOLUTELY DO NOT TAKE ANY OF THE INTERFACE DURING THIS EXTRACTION **!**
(8) Bring volume to 5 ml with double-distilled water and add 100 μl 5 M NaCl. Invert tube, and then add 10 ml − 20°C 100% ethanol. Invert several times. The solution may be stored at −20°C for later use.
(9) Pour solution into 15 ml centrifuge tube (specifically for the Sorvall SS-34 rotor) and pellet DNA at 15 000 r.p.m. for 30 min at 4°C. Pour off ethanol; aspirate excess with a Pasteur pipette—take care not to aspirate the pellet. Circle pellet with a marker pen, because it will disappear upon drying. Dry pellet in desiccator.
(10) Using a 200 μl pipette, add 100 μl of TE plus 5μl RNAase (stock of 1 mg/ml) directly on top of

Table 16.1

Number of plates	*HSV DNA* (μl)	2.6 M $CaCl_2$ (μl)	*TNE* (μl)	*Total volume*
1	10	25	215	250
5	50	125	1075	1250

the circled pellet, scrape with pipette tip and pipette up and down until the pellet is resuspended. Store at −20°C.

Protocol #88: Preparation of Rabbit Skin Cells for Transfection of HSV DNA

See Graham and Van der Eb (1973); Stow and Wilkie (1976).

(1) Pass one 3-day-old 16 oz bottle of rabbit skin cells into three bottles containing 5% CS MEM at 37°C.
(2) Pass one of these bottles 24 h later into 20 60 mm Petri plates containing 5% CS MEM, 37°C.
(3) After 24 h replace the 5% CS MEM with 1.5% FCS MEM and incubate at 31°C.
(4) After 24 h at 31°C the cells are ready for transfection (cells should be about 50% confluent).

Protocol #89: Preparing the Transfection Cocktail

(1) Transfections normally require 10 μl of HSV transfection DNA per plate (empirically determined by titration to obtain the maximum number of plaques).
(2) Assume the DNA requires 10 μl HSV DNA/plate. Make 250 μl of transfection cocktail for each plate (or tube above containing 2 × HEPES) in a single 5 ml polypropylene tube. Use Table 16.1 as an example.
(3) Order of mixing (in a polypropylene falcon tube): TNE, $CaCl_2$, HSV DNA. Use wide-mouthed plastic pipettes for HSV DNA and mix gently.

In marker rescue experiments the rescuing DNA is added to 10-fold mass excess (by analysis on a mini-gel) compared to the unit-length HSV DNA.

Protocol #90: Transfection of HSV-1 DNA

(1) Add 250 μl 2 × HEPES buffer to the same number of 5 ml polypropylene tubes as plates to be transfected.
(2) Slowly add 250 μl of the transfection cocktail prepared in Protocol #89 to each tube, while gently bubbling the solution with a Pasteur pipette. This produces the transfection mix.
(3) Let tubes sit 20 min at room temperature.
(4) Remove the 1.5% FCS MEM from the transfection plates by aspiration, then pour on 0.5 ml transfection mixture, rotate, and allow to sit on the cells for 20–30 min at room temperature.
(5) Add 5 ml 1.5% FCS MEM and incubate at 37°C for 4 h.
(6) After 4 h, aspirate medium, wash in 5 ml 5% CS MEM, remove wash then subject cells **briefly** (1–2 min) to hypertonic shock in 1–2 ml hypertonic shock buffer.
(7) Remove buffer by aspiration and wash again in 5 ml 5% CS MEM. Remove wash and feed with 5 ml 5% CS MEM. Incubate at 37°C in CO_2.

Protocol #91: Mini-viral DNA Preparation for Southern Blot Analysis

(1) Infect a 60 mm dish of chosen cells at a MOI of 10 p.f.u./cell.
(2) When cells have been destroyed, pellet the cells (saving supernatant).
(3) Resuspend in 200 μl 50 mM TES.
(4) Add 200 μl 2% SDS and 100 mM ME. Allow to stand on ice for 30 min.
(5) Incubate with 10 μl proteinase K overnight at 55°C.
(6) Extract twice with phenol/chloroform (1 : 1) then once with chloroform : isoamyl alcohol (24 : 1).

(7) Precipitate DNA by adding 75 μl 7.5 M NH_4OAc and 2.5 volumes of ice-cold 95% ethanol.
(8) Rock at room temperature, dry briefly (do not dry too thoroughly or the pellet will be difficult to resuspend).
(9) Resuspend in 50 μl double-distilled water.
(10) Cut 10 μl in a total reaction volume of 30 μl. This will be enough to run two gels if required. Run 15 μl in mini-well of gel.

4 NOTES AND TROUBLESHOOTING

4.1 Constructing a Recombinant HSV-1 Virus Containing the Required Promoter Driving the *lac*Z Gene

The recombinant viruses described in this chapter will contain deletions of essential immediate–early genes, so will be defective in viral growth and may be used to test the acute and latent activity of the promoter in neurons of the peripheral and central nervous system *in vivo*. The advantage of using this reporter system is that promoter activity is easily assessed by staining neuronal sections or whole mounts of ganglia with X-gal to observe blue neurons. The staining pattern observed helps to determine the number of neurons infected. If a suitable system is obtained, the *lac*Z gene may be replaced by the cellular gene of choice.

The first step is to choose a promoter element to pair with the LTR. The promoter should contain DNA binding sites for the transcription factors of the targeted neuron. The HSV-1 LAT promoter is highly active in neurons of the peripheral nervous system, but is much less active in neurons of the central nervous system. The expression obtained from the vector in each neuronal site will depend partly on the activity of the promoter in those cells.

The selected promoter should be joined to the LTR–*lac*Z. Do not include the TATA box of the neuronal promoter in this plasmid construction; the idea is to provide the upstream activation sequences for the targeted neuron and that transcription will initiate from within the LTR. It is a very good idea to test the construct for promoter activity by performing transient assays for β-galactosidase activity, ideally in neurons similar to those targeted *in vivo*. Everything possible should be done to make sure that the recombinant virus will express the *lac*Z gene in the animal.

To insert this construct into the virus it is necessary to add DNA sequences both 5′ and 3′ of the construct to facilitate homologous recombination. These sequences need not be contiguous on the virus; in the following example the ICP4 gene is deleted. The promoter–LTR–*lac*Z construct should be cloned into a portion of the HSV-1 genome from which the ICP4 gene and flanking sequences have been deleted (Fig. 16.1). In this particular construction there are two considerations of importance. One is that the plasmid construct just made must be cleaved on both flanks before cotransfection with viral DNA (i.e. linear DNA will be transfected). This means that the construct must contain at least one restriction site on the 5′ HSV-1 side and one on the 3′ HSV-1 side not contained in the insert. In our case, *Sac*I or *Sph*I can be used if they are not present in the promoter-LTR-*lac*Z construct. It is therefore absolutely essential that no restriction sites that are to be used to linearize the final plasmid are inserted.

The second consideration is that no DNA sequences from the ICP4 gene which overlap with those present in the host range cell should be left in the virus. In earlier examples, we deleted only part of the ICP4 gene. This left flanking sequences on both ends of the viral DNA that matched the sequences present in the integrated copies of the ICP4 gene in the E5 cells. The result of this overlap was that no matter how many times the recombinant virus was plaque purified, a wild-type contaminant remained in the viral population. Although such contaminants may be present at a very low frequency (10^{-6}–10^{-8}), they can be lethal when injected directly into the central nervous system. These steps are represented in Fig. 16.1.

Cotransfect the linearized plasmid DNA with wild-type virion DNA, made as described in Protocol #90. The frequency of recombination of the plasmid DNA into the viral DNA will depend largely on the amount of flanking sequences—the larger the overlap, the greater the frequency of recombination. It is also possible to make recombinant viruses by first transfecting in the linear plasmid and then superinfecting the cells the next day with wild-type virus; however, this approach is not recommended. Production of high-quality DNA is time consuming, but it is far

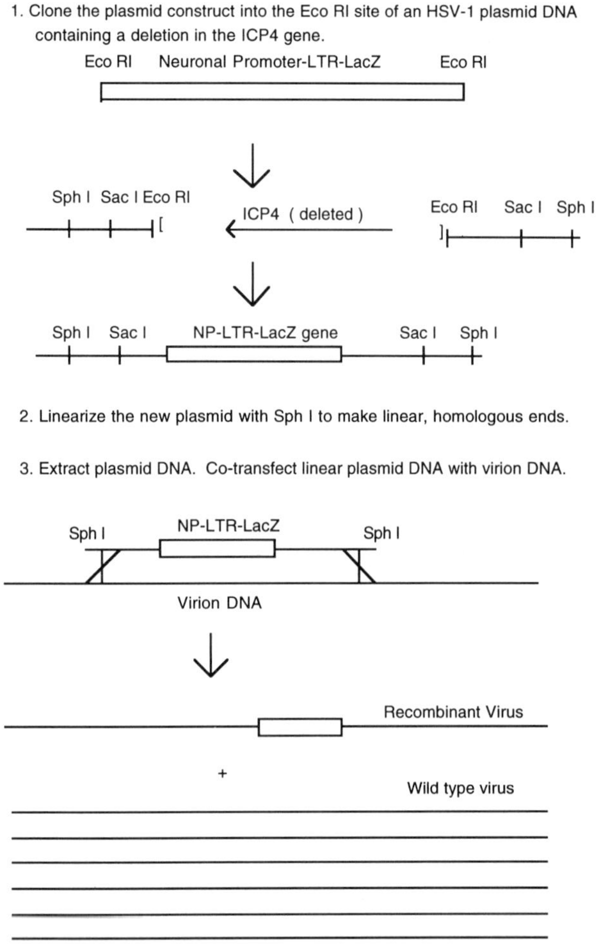

Figure 16.1 Making the recombinant virus by cotransfection. Note that the ICP4 gene has been deleted and the LTR construct inserted into the plasmid, leaving HSV-1 DNA sequences on either side

easier in the long term to make a recombinant virus if viral DNA is used in cotransfection rather than in superinfection. Although the second method works, the frequency of recombination is far lower than obtained using cotransfected cells.

4.2 Isolating Recombinant Virus

Within 2–3 days of transfection plaques will be visible on the monolayers. These appear as a small group of 4–8 cells that have rounded up or have fused. These foci progressively enlarge and the released virus begins to cause new areas of degeneration all over the plate. By 5–7 days the virus is ready to harvest by scraping or pipetting the cells into a tube, quick freezing them in dry ice and ethanol and storing at −70°C. As the number of plaques and growth of the virus will vary considerably in the initial transfection, the virus should be passed onto E5 cells for two reasons: (1) it is easier to standardize the titer by one passage under more uniform conditions; (2) the recombination event actually occurs in two sites on the viral DNA because the ICP4 gene is in the short repeat sequences. Initially it will occur at only one of these sites, and the virus isomerizes the repeat sequences as it replicates, producing either a two-sided recombinant or a wild-type virus depending on which of the repeats is used as a template. By passing the initial virus transfection the virus is forced into many new rounds of replication and the chances of obtaining a two-sided recombinant increase. The tube from the freezer should be thawed in a 37°C water bath, and 10 μl applied to a 60 mm dish of E5 cells. This new inoculum will grow and kill the E5 cells in 2–3 days, when the virus can be harvested as before. For a 60 mm dish containing 5 ml medium, the titer is 1×10^7 p.f.u./ml.

4.3 Screening for Recombinant Viruses

The mixture of wild-type and recombinant virus in a ratio of approximately 100:1 should be separated and the viruses containing the promoter–*lacZ* construct identified by plaque purification. The tube containing the passed virus at 1×10^7 p.f.u./ml is thawed and the cell debris is spun down in a microfuge for 20 s at a low speed. Do **not** spin at a high speed; this will cause the herpesviruses themselves to spin down, leaving very little in the supernatant. The supernatant, containing the virus, is diluted in medium to 1×10^{-3}, 10^{-4} and 10^{-5} p.f.u./ml, and 100μl is applied to a 60 mm dish in 1 ml of medium for 1 h to allow the virus to enter the cells. Following this adsorption period, the virus inoculum replaced with an overlay of 3 ml agarose made by combining 1.4% agarose in water with 2 × medium, cooling to about 47°C. If the overlay is too hot the cells will die; if it is too cold the agarose will solidify. The overlay should look relatively clear, and will harden within 5 min, after which the plates are incubated for 3 days at 47°C. On the third day individual plaques, representing the progeny of a single virus, should be visible. Be sure that you are visualizing plaques, and not deformities in the monolayer, by checking that the titer makes sense—there should be a hundredfold difference in the titers between the 10^{-3} and the 10^{-5} plates. If necessary, the plaques can be enhanced visually by staining with a 0.1% solution of neutral red in PBS, 2 ml of which is added to the top of the agarose for 2 h at 37°C. After removing neutral red the plaques can be picked with a Pasteur pipette or with an Eppendorf fitted with a yellow tip. Pick each plaque directly into one well of a 96-well culture of confluent E5 cells. These viruses will grow out over the next 3 days.

4.4 Assaying for Recombinant Viruses

Once the plaques in each well have produced their characteristic cytopathic effect, the virus is ready for assay. This is done by removing 50 μl from each well with an 8-channel Eppendorf pipette and applying it to a 96-well dot-blot apparatus (Fig. 16.2) which should have the same configuration as the 96-well plate. A piece of Whatmann 3 mm filter paper and a sheet of nitrocellulose should be sandwiched between the top and bottom. The 96 wells are essentially replica plated onto the nitrocellulose, on top, baked at 80°C for 2 h, denatured in alkali (e.g. 0.1 N NaOH) and baked again. The nitrocellulose strip can be probed with any DNA sequence which is newly inserted into the virus, e.g. the upstream promoter, the LTR or the *lacZ* gene. The nitrocellulose can be probed essentially as a Southern blot, using ^{32}P-labeled DNA and hybridizing in Denhardt's solution. A wild-type virus inoculated into one well serves as a negative control, and plasmid DNA on one spot as a positive control. In this first screening three 96-well plates should be analysed to give several putative recombinants. The nitrocellulose should be washed stringently, in 0.1 × SSC at 65°C for 2 h, with three changes. When analysing the film look for dark circles appearing after only an overnight exposure, most of the circles remaining blank. If most of the circles are dark, the filters must be washed more stringently, because only about 1% of the wells should contain recombinant virus capable of hybridizing with the probe. The putatively positive wells will not be as dark as the positive control containing only plasmid DNA, even if only 100 ng is placed onto the paper.

Consider the two darkest spots. The virus in these two wells are unlikely to be pure recombinant, even though they are plaque purified, and they are also unlikely to be two-sided recombinants. Remove 10 μl from each well and refreeze the plate at −70°C, place the 10 μl into a new 60 mm dish of E5 cells and grow for 3 days, again producing a titer of 1×10^7 p.f.u./ml. The objective is to isolate a recombinant virus which has not stuck to another wild-type virus and which is a double-sided recombinant. A second round of plaque purification and picking the plaques into wells containing E5 cells is carried out. This time it will be necessary only to pick

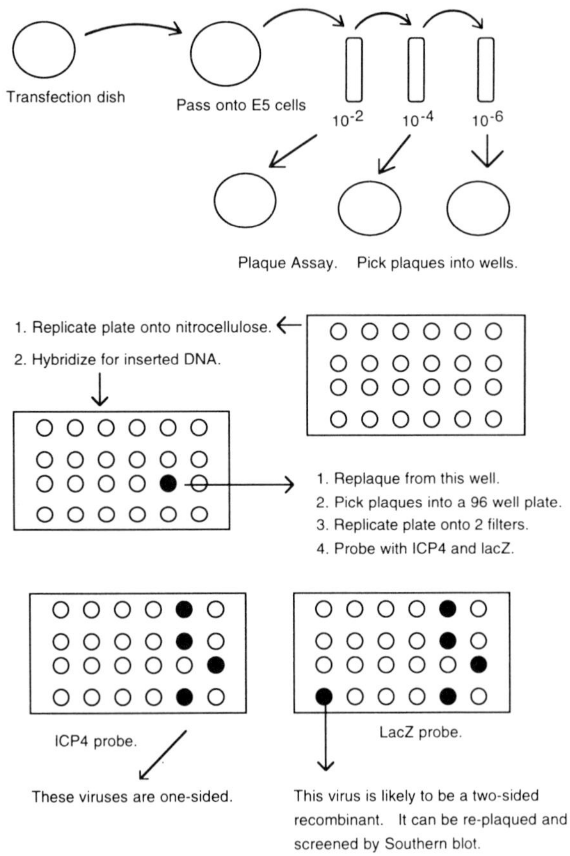

Figure 16.2 Assaying for recombinant viruses

40–50 of each of the two plaque types.

Probe the nitrocellulose filter with labeled ICP4 gene, develop the film, rehybridize, without stripping, for the *lac*Z gene, develop a second film and compare with the first. The desired recombinant should be negative for the ICP4 gene and positive for the *lac*Z gene. Variation among the 96 wells for these two properties is likely to be considerable. Wells that are positive for both probes may contain either two types of virus not yet separated or a single virus which is one-sided for each gene. Note how many wells are positive for *lac*Z and negative for ICP4: this may be only 10–20% of the total. Pick virus from the well which is most negative for ICP4 and most positive for the *lac*Z gene, make new plaques from them and repeat the probing with the ICP4 and *lac*Z probes as above.

On the third round of plaque purification, the percentage of *lac*Z-positive plaques should increase to approximately 100%. If several plaques appear to be negative for hybridization to the ICP4 gene and positive for the *lac*Z gene, it may be time to analyse the viruses by Southern blot. Pick viruses from each of six wells with these properties and inoculate a 60 mm dish with 100 μl. After overnight growth, perform a Southern blot. For a DNA insertion such as this, the Southern blot will verify not only that the insertion is in the correct location but also that both copies of the short repeat contain the recombinant DNA. This is very important, as a one-sided virus will be essentially wild-type because it contains the ICP4 gene.

Choose an enzyme such as *Hin*dIII, which does not cut in the repeats, or one such as *Xho*I, which cuts in the long but not the short repeat. These enzymes will generate two bands in a Southern blot, each band being positive for the *lacZ* gene and negative for the ICP4 gene. If only one band hybridizes to each probe, the virus has not yet isomerized and may be unstable; it requires further viral growth and plaque assay to identify completely two-sided recombinants.

REFERENCES

Bloom, D.C., N.T. Maidment, L.T. Feldman and J.G. Stevens. 1994. Long term expression of a reporter gene from latent HSV in the rat hippocampus (manuscript in preparation).

DeLuca, NA., A.M. McCarthy and P.A. Schaffer. 1985. Isolation and characterization of deletion mutants of herpes simplex virus type 1 in the gene encoding immediate-early regulatory protein ICP4. *J. Virol.* **56**:558–570.

Graham, F.L. and A.J. van der Eb. 1973. A new technique for the assay of infectivity of human adenovirus 5 DNA. *Virology* **52**:456–467.

Read, G.S., M. Karr and K. Knight. 1993. Isolation of a herpes simplex virus type 1 mutant with a deletion in the virion host shutoff gene and identification of multiple forms of the vhs (UL41) polypeptide. *J. Virol.* **67**: 7149-87160.

Sandri-Goldin, R.M. and G.E. Mends. 1992. A herpesvirus regulatory protein appears to act post-transcriptionally by affecting mRNA processing. *Gene Dev.* **6**:848–863.

Stow, N.D. and N.M. Wilkie. 1976. An improved technique for obtaining enhanced infectivity with herpes simplex virus type 1 DNA. *J. Gen. Virol.* **33**:447–458.

CHAPTER 17

Herpes Simplex Virus Latency in Tissue Culture Cells

CHRIS M. PRESTON*, JACKIE RUSSELL†, RUTH A. HARRIS† AND D.R. STUART JAMIESON†

*MRC Virology Unit, †Institute of Virology, Glasgow G11 5JR, UK. Tel: 0141 339 8855 Extension 4635 or 4630; Fax: 0141 337 2236; Email:cpreston@vir.gla.ac.uk

1 INTRODUCTION

This chapter describes tissue culture systems for latency *in vitro* with HSV, involving methods used almost exclusively in our laboratory. Although HSV can replicate in sensory neurons, it can also establish latency, a long-term interaction in which the host cell survives and most viral gene expression is repressed (see Chapter 10). The use of animals to study latency, although providing good models for the phenomenon in humans, suffers from experimental limitations. Laboratory animals are expensive and inevitably vary in their response to virus infection. Replication and latency of HSV in neurons is preceded by virus replication at the site of inoculation, providing a gradual and immeasurable supply of virus to the nerve endings. As a consequence it is not possible to determine accurately the effective inoculum or to achieve a synchronous infection at the ganglion. In addition, immune responses affect the interaction of HSV with the host. At the biochemical level, the study of latency is hindered by the low number of cells within a ganglion harboring latent virus: at best, only 1% of ganglion cells (approximately 20% of neurons) contain HSV genomes as judged by *in situ* hybridization using probes specific for the latency-associated transcripts (LATs). Many of the problems associated with the use of experimental animals could be overcome by developing tissue culture systems which reproduce latency. Infection of permissive cells, however, invariably leads to cell death, and methods must be developed to prevent this outcome before any possibility exists of detecting latency.

The first system described involves incubating infected cells at 42° to suppress virus replication and promote latency. The second system takes advantage of the properties of the HSV-1 mutant *in*1814, which has a 12 base pair insertion in the coding sequences for the virion protein Vmw65 (also named VP16 or α-TIF) (Ace et al., 1989). Protein Vmw65 normally activates transcription of immediate–early (IE) genes by forming a multiprotein complex with the cellular factors Oct-1 and HCF (O'Hare and Goding, 1988; Preston et al., 1988; Stern et al., 1989; Wilson et al., 1993). Oct-1 binds to the DNA element TAATGARAT (R is a purine) present in one or more copies upstream of all IE promoters, then HCF and Vmw65 assemble on the DNA-bound Oct-1. As a consequence of these interactions, a highly acidic region at the C-terminus of Vmw65 is brought into proximity with the transcription preinitiation complex and initiation of IE transcription is stimulated (Sadowski et al., 1988; Triezenberg et al., 1988). The insertion in *in*1814 results in a four-amino acid addition in a domain of Vmw65 crucial for interaction with Oct-1 and HCF; thus the multiprotein

Protocols for Gene Transfer in Neuroscience: Towards Gene Therapy of Neurological Disorders
Edited by P.R. Lowenstein and L.W. Enquist

complex cannot be formed and transcription of IE genes is impaired. The reduction in transcription facilitates the establishment of latency *in vitro*.

The overall aims must be carefully considered before investigations using the approaches described in this chapter are undertaken. If a study of latency is envisaged the opinions expressed in the two most widely quoted reviews on this subject (Roizman and Sears, 1987; paraphrased in Stevens, 1989) must be considered: "The mimicry of tissue culture systems to latency *in vivo* is likely to be insignificant with respect to the mechanism of latency but significant with respect to our understanding of gene expression in non-permissive cells." Unless you are prepared to question this view, and to defend your decision to question it, you should abandon the project or use the methodology described in Chapter 18. Many eminent workers in the field consider HSV latency to be critically dependent upon the infection of **neurons** by HSV, arguing that specific properties of the neuron, probably involving the profile of transcription factors present, are crucial for latency. The counter argument, upon which any attempts to reproduce latency in non-neuronal cells are based, states that the specific contribution of the neuron is limited and that most aspects of latency can be reconstructed by careful manipulation of the interaction of HSV with the host cell. At present there is insufficient information for a definitive judgment to be made on this issue.

Notwithstanding these caveats, there are reasons why the study of latency in tissue culture cells, especially using *in*1814, is interesting and informative. The justifications that we use for pursuing this line of research are as follows. First, study of *in*1814 is the best way to understand the biological importance of transactivation of IE transcription by Vmw65, because no other equivalent mutants are available and specific means of preventing Vmw65 activity *in vivo* are not known. Second, latency that can be established in tissue culture cells after infection with *in*1814 is, in many ways, very similar to the interaction that occurs in neurons after infection with wild-type HSV-1. Suspicion is growing that the normal route to latency involves repression of IE transcription in neurons (Roizman and Sears, 1987; see Chapter 10). If this is the case, it is reasonable to propose that the artificial block imposed by the mutation present in *in*1814 reproduces the "natural" block that occurs in neurons. The third justification for studying latency *in vitro* is particularly relevant to the context of this book: for gene therapy, an HSV vector arrested as early as possible in the replication cycle is desirable since expression even of IE gene products can be cytotoxic. *in*1814 is the earliest mutant available that is able to uncoat its genome and enter the cell nucleus; if it can be engineered to retain its ability to establish latency and to express stably the product of an inserted gene, it should form the basis for a useful vector.

2 MATERIALS AND EQUIPMENT

(1) Human fetal lung (HFL) fibroblasts.
(2) EF10 and EF5 media for growth of HFL cells: × Eagle's medium (Glasgow modification) containing 4 mM L-glutamine, 100 units/ml penicillin, 100 μg/ml streptomycin, 1 × non-essential amino acids, 10% or 5% (v/v) fetal calf serum.
(3) Virus stocks: stocks of wild-type HSV-1 or HSV-2 are widely available, but it is best to start with one of the commonly used strains such as KOS, 17, F and SC16 for HSV-1 and G, HG52 and 186 for HSV-2. Seed stocks should be obtained from a laboratory specializing in the use of that strain. The HSV-1 (strain 17) mutant *in*1814 can be obtained from the Institute of Virology, Glasgow, or from Professor N.W. Fraser at the Wistar Institute, Philadelphia, USA.
(4) Cells for propagation of HSV: many tissue culture cells are satisfactory hosts for HSV-1. Strain 17 is normally grown in BHK-21 clone 13 cells, available from ATCC.
(5) ETC10 medium for growth of BHK cells: 1 × Eagle's medium (Glasgow modification), 4 mM L-glutamine, 100 units/ml penicillin, 100 μg/ml streptomycin, 10% newborn calf serum, 10% (v/v) tryptose phosphate.
(6) Hexamethylene bisacetamide (HMBA): prepare fresh as a 100 mM stock in EF10 or ETC10 (incubate at 37° for approximately 60 min to dissolve) and sterilize by passage through a 0.22 μM filter.
(7) EHu5 medium for neutralizing HSV released from cells: 1 × Eagle's medium (Glasgow

modification), 4 mM L-glutamine, 100 units/ml penicillin, 100 μg/ml streptomycin, 5% human serum. Purchase pooled human serum known to be negative for HIV and hepatitis B virus. Avoid exposure to human serum.

(8) Tissue culture incubators set to 31, 37 and 42°C.

(9) A sterile hood located as close as possible to the 42°C incubator.

3 THE PROTOCOLS

Protocol #92: Setting up HFL Cell Monolayers to Measure HSV-1 Latency after Infection at 42°C

(1) Prepare a cell suspension by trypsinizing larger cultures, for example in 800 cm^3 flasks, and seed 5×10^5 cells per 35 mm Petri dish in 2 ml EF10. The experiment can be scaled up for 50 mm plates by seeding 1.25×10^6 cells in 5 ml EF10 or 90 mm diameter plates by seeding 4×10^6 cells in 15 ml EF10.

(2) Incubate cells at 37°C overnight. The monolayers should be almost confluent, with no overlaps but few gaps. If monolayers are too sparse, incubate further at 37° until the cells are almost confluent; if they are too dense, discard them.

Protocol #93: Infecting HFL Monolayers

(1) Prewarm EF5, allowing 2 ml per plate plus a little extra, to 42°C in an incubator or water bath. Note that water baths are common sources of contamination, so wipe the bottle with a tissue, spray with ethanol and wipe again before taking it near to cells.

(2) Make up a virus suspension in EF5, such that the desired quantity of inoculum for each plate is contained in 0.2 ml.

(3) Transfer plates, one tray at a time (each tray holding ten 35 mm plates) from the 37°C incubator to a sterile cabinet.

(4) Remove the culture medium by aspiration through a Pasteur pipette, and add 0.2 ml EF5 containing virus.

(5) Incubate at 37°C for 1 h, rocking gently every 20 min to prevent cells drying out.

(6) Remove the virus inoculum by aspiration and add 2 ml of EF5 prewarmed to 42°C.

(7) Incubate at 42°C. This procedure, and subsequent medium changes, are best performed with one tray of plates at a time.

(8) Leave cultures at 42°C for 2 days, then remove the medium and replace with 2 ml EF5, prewarmed to 42°C.

(9) Change medium again after a further 2 days, and 2 days later (i.e. 6 days after infection) inspect cultures. Cells should be morphologically normal, with no evidence of viral cytopathic effect or plaques. Use uninfected but mock-treated cultures for comparison.

(10) The period at 42°C should have resulted in the establishment of latency, such that no virus can be detected by titration of culture medium or sonicated cell extracts on permissive cells. Cultures may now be returned to 37°C.

(11) After 6 days at 42°C, change the EF5 and incubate at 37°C.

(12) After 2 days, change EF5 and incubate for a further 2 days. Inspect each plate carefully, preferably using a plate microscope under dark field illumination. Discard any plates showing viral plaques.

(13) At this stage (10 days after infection) a number of infected HFL monolayers, showing no evidence of free virus or viral replication, will be available.

Protocol #94: Reactivation by Superinfection

(1) To demonstrate that latent virus is present in the monolayers, it must be reactivated by superinfection of cells with wild-type or mutant HSV-1 or HSV-2. The HSV-1 temperature sensitive (ts) mutant *ts*K (available from the MRC Institute of Virology, Glasgow, UK; see Chapter 14) is a convenient conditional lethal mutant to use, although others can be

substituted (Russell and Preston, 1986).

(2) Take latently infected cultures, remove medium by aspiration and add 0.2 ml of EF5 containing the required amount of *ts*K.

(3) Place cells in an incubator set at 37°C or higher: *ts*K is convenient because it remains temperature sensitive at 37°C. If an alternative mutant is used, superinfection must be carried out at a temperature known to be non-permissive for that mutant (usually 38°C or above).

(4) Incubate at 37°C for 1 h, rocking plates every 20 min. Add 2 ml EHu5 and incubate at 37° for 2 days.

(5) In parallel, dilute the *ts*K stock used for superinfection to 250 p.f.u./ml and add 0.2 ml to duplicate plates of HFL cells not initially infected but carried through the 10-day 42°/37° regimen: if such monolayers are not available, use fresh HFL monolayers. Incubate these cultures at 31°C, the permissive temperature for *ts*K, for 1 h with rocking every 20 min, then add 2 ml EHu5 and continue incubation at 31°C. This procedure is included to check the MOI of *ts*K applied during superinfection.

(6) After 2 days, remove EHu5 and add approximately 1 ml Giemsa stain. Leave at room temperature for 30–60 min.

(7) Wash plates under running water, dry and count plaques under a plate microscope.

(8) Calculate the reactivation efficiency by extrapolating from results obtained at low multiplicity of superinfection as follows: if 10^3 p.f.u. of HSV-2 were first applied to monolayers, and superinfection with 0.1 p.f.u. of *ts*K per cell yielded 50 plaques, the efficiency of reactivation will be approximately 50%, because only 10% of cells received *ts*K.

Protocol #95: Infection with HSV-1 *in*1814

(1) Prepare HFL cell monolayers and infect them with *in*1814, using Protocols 92 and 93.

(2) Incubate for 1 h at 37°C, rocking every 20 min, then remove virus inoculum and add EF5 containing an inhibitor of DNA replication. We routinely use 50 μg/ml cytosine arabinoside, but alternatives are 5 μg/ml aphidicolin or 5 μM acycloguanosine.

(3) Maintain cultures at 37°C for 2–3 days.

(4) Remove EF5 by aspiration, add and immediately remove 2 ml EF5.

(5) Add a further 2 ml EF5 and incubate at 37°C.

(6) After 1–2 h, replace EF5 with 2 ml fresh EF5.

(7) Analyse cells immediately or reactivate latent virus by superinfection, for example with *ts*K, as described in Protocol #93.

4 NOTES AND TROUBLESHOOTING

4.1 On Protocol #92: Setting up HFL Cell Monolayers to Measure HSV-1 Latency after Infection at 42°C

The techniques described in this chapter are relatively straightforward, requiring no sophisticated equipment or special materials, apart from mutant *in*1814. Adaptation of the techniques to address specific questions, however, requires careful thought.

No problems other than those commonly associated with maintenance of cell cultures should arise when following the protocols described above. Occasionally we have found that incubation of infected cells at 42°C has not converted the virus to latency, with the consequence that viral cytopathic effect was observed upon downshift to 37°C. If this occurs the experiment should be abandoned. Repeat the calculations to ensure that the input MOI was not too high and check that the incubator temperature has not fallen below 42°C. If these tests do not reveal the cause of the problem, discard the cells and begin a new HFL cell culture.

HFL fibroblasts can be obtained by direct culture from an aborted human fetus, provided that it is carried out by a properly qualified individual who has obtained the necessary ethical permission. Commercial cultures are available. We use Flow 2002 cells, requesting "lowest pass available". This approach normally ensures a supply of cells at pass 16 or 17, which can be used for approximately eight passages before exhibiting slow growth and, sometimes, abnormal (less elongated) morphology. HFL cells can readily be passaged at a 1:4 subculture ratio, so it is possible to produce a relatively large quantity after two successive subcultures. It is advisable to produce a backup supply by storing cells at −140°C at this stage (pass 18 if the cells were supplied at pass 16). Human foreskin fibroblasts produce equivalent results.

4.2 On Protocol #95: Infecting With HSV-1 *in*1814

The particle:p.f.u. ratio for *in*1814 on HFL cells is approximately 1000 times that of a wild-type virus or of *in*1814 titrated in the presence of HMBA. Infection of HFL monolayers with 1000 p.f.u. (+HMBA titer) in the absence of HMBA will result in one plaque plus 999 cells receiving a virus that does not replicate. If measures are taken to prevent the one potentially active virus/cell interaction from resulting in virus replication (and hence amplification), monolayers can be maintained harboring 999 genomes which do not replicate. This is achieved by adding an inhibitor of viral DNA synthesis. At the biochemical level, the background contributed by non-latent genomes will be only 0.1%. The retention of the 999 genomes in a latent state for 2 days or more can be demonstrated by their reactivation after superinfection with *ts*K (Harris and Preston, 1991). Increasing the initial MOI will maintain the 999:1 ratio, so the genome number can be increased until cytotoxicity is observed. In practice, this point is reached at 2×10^5 p.f.u. (+HMBA titer) per culture, which results in 10–20% of cells receiving a genome that can be reactivated by superinfection.

4.3 General Comments and Safety Aspects Regarding Work with HSV-1

When using HSV gloves, laboratory coat and eye protection should be worn. Immediately a virus seed stock is received it should be grown to a larger stock of reasonably high titer (10^7–10^8 p.f.u./ml), and stored in aliquots. This stock should be used whenever a high titer virus preparation is being grown. A virus stock should not be repeatedly passaged, as mutations may accumulate in genes not essential for growth in tissue culture. Samples of *in*1814 (or any mutant obtained from another scientist) should never be given to a member of a different laboratory without permission from the supplier of the mutant. A mutant should never be renamed without permission from the supplier.

4.4 Notes on Calculation of Reactivation Efficiency

This calculation is performed by extrapolating from the results obtained at low MOI because at 1 p.f.u. or more *ts*K per cell all cells are infected and plaques cannot form. The calculation will be an underestimate if non-infectious particles in the *ts*K stock are able to reactivate latent HSV-2. It is difficult adequately to address this problem, although we have made an attempt by studying a variant of *ts*K containing an insertion of *lacZ* under immediate–early control (*ts*K/β-gal; see Chapter 14). This virus was titrated at 38.5 and 31°C, and plaques (at 31°C) or β-gal-expressing cells (at 38.5°C) counted. The "titer" at 38.5°C was approximately 1.5 times that at 31°C, suggesting that the calculation may overestimate the reactivation efficiency by a factor of 1.5.

4.5 On Titration of HSV-1 Mutant *in*1814

When titrated on cells permissive for HSV-1, *in*1814 preparations exhibit low titers compared to the number of particles present. The particle:p.f.u. ratio is typically $2–3 \times 10^3$ on BHK cells and $1–5 \times 10^4$ on HFL cells, whereas wild-type HSV-1 stocks exhibit ratios of 10–50 on both cell types. This causes difficulties in designing experiments using *in*1814 based on p.f.u., so in initial experiments particle concentrations were used as the basis for normalizing infections.

Inclusion of 3–5 mM HMBA in the EHu5 overlay during titration results in a large increase in titer of *in*1814, yielding a particle:p.f.u. ratio of 100, close to that observed for wild-type HSV-1 (McFarlane et al., 1992). The titer on BHK cells in the presence of 3 mM HMBA is the most reliable value to use as a basis for quantifying *in*1814 stocks.

4.6 Limitations

Establishment of latency by incubation at 42°C is not absolute: approximately 1 in 5×10^5 genomes remain potentially active and form plaques upon return to the permissive temperature of 37°C (Russell and Preston, 1986) (this proportion may vary depending on virus strain and cells used). One plaque on a plate will ruin that plate as experimental material. Clearly if a low MOI (e.g. 10^3 p.f.u.) were initially applied the problem will be insignificant, affecting 1 plate in 500, but at higher MOI a greater proportion of plates will contain "non-latent" virus.

At the current stage of development there is always a background of virus that is not converted to a latent form. This constitutes only approximately 0.01–0.1% of the potentially infectious virus added to HFL cells, but if allowed to replicate the non-latent genomes will quickly be amplified and overrun the cultures. It cannot be emphasized too strongly that this must be considered and quantified in each experiment. To circumvent the problem of non-latent virus an initial MOI should be used at which no active virus would be expected on a plate, or inhibitors of viral DNA synthesis should be added to prevent amplification of non-latent genomes. An additional consideration is that the proportion of the input virus that remains non-latent varies with cell type and the metabolic state of cell cultures. It has been shown that *in*1814 forms plaques more efficiently on cells in G1 phase than in G2 (Daksis and Preston, 1992). Incubation at 42°C to block virus replication is successful for the methods described in this chapter because human fibroblasts readily withstand culture at the supraoptimal temperature. Other cell types may not survive prolonged incubation at 42°C.

At present it is not possible to establish latency in all cells of a culture because monolayers may be destroyed at MOI of *in*1814 greater than 0.2 p.f.u. per cell at 37°C or 0.03 p.f.u. of wild-type HSV-1 or HSV-2 per cell at 42°C. Further measures to reduce IE transcription might reduce cytopathic effect, as suggested by Johnson et al. (1992).

The population of latently infected cells cannot be expanded, because the viral genome does not coreplicate with the host cell upon subculture of monolayers.

Although, as described in the introduction, there are good reasons for studying HSV latency *in vitro*, there is not yet universal acceptance that the phenomenon is relevant to latency *in vivo*.

4.7 Future Perspectives

Further investigation of HSV latency in tissue culture cells might proceed in several ways.

Studying the structure of the latent genome and the changes that occur on reactivation by superinfection. The latent viral genome is sequestered as a non-linear, probably circular, molecule (Harris and Preston, 1991; Preston and Russell, 1991) but it is not clear whether it is supercoiled or relaxed, methylated or unmethylated. Furthermore, it is not known whether the latent genome adopts a chromatin structure similar to that of the host cell. Studies to address these questions should be possible, especially as very sensitive methods, some using the polymerase chain reaction, are available to study chromatin assembly.

Investigation of viral gene expression during latency. We have found no tk mRNA or LATs in cultures latently infected with *in*1814, but other genome regions have still to be analysed. The fact that virus replication does not occur in latently infected cells suggests a block to gene expression, probably at the level of IE transcription for *in*1814, but it is not clear whether the block is absolute or selective. Further study of gene expression by reverse transcription and polymerase chain reaction, *in situ* hybridization, immunoprecipitation, protein blotting or immunofluorescence should be undertaken. Alternatively, viral or heterologous promoters regulating the expression of an easily detectable reporter protein, for example β-galactosidase, could be introduced into one of the many non-essential loci in the *in*1814 genome.

Studying reactivation of latent HSV. We have shown that the superinfecting virus must express the HSV-1 IE protein Vmw110, or a human cytomegalovirus functional homologue, for reactivation to occur (Russell et al., 1987; Harris et al., 1989; Harris and Preston, 1991). Vmw110 is an activator of gene expression from a wide range of viral and cellular promoters but its mode of action is currently unclear (Everett et al., 1991). Further study of reactivation of latent virus may provide clues to the mode of action of Vmw110. So far, all of our attempts to induce reactivation of latent HSV-1, HSV-2 or *in*1814 by manipulation of cell culture conditions have failed, but success in this endeavor would open the way to new approaches to the study of reactivation.

Development of mutant in*1814 as a vector for gene transfer into neurons*, because the very early block to gene expression permits survival of cells after infection. The problem to be overcome is that of attaining long-term expression of genes inserted into the latent *in*1814 genome. Portions of promoters controlling the HSV LAT or other neuron-specific elements would be good starting points for these studies.

REFERENCES

Ace, C.I., T.A. McKee, J.M. Ryan, J.M. Cameron, and C.M. Preston. 1989. Construction and characterization of a herpes simplex virus type 1 mutant unable to transinduce immediate-early gene expression. *J. Virol.* **63:** 2260–2269.

Daksis, J.I., and C.M. Preston. 1992. Herpes simplex immediate early gene expression in the absence of transinduction by Vmw65 varies during the cell cycle. *Virology* **189:** 196–202.

Everett, R.D., C.M. Preston, and N.D. Stow. 1991. Functional and genetic analysis of the role of Vmw110 in herpes simplex virus replication. In *Herpesvirus Transcription and its Regulation*, pp 49–76. Edited by E.K. Wagner. Boca Raton: CRC Press.

Harris, R.A., and C.M. Preston. 1991. Establishment of latency *in vitro* by the herpes simplex virus type 1 mutant in1814. *J. Gen. Virol.* **72:** 907–913.

Harris, R.A., R.D. Everett, X. Zhu, S. Silverstein, and C.M. Preston. 1989. Herpes simplex virus type 1 immediate-early protein Vmw110 reactivates latent herpes simplex virus type 2 in an *in vitro* latency system. *J. Virol.* **63:** 3513–3515.

Johnson, P.A., A. Miyanohara, F. Levine, T. Cahill, and T. Friedmann. 1992. Cytotoxicity of a replication defective mutant of herpes simplex virus type 1. *J. Virol.* **66:** 2952–2965.

McFarlane, M., J.I. Daksis, and C.M. Preston. 1992. Hexamethylene bisacetamide stimulates herpes simplex virus immediate early gene expression in the absence of trans-induction by Vmw65. *J. Gen. Virol.* **73:** 285–292.

O'Hare, P., and C.R. Goding. 1988. Herpes simplex virus regulatory elements and the immunoglobulin octamer domain bind a common factor and are both targets for virion transactivation. *Cell* **54:** 435–445.

Preston, C.M., M.C. Frame, and M.E.M. Campbell. 1988. A complex formed between cell components and an HSV structural polypeptide binds to a viral immediate early gene regulatory sequence. *Cell* **52:** 425–434.

Preston, C.M., and J. Russell. 1991. Retention of non-linear viral DNA during herpes simplex virus latency *in vitro*. *Intervirology* **32:** 69–75.

Roizman, B., and A.E. Sears. 1987. An inquiry into the mechanisms of herpes simplex virus latency. *Annu. Rev. Microbiol.* **41:** 543–571.

Russell, J., and C.M. Preston. 1986. An *in vitro* latency system for herpes simplex virus type 2. *J. Gen. Virol.* **67:** 397–403.

Russell, J., N.D. Stow, E.C. Stow, and C.M. Preston. 1987. Herpes simplex virus genes involved in latency *in vitro*. *J. Gen. Virol.* **68:** 3009–3018.

Sadowski, I., J. Ma, S.J. Triezenberg, and M. Ptashne. 1988. GAL4-VP16 is an unusually potent transcriptional activator. *Nature* **335:** 563–564.

Stern, S., M. Tanaka, and W. Herr. 1989. The oct-1 homeodomain directs formation of a multiprotein-DNA complex with the HSV transactivator VP16. *Nature* **341:** 624–630.

Stevens, J.G. (1989). Human herpesviruses: a consideration of the latent state. *Microbiol Rev.* **53:** 318–332.

Triezenberg, S.J., R.C. Kingsbury, and S.L. McKnight. 1988. Functional dissection of VP16, the trans-activator of herpes simplex virus immediate early gene expression. *Genes Dev.* **2:** 718–729.

Wilson, A.C., K. LaMarco, M.G. Peterson, and W. Herr. 1993. The VP16 accessory protein HCF is a family of polypeptides processed from a large precursor protein. *Cell* **74:** 115–125.

CHAPTER 18

Studies of Herpes Simplex Virus 1 Latency Using Primary Neuronal Cultures of Dorsal Root Ganglion Neurons

RODERIC L. SMITH AND CHRISTINE L. WILCOX*

Department of Neurology, University of Colorado Health Sciences Center, Denver, CO USA

**Department of Microbiology, Colorado State University, Fort Collins, CO 80523, USA. Tel: 303 491 2552; Fax: 303 491 1815; Email: cwilcox@vines.colostate.edu*

1 INTRODUCTION

Herpes simplex virus (HSV) infections cause diseases in humans that range in severity from the common cold sore to lethal encephalitis (Price, 1986). An essential feature of the human disease is the ability of the virus to establish latent infection in neural crest-derived neurons of the peripheral nervous system (Hill, 1985; Price, 1986; Stevens, 1989). The episodic reactivation and retrograde transport of virus from these neurons to cause recurrent mucocutaneous disease is the essential strategy of transmission of HSV infection. Animal models have been valuable in understanding the neurobiology of HSV infection and allow aspects of the immune response to be examined. However, the efficiency of establishing latency is limited to a small fraction of the neurons in a ganglion (Hill, 1985; Stevens, 1989). Although many excellent animal models are capable of stimuli-triggered reactivation, these models are limited by the relatively few neurons harboring latent HSV in the innervating ganglion and the low frequency of inducible reactivation. For many studies these limitations do not pose a problem but for studies directed towards understanding the molecular events that control latency animal models have a limited number of neurons that harbor latent virus in a ganglion, problems in timing the stages of the infection, and limitations resulting from the lack of *in vivo* controlled reactivation stimulus.

We have developed an *in vitro* model of HSV latency in neurons that mimics many of the *in vivo* aspects (Wilcox and Johnson, 1987, 1988; Wilcox, et al. 1990). Using this model we have demonstrated that HSV-1 or HSV-2 establish latent infections *in vitro* in the same populations of neurons that harbor latency in humans. We have produced latent HSV infections in neuronal cultures from ganglia of rodents and primates (Wilcox et al., 1990). In all cases the neurotropin nerve growth factor (NGF) is required to maintain the latent infections (Wilcox and Johnson, 1987, 1988; Wilcox et al., 1990). Depending on infection conditions, latency can be established in essentially all of the primary sensory or sympathetic neurons in tissue culture (Wilcox and Johnson, 1988; Smith et al., 1994). To achieve this high efficiency an antiviral agent (e.g. acyclovir)

Protocols for Gene Transfer in Neuroscience: Towards Gene Therapy of Neurological Disorders
Edited by P.R. Lowenstein and L.W. Enquist

is added to the neuronal cultures during the first week after inoculation with a high multiplicity of infection (MOI). An often misunderstood aspect of the *in vitro* neuronal model of latency is the assumption that an antiviral is required to establish latency: this is not the case (Wilcox and Johnson, 1987, 1988). However, in the absence of antivirals the MOI must be very low and the resulting frequency of latency is also low. At least one of the actions of the antiviral agent is to prevent amplification of the virus in the non-neuronal cells in the culture at the outset of infection (Smith et al., 1994). Virus infection of the non-neuronal cells in the presence of acyclovir prevent virus replication and results in the death of the non-neuronal cells. Latency is maintained in neurons in culture for as long as 10 weeks in the presence of NGF. Viral antigens associated with the productive infection are not detected during the latent infection (Wilcox and Johnson, 1988; Wilcox et al., 1990; Doerig et al., 1991). Viral transcription is restricted to the latency-associated transcripts (LAT) during latent infection (Doerig et al., 1991). Using *in situ* hybridization methods, LAT-region transcription is detected in the nuclei of 80–90% of the neurons in culture by 3 weeks (Smith et al., 1994). If NGF is removed from the medium, for as brief a time as 1 h, latent virus is reactivated (Wilcox et al., 1990) and viral antigens associated with the productive infection and infectious virus can be detected 48–72 h after NGF deprivation.

The *in vitro* model is well suited for molecular studies of the regulation of latency and cellular signaling because it can produce a population of neurons with a very high frequency of latent virus and establishment and reactivation of latency are controlled, synchronous events. The model also allows manipulation using pharmacological methods and has the potential for examination of signaling pathways in individual neurons using microinjection methods. Initial studies of the cellular signaling pathways involved in the regulation of reactivation demonstrated that stimulation of cAMP-dependent pathways or activation of protein kinase C reactivates latent virus even in the presence of NGF (Smith et al., 1992).

The best characterized system currently used in our laboratory is prepared from dorsal root ganglia (DRG) obtained from embryonic day 15 (E15) rats. The development of this system has been driven by both practical and biological considerations. The DRG neurons are a natural site of HSV latency in humans (Baringer, 1974), there are 50 DRG per animal, they are easy to identify and remove from the fetus and their neurobiology has been well studied. With minor changes the methods described here for DRG could be adapted for isolation and maintenance of neurons from other sources.

Highly sophisticated equipment or techniques are not needed, although careful dissection, meticulous adherence to sterile technique and constant attention to the needs of neuronal cultures are vital. Attention to these details provides a highly reproducible and easily manipulated model system for studies of many aspects of HSV latency. Unfortunately, the system is unforgiving of bad technique, which, considering that the average experiment extends over at least a month, can undo a great deal of hard work.

2 MATERIALS AND EQUIPMENT

2.1 Collagen Preparation

(1) Tails from two large rats for a 200 ml preparation of collagen stock solution. Tails can be wrapped and frozen until needed.
(2) Sterile instrument tray containing two large hemostats, large scissors, heavy forceps.
(3) Sterile labware: beaker (500 or 600 ml), large Petri dish.
(4) Sterile solutions: autoclaved distilled water (100 ml for rinsing tendons), 10% acetic acid in distilled water, sterilized by filtration through 0.2 μm membrane filter.
(5) Dialysis tubing, 1 l glass flask, fitted with two-hole stopper with glass tubing in the holes, one long, one short.

2.2 Collagen Coating of Tissue Culture Dishes

(1) Dialysed collagen stock solution.
(2) Ammonium hydroxide (30%).

(3) Tissue culture multiwell cluster dishes.
(4) Sterile pipettes.
(5) Sterile spreaders (glass rods with bent tips).
(6) Biosafety cabinet.

2.3 Dissection of DRG

(1) Sterile tissue culture dishes, plastic coverslips for *in situ* hybridizations or immunohistochemistry, tubes, pipettes, including cotton-plugged Pasteur pipettes.
(2) Water-jacketed CO_2 incubator to maintain 35–37°C, 5% CO_2.
(3) Dissecting microscope that can be used in either a horizontal, laminar flow hood, or a clean dead-air space.
(4) Timed-pregnant, pathogen-free rat(s), embryonic day 15 (E-15). E15 is the easiest time to isolate the DRG, with the best recovery of viable neurons. Later in pregnancy, even only 1 day, many of the ganglia remain embedded between the vertebrae, making the dissection much more difficult and less efficient. Earlier than E15, the anatomic landmarks are less distinct and the tissue is very fragile.
(5) Collagen-coated tissue culture dishes: A single layer of ammonium-vapor polymerized dialysed collagen should be applied to tissue culture dishes before starting dissection. These can be prepared the day before as long as sterility is maintained.
(6) Instruments (sterile): three large scissors, three large forceps, two jeweler's forceps (e.g. Dumont pattern #5). Back-up sets of sterile instruments are recommended, especially the jeweler's forceps.
(7) Leibovitz's L-15 medium (L-15) + 10% calf serum (CS) + 2 × penicillin/streptomycin (P/S).
(8) Collagenase A (Boehringer Mannheim, Indianapolis, IN, USA), 3 mg/ml in L-15 + 10% CS + 2 × P/S. Filter sterilize through 0.22 mm syringe filter. Prepare immediately before use.
(9) AM-100 culture medium (see below).

2.4 Media and Stock Solutions for Preparation and Maintenance of DRG Neuronal Culture

(1) L-15 for use outside the CO_2 incubator. This is a balanced salt solution containing nutrients but no $NaHCO_3$. The dissection is performed in this medium with the addition of 10% CS and 2 × P/S (see Steps 3 and 6).

! DO NOT USE L-15 IN A CO_2 INCUBATOR !

(2) Dulbecco's Modified Eagle's Media (DMEM). This is used to prepare the neuronal media, F-100 and AM-100.
(3) Calf serum (CS), final concentration 10% for neuronal media. Serum must be heat-inactivated before use. Lots of serum must be tested for compatibility with the neuronal cultures. It is recommended that a 1-year supply is purchased after testing to ensure reproducibility.
(4) 2.5S mouse nerve growth factor (NGF) (Harlan Bioscience for Science, Indianapolis, IN, USA). NGF binds to many surfaces and is best prepared and stored in plastic containers: avoid using glass containers. For a 100 × stock solution, prepare NGF at 0.01 mg/ml (1 mg NGF per 100 ml of L-15 + 10% CS). Filter sterilize (0.22 μm acetate membrane filter), aliquot and store below 0°C. The final concentration of NGF is 100 ng/ml.
(5) Antimitotic stock solution: FUdR + uridine. For a 100 × stock solution, prepare solution of 2×10^{-3} M FUdR and uridine (0.05 g FUdR and 0.05 g uridine per 100 ml L-15 + 10% CS). Filter sterilize (0.22 μm). Final concentrations of FUdR and uridine 2×10^{-5} M.
(6) Penicillin and streptomycin (P/S). Final concentration in a 2 × solution 200 mg/ml streptomycin + 200 mg/ml penicillin.
(7) Acyclovir (ACV), 5 mM stock (50 ×). Dissolve 11.5 mg acyclovir at 37°C in 10 ml L-15 and filter sterilize (0.22 μm).
(8) Supplemental glutamine is not required if medium is purchased containing glutamine and is used before expiration date. Otherwise media must be supplemented with glutamine at a final

concentration of 1.4 mM.

(9) Standard maintenance medium (F-100): 100 ng/ml NGF, 10% CS, 90% DMEM.

(10) Antimitotic medium used for the first 1–2 weeks after preparing the cultures to reduce the non-neuronal cell population (AM-100): 100 ng/ml NGF, 10% CS, 2×10^{-5} M FUdR and uridine.

(11) The number of the medium denotes the concentration of NGF in ng/ml; 100 ng/ml is the standard concentration. Prepare the media in a sterile plastic container. These media can be stored either frozen or refrigerated, depending on duration of use: if it will be used within 2 weeks store refrigerated; otherwise aliquot and freeze.

3 THE PROTOCOLS

Protocol #96: Preparation of Rat Tail Collagen

! STERILE TECHNIQUE MUST BE USED THROUGHOUT THE PREPARATION !

(1) Thaw rat tail(s) which had been stored frozen.

(2) Wash tails with disinfectant, rinse well with distilled water, then soak in 70% ethanol for 30 min.

(3) In the laminar flow hood, prepare 0.1% acetic acid by adding 1 ml sterile 10% acetic acid to 100 ml sterile distilled water in a capped sterile flask. This is the solution in which the collagen in the tendons will dissolve.

(4) With sterile forceps remove the tail(s) from the 70% ethanol, place in a large Petri dish and dry in a laminar flow hood. Clamp a hemostat securely to the tip of the tail.

(5) A second hemostat is positioned away from the tip (about 2 cm from the first) and clamped to hold the tail fairly tightly.

(6) The tail is then repeatedly flexed between the hemostats until the bone and skin gives way, leaving only tendons connecting the tip to the remainder of the tail.

(7) The hemostat with the tip attached is then pulled away from the second hemostat. As the tip is pulled, the attached white tendons will be pulled from the body of the tail.

(8) The tendons are then cut with scissors from the tail tip so that they fall into the beaker containing distilled water.

(9) After pulling all tendons, any debris (bone chips, blood vessels, etc.) should be removed.

(10) The mass of tendons is then picked up out of the water with the forceps and placed into the flask of 0.1% acetic acid, sealed and refrigerated for a minimum of 5 days to allow the tendons to dissociate into collagen. The collagen is stable in this solution for 6 months at 4°C.

Protocol #97: Using Collagen Stock in Neuronal Cultures

(1) Dialyse the collagen solution against distilled water overnight under sterile conditions using a 1 l flask fitted with a two-holed cork with two glass tubes; tie the dialysis bag to one tube and use the other for a vent.

(2) Place into the flask containing distilled water (tissue culture grade).

(3) Cover with foil and autoclave.

(4) Cool to 4°C and add collagen solution that has been cleared of undissolved tendons by centrifugation at 10 000*g* for 30 min at 4°C.

(5) Pipette the collagen supernatant into the dialysis bag and refrigerate overnight without stirring.

(6) Aliquot collagen into tubes.

(7) Store at 4°C (do not freeze). The solutions should be clear, slightly viscous and will be stable after dialysis for 2–3 weeks.

Protocol #98: Collagen Coating of Tissue Culture Dishes for Preparation of DRG Neurons

(1) Add 1 drop of dialysed collagen solution to each well of a 12-well or 24-well dish (sterile plastic

coverslips can be placed in wells then coated with collagen for *in situ* hybridization or immunohistochemistry studies).

(2) Rotate a sterile glass rod with a 90° bend of appropriate size in each well to spread the collagen solution evenly on the plastic surface, making sure the edges are coated.

(3) Ammoniate the collagen by placing a drop of NH_4OH in the space between wells near both ends of the cluster plate or on the lid.

(4) Carefully replace the lid, leaving it slightly ajar to allow ammonia to penetrate to all the wells.

(5) After 5 min open lids in a biosafety cabinet and dry the collagen completely before use. The opened culture dishes can be exposed to UV irradiation: this may facilitate further crosslinking of collagen but is not required. The collagen will require about 1 h to dry.

Protocol #99: Preparation of DRG Neurons

The initial steps of the dissection (Steps 1–4) should be performed on a clean bench top using good aseptic technique. The remainder of the dissection is performed in a horizontal flow tissue-culture hood. Steps 7–17 are best performed using a stereomicroscope in a horizontal flow tissue-culture hood.

(1) Decapitate an anesthetized rat and cleanse the abdomen with bactericidal soap, followed by 70% ethanol.

(2) Use one pair of scissors and forceps to remove the skin exposing the abdominal wall.

(3) Use a second set of instruments to cut through the abdominal muscles, taking extreme care to avoid nicking the large bowel.

(4) Lift the uterus (two horns, which should contain fetuses in their amniotic sacs, each with a placenta) carefully with the forceps and cut free at any sites of attachment and at the point of bifurcation in the lower part of the uterus.

(5) Remove the uterus with fetuses and place into a large sterile Petri dish. The uterus is fragile and can tear, thus dropping the fetuses on a non-sterile surface.

(6) Remove the fetuses by first cutting to separate the enlarged regions of uterus containing individual fetuses. In many cases this is sufficient to allow the fetuses to separate from the uterus. However, an additional short scissors cut along the uterus may be needed.

(7) Use the scissors to cut between the placenta and fetus, using the forceps to peel away any remaining amniotic membrane.

(8) Place fetuses in a Petri dish containing sufficient L-15 + 10% CS + 2 × P/S to cover.

(9) Individual fetuses are dissected in 35 mm Petri dishes containing L-15 + 10% CS + 2 × P/S.

(10) Dissect the fetus with a jeweler's forceps in each hand. Because the fetus is young the forming bones are soft, which makes cutting with forceps possible. The delicate forceps must be handled with extreme care and maintained in good condition to allow the points to come into smooth contact.

(11) Cut off head and tail with forceps.

(12) Cut laterally to remove the viscera from the back (see Fig. 18.1A, B).

(13) With the ventral surface of the back up, remove any remaining viscera and cut through the ventral surface of the vertebrae on both sides of the spinal cord, cutting through only the ventral surface of the vertebrae (Fig 18.1B, C).

(14) Peel sheet of cut vertebrae section off (arrow in Fig. 18.1C) to expose the spinal cord (more white than surrounding structures).

(15) Gently pull the spinal cord out of the remains of the back, starting at anterior end and lifting the spinal cord out. The DRG should remain attached to the spinal cord (Fig. 18.1D).

(16) Collect spinal cords with DRG attached in a separate 35 mm Petri dish containing L-15 + 10% CS + 2 × P/S.

(17) Pull off the DRG from the spinal cord, several at a time, with the jeweller's forceps, discarding the spinal cord.

(18) After all ganglia are freed from the spinal cords, transfer them to a 17 × 100 mm sterile plastic test tube with a sealable top using a 5 ml pipette. The Petri dish may be rinsed with a small volume of additional medium to recover any remaining ganglia.

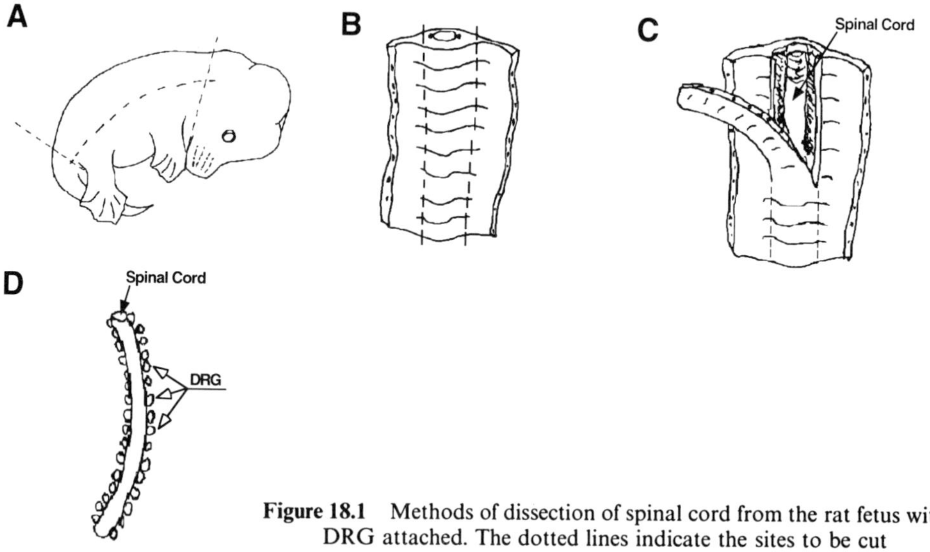

Figure 18.1 Methods of dissection of spinal cord from the rat fetus with DRG attached. The dotted lines indicate the sites to be cut

(19) Allow ganglia to settle in bottom of the tube and carefully aspirate medium.
(20) Add 1–3 ml (depending on number of ganglia) of 3 mg/ml collagenase A. Generally, 1 ml for the ganglia from each timed-pregnant rat, assuming 10 fetuses per rat, is a reasonable volume.
(21) Incubate 60 min at 37°C, periodically agitating gently.
(22) Remove collagenase and rinse four times with L-15 + 10% CS + 2 × P/S (ganglia will settle by gravity; remove supernatant carefully so as not to lose ganglia).
(23) Add 1–2 ml of AM-100 and triturate with a sterile constricted-bore Pasteur pipette plugged with cotton wool (reduce the bore by placing pipette tip in flame, allow to cool before use). Ganglia should dissociate readily (approximately 10–20 triturations).
(24) For 24-well dishes, add enough amount of medium to ensure 0.1 ml neuron-containing medium can be added to each well of a 24-well dish.
(25) Let cells attach to collagen in the drop for 1–3 h, then add 0.5 ml of AM-100 medium per well of the 24-well dish. For 12-well dishes, add an appropriate volume to add 0.5 ml of neuron-containing medium to each well.
(26) Let cells attach overnight, then replace medium to 1 ml per well of the 12-well dish (0.5 ml per well of 24-well dish).

Protocol #100: Establishment of HSV-1 Latency *in vitro*

An overview of the scheme is shown in Fig. 18.2.

(1) On the day before infection, change neuronal culture media to AM-100 containing ACV at a final concentration of 100 μM.
(2) On the day of infection carefully remove medium and replace with medium containing up to 10 p.f.u. of virus per neuron in culture in a volume of 0.2 ml/well of a 24-well cluster dish, 0.5 ml/well of a 12-well cluster.
(3) Allow virus to absorb for 1 h, gently rocking the dish every 15 min.
(4) Remove the inoculum and replace with AM-100 + 100 μM ACV. This medium is used for all feedings for the first week after infection. Incubate at 35–37°C, 5% CO_2 for 1 week.
(5) After 1 week, feed the cultures using F-100 without ACV. The neurons harboring latent virus should look like mock-infected controls, with normal morphology. We generally do not use cultures for reactivation or latency studies until 2 weeks after establishment of latency.

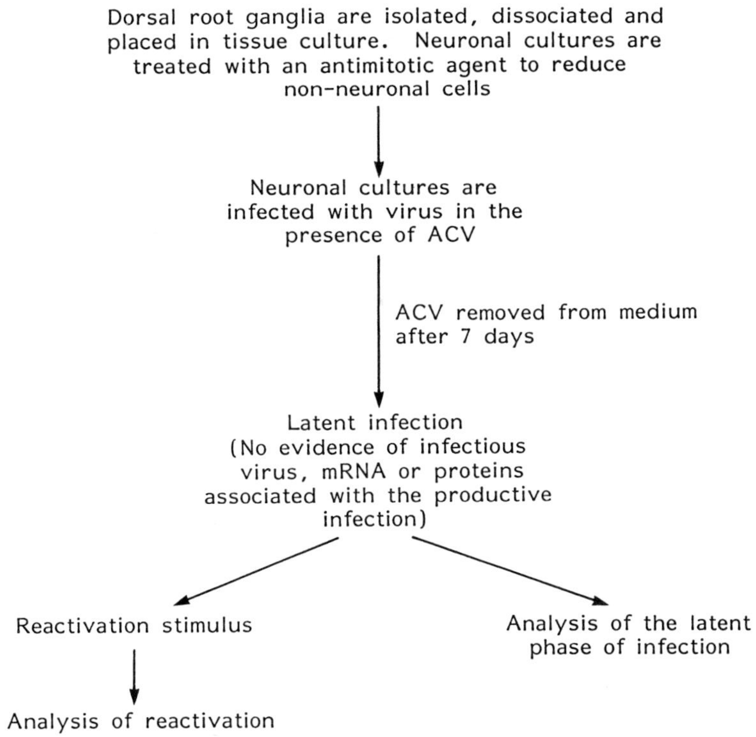

Figure 18.2 Schematic outline of the preparation of neuronal cultures for HSV latency

However, they can be used earlier if appropriate to the experiment, such as study of the initial events in the establishment of latency.

4 NOTES AND TROUBLESHOOTING

4.1 On Protocol #96: Preparation of Rat Tail Collagen

Neurons have special requirements for an attachment matrix for neuronal survival and neurite outgrowth. Many attachment matrices are available but we have found that rat tail collagen is the most enduring and most economical. An ammoniated rat-tail collagen layer is the only substrate that we have found is able to remain attached to the plastic tissue culture dishes for cultures of longer than about 1 week. The preparation of the collagen is time consuming and freshly dialysed collagen must be prepared within several weeks of use for long-term cultures. Some of the commercial preparations have been tested for their ability to support neuronal growth and differentiation; none was satisfactory for the long-term cultures used in establishment of HSV latency. Perhaps some of the new substrates will function as well or better than the preparation currently used. However, problems with the matrix are frequent causes of failure in growth of neurons and the only matrix that has been successfully used in this laboratory is the one described here.

4.2 On Protocol #99: Preparation of DRG Neurons

Generally, three or four 24-well plates can be prepared from 10–12 fetuses (assuming a harvest of 20–30 ganglia per fetus), providing a density of approximately 10^3 neurons/well. The largest size dishes currently in use are 12-well clusters. Two of these can be plated from 10–12 fetuses. Pooling the neurons in each 12-well plate provides sufficient material for 1–2 lanes on a Northern blot.

Larger dishes lead to excessive losses of cultures from problems related to peeling of collagen, evaporation, and increased need for feeding because of the density of neurons.

4.2.1 Dissection

Dissection of DRG from fetal rats is a learned motor skill—the first attempts are expected to be slow and clumsy. The authors vary greatly in their speed of performing the dissection: CLW is able to dissect four timed-pregnant rats in about 4 h; RLS can dissect two in a similar time. A beginner, after a few practice dissections, will take 4–6 h to complete one dissection.

4.2.2 Maintenance of DRG Cultures

Any cultures with the slightest hint of contamination should be immediately destroyed. Incubators must be maintained clean and well-humidified at all times, because the neurons are grown in a small volume and are very sensitive to evaporation.

The neurons may not be obvious until they start to develop neurites. Many non-neuronal cells (fibroblasts and Schwann cells) will be present in the cultures. In the first few days (the earlier, the better) the cultures should be treated with the FUdR to reduce the non-neuronal cell population. This is done by growing cultures in AM-100, as described above. It usually takes 5–7 days after starting treatment for non-neuronal cells to significantly decrease in numbers. Cycling between AM-100 and F-100 is often more effective.

Medium should be changed every 3–4 days, more frequently if the neurons are plated at a high density. At 2 weeks after plating, neuronal metabolism seems to increase, and you may need to replace the medium more often. It is not advisable to remove all the medium from cultures during feeding; this could damage the collagen matrix. It is more important that a consistent routine of feeding is maintained.

For investigators interested in studying HSV latency in sympathetic neurons, Johnson and Argiro (1983) provide a very detailed discussion of the preparation of superior cervical ganglia neuron cultures.

4.3 On Protocol #100: Establishment of HSV-1 Latency *in vitro*

4.3.1 Reactivation of Latent HSV

A major advantage of the *in vitro* latency system is the ability to trigger a temporally synchronized reactivation from essentially all of the neurons in culture (Wilcox and Johnson, 1988).

Stimuli Used for Reactivation

A relatively large number of stimuli are effective in producing reactivation and the decision of which to use will depend on the experimental questions being addressed (Wilcox et al., 1990; Smith et al., 1992). The following notes are intended to summarize some of the stimuli that have been used in our laboratories. NGF deprivation is the only stimulus that we have examined to determine that reactivation occurs in essentially all of the neurons; this analysis has not yet been performed for other stimuli. One major caution is that ACV and antimitotic agents must be removed completely before initiating reactivation.

NGF Deprivation.
NGF is a relatively "sticky" molecule and can be difficult to remove from culture by replacement of NGF-minus medium alone. Therefore, high-titer anti-NGF serum is usually included (1% serum with a neutralizing titer of 1/25 000 or higher, as measured in the chick dorsal root ganglia neurite outgrowth bioassay (Fenton, 1970)). Antisera are available from several commercial sources.

cAMP Agonist.
Several pharmacological approaches to activating cAMP systems are effective (Smith et al., 1992).

A convenient approach is to use a membrane-permeable cAMP analog, Chlorophenyl-thio-cAMP, at a concentration of 0.5–1 μM for as brief a period as 1 h (Smith et al., 1992).

Protein kinase C (PKC) Activation.
The phorbol ester PMA is a potent reactivator of latent HSV-1 which produces reactivation at a concentration consistent with the activation of PKC (10^{-9}–10^{-10} M PMA) (Smith et al., 1992).

Problems Related to Establishment of Latency and Reactivation

Inability to Establish Latency with High Efficiency.
This problem can have a variety of causes, including HSV neutralizing antibodies in serum, inaccurate titers of virus, poorly dispersed neurons that are present in clumps and unhealthy neurons.

Spontaneous Reactivation of Virus.
Possible causes for this include inaccurate viral titers; latency is generally not established at titers greater than 20 p.f.u./neuron and results in neuronal death. Insufficient NGF or other conditions leading to unhealthy cultures can lead to reactivation.

Inability to Reactivate Virus.
Cytopathic effects in neurons look very different from cytopathic effects in cell lines. Virus replication in a neuron is slower than in a replicating cell, so patience is needed. If using anti-NGF, NGF must be adequately removed from medium and antibodies of sufficient titer are required. If viral antigens are detected but virus is not recovered, it is likely that ACV or antimitotic has not been removed, or infectious virus is being inactivated by handling.

4.3.2 Special Methods for the Analysis of HSV Infections in Neurons in Tissue Culture

Some routine methods such as Northern or Southern blot analysis can be directly applied to neurons in culture as for any biologic sample. The only caution in using these methods is that a relatively large amount of culture material may be required. This limitation has led us to use histologic methods together with methods that require more culture material. It is beyond the scope of this chapter to describe in detail the immunohistochemistry and *in situ* hybridization methods. The comments below are included to note areas where the neuronal system requires modification, and to provide a rationale to assist other investigators.

Immunohistochemistry and *in situ* hybridization methods that work on tissue sections must be modified to achieve similar results on neurons in culture. Some of the technical problems we encountered were related to the extensive cytoskeleton of neurons. This can lead to loss of antigenicity with the use of cross-linking fixatives and similar problems limiting penetration of probes used for *in situ* hybridizations. We have used two immunohistochemical approaches successfully. Optimally, very brief fixation (1 min) can be used with 4% paraformaldehyde (phosphate buffered). If longer fixation is required, as would be routine for tissue that will be analysed by both *in situ* hybridization and immunohistochemistry, antigenicity can be restored by treatment after fixation by lightly digesting with protease (1–5 μg/ml proteinase K for 20 min, 37°C) followed by extensive rinsing and dehydration.

For *in situ* hybridization analysis the effective methods are constrained by the nature of the cultures. The neurons grow in small groups that are elevated above the level of the collagen matrix and neurites. The three-dimensional cell groups limit the utility of radioactive methods that involve detection of signal by an emulsion. This is particularly true for localization of RNAs that have a specific cellular localization such as the nuclear LAT. For these reasons we use indirect detection methods that generate a signal at the site of the hybridization within the structure of the neuron. At present we use digoxigenin-labeled riboprobes for detection of RNA by *in situ* hybridization (Smith et al., 1994). Other groups have successfully used digoxigenin-labeled oligonucleotide probes for detection of cellular transcripts in DRG neurons in tissue sections (Sohrabji et al., 1994).

Even with indirect detection methods, several additional modifications of *in situ* hybridization protocols may be required. In comparing the digoxigenin-labeled riboprobes in tissue sections and in neurons in culture, two striking differences were noted. First, the neurons in culture required more extensive protease treatment to achieve the same sensitivity of hybridization. Secondly, the inclusion of sodium dodecyl sulfate in the hybridization mixture at a concentration of 0.1–0.2% greatly increased the sensitivity.

4.4 General Problems

4.4.1 Contamination

Overt infection of cultures with bacteria or fungi is uncommon, provided that routine aseptic practices are followed and solutions are tested. However, poorly characterized low-grade contamination is noted even in laboratories that have extensive experience with culture of neurons. This is an area of great concern. If the problem is not recognized, spurious results will be obtained and much hard work will be wasted. As a general rule, any cultures demonstrating unexplained morphologic changes or dying neurons must be discarded. This problem can generally be improved by a review of aseptic techniques; occasionally it may be necessary to change suppliers of rats.

4.4.2 Collagen Matrix

The collagen matrix used to support neuronal growth is critical for long-term culture of neurons. The ammoniation of collagen causes association of the collagen monomers, forming a durable matrix for neuronal growth.

The collagen can detach if the initial coating of tissue culture plates or coverslips is performed with collagen of excess viscosity or out of date. Superior cervical ganglia neurons are reported to grow much better on a double layer of collagen: an ammoniated layer prepared the day before dissection below an air-dried layer prepared just before starting dissection. The upper layer should be dry before adding dissociated neurons.

4.4.3 Neurons Poorly Dispersed or Present in Large Clumps

The neurons will normally tend to form small clusters. However, if the ganglia were not initially dispersed well, resulting large clumps of tissue can present problems for efficient establishment of latency. This problem is common and is usually seen in cultures prepared by inexperienced workers. The solution is usually to triturate more aggressively or further restrict the bore of the pipette. Occasionally the problem is related to insufficient or deteriorated collagenase.

4.4.4 Medium Acidifies in One or Two Days

Contamination of cultures is a rare cause of this problem, which is usually related to plating neurons at too high a density. It reflects the high metabolic needs of the large number of neurons in a small volume. The problem may be resolved by frequently replacing medium, but will be avoided if cultures are plated at lower density.

ACKNOWLEDGMENTS

This work is supported by National Institutes of Health grants NS 01741 (RLS) and NS 29046 (CLW).

REFERENCES

Baringer, J. R. 1974. Recovery of herpes simplex virus from human sacral ganglions. *N. Engl J. Med.* **291:** 828–830.

Doerig, C., L. I. Pizer, et al. 1991. Detection of the latency-associated transcript on neuronal cultures during

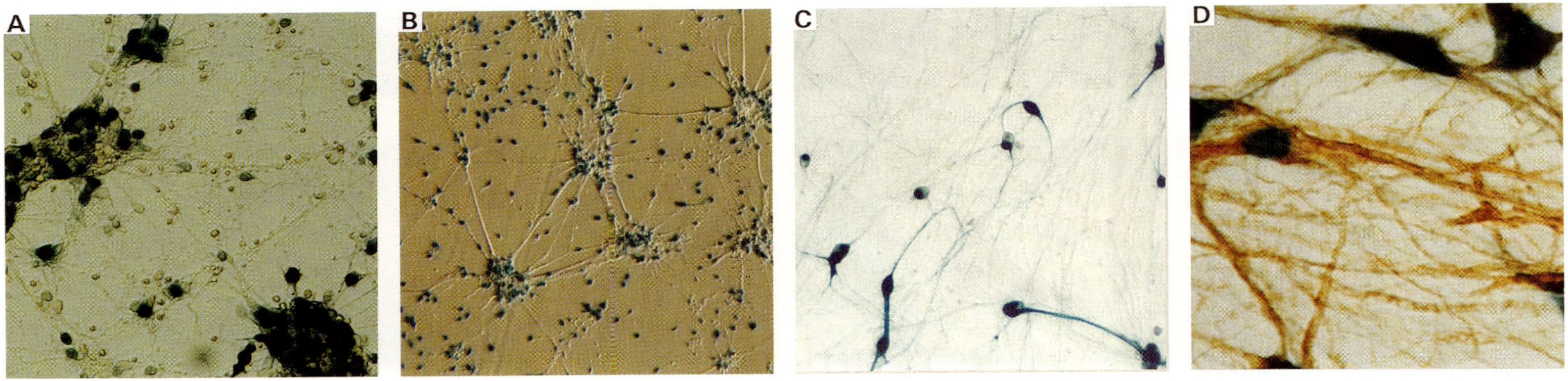

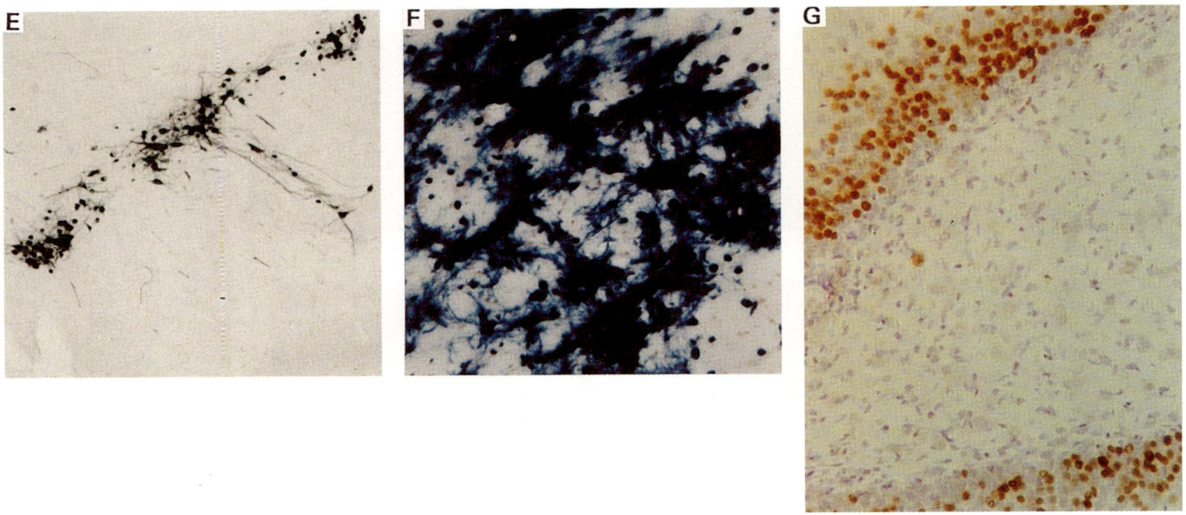

Figure 7.2 Examples of *in vitro* (A–C) and *in vivo* (D–G) infection of neural cells using Adßgal. (A) Superior cervical ganglia neurons; (B) astrocytes; (C) granular cerebellar neurons; (D) substantia nigra. Brain slices were stained for galactosidase expression using Xgal histochemistry (blue), and for TH expression by immunohistochemistry (brown). The photographs show expression of galactosidase in dopaminergic neurons 5 days after injection. (E) *In vivo* retrograde transport of Adßgal-infected rat striatum; expression of ß-galactosidase in dopaminergic neurons of substantia nigra 2 days after injection. (F) Rat striatum 3 days after infection with Adßgal. (G) Infected rat granule cells of the dentate gyrus of the hippocampus. ß-Galactosidase expression was revealed by immunohistochemistry 1 month after injection

Plate I

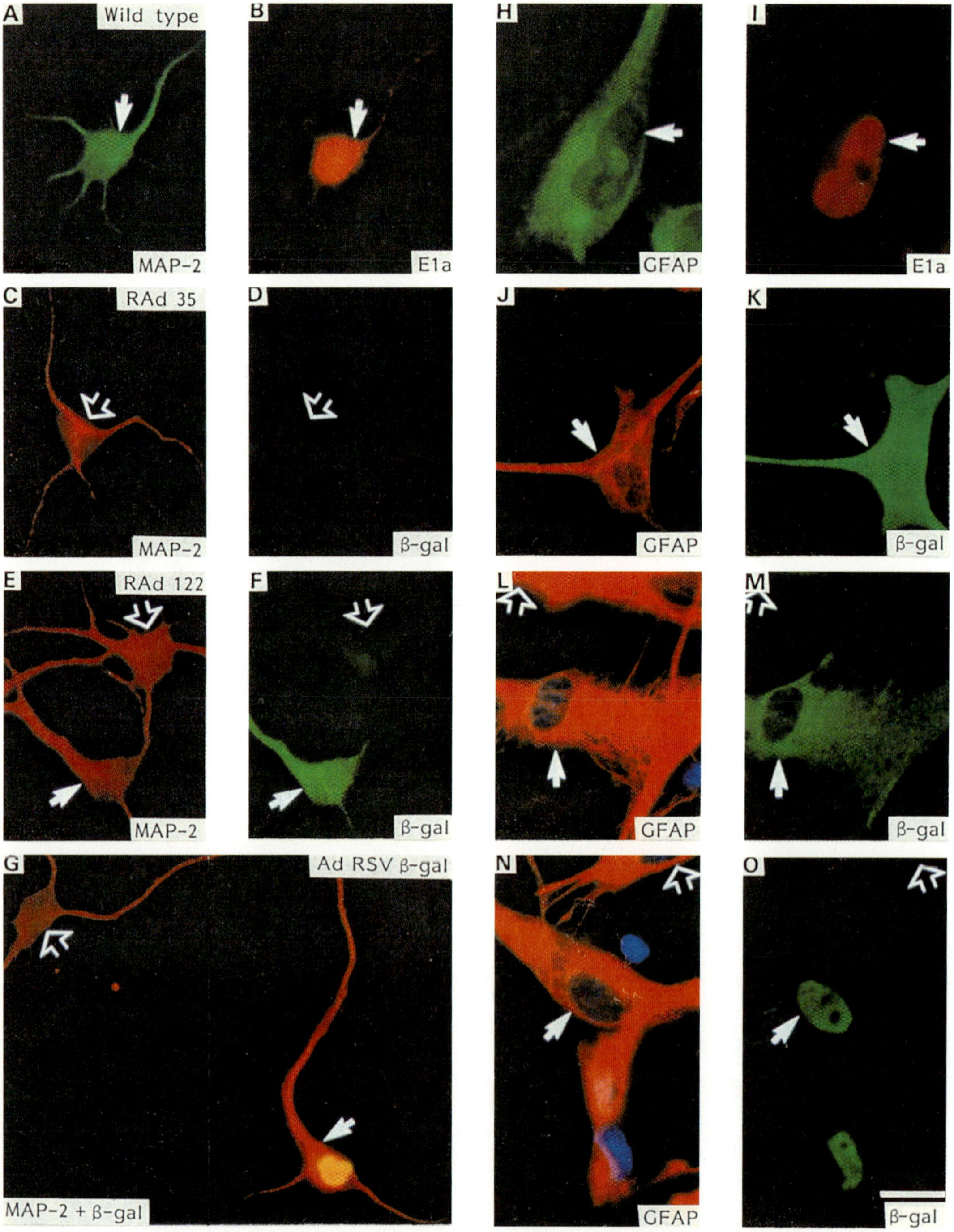

Figure 8.4 Expression from adenovirus and adenovirus recombinants. Primary cultures of neurons or glial cells were infected for 3 days with wild-type adenovirus, RAd 35, RAd 122 and AD RSV ß-gal, all with a MOI of 10. Expression from wild-type adenovirus type 5 was detected by immunoreacting cells with antibodies against E1a proteins; expression from the three other recombinants was detected by immunoreacting cells with antibodies recognizing ß-galactosidase. A–G show neuronal cultures immunoreacted for the neuronal marker MAP-2 (A, C, E, G) and ß-gal (B, D, F, G) (G is a double exposure, showing cytoplasmic MAP-2 and nuclear ß-gal). H–O show glial cultures immunostained for GFAP (H, J, L, N) and ß-gal (I, K, H, O). Similar arrows indicate the same cell under both the astroglial marker fluorescence channels. Blue staining in (L) and (N) indicates nuclear staining with DAPI. Scale bar, shown in (O), represents 20 μm

Plate II

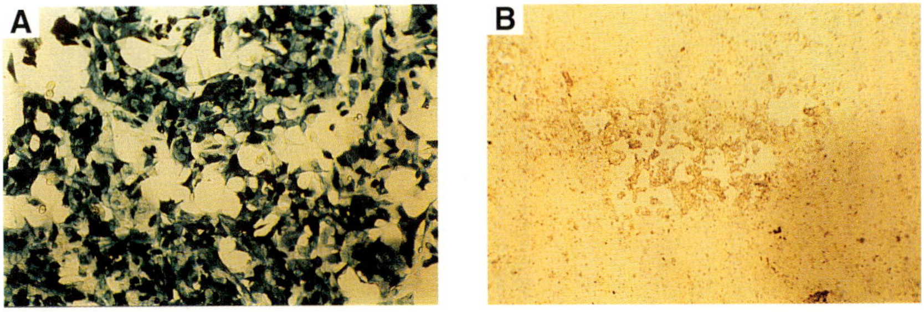

Figure 8.3 (A) 293 cells can be transfected very efficiently by lipofection or calcium phosphate-mediated transfection. This photograph shows 293 cells transfected using calcium phosphate with a plasmid encoding the ß-galactosidase gene under the control of the CMV IE promoter and stained after 46 h with X-gal. As a rough guide, a transfection efficiency above 20% can generate recombinant viruses. (B) A recombinant adenovirus plaque developing in a monolayer of 293 cells following DNA transfection. It is easy to mistake holes in the monolayer for virus plaques until familiar with the system. Plaques will increase significantly in size from day to day, spreading right through the monolayer

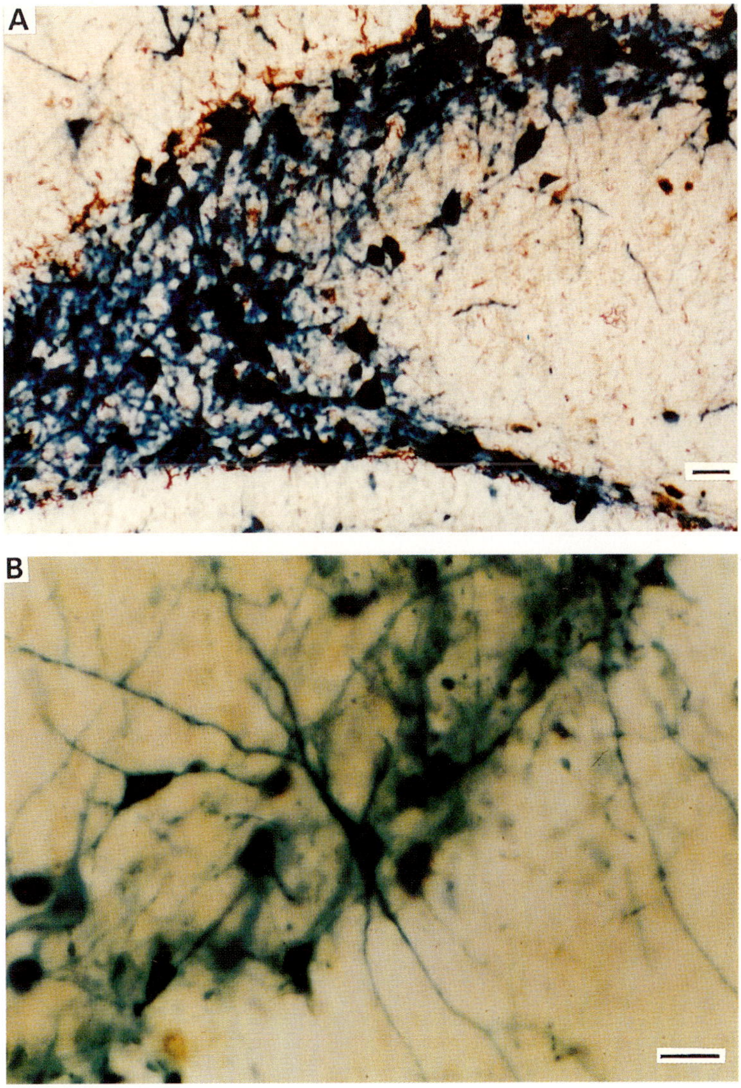

Figure 9.3 Detection of transgene expression in rat brain mediated by a recombinant AAV virus containing a ß-galactosidase marker gene. Gene expression, assayed by ß-galactosidase activity, is shown 7 days after infection with recombinant virus.(A) Longitudinal section through the hippocampus processed for X-gal activity, demonstrating ß-galactosidase activity in a large number of neurons; (B) five-fold magnification of a region of (A), showing individual neurons expressing the transduced gene. Scale bars: 50 μm

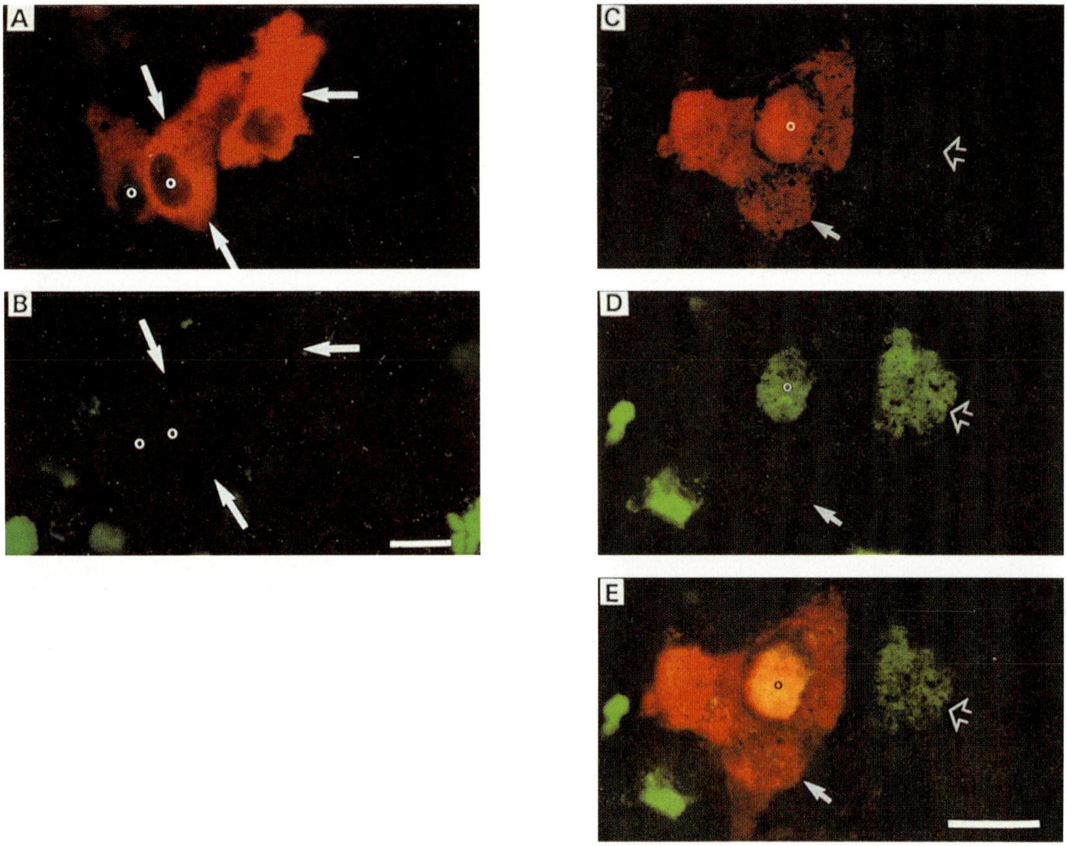

Figure 13.2 Primary cultures of neocortical glial cells infected with pA-SF1/wt. Cells were immunoreacted with rabbit antibodies against ß-galactosidase (detected with secondary anti-rabbit rhodamine-labelled antibodies) (A, C, E), or mouse monoclonal antibodies raised against UL42 (detected with secondary anti-mouse fluorescein-labeled antibodies (B, D, E). Three cells, indicated by large arrows in (A) and (B), became infected only by pA-SF1, but not by helper wt virus: note that their nuclei, indicated by small circles in (A) and (B), are devoid of ß-galactosidase immunoreactivity. The distribution of ß-galactosidase in a cell infected by both viruses is shown in (C–E) (left cell indicated by a straight white arrow, and its nucleus is indicated by a small circle); another cell infected only by wt HSV-1 and displaying the typical nuclear UL42 immunoreactivity is shown to the right in (C–E). (E) is a double exposure through both the fluorescein and rhodamine filters; thus the nucleus of the double-infected cell appears yellow. Scale bars: (A, B) 6.6 μm; (C–E) 17.7 μm

---

Figure 13.3 Primary cultures of neurons infected with either pA-SF1/wt (A, C, D, E, F, H, I, J) or pA-TT1/wt (B, G), or 1321NI astrocytoma cells infected with pA-TT1/CgalΔ42 (K–O). (A) and (F), (B) and (G) show that both amplicons pA-SF1 (A) and pA-TT1 (B) expressed transgenic proteins within infected neurons, as infected cells were immunopositive for MAP-2 (arrows in A, B indicate infected cells expressing transgenes; corresponding arrows in F, G indicate MAP-2 immunopositive neurons using either a mouse monoclonal (F) or a rabbit polyclonal (G) antibody specific to the neuronal specific protein MAP-2). In (A), ß-galactosidase was detected using a rabbit polyclonal antibody and TIMP was detected in (B) using a mouse monoclonal antibody, In (A), ß-galactosidase immunoreactivity can be seen within the cell body and its processes; a large white arrow indicates the cell body of an infected neuron in (A), which is immunopositive for MAP-2 (F), while a shorter white arrow indicates a long process immunoreactive for ß-galactosidase, which is only partially immunoreactive for MAP-2 and possibly corresponds to the neuronal axon. Two further MAP-2 immunoreactive neurons, not expressing ß-galactosidase, are seen in (F). (C–E, H–J) Individual neurons which have been infected by pA-SF1 alone (C–E) or both pA-SF1 and wt (H–J). (C), (D) and (E) show a neuron exposed to pA-SF1/wt, which is immunoreactive for ß-galactosidase (C, long arrow) but not for the HSV-1 protein UL42 expressed by the helper wild-type HSV-1 (D, long white arrow). Note in (C) that ß-galactosidase immunoreactivity extends from the cell body (indicated by a long thick white arrow), throughout the axon (small thin white arrows). A second cell, possibly non-neuronal, which is immunoreactive for both ß-galactosidase (C) and UL42 (D) is indicated by a medium white or black arrow in (C–E). The phase image of these cells is shown in (E). A neuron immunoreactive for both ß-galactosidase (H) and UL42 (I) is shown in (H), (I) and (J) (long and short white arrows). A double exposure of this cell taken through both the rhodamine and fluorescein filters is shown in (J); the nucleus thus appears yellow (indicated by

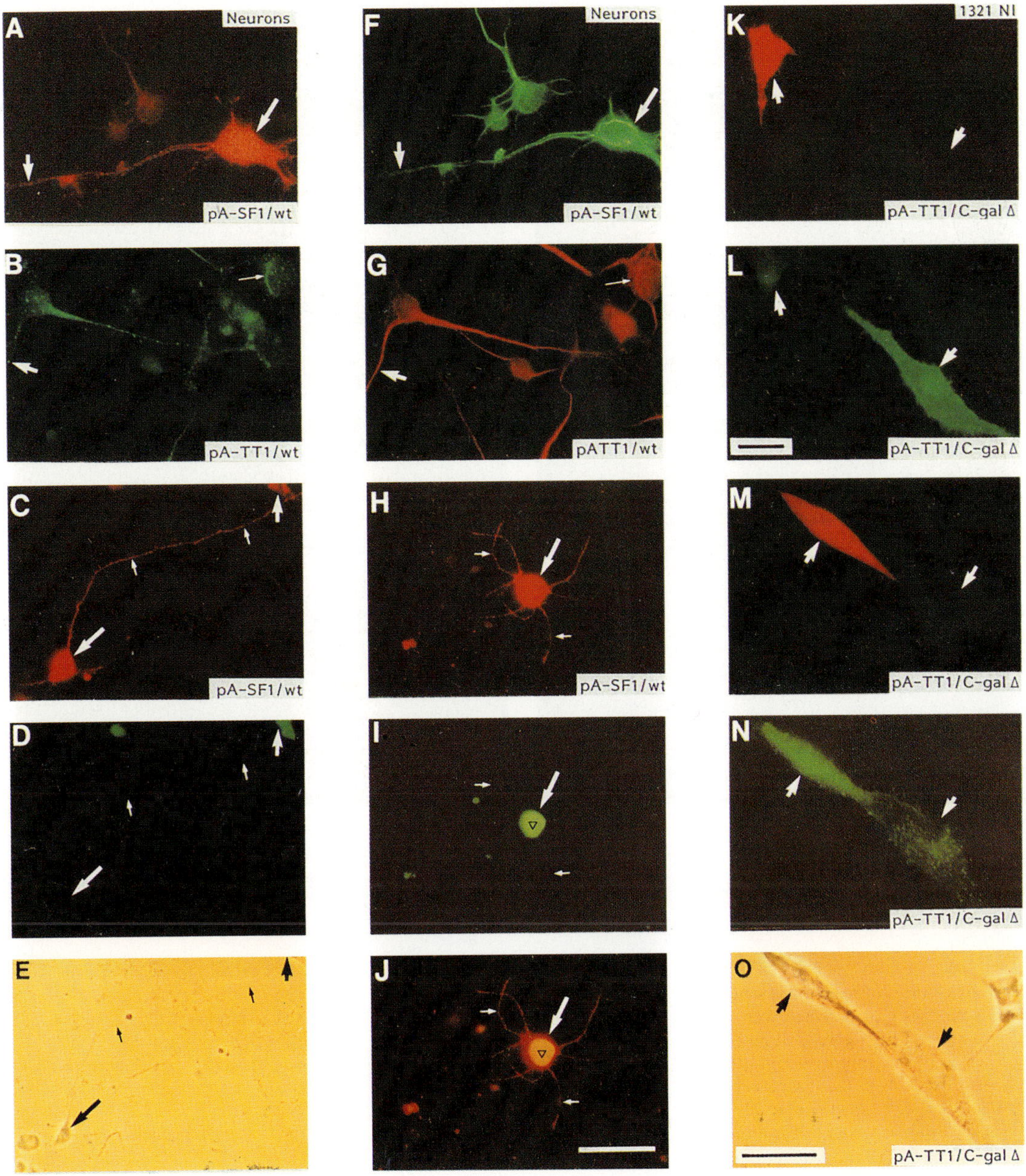

a black triangle in I, J). Small fine arrows indicate this cell's processes. (K–O) Astrocytoma cells from the glial cell line 1321NI after infection with pA-TT1/CgalΔ42. The field shown in (K) and (L) illustrates two astrocytoma cells: one is immunoreactive only for ß-galactosidase expressed by the helper CgalΔ42 (K), another (L) is immunoreactive only for TIMP expressed by pA-TT1; short thick white arrows indicate the positions of the cells in both (K) and (L). The field shown in (M–O) shows a cell infected with both CgalΔ42 (ß-galactosidase immunoreactive; (M), upper left) and pA-TT1 (TIMP/Thy1 immunoreactive, (N)) and, to the right in (N), another cell only infected by pA-TT1. A group of cells not infected by either viral particle can be seen in the upper right-hand corner in (O). Scale bar for (A–J) shown in (J); for (K–L) shown in (L); for (M–O) shown in (O). All scale bars: 17.7 μm

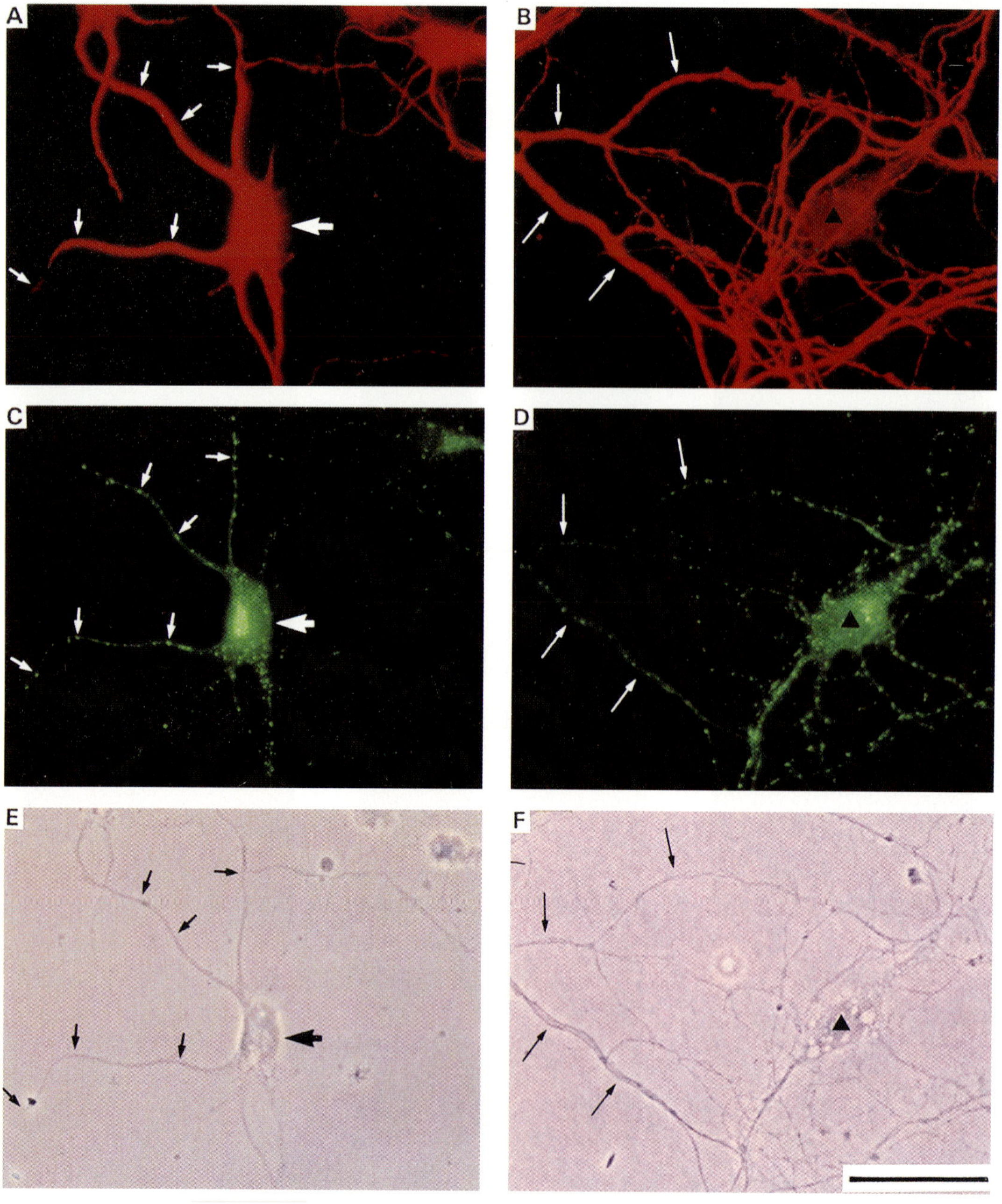

Figure 14.5 Neocortical neurons were infected with a tsK-derived recombinant expressing TIMP/Thy1. (A) Shows neurons immunostained for Map2, (C) the same field immunostained for TIMP and (E) the phase-contrast image; note that most of the TIMP (C) is located on the dendrites (A). Small arrows indicate similar areas of the processes under phase-contrast or after immunostaining in all three panels; the larger arrow indicates the origin of the axon, which remains unstained in this neuron, indicating that TIMP is preferentially targeted to dendritic processes. (B) Neurons immunostained for tau, (D) the same field immunostained for Thy1, (F) the phase-contrast image. Fine arrows indicate the same processes in all three panels. Note that some, but not all, tau immunoreactive processes are immunostained. Many of the dendrites originating from the cell body can be identified in (F) as thick processes, which do not display TIMP immunoreactivity. This shows that in some neurons TIMP immunoreactivity can also be target to axons. Examination of many neurons demonstrates that TIMP-Thy1 is mainly targeted to dendrites but can also be found in a minority of axonal processes. Scale bar = 20 μm

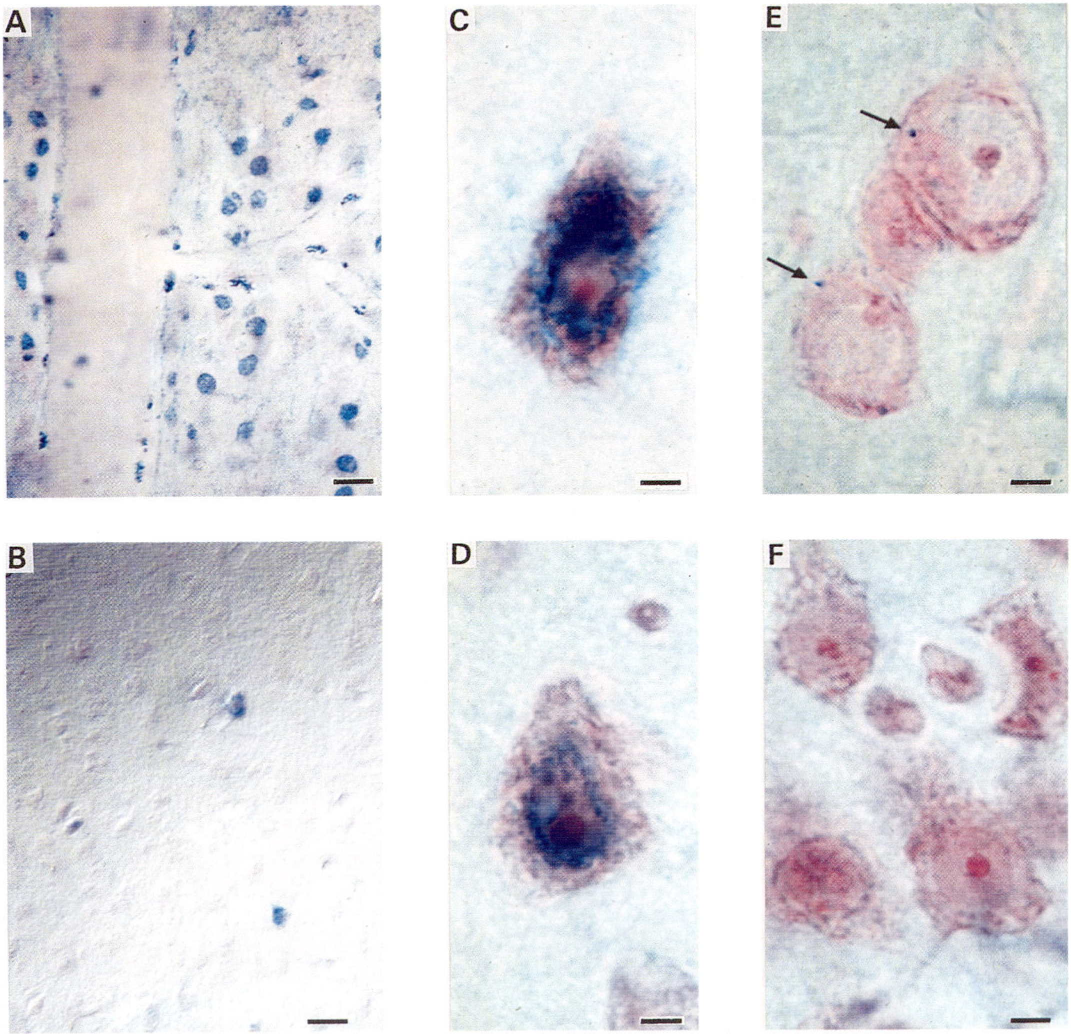

Figure 21.3 Histochemical staining for acidic α-mannosidase. (A) Normal cat cerebral cortex, showing widespread neuronal and perivascular cell labelling (blue stain). Bar = 25 μm. (B) A 1-year-old cat with α-mannosidosis that received BMT at 2 months of age, showing positively labelled cells scattered throughout the cortex. Bar = 25 μm. (C–D) Higher powered photomicrographs of neurons in (A) and (B), respectively. Bars = 4 μm. (E) Photomicrograph of strongly labelled cortical neurons in the cat shown in (B), illustrating that low-level staining (arrows) was often present and visible only at high magnification. Bar = 4 μm. (F) Histochemical staining of an affected untreated cat, showing complete lack of histochemical reaction product. Bar = 4 μm

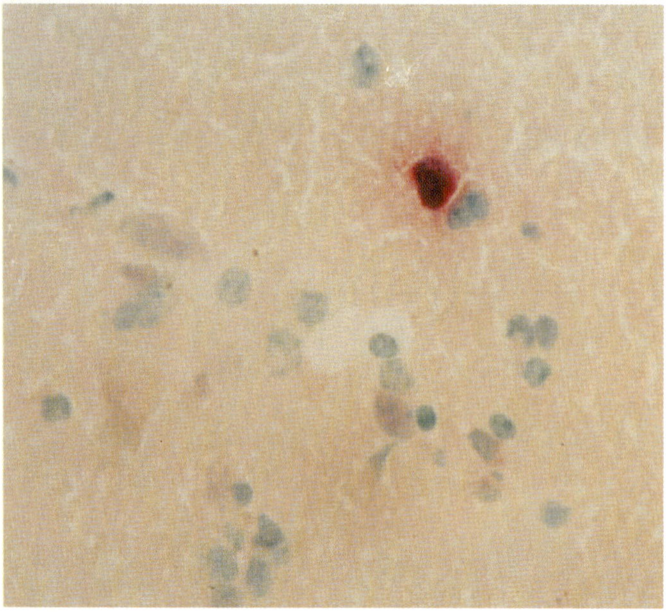

Figure 20.2 A single GUSB-positive cell, derived from transplanted normal bone marrow, in the cortex of an MPS VII mouse. Note the red reaction product surrounding the cell which may be cross-reactive enzyme released by the positive cell. The section is counterstained with methyl green. Original magnification × 200

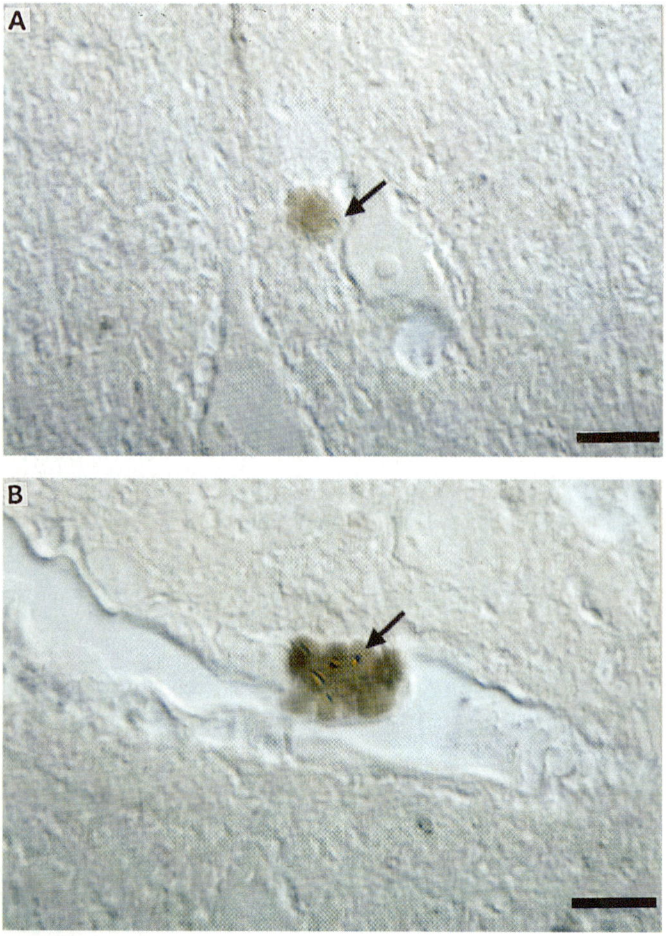

Figure 21.4 Histochemical staining of parenchymal (A) and perivascular (B) microglial-like cells in a cat with α-mannosidosis that was given BMT. These cells contained lipid material and were histochemically positive for acidic α-mannosidase (reaction product, arrows). Scale bar (A) = 24 μm; (B) = 12 μm

the latent infection with herpes simplex virus type 1. *Virology* **183:** 423–426.

Fenton, E. L. 1970. Tissue culture assay of nerve growth factor and of the specific antiserum. *Exp. Cell Res.* **59:** 383–392.

Hill, T. 1985. Herpes Simplex Virus Latency. In *The Herpes Viruses* Ed. B. Roizman. NY, Plenum Press. 175–240.

Johnson, M. I. and V. Argiro 1983. Techniques in the tissue culture of rat sympathetic neurons. *Meth. Enzymol.* 334–337.

Price, R. W. 1986. Neurobiology of human herpesvirus infection. *CRC Crit. Rev. Clin. Neurobiol.* **2:** 61–123.

Smith, R. L., J. L. Escudero, et al. 1994. Regulation of the herpes simplex virus latency-associated transcript during establishment of latency in sensory neurons *in vitro. Virology* **202:** 49–60.

Smith, R. L., L. I. Pizer, et al. 1992. Activation of second-messenger pathways reactivates latent herpes simplex virus in neuronal cultures. *Virology* **188:** 311–318.

Sohrabji, F., R.C. Miranda and C.D. Toran-Allerand 1994. Estrogen differentially regulates estrogen and nerve growth factor receptor mRNAs in adult sensory neurons. *J. Neurosci.* **14:** 459–471.

Stevens, J. G. 1989. Human herpes viruses: A consideration of the latent state. *Microbiol. Rev.* **53:** 318–332.

Wilcox, C. L. and E. M. Johnson 1987. Nerve growth factor deprivation results in the reactivation of latent herpes simplex virus *in vitro. J. Virol.* **61:** 2311–2315.

Wilcox, C. L. and E. M. Johnson Jr. 1988. Characterization of nerve growth factor-dependent herpes simplex virus latency in neurons *in vitro. J. Virol.* **62:** 393–399.

Wilcox, C. L., R. L. Smith, et al. 1990. Nerve growth factor-dependence of herpes simplex latency in peripheral sympathetic and sensory neurons *in vitro. J. Neurosci.* **10:** 1268–1275.

SECTION 5

Protocols for Gene Delivery Using Cells

CHAPTER 19

Delivery of Gene Products to the Central Nervous System by Grafting Retrovirally Engineered Neuronal and Non-neuronal Cells

THEO D. PALMER AND FRED H. GAGE

Laboratory of Genetics, The Salk Institute, La Jolla, CA 92037, USA.
Tel: 619 453 4100; Fax: 619 597 0824

1 INTRODUCTION

Many of the complexities of the vertebrate central nervous system (CNS) were recognized well before the turn of the century and, while the 19th century view of brain architecture remains amazingly accurate, we are just beginning to understand how the complex processes of thought, memory and behavior are regulated at the genetic level. The ability to perturb the normal workings of the brain by introducing an active gene provides a powerful tool for examining molecular mechanisms in the developing and adult brain. The potential for genetically altering specific cellular populations within the adult CNS provides a promising approach for intervening in these processes when they go awry in human neurological disease.

A wide variety of gene transfer methods is being applied to the restoration of neurological function and, although diverse vector systems are used, many clinical objectives are held in common. In an ideal setting, administration of therapeutic genes would employ vectors that target specific populations of cells and provide appropriately regulated, long-term expression of the gene product. Although the current generation of gene transfer vehicles falls short of this ideal, the recent clinical use of viral vectors demonstrates the utility of even a rudimentary ability to transfer and express therapeutic genes *in vivo* (Suhr and Gage, 1993; Mulligan, 1993; Anderson, 1992; Miller, 1992; Verma, 1990; Gage et al., 1990).

The current generation of adenovirus and herpes simplex virus-based vectors offer the first evidence that post-mitotic CNS cells can be efficiently manipulated *in situ*. Albeit transiently, these vectors efficiently express episomally maintained transgenes and can provide readily detectable physiological changes to a targeted brain region (Boviatsis et al., 1994; Chen et al., 1994; Glorioso et al., 1994; Akli et al., 1993; Davidson et al., 1993; Ho et al., 1993; Kozarsky and Wilson, 1993; Le Gal La Salle et al., 1993; Fink et al., 1992; Freese et al., 1990; Geller et al., 1990; Chiocca et al., 1990). Unfortunately, there is little specificity in the types of cells transduced and the cellular toxicities associated with wild-type virus infections have not been completely resolved (Alton and Geddes, 1994; Crystal et al., 1994; Engelhardt et al., 1994; Yang et al., 1994; Kozarsky and Wilson, 1993; Simon et al., 1993; Johnson et al., 1992). Retroviral and adeno-associated viral (AAV) vectors may provide some improvement in long-term expression since these vectors stably integrate into the cellular genome and, therefore, are maintained for the life of the cell (Kaplitt et

Protocols for Gene Transfer in Neuroscience: Towards Gene Therapy of Neurological Disorders
Edited by P.R. Lowenstein and L.W. Enquist

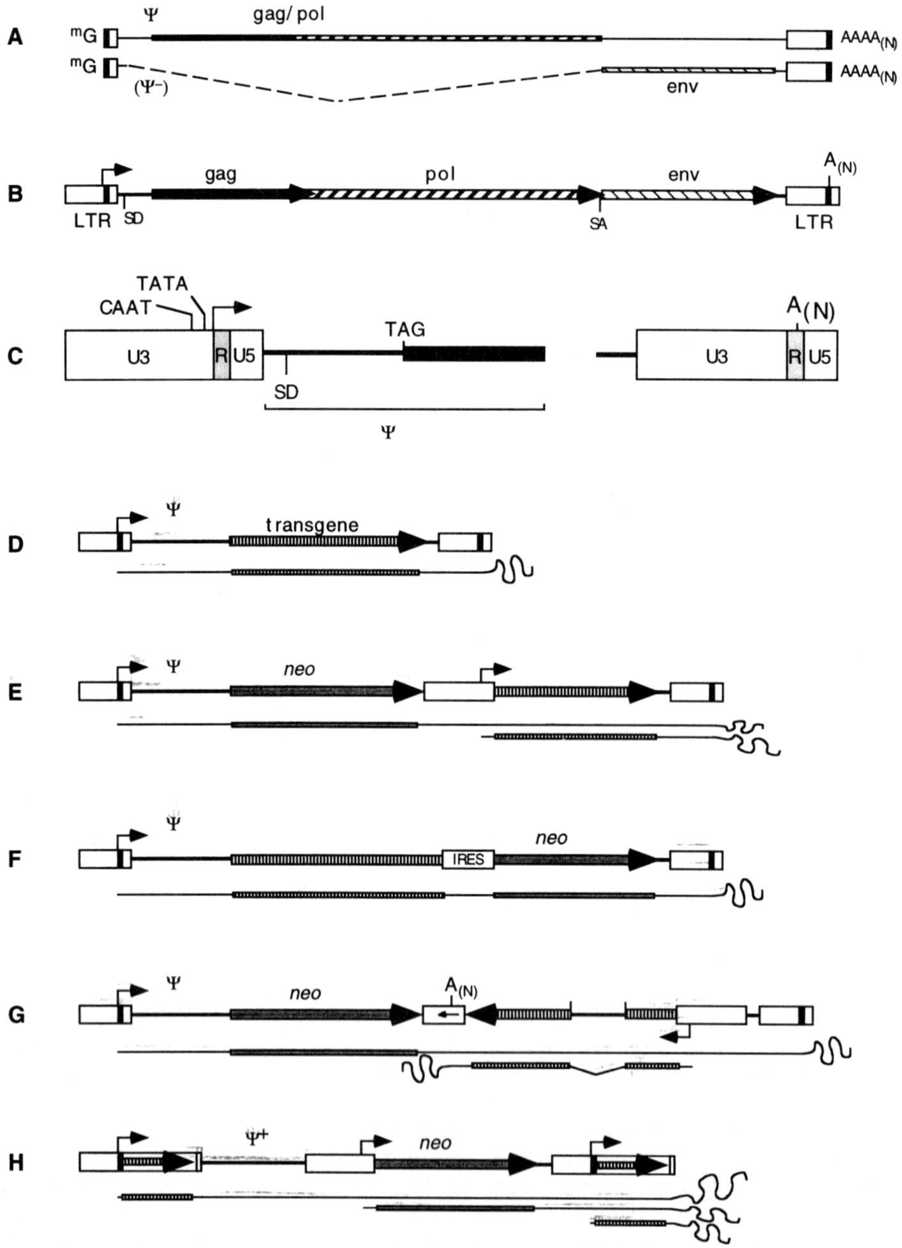

Figure 19.1 Organization of wild-type and replication-defective proviral sequences. The wild-type MoMLV proviral genome (B) produces two transcripts (A). The spliced transcript does not contain the packaging signal, Ψ or Ψ^+, and is not packaged. Proviral sequence elements essential for transcription and packaging of a vector RNA (C) are contained in and near the viral LTR. The viral enhancer and the promoter's CAAT and TATA box consensus are located in the viral LTR's U3 region. Deletion of the viral protein encoding sequences conserves these sequences and allows transgenes to be inserted in the analogous location (D–H). Transcripts for each recombinant vector are shown below the provirus and, although a transcript may contain open reading frames of two or more genes, only the first gene is translated (shown as a boxed zone on the transcript). Only those transcripts from the vector that contain the Ψ signal are packaged. Arrows indicate promoters, $AAAA_{(N)}$ indicates polyadenylation signals and the adenylated portion of the transcript is represented as a recurved line

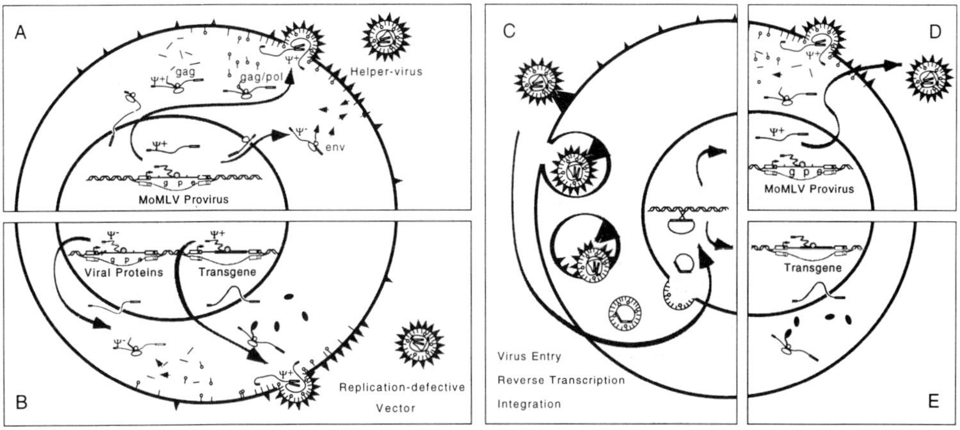

Figure 19.2 Retroviral-mediated gene transfer and helper-free packaging cells. The wild-type retroviral particle produced from an infected cell (A) carries viral protein encoding sequences on its RNA genome, allowing the packaging function to be transmitted to additional cells (D). Helper virus-free packaging cell lines (B) contain two or more integrated plasmid constructs which complement each other to assemble viral particles containing only the recombinant vector RNA which has a packaging signal Ψ^+ (C). The viral protein-encoding genes are not packaged, so the integrated vector genome produces only the transgene product only in target cells (E) and vector sequences do not spread to additional cells

al., 1994; Boris-Lawrie and Temin, 1993; Miller et al., 1993; Samulski, 1993; Muzyczka, 1992; Jolly and Warner, 1990; Cepko, 1988; Miller et al., 1986b). Since vector integration depends on cell replication (Russell et al., 1994; Roe et al., 1993; Miller et al., 1990), retroviral and AAV vectors are poor choices for targeting post-mitotic neurons *in situ*, but can be effectively used to engineer proliferating cells in culture.

Although the process of culturing and grafting cells introduces additional complexity in comparison to the direct injection of gene transfer vectors, manipulation of purified cells in culture is presently the only method that allows a specific cell type to be targeted exclusively. *In vitro* transduction also allows selection for an appropriate level of transgene expression which, in combination with the ability to adjust the number of cells grafted, provides considerable control over the subsequent *in vivo* outcome.

Both *in vivo* and *ex vivo* gene transfer models often evaluate the biological impact of a candidate transgene by first using grafts of established cell lines that are easily grown and transduced (Uchida et al., 1989; Geller, 1991; Ridoux et al., 1994; Calliaud et al., 1993; Wolff et al., 1989). Once a physiological effect is confirmed, the long-term efficacy can be evaluated using grafts of primary cell cultures. The use of non-immortalized cells avoids the complicating tendency of transformed cell lines to form tumors and allows a more accurate prediction of cell survival and expression phenotypes that would be seen using freshly isolated human primary cells. This issue may seem trivial but several studies using peripherally transplanted cells demonstrate that immortal cell lines exhibit quite different post-grafting expression characteristics in comparison to similarly grafted primary cell populations (Roman et al., 1992; Dhawan et al., 1991, Palmer et al., 1989, 1991).

Both peripheral and CNS-derived cell types can be isolated from normal tissues and serially propagated as proliferative cell strains (Ray and Gage, 1994; Sensenbrenner et al., 1994; Kilpatrick and Bartlett, 1993; Mayer et al., 1993ab; Ray et al., 1993; Shahar et al., 1993; Louis et al., 1992; Noble and Wolswijk, 1992; Reynolds et al., 1992; Reynolds and Weiss, 1992; Wren et al., 1992; Noble et al., 1990; Perraud et al., 1990). Although cells from peripheral tissues, such as skin fibroblasts or myoblasts, are clearly out of place in the brain, genetically modified non-neural grafts can provide an effective source of therapeutic trophic factors or neurotransmitters (Fisher et al., 1993ab; Chen et al., 1991; Horellou et al., 1991; Stromberg et al., 1990; Jiao and Wolff, 1992; Jiao et al., 1993, Gage and Fisher 1991; Gage et al., 1990a). Alternatively, proliferative primary cultures of fetal neurons can be recovered and propagated as non-immortalized cultures from a variety of brain regions (Mayer et al., 1993a; Reynolds and Weiss, 1992; Kilpatrick and Bartlett, 1993; Ray and Gage, 1994; Ray et al., 1993; Sensenbrenner et al., 1994) and, although the potential for modifying these cells to improve a therapeutic effect has not been fully explored, grafting naive fetal cells to the adult brain has shown promise in primate models and in the clinical treatment of Parkinson's disease or Parkinson's-like symptoms induced by MPTP toxicity (Redmond et al., 1993; Widner et al., 1993; Freed et al., 1992; Spencer et al., 1992; Widner et al., 1992; Dunnett, 1991a, b; Taylor et al., 1991; Bankiewicz et al., 1990).

Both dermal fibroblasts and fetal neurons have proven effective as grafting cell populations in our laboratory (Tuszynski et al., 1994; Fisher et al., 1993; Fisher and Gage, 1993; Shimohama et al., 1993; Kawaja and Gage, 1992; Gage and Chen, 1992; Kawaja et al., 1991; Chen et al., 1991; Gage and Fisher, 1991; Gage et al., 1990a; Schinstine et al., 1991; Tuszynski et al., 1990; Fisher et al., 1991; Fisher et al., 1990). Although we have used these cell types to address the relatively separate issues of protein delivery vs. neuronal reconstitution, we are beginning to combine these approaches to determine if neuronal replacement can be improved when mixed grafts are carefully tailored for a specific functional outcome. For instance, fetal neurons engineered to exhibit a particular transmitter phenotype might be cografted with fibroblasts or astrocytes that produce a trophic factor. In this way, a neuronal graft would have high functional activity and yet be protected from potential degenerative insults in the host (Takayama et al., 1995).

At present, retroviral vectors provide an efficient method for introducing genes into proliferating cells, yet despite promising results in rodent models (Shimohama et al., 1993; Fisher and Gage, 1993; Fisher et al., 1993b; Cepko, 1988), retrovirally transferred genes are often transcriptionally downregulated after grafting, presumably due to cell differentiation or transition from the proliferative to a quiescent state (McLachlin et al., 1993; Kang et al., 1993; Ramesh et al., 1993; Schinstine and Gage, 1993; Palmer et al., 1991; Palmer et al., 1987; Emmerman and Temin, 1986). In many instances, nevertheless, the reduced production of transgene product is still sufficient for maintaining a biochemical or behavioral phenotype *in vivo* (Tuszynski et al., 1994; Fisher et al., 1993a; Shimohama et al., 1993; Chen et al., 1991).

Post-grafting regulation of transcriptional activity appears to be cell type-specific because some cell types demonstrate long-term expression with vectors that are downregulated in fibroblasts (Kaleko et al., 1991; Clowes et al., 1994; Lynch et al., 1992). In other cases, transcription has been maintained in a refractive cell type by using cellular promoters to drive the transgene or by increasing the number of vector copies each cell carries (Dai et al., 1992; Nakajima et al., 1993; Moolten et al., 1992; Scharfmann et al., 1991; Taketo and Tanaka, 1987). Whether or not transgene expression levels will be an issue in transduced fetal neurons remains to be demonstrated; however, transduction of cells *in situ* in the developing CNS demonstrates that a variety of neuronal and glial cell types can express retrovirally transferred genes (Luskin, 1993, 1994; Ryder and Cepko, 1994; Walsh and Cepko, 1993; Cepko et al., 1993; Levison et al., 1993; Levison and Goldman, 1993). Although these observations cannot be directly extrapolated to the expression potential of cultured and grafted CNS cells, it may be possible to use retroviral vectors to improve reconstitution of the damaged brain with grafted neuronal populations.

1.1 Retroviral Biology and Vector Systems

Retroviral vectors are derived from an RNA virus that carries two copies of viral mRNA as a genome (Weiss et al., 1985). Upon entering a target cell, one or both copies of mRNA is reverse transcribed into double-stranded DNA and integrated into the host cell's genome. The integrated proviral sequence produces two mRNA transcripts, a full-length transcript that encodes the viral *gag* and *pol* gene products, and a spliced message that encodes the *env* gene product (Fig. 19.1A, B). The newly made viral proteins assemble at the cell membrane and package two full-length *gag*/*pol* encoding transcripts (Fig. 19.2A) which, upon entry into a new target cell (Fig. 19.2C), are reverse transcribed, integrated, etc.

The sequences necessary for transcription, packaging, reverse transcription and integration are restricted to a relatively small section at each end of the proviral sequence which includes the viral long terminal repeats (LTR) (Fig. 19.1C). If viral proteins are provided by a separate wild-type virus (helper virus), or by a non-viral expression plasmid (as found in retroviral packaging cells; Fig. 19.2B), the viral protein encoding sequences can be replaced by a useful transgene (Fig. 19.1D–H). Because none of the viral protein encoding sequences are present in the recombinant vector, cells transduced by the vector can not repackage the vector mRNAs and instead use the mRNAs only for production of transgene product (Fig. 19.2E). If helper virus subsequently infects the target cell, it can provide the viral proteins in *trans* and the vector sequences would be packaged and passed on to a new target cell (Fig. 19.2D).

Retroviral packaging cells are derived from immortal cell lines, such as mouse 3T3 cells, which have been transfected with a plasmid that encodes the viral *gag*, *pol* and *env* proteins (see Miller, 1990 for a comprehensive review). Transcripts from these plasmids do not contain the viral sequences necessary for packaging and therefore assembled viral particles contain only randomly packaged cellular RNAs and virus-like 30s RNAs (Torrent et al., 1994; Arnof and Linial, 1991; Hatzoglou et al, 1990). If a recombinant vector plasmid (Fig. 19.1D–H) is introduced into these cells its mRNA, which contains a packaging signal (Ψ), is packaged at much higher efficiency and many of the viral particles secreted into the medium carry the vector transcript.

Various wild-type retroviruses use different envelope genes, each of which mediates viral entry through a different cellular receptor (Weiss et al., 1985). This receptor specificity is divided into separate tropisms based on the relative ability of each envelope to mediate entry into cells of different species. The two most commonly used envelopes in packaging cell lines, ecotropic and amphotropic, recognize respectively an amino acid transporter on rodent cells (Kim et al., 1991; Wang et al., 1991) or a phosphate transporter present on cells from a variety of species (Kavanaugh et al., 1994; Miller et al., 1994). A number of packaging cell lines have been recently reviewed elsewhere (Miller, 1990).

As retroviral vectors can transduce human cells there is often a question of safety in the laboratory (Boris-Lawrie and Temin, 1994). The wild-type Moloney murine leukemia virus (MoMLV) can cause tumors in newborn or immune-compromised mice, presumably by insertional mutagenesis (Weiss et al., 1985). To determine the effects of wild-type virus in primates, several studies have introduced replication-competent helper virus into either normal monkeys (Cornetta et al., 1993; Cornetta et al., 1991) or monkeys immune compromised by total bone marrow ablation (Donahue et al., 1992). There were no apparent ill effects in the normal monkeys but some of the animals undergoing bone marrow transplant eventually developed T-cell lymphomas, presumably as a result of unchecked spread of replication-competent helper virus and insertional mutation of a proto-oncogene. In the absence of helper virus, the risk of acquiring a disease-causing insertional mutation is remote. Human complement inactivates murine retroviruses (Welsh et al., 1975, 1976). If, in spite of this inherent safety, an additional level of precaution is desired, retroviral experiments could be limited to rodent models in which ecotropic vectors can be used. Ecotropic vectors are presumably safe even in the presence of helper virus because ecotropic viruses transduce non-rodent cells with very low efficiency (Weiss et al., 1985). For laboratories in the USA, the commonly used helper virus-free ecotropic and amphotropic vectors are considered class 1 agents and should be handled under biosafety level 1 containment (see "Guidelines for research involving recombinant DNA molecules," *The Federal Registrar* 1986, 51(88): 16958–16985, section III, part III-B-3, and III-C).

1.2 Plasmids for Constructing Vectors

Plasmids are available which contain the necessary viral sequences, a selectable marker gene and convenient cloning sites for the introduction of transgene sequences (Miller and Rosman, 1989; Stockschlaeder et al., 1991; Jaffee et al., 1993; Cone and Mulligan, 1984, 1992; Morgenstern and Land, 1990; Ray and Gage, 1992; Danos and Mulligan, 1988). We have had good success with the pLN derived plasmids which contain a dominant neomycin phosphotransferase-selectable marker (*neo*) (Miller and Rosman, 1989). Similar plasmids are available with a histidinol dehydrogenase selectable marker, which is more effective in some cell types (Stockschlaeder et al., 1991).

Most retroviral vectors follow a common design, which uses the promoter within the viral LTR to transcribe one transgene sequence (Fig. 19.1D) and/or an exogenous promoter placed within the vector to drive the second transgene (Fig. 19.1E). Transcripts from both promoters are terminated by the same polyadenylation signal in the 3′ LTR. Most of the commonly available plasmids can be used directly by placing a coding sequence into a multiple cloning site downstream of the LTR or downstream of an internal promoter. Although this is a simple "cut-and-paste" step, several design options and obscure pitfalls must be considered.

1.3 Size Limitations

The upper limit for efficient packaging of a vector mRNA is about 10–12 kb (Weiss et al., 1985). Vectors that generate an mRNA genome of less than 7–8 kb seem to work most efficiently. In the pLN-series plasmids, the space taken up by the viral elements and the selectable *neo* gene leaves roughly 3–4 kb of useful space for transgene sequences. If a selectable marker is not required, then the transgene sequences can be slightly larger.

1.4 Splice Sites

The wild-type viral mRNA produces *gag* and *pol* gene products from a non-spliced message and the *env* gene product is produced from a spliced transcript (Fig. 19.1A). The 5′ splice donor adjacent to the 5′ LTR is still present in most common vectors. Consequently, if a sequence containing a functional splice acceptor is placed into the vector, splicing can remove the intervening sequences. If this process is efficient, most of the mRNA produced in packaging cells would not contain Ψ and therefore would not be packaged. On the other hand, if splicing is only moderately efficient, the apparent viral titers may not be significantly affected. In fact, a splicing event may improve transgene expression and some vectors have been designed to retain functional splice signals (Jaffee et al., 1993; Cone and Mulligan, 1992). However, as presently designed these vectors carry only a single gene and hence the absence of a selectable marker can make the generation and characterization of virus-producing cell lines more difficult.

1.5 Introns

As the viral genome is mRNA, packaging cells will dutifully excise the introns from a transgene and provide processed cDNAs for integration into the target cell (McIvor, 1990; Dornburg and Temin, 1990). Intron removal can be disconcerting if a desired phenomenon depends on alternate splicing or if necessary regulatory elements are contained in intronic sequences (Gelinas and Novak, 1990). Placing the transgene elements in the reverse orientation with respect to normal viral transcription may solve this problem (Fig. 19.1G). However, the transgene must then be introduced on a complete reverse-orientation expression cassette which includes a dedicated promoter and polyadenylation signal.

1.6 Polyadenylation Signals

The viral elements at both ends of the vector's genomic RNA are required for reverse transcription and integration, so transgene sequences that contain polyadenylation (poly-A) signals within the vector's transcribed strand can prematurely terminate the vector RNA and subsequently prevent reverse transcription in the target cells. A rapid screen for the poly-A consensus signal, AATAAA, can save frustration later. The most commonly used SV40 poly-A sequence contains functional poly-A signals in both orientations and precludes its use in reverse-orientation cassettes.

1.7 Repeated Sequences

During synthesis of the first DNA strand in the target cells reverse transcriptase performs a strand-transfer step from the 5′ R region to 3′ R region (Weiss et al., 1985; Gilboa et al., 1979; Whitcomb and Hughes, 1992). This process is relatively permissive and tandemly repeated sequences within the RNA genome can act as illegitimate transfer sites (Pulsinelli and Temin, 1991; Hu and Temin, 1990a, b; Zhang and Temin, 1993, 1994; Temin, 1993; Olson et al., 1992; Otto et al., 1994). Depending on how efficiently reverse transcriptase transfers between these sequences, many of the integrated proviral sequences in a target cell population may be missing the sequences between the repeats.

1.8 Upstream ATGs

Ribosomes assemble at the 5′ cap structure of the viral mRNAs and then scan for the first ATG codon that is in an optimal surrounding sequence (i.e. in good context; Kozak, 1986, 1987, 1991, 1992). Although several ATGs are present between the 5′ LTR and the commonly used cloning site downstream of Ψ, translation initiates poorly from these ATGs and generally initiates at the first "good" ATG within the transgene sequences. ATGs in the transgene sequences that are in good context and upstream of the desired start codon can produce unexpected fusion proteins or non-sense proteins, and greatly reduce initiation at the authentic ATG.

1.9 Transgene Products

The vector RNAs that are packaged are also translated in packaging cells and the transgene product must be compatible with normal cell biology. Some gene products (transcription factors, proteins controlling cell replication, cellular toxins, etc.) may not be compatible with generating stable virus-producing cell lines. Even if normal levels of expression are tolerated by cells, the robust expression offered by most promoters used in retroviral vectors may pose overexpression-related problems. Some vectors have been specifically designed to provide low but stable expression *in vivo* and have used cellular housekeeping gene promoters (Hawley et al., 1989; Taketo and Tanaka, 1987; Scharfmann et al., 1991). If the transgene product is not well tolerated, this low level of expression may be adequate for function yet low enough to prevent toxicity.

1.10 Selectable Markers

Although the protocols listed below describe the use of vectors carrying the *neo* gene, there are many alternative marker genes that can be used to select for or against expression of the gene product (Eglitis, 1991). Drug resistance genes are useful for eliminating non-transduced cells, although some target cells are particularly sensitive to the drugs used for a given marker gene. Simply switching selectable markers may suddenly resolve difficulties in transducing a given cell type (Stockschlaeder et al., 1991). If geneticin sulfate (G418) selection for the *neo* gene does not work well, vectors using one of the following gene/drug combinations should be used: histidinol dehydrogenase/histidinol (Stockschlaeder et al., 1991; Barnes, 1981); hygromycin phosphotransferase/hygromycin-B (Palmer et al., 1987; Gritz and Davies, 1983); mutant dihydrofolate reductase/methotrexate (Miller et al., 1985; Haber et al., 1981). Some gene/drug combinations select against transduced cells *in vitro* and *in vivo*. For example, herpes simplex thymidine kinase/ganciclovir selection is currently being used in a variety of CNS and peripheral antitumor applications (Ram et al., 1994; Ezzeddine et al., 1991; Moolten and Wells, 1990; Culver et al., 1994; Boviatsis et al., 1994; Moolten, 1986).

1.11 Promoters, Regulatory Elements and Unconventional Designs

While many of the common vectors contain strong viral promoters for driving transgene expression, the characteristics of the target cell can play a role in the choice of enhancer or promoter elements used. Of the promoters in the pLN-series vectors, the viral LTR is most active in rodent cells whereas the CMV promoter seems to be stronger in primate and human cells. The SV40 promoter appears to be less efficient than either the LTR or CMV promoters (Palmer et al., 1987, 1989; Hock et al., 1989). Many vectors are downregulated following transplantation in some cell types. Cellular promoters that are active in the cells of interest may improve expression; however, it is difficult to predict the expression phenotype of modified vector designs *a priori*.

Vector designs generally insert transgenes or promoter elements into the location previously occupied by the viral protein-encoding genes; however, several unconventional formats expand the versatility of the retroviral vector systems. For example, sequences placed within the R or U5 region of the 5′ viral LTR are duplicated during reverse transcription and the resulting proviral genome contains two copies of the inserted gene, one in each LTR (Faustinella et al., 1994; Hantzopoulous et al., 1989; Sullenger et al., 1990a, b) (Fig. 19.1H). As both LTRs are active, both copies of the gene are transcribed and translated. Another interesting design eliminates internal promoters and uses internal ribosome entry sites or IRES elements (Morgan et al., 1992; Ghattas et al., 1991; Adam et al., 1991) (Fig. 19.1F). These elements direct assembly of ribosomes at the IRES site within the mRNA as well as the normally used 5′ cap structure. This allows a second open reading frame to be efficiently translated from a polycistronic message. Promoters used in retroviruses need not be limited to those transcribed by RNA polymerase II. One interesting design utilizes a tRNA *pol* III promoter within the LTR to drive expression of an RNA intended to inhibit HIV replication (Faustinella et al., 1994; Sullenger et al., 1990a, b).

A word of caution for those interested in inserting or substituting sequences in the LTR: modifications placed outside of the transcribed region of the plasmid will not be transferred to target cells. In some instances, this phenomenon can be put to practical use. Deletion of the promoter elements in the plasmid 3′ LTR results in a vector that integrates into target cells as a promoterless provirus. Subsequently, transgene sequences are only expressed when integrated downstream of an active cellular promoter (Flamant et al., 1993; Soriano et al., 1991; Marty et al., 1990; Friedrich and Soriano, 1991). LTR sequences that are carried into target cells are the U5 region of the 5′ LTR, the U3 region of the 3′ LTR and both R regions. Sequences that are to be functional only in the original plasmid should be placed in the 5′ U3 or 3′ U5 regions.

2 MATERIALS AND EQUIPMENT

2.1 Plasmid Vectors

(1) pLNSX, pLNCX, pLXSN (Miller and Rosman, 1989).
(2) pLHDSX, pLHDCX, pLXSHD (Stockschlaeder et al., 1991).
(3) Any equivalent retroviral plasmid.

2.2 Tissue Culture Reagents

(1) Amphotropic PA317 packaging cells, ATCC#CRL 9078, ECACC# 89032007 (Miller and Buttimore, 1986).
(2) Ecotropic Ψ2 packaging cells (Mann et al., 1983).
(3) Immortal mouse fibroblast line, NIH 3T3, ATCC #CRL 1658.
(4) Dulbecco's Modified Eagle's Medium (DMEM), containing 4.5 g/l glucose.
(5) DMEM/F12 (1:1).
(6) Phosphate-buffered saline (PBS), sterile filtered.
(7) Fetal bovine serum.
(8) N2 tissue culture supplement (Gibco/BRL).
(9) 100 × penicillin/streptomycin supplement (Gibco/BRL).
(10) Amphotericin B (Fungizone) (Gibco/BRL).
(11) Trypsin/EDTA solution (Gibco/BRL).
(12) Tissue-culture dishes, 60 mm and 100 mm diameter.
(13) Geneticin (G418-sulfate) (Gibco/BRL).
(14) Polybrene (Sigma).
(15) Glass coverslips.
(16) Poly-L-ornithine, M_r 30 000–70 000 (Sigma).
(17) Mouse laminin (Gibco/BRL).
(18) FGF-2 (basic FGF) (Gibco/BRL).

3 THE PROTOCOLS

Ex vivo gene transfer protocols proceed in three phases. First, the vector is designed and constructed using standard plasmid subcloning techniques. Second, a clonal virus producing line is generated and characterized. Finally, virus from this producer line is used to transduce the grafting population of target cells which are then transplanted directly or further propagated *in vitro* to characterize transgene expression. As the methods for subcloning cDNAs into plasmids are well described elsewhere (Sambrook et al., 1989), the following protocols skip the "cut-and-paste" portion of vector design and begin with the generation and characterization of virus-producing cell lines.

Protocol #101: Generation of Retrovirus-producing Cell Lines

Culture Ψ2 cells in high glucose DMEM (4.5 g/l) containing either 10% fetal bovine serum or 10% newborn calf serum. Make sure the cells are fully adapted to the medium and serum being used. PA317 cells are grown in high glucose DMEM containing 10% fetal bovine serum. Antibiotic supplements are optional.

Day 1: Prepare Ψ2 Packaging Cells for Transfection

Plate 5×10^5 log phase Ψ2 cells per 60 mm plate, one plate per plasmid plus one negative control plate.

Day 2: Transfect Ψ2

Transfect the Ψ2 cells using any common transfection protocol. We typically use lipofection or calcium phosphate precipitation (SEE CHAPTER 2). Leave the negative control plate untransfected.

Day 3: Plate PA317 Targets for Transduction

(1) Replace medium on transfected Ψ2 with 4 ml fresh medium.
(2) Plate 5×10^5 PA317 cells per 60 mm plate, two plates per Ψ2 transfection plus one negative control.

Day 4: Harvest Ψ2 Virus and Transduce PA317 Cells

(1) Collect medium from Ψ2 and remove cells by centrifugation for 5 min at 5000*g* or by filtering through a 0.45 μm filter.
(2) Replace medium on PA317 targets with 4 ml fresh medium containing 4μg/ml polybrene. Polybrene increases the transduction efficiency roughly tenfold.
(3) Add 100 μl or 1 ml of cell-free Ψ2 supernatant to the medium on the PA317 cells and swirl to mix.
(4) To determine the success of the transfection, treat Ψ2 cells with trypsin and re-plate 10% of the cells in a 60 mm dish in 4 ml medium containing 500μg/ml active concentration of G418. Likewise, plate cells from the negative control plate (non-transfected) into drug to ensure that the selection conditions are working.

Day 5: Passage Transduced PA317 Cells into Selective Medium

Treat PA317 cells with trypsin and re-plate 10% into a 100 mm dish using 10 ml G418-containing medium as above.

Days 6–14: Monitor Cultures for Drug-resistant Colonies and Isolate Individual Clones of Transduced PA317 Cells

(1) Observe cultures for cell survival and replace medium with fresh G418 medium as needed to reduce cellular debris.
(2) Determine the approximate number of G418-resistant colonies in the Ψ2 and PA317 dishes. If the colonies are big enough, they can be seen by eye; otherwise, an estimate under low-power magnification is sufficient.

(3) Pick colonies of PA317 cells from a plate that has well separated colonies and transfer into a 24-well dish. A simple isolation method involves the use of glass cloning rings. Briefly, coat the end of a cloning ring with silicon high-vacuum grease and place the ring over an individual colony. Place a drop of trypsin into each cloning ring and transfer detached cells into individual wells of a 24-well dish.

Day 15: Characterize PA317 Clones for Later Use

(1) Determine the viral titer produced by each clone (see Protocol #102). Titers lower than 10^4 colony forming units/ml (c.f.u./ml) are marginally useful. Many vector constructs will commonly produce titers of 10^5 c.f.u./ml, although titers of 10^6 c.f.u./ml or more can be generated with some vectors. Eliminate low-titer clones and continue with characterization.
(2) Check for gross rearrangements of the vector sequences by Southern blot analysis. Restriction enzymes that cut only in the LTRs (e.g. *Kpn*I, *Xba*I, *Sac*I) allow the overall size of the vector to be evaluated. This verification is often sufficient if the vector functions as expected.
(3) Confirm that the gene of interest is being expressed in cells transduced by PA317 virus. Evaluation of the target cells by Northern analysis will determine if the transgene is being transcribed and Western blots or bioassays will determine if the protein is being produced.
(4) Screen supernatant from PA317 clones for the presence of helper virus. Helper virus can be generated through recombination between the vector plasmid sequences and the viral protein-encoding sequences of the packaging cell line (Otto et al., 1994; Miller and Buttimore, 1986; Danos and Mulligan, 1988).

Protocol#102. Measuring Retroviral Titer

Day 1: Prepare Packaging Cells

Plate 5 × 10^5 packaging cells (Ψ2 or PA317) into a 60 mm dish.

Day 2: Prepare Target Cells

(1) Plate 5 × 10^5 3T3 cells into a 60 mm dish, two dishes per clone to be titered plus one dish for a positive control (to be transduced with an aliquot of virus with known titer) and one dish for a negative control which receives no virus.
(2) Replace the medium on the producer cells with fresh medium.

Day 3: Harvest Virus and Transduce Target Cells

(1) Harvest virus containing medium from producer cells and remove floating cells by centrifugation (5000*g* for 5 min) or filtration (0.45 μm syringe filter). Virus-containing medium can be frozen in small aliquots at −70°C and thawed once with no loss of titer.
(2) Replace the medium on 3T3 cells with fresh medium containing 4 mg/ml polybrene. Add 0.1 μl or 10 μl of virus containing medium to each 3T3 dish and swirl to distribute. A 1:10 or 1:100 dilution of supernatant can be used to accurately measure volumes equivalent to 0.1 μl of neat supernatant.

Day 4: Passage Transduced 3T3 Cells into Selective Medium

Treat 3T3 cells with trypsin and redistribute 10% of the cells into a 60 mm dish containing 4 ml medium supplemented with 500 μg/ml active G418. Plate the remaining 90% of the cells onto a 100 mm dish in 10 ml G418-containing medium.

Days 5–12: Monitor Cells for Survival and Colony Formation

(1) Replace medium with fresh G418-containing medium as needed to remove cellular debris and continue selection until all cells on the negative control plate are dead.

(2) Fix and stain colonies with any agent that will facilitate visualization. A brief rinse with PBS and subsequent incubation with a solution of Coomassie blue (Brilliant Blue-G, 1 g/l, Sigma) in 75% methanol/5% acetic acid/20% H_2O works well. Allow colonies to stain for 5–10 min and rinse plates gently with tap water.

Protocol #103: Detection of Replication-competent Helper Retrovirus (Neo Marker Rescue Assay)

Day 1: Prepare Marker Cells

SEE SECTION 4.3 for suitable "marker" cells. Plate 10^5 marker cells into a 60 mm dish. Plate one dish per PA317 clone to be assayed plus one dish as a negative control.

Day 2: Transduce Marker Cells with Supernatant from PA317 Clones to be Tested

(1) Replace the medium on the marker cells with fresh medium containing 4μg/ml polybrene.
(2) Add 1 ml of cell-free supernatant from a PA317 producer clone to the marker cells and incubate overnight. PA317 supernatant should be prepared as for measuring titers. We often assay titers and screen for helper virus using the same viral preparation (either fresh or frozen).

Days 3–14: Passage Transduced Marker Cells

Do not select the transduced marker cells as they are already G418 resistant. Instead, passage them as needed to maintain the cells at log phase and at relatively high density. This improves the spread of replicating helper virus throughout the culture.

Day 14: Measure G418 Titers on Transduced Marker Cells

Treat the infected marker cells as if they were virus-producing cell lines and determine the titers on naive 3T3 cells. The generation of G418-resistant 3T3 colonies indicates the presence of helper virus.

Protocol #104: Isolation of Rat Dermal Fibroblasts (Cell Outgrowth Method)

Day 1: Culture Initiation

(1) Shave skin over the biopsy site, scrub with iodine solution and rinse with 70% ethanol. Allow to air dry.
(2) Remove a small section of full-thickness skin (1–2 cm^2) with scissors or scalpel blade.
(3) Rinse the skin in PBS supplemented with antibiotic solution.
(4) Remove fatty connective tissue from the underside of the skin.
(5) Dice the skin into pieces smaller than 1 mm^2 with scissors or a scalpel blade, place 10–20 of these pieces under a glass coverslip in a tissue culture dish.
(6) Carefully instill culture medium under the coverslip, adding just enough to wet the bottom of the dish. If the top of the coverslip is kept dry and the depth of medium is slightly lower than the top of the coverslip, surface tension will hold the coverslip down and cell outgrowth will nucleate more rapidly.

Days 2–14: Monitor Cell Outgrowth

(1) Incubate the tissues for 1–2 weeks, replacing medium every 2–4 days. After several days the glass coverslips may be well adhered to the tissues and larger volumes of medium can be used with less frequent feedings.
(2) Monitor cell outgrowth and when small areas of cell monolayers are well established on either the glass coverslip or the underlying tissue culture dish, treat with trypsin and redistribute the

cells onto a new tissue culture dish. Consider this passage 1. The tissue can be discarded or replated under coverslips to recover additional cells.

Protocol #105: Fetal Hippocampal Neuron Cultures

This protocol requires knowledge of fetal rat brain anatomy as well as skill in fetal brain removal and microdissection. These methods are described in detail elsewhere (Shahar et al., 1993; SEE ALSO CHAPTERS 6 AND 14) and the following protocol starts with a dissected hippocampal formation from a fetal brain. Culture medium consists of DMEM/F12 (1:1) containing 1 × N2 supplement and 20 ng/ml FGF-2. The cells are maintained in a 5% CO_2 humidified atmosphere at 37°C.

Day 1: Dissect and Prepare Hippocampal Cells

(1) Carefully remove meninges and vascular adhesions from the hippocampal formation and gently dice into small pieces using a sharp scalpel or scissors. Resuspend in 5 ml DMEM/F12 containing N2 supplement.
(2) Very gently pass the tissue through a flame-polished Pasteur pipette (pass the end of a glass Pasteur pipette through a flame to round the sharp edges and to introduce a slight restriction at the end of the pipette). Use increasingly smaller restrictions at the end of the pipette until the tissues are dissociated into a suspension of single cells.
(3) Determine the number of viable trypan blue excluding cells and plate 3–5 × 10^6 cells per 100 mm polyornithine–laminin coated dish in complete culture medium. Sufficient viable cells should be recovered for approximately one 100 mm dish per fetus.

Day 2 and Onwards: Monitor Cell Growth, Feed and Passage

(1) Replace half of the medium with fresh N2 supplemented medium containing twice the normal concentration of FGF-2 (40 ng/ml) every 3–4 days. Avoid dislodging the poorly adherent cells.
(2) Passage the cells as they reach confluence by gently rinsing with warm PBS and immersing them in 2 ml of warm trypsin solution for 1 min or less. Remove the trypsin and dislodge the less adherent neuronal cells by tapping the plate and dilute the floating cells in 4 ml DMEM/F12. Some of the more adherent non-neural cells will remain attached. Pellet the cells by centrifugation at 700*g* for 5–10 min.
(3) Resuspend the cells in several ml DMEM/F12 and pellet again to completely remove the trypsin. Re-plate the cells in fresh DMEM/F12 containing N2 supplement and FGF-2.

Protocol #106: Coating Dishes with Poly-L-ornithine and Laminin

Tissue culture dishes or glass coverslips are coated in a two-step process: first with poly-L-ornithine, and then laminin.

Day 1: Poly-L-ornithine Coating

Dissolve poly-L-ornithine in sterile double-distilled water to a final concentration of 10 μg/ml (use 50 μg/ml if coating glass) and cover the bottom of the tissue culture dish (about 3–4 ml per 100 mm dish). Leave at room temperature overnight.

Day 2: Laminin Coating

(1) Wash the poly-L-ornithine coated dish twice with sterile double-distilled water.
(2) Dilute laminin to a final concentration of 5 μg/ml in sterile PBS and cover the bottom of the dish. Leave in a humidified incubator at 37°C overnight.

Day 3: Rinse and Store Coated Dishes

Rinse the dishes twice with sterile PBS. Do not allow the dishes to dry. Use immediately or freeze at −20°C with PBS covering the bottom of the dish.

Protocol #107: Transducing Cells for Transplantation with Retrovirus

The best gene transfer efficiencies are observed when the target cells are at log phase and cell density is just subconfluent.

Day 1: Prepare Target Cells

Plate dermal fibroblasts at approximately 10^6 cells per 100 mm dish. Plate fetal neurons at approximately 5×10^6 cells per 100 mm dish. Include a negative control plate for the selection step.

Day 2: Transduce Target Cells

Replace the medium on the target cells with fresh medium containing 4μg/ml polybrene and add approximately 10% volume cell-free virus-containing medium prepared as if for titering. Swirl the dishes to distribute the virus.

Day 3: Select Transduced Cells with G418-containing Medium

Passage fibroblasts into four 100 mm dishes using G418-containing medium (400 μg/ml, active concentration).

Neurons may either be passaged as above into two dishes (rather than four) or selected *in situ* by replacing the medium with fresh medium containing G418 (100 μg/ml).

Day 4 Onwards: Monitor and Passage as Needed

Monitor cell survival and passage transduced cells as needed to keep cells at log phase during selection. Non-transduced cells do not die when the cultures are dense and cells are stationary. Continue selection for 7–14 days and confirm that the selective conditions were sufficient to kill all non-transduced cells in the negative control population.

Protocol #108: Intracranial Transplantation

Many of the methods used for stereotactic injections have been reviewed in detail elsewhere (Kawaja et al., 1991; Gage and Fisher, 1991; Gage et al., 1990a). The following protocol covers specific details regarding cell preparation and suggested graft sizes and volumes.

(1) For either fibroblasts or neurons, rinse the cells with warm PBS and treat with warm trypsin solution just long enough to generate a single-cell suspension. Tap the dish to dislodge all cells.
(2) Add two volumes of PBS containing 4.5 g/l glucose (PBS-G) and pellet the cells by centrifugation at 700*g* for 5 min. Resuspend and pellet the cells twice more using PGS-G to remove the last traces of trypsin.
(3) Resuspend the cells at a final concentration of 50 000–100 000 cells per μl in PBS-G. Keep the cell suspensions at room temperature.

Prepare the Rat

(1) Anesthetize the animal by intraperitoneal or intramuscular injection. We use a mixture of ketamine, xylezine and acepromazine. Consult the institutional veterinarian for recommended doses and administration routes.

(2) Shave the hair from the top of the head using electric clippers and decontaminate the skin with iodine solution.
(3) Apply ophthalmic ointment to the eyes to prevent drying of the cornea and subsequent loss of visual acuity (boric acid or mithramycin ophthalmic ointments are commonly used). This step is critical if vision-dependent behavior is to be monitored after grafting.
(4) Place the animal into a Kopf stereotactic device or equivalent. For most applications using 170–200 g rats, we set the nose bar to −3.3 mm relative to the ear bars.
(5) Open a skin incision along the rostral–caudal midline of the head. One bold cut is better than several small slices. Separate the skin laterally and anchor with hemostats or small clips to provide an open field over the skull.
(6) Make both lateral and longitudinal incisions (a cross) in the translucent connective tissue over the skull and expose the bone by swabbing with sterile gauze or cotton swab.
(7) Position a Hamilton syringe over the recommended distance from bregma to locate the injection site.
(8) Drill a small hole in the skull at the tip of the syringe using a small caliber burr and Dremel tool. Carefully drill to expose the dura, making sure that the hole allows clear needle access past the bone.
(9) Resuspend the cells by flicking the tube with a finger and draw up the desired volume of cells into the syringe.
(10) Lower the syringe to touch dura and then lower evenly into the brain to the lowest desired coordinate.
(11) Inject the cells at a rate of 1 μl/min. Raise the syringe to the next coordinate and inject again if needed. We generally make multiple deposits of 0.5–1 μl along a short injection tract and rarely exceed 3–5 μl total per tract. We have found that deposits of 0.5–1.0 μl at a density of 50–100 000 cells/μl provide optimum survival of the grafted cells. Injection rates faster than 1 μl/min can induce a displacement injury at the injection site.
(12) Raise the syringe 1 mm above the last coordinate and wait 2 min to allow the injection volumes to be absorbed. This prevents ejection of the cell suspension along the needle tract.
(13) Raise the syringe and remove the animal.
(14) Apply a generous dusting of antibiotic powder to the open incision. Close the wound with wound clips and return the animal to a clean cage. Monitor the animal's recovery during the next 24 h.

4 NOTES AND TROUBLESHOOTING

4.1 On Protocol #101: Generation of Retrovirus-producing Cell Lines

The goal of this protocol is to generate clonal amphotropic PA317 packaging cell lines by first transiently transfecting ecotropic Ψ2 packaging cells and then using the transiently expressed ecotropic virus to transduce PA317 cells (Miller and Buttimore, 1986). If permanent cell lines producing ecotropic vector are desired, reverse the Ψ2 and PA317 cells at each step. Comparisons should be made between the newly constructed and the parental plasmids. Although many plasmids can be used in these cell lines, the pLN-series (Miller and Rosman, 1989) have been specifically designed to prevent helper virus formation when used in the PA317 packaging cell line. Accordingly, Protocols 101–104 discuss generation of packaging lines using G418 selection for the *neo* gene carried by the pLN-series plasmids.

The presence of numerous drug-resistant Ψ2 colonies indicates successful transfection. Drug-resistant colonies in transduced PA317 cells indicate successful vector packaging and integration. The control vector, for example pLN, pLXSN, pLNCX or pLNSX, should give approximately 50–100 G418-resistant colonies in the plate containing 10% of the PA317 cells transduced with 1 ml of cell-free Ψ2 medium (equal to a rough titer of 500–1000 c.f.u./ml from the transient expression of the plasmid in Ψ2 cells).

4.1.1 What to Look for by Southern Analysis

Southern blots are used to determine if the integrated provirus contains large deletions or insertions. Genomic DNA prepared from a clone with an acceptable titer can be digested with restriction enzymes that cut once in each LTR. There should be a single band when the blot is probed for *neo* sequences and it should be of the size predicted by the plasmid map. For comparison, a control band can be generated from about 15 pg of the vector plasmid digested with the same enzymes. Those using pLN series vectors should be aware that some restriction sites in the 5′ LTR will differ between the plasmid and the integrated provirus due to the presence of MoMSV (rather than MoMLV) sequences in the plasmid 5′ LTR that are not transcribed and therefore not present in the integrated proviral DNA. An *Xba*I site present only in the plasmid 3′ LTR becomes duplicated during reverse transcription and is present in both integrated proviral LTRs.

4.1.2 What to Look for by Northern Analysis

Generally the size of a given transcript can be predicted from the plasmid map by calculating the distance from the +1 site to the polyadenylation signal and then adding 200–400 bases for the poly-A tail. There should be one genomic LTR transcript: any additional transcripts are dependent on splicing or internal promoters. For example, vectors similar to LXSN, LNSX and LNCX would produce two transcripts (Fig. 19.1E)—the LTR transcript and the transcript from the internal promoter. Although transgene sequences placed downstream of the internal promoter would be present on both transcripts, only the internal promoter transcript contributes to the production of the downstream open reading frame. With few exceptions (e.g. messages containing IRES elements; Fig. 19.1F), only the first coding sequence on a transcript will be translated. Inclusion of RNA from non-transduced cells helps to differentiate between endogenous and viral-derived messages. Avoid including viral sequences in the probe: these will hybridize with a variety of cellular transcripts in rodent cells and generate misleading bands. Significant discrepancy from the predicted transcript size suggests either rearrangements in the provirus (which can be confirmed by Southern blot) or the presence of cryptic splice sites or polyadenylation signals.

4.1.3 Why Two Packaging Cell Lines?

Producer lines can be generated simply by transfecting packaging cells and isolating virus-producing clones. However, transfected plasmid DNA often integrates as multiple rearranged copies and clones isolated in this manner often produce mixtures of virions containing not only the expected vector genome but also rearranged genomes. Infecting a second packaging cell line with limiting dilutions of the rescued virus provides clones containing a single integrated proviral genome that can be confirmed as unrearranged and functional. Two cell lines of different tropisms are used because the envelope protein produced by each packaging cell line saturates the receptors for vectors of the same tropism. Transduction of packaging cells with vectors of the same tropism is more than 1000 times less efficient than transduction with vectors of a different tropism.

4.2 On Protocol #102: Measuring Retroviral Titer

Several methods are available for measuring titer (Miller and Buttimore, 1986; Weiss et al., 1985; Mann et al., 1983) and, although each method may provide slightly different absolute values, consistent use of a single method allows useful comparisons to be made between vectors generated within a given laboratory.

4.2.1 Calculating Titers

Titers are traditionally calculated by dividing the number of drug resistant colonies produced per milliliter of virus used. This value is corrected for the dilution of cells plated into G418. For example, if 30 colonies were generated when 3T3 cells were transduced with 0.1 μl of virus and then passaged 1:10 into G418, the calculation would be (30 colonies/0.0001 ml) $\times$ 10 = 3 $\times$ 10^6 c.f.u./ml. For a single vector design, titers from individual clones can range over many orders of magnitude (from 10^7 to less than 1 c.f.u./ml). Titers below 10^4 c.f.u./ml are not very useful because the transduction efficiency in primary cells will be quite low. Titers above 10^7 may indicate the presence of a replication-competent helper virus.

4.2.2 Short-cuts for Screening Numerous Packaging Cell Clones

After clones of PA317 cells are transferred into 24-well dishes, virus can be harvested from each well as it becomes confluent by exposing a fresh 1 ml aliquot of medium to the cells overnight. This medium can be immediately used to transduce 3T3 cells or frozen at -70°C until medium has been collected from several clones. Although the titers will not be accurate, low-titer clones can be rapidly eliminated and the remaining clones can be subsequently evaluated in more detail.

4.3 On Protocol #103: Detection of Replication-competent Helper Retrovirus (Neo Marker Rescue Assay)

Recombination between the retroviral vector and packaging sequences will occasionally generate replication-competent helper virus (Otto et al., 1994; Miller and Buttimore, 1986; Danos and Mulligan, 1988). When present in grafted cells, this helper virus can cause the spread of the transgene sequences to the surrounding host tissues. This not only can inflate the apparent production of transgene product but complicates the evaluation of engraftment and survival of the engineered cells.

The marker rescue assay is based on the ability of helper virus to package a replication-defective vector RNA and transfer it to a naive target cell (Miller and Rosman, 1989; Danos and Mulligan, 1988). Any clonal line of 3T3 cells transduced with a helper-free vector containing a selectable marker can be used for this assay. LN or LNCX containing 3T3 cells work well. Test that these "marker cells" have not been contaminated with helper virus by measuring titer from the marker cells as if they were packaging cells, e.g. use 1 ml of cell-free supernatant from the marker cells to "infect" a naive population of 3T3 cells and then select for G418-resistant cells. There should be no colonies (less than 1 c.f.u./ml).

G418-resistant colonies detected in transduced 3T3 cells indicate helper virus was present in the original PA317 producer clone. The absence of colonies demonstrates that there was less than one helper virus per ml of the original PA317 supernatant.

While the marker rescue method detects helper virus of several tropisms, packaging cell lines contain defective genomes from a wide variety of retroviruses and it is possible that activation or recombination of endogenous viral sequences could generate helper virus that is not able to infect rodent cells and would not be detected in the marker rescue assay (e.g. xenotropic virus—Weiss et al., 1985; Battini et al., 1992). If this possibility poses a safety issue, helper virus detection methods that use non-rodent cells can be used in addition to the marker rescue assay (Anderson et al., 1993; Muenchau et al., 1990; Danos and Mulligan, 1988, Miller and Rosman, 1989; Miller et al., 1986).

4.4 On Protocol #104: Isolation of Rat Dermal Fibroblasts (Cell Outgrowth Method)

If using syngeneic animal strains, such as Fischer 344 rats, a single animal can be killed and the skin used in multiple experiments. If an outbred strain is to be used, autologous cells can be recovered from a small biopsy sample from an anesthetized animal. The culture medium used for primary fibroblasts is high-glucose DMEM supplemented with 10% FBS, penicillin/streptomycin and Fungizone. Cells are maintained at 37°C in a humidified 10% CO_2 atmosphere.

Cell cultures from young animals can be established more readily than those from older animals. Cell outgrowth from aged animal tissues tends to be slow and there may be a significant crisis stage, from which few cells survive. Cells from newborn or fetal skin can be recovered easily and should be used if the model is not intended to represent autologous adult-derived cell transplantation. Cells from young adult animals can be expanded for up to 10–15 passages with a 2–4-fold dilution at each passage. Cells may undergo a mild crisis at 2–4 passages, after which a subpopulation of cells will rapidly recover and continue to proliferate. Freeze stocks of the earliest passages for later use. Extensive passaging may select for rare spontaneously immortalized cells which, if used in grafting experiments, may not accurately represent the survival or transgene expression characteristics of early passage normal diploid fibroblasts.

4.5 On Protocol #105: Fetal Hippocampal Neuron Cultures

Several cell morphologies will be represented in the primary plating and proliferative populations should be apparent within the first week. Neuronal progenitors are selectively cultured from this mixture by differential trypsinization and rapid growth in the presence of FGF-2. These cultures initially grow at a moderate rate but will grow very rapidly when a critical minimum density is reached. Doubling time of established cultures is typically 36 h. The neuronal progenitors seem to be more sensitive to neglect than the non-neuronal cells and require conscientious feeding. Cultures can be evaluated via immunocytochemical techniques for the presence of neurons and/or glia (Bock et al., 1980; Iwanaga et al., 1989; Isobe et al., 1989; Yang et al., 1994ab; Walker et al., 1984; Hansson et al., 1984). Typical markers for glial lineages include galactocerebroside and glial fibrillary acidic protein. Commonly used markers for neurons include neuron-specific enolase and neurofilament proteins. Immature cells of the oligodendroglial lineage often express ganglioside markers recognized by the A2B5 and/or O4 monoclonal antibodies (for a variety of characterization strategies see Ray and Gage, 1994; Sensenbrenner et al., 1994; Kilpatrick and Bartlett, 1993; Mayer et al., 1993ab; Ray et al., 1993; Shahar et al., 1993; Louis et al., 1992; Noble and Wolswijk, 1992; Reynolds et al., 1992; Reynolds and Weiss, 1992; Wren et al., 1992; Noble et al., 1990; Perraud et al., 1990).

4.6 On Protocol #107: Transducing Cells for Transplantation

Under the conditions outlined in this protocol, vector preparations with titers above 10^5 c.f.u./ml should transduce roughly 10–50% of a fibroblast population and 1–10% of a neuronal population. Although higher concentrations of virus can be used, elevated concentrations of viral envelope can cause cell fusion. The resulting cell loss negates the potential gains in increased transduction efficiency. Repeated exposures to virus over several days may increase transduction efficiency; however, passaging may be required to maintain the target cells at log phase and, in the case of neurons, the repeated exposure to serum can encourage astrocyte proliferation.

Continual maintenance of the transduced cells in G418 can reduce the clonal diversity of a population since cells expressing higher levels of the *neo* gene product will grow more readily than those less resistant to G418 (Paludan et al., 1989). This can pose problems if transgene expression is to be compared between vectors. Since vector expression is influenced by both cellular flanking sequences and elements within the vector, expression should be evaluated in bulk oligoclonal populations where position effects are averaged over many integration sites. This will more accurately reflect vector intrinsic expression characteristics.

4.7 On Protocol #108: Intracranial Transplantation

Most animals should begin to recover within 2 h of injecting anesthetic. If for some reason the animal has not fully recovered by the next morning, it may need hydration by subcutaneous injection of saline or dextrose solution until fully recovered. Consult a veterinarian for appropriate volumes and dosing schedules.

4.8 Common Questions

4.8.1 What does "Titer" Measure and When Can Selecting for High Titer be Problematic?

Virus titer is a combined measurement of (1) the number of infectious particles secreted by producer cells (which correlates most strongly with abundance of vector mRNA in producer cells), (2) the susceptibility of target cells to virus entry and integration (dependent on receptor levels and the fraction of cells undergoing mitosis while virus is present) and (3) the strength of marker gene expression in the target cells (which is dependent on the activity of the enhancer/promoter driving the selectable marker and the stability and translation efficiency of the marker transcript). If the transgene or regulatory elements introduced into a vector affect any of these aspects, it will be reflected as a relative change in titer. If a transgene sequence dramatically reduces the abundance of viral transcripts for any reason, selecting producer clones on the basis of high titer may yield only cells that contain rearranged proviruses that are missing the offending transgene sequences (Lynch et al., 1993).

4.8.2 At What Steps are Mutations or Rearrangements Most Likely to Occur?

Most mutations or rearrangements are introduced during transfection of the plasmid into the producer cells. Nicks and double strand breaks are efficiently repaired in mammalian cells. This results in integration of concatamerized, rearranged or deleted plasmid. Any rearranged mRNA containing the Ψ signal can be packaged (Aronuff and Linial, 1991; Adam and Miller, 1988) and if the LTR elements are intact, or if two LTRs are simply present on a transcript that reads through several concatamers, the RNA can be reverse-transcribed and integrated into a target cell's genome.

The second most likely step at which mutations may occur is during reverse transcription. Reverse transcriptase often undergoes illegitimate strand transfer events and these can lead to deletions or inclusions that interrupt the transgene sequences (Pulsinelli and Temin, 1991; Hu and Temin, 1990a, b; Zhang and Temin, 1994; Temin, 1993; Zhang and Temin 1993; Olson et al., 1992; Otto et al., 1994). In addition, MoMLV reverse transcriptase itself exhibits a relatively low fidelity in its polymerase function, with approximately one misincorporation per 10^5 bases (Bakhanashvili and Hizi, 1993; Bakhanashvili and Hizi, 1992). By extrapolation, one of every ten 10 kb vectors will contain at least one misincorporated base. Although the high rate of mutation can pose problems, careful screening of individual packaging cell clones assures that the proviral template for producing vector RNA genomes is intact and functional.

4.8.3 Why Generate a Characterized Packaging Cell Clone if Some of the Vectors in a Bulk Transfected Population are Functional?

A common and often acceptable short-cut is to transfect and directly select for bulk drug-resistant populations or clones. Often a low proportion of the drug-resistant target cells make the desired gene product due to a high frequency of rearranged vector. If transgene sequences negatively affect titer or expression of the drug resistance gene it is likely that a small number of rearranged proviruses (which are missing the offending sequence) contribute to most of the transduction events scored in the target cells. To a certain extent the relative "toxicity" of a transgene sequence is indicated by the frequency that rearranged proviral sequences are observed in target cells. This is largely due to the fact that selection for drug resistance most efficiently isolates those cells expressing the highest levels of the drug resistance gene (Paludan et al., 1989). Some sequences so severely affect accumulation of vector RNA (for example, clotting factor VIII sequences) that few, if any, G418-resistant target cells contain an intact transgene.

4.9 Problems and Possible Solutions

4.9.1 Neither the Experimental nor the Control Plasmid Produces Virus in Transfected Ψ2 Cells

The most probable cause is poor transfection efficiency. Optimize the transfection protocol or try another physical transfection method such as lipofection or electroporation.

A less likely reason for a lack of virus production is that the producer line no longer has packaging function. Cells may have been inadvertently swapped with another cell line, or genetic drift over several months or even years of passaging has selected against expression of the viral protein-encoding genes. Thaw an earlier passage of packaging cells or reorder the cells from ATCC.

4.9.2 Only the Control Vector Produces Virus in Transfected Ψ2 Cells

If the transfections are successful the transfected Ψ2 cells should be G418 resistant. If they are not, it is likely that the experimental plasmid preparation is contaminated with something that interferes with transfection or the experimental vector's transgene is directly toxic to cells. Makc sure that the cells survive transfection to rule out transgene toxicity or try a plasmid preparation from another bacterial clone to rule out small deletions or point mutations that make the *neo* gene non-functional.

If the Ψ2 cells become G418 resistant yet still produce no virus, determine if the vector's genomic RNA is made in the transfected producer cells. If this RNA is shorter than expected, check the sequence of the transgene for potentially incompatible elements such as polyadenylation signals or cryptic splice acceptor sites that may interfere with packaging or subsequent reverse transcription. Redesign the subcloning strategy or alter the offending sequence via site-specific mutation.

If the genomic mRNA is the correct size but low in abundance it is probable that the introduced elements downregulate transcription, destabilize the mRNA, or encode a protein incompatible with cell survival, so that only cells expressing low levels of transgene product survive. If the transgene sequences destabilize the vector's genomic RNA (shorten the half-life), inverting the transgene expression cassette within the vector may remove the destabilizing effect. This places the transgene's antisense strand (rather than the sense strand) into the vector's genomic RNA. Although viral titers may improve, the transgene transcript itself may still be unstable in target cells and may yield very little transgene product.

4.9.3 G418-resistant PA317 Clones were Successfully Generated and the Virus Confers G418 Resistance to Target Cells but Detectable Protein Product is Expressed from the Transgene

Confirm that the integrated proviral sequences are unrearranged and that the transgene mRNA is present and of the expected size in the target cells. If mRNA is detectable by Northern analysis, confirm that the original transgene sequences were functional by evaluating protein production from a transiently transfected cDNA carried in a simple plasmid expression vector. If the retroviral vector makes RNA and the plasmid expression vector makes protein, a minor defect is probably present in the vector design or there is a mutation in the transgene coding sequences. Test an alternate bacterial clone of the vector plasmid and re-evaluate the subcloning strategies to confirm that the transgene's start codon is present and retains a consensus translational initiation context (Kozak, 1986, 1987, 1991, 1992). Also confirm that the cloning strategy did not introduce upstream ATGs in good "Kozak" context.

4.9.4 None of the Cells Die under Selection, Even the Non-transduced Cells

Confirm that the selective drug is the correct drug for the model system. It is surprising how frequently this problem has been traced to the use of gentamicin sulfate or neomycin sulfate instead of the correct neomycin analog geneticin (G418) sulfate.

4.9.5 An Originally High-titer Packaging Cell Clone Now has Reduced Titers

The most probable cause is that continuous culturing for many cell generations has produced some genetic drift in the once clonal population. This may select cells that have lost vector expression or packaging function and can often be corrected by reselecting for the vector's drug resistance marker. Alternatively, the packaging cells can simply be subcloned to isolate cells that are still functional.

4.9.6 A Once Functional Packaging Cell Clone Retains the Ability to Confer G418 Resistance to Target Cells but Few Target Cells now Express the Transgene

This problem is not common but continual maintenance of packaging cells in G418 may increase the likelihood of enriching for cells that contain a mutant vector. Although resistant to infection by their own virus, packaging cells are continually reinfected at a low rate. Occasionally one of these newly integrated genomes deletes a portion of the transgene sequence. If the loss of transgene sequences improves the expression of the *neo* gene product, continual drug selection can rapidly enrich the culture for cells expressing the mutant vector sequences. Maintaining producer clones in the absence of selection will avoid this problem and, if it is suspected that vector sequences have been lost from some of the packaging cells, a brief period of selection in G418 should be sufficient to eliminate non-expressing cells. Frequent reinitiation of cultures from early passage frozen stocks can also prevent gradual changes in packaging cell clones.

4.9.7 The Transgene Product is Detected in Transduced Target Cells but is Absent in Later Passages of the Same Cells or Several Weeks After Grafting

Unfortunately, this is common with many vector systems (not only retroviral vectors). To a large extent the phenomenon can be attributed to selection for low expression levels (i.e. cells expressing less transgene product grow more quickly or more readily survive grafting) or to gradual transcriptional downregulation. It is difficult to distinguish between these two processes. If differential growth selects for lower expression, grafting early passage transduced cells can avoid some loss of expression. If the transgenes are transcriptionally downregulated, the only cure is to develop vectors that remain transcriptionally active in specific target cell populations.

Post-grafting downregulation could be due to changes in the local graft environment (e.g. wound healing) or to cell-intrinsic changes such as differentiation or transition from a proliferative to quiescent state. Many experimental approaches address these issues and, although transcriptional downregulation is often a suggested culprit (Palmer et al., 1991; Scharfmann et al., 1991; Dai et al., 1992), non-CNS grafts placed into immune-deficient animals are thought to express transgenes much longer than similar grafts in immune-competent animals (Palmer et al., 1989; Dai et al., 1992). This suggests that immune selection against cells overexpressing transgenes may also play a rọle in experimental outcome.

The extent to which transgene expression can be regulated in the CNS with the present vector systems remains to be seen; however, the most elegant solutions will probably involve a combination of approaches that include modifying or combining vector systems as well as developing a better understanding of regulatory sequences that function in a predictable fashion within the restricted confines of a vector genome.

REFERENCES

Adam MA; Miller AD. Identification of a signal in a murine retrovirus that is sufficient for packaging of non-retroviral RNA into virions. *Journal of Virology*, 1988, **62**:3802–6.

Adam MA; Ramesh N; Miller AD; Osborne WR. Internal initiation of translation in retroviral vectors carrying picornavirus 5′ non-translated regions. *Journal of Virology*, 1991, **65**:4985–90.

Akli S; Caillaud C; Vigne E; Stratford-Perricaudet LD; Poenaru L; Perricaudet M; Kahn A; Peschanski MR. Transfer of a foreign gene into the brain using adenovirus vectors. *Nature Genetics*, 1993, **3**:224–8.

Alton E; Geddes D. A mixed message for cystic fibrosis gene therapy. *Nature Genetics*, 1994, **8**:8–9

Anderson WF. Human gene therapy. *Science*, 1992, **256**:808–13.

Anderson WF; McGarrity GJ; Moen RC. Report to the NIH Recombinant DNA Advisory Committee on murine replication-competent retrovirus (RCR) assays. *Human Gene Therapy*, 1993, **4**:311–21.

Aronoff R; Linial M. Specificity of retroviral RNA packaging. *Journal of Virology*, 1991, **65**:71–80.

Bakhanashvili M; Hizi A. Fidelity of the RNA-dependent DNA synthesis exhibited by the reverse transcriptases of human immunodeficiency virus types 1 and 2 and of murine leukemia virus: mispair extension frequencies. *Biochemistry*, 1992, **31**:9393–8.

Bakhanashvili M; Hizi A. The fidelity of the reverse transcriptases of human immunodeficiency viruses and murine leukemia virus, exhibited by the mispair extension frequencies, is sequence dependent and enzyme related. *FEBS Letters*, 1993, **319**:201–5.

Bankiewicz KS; Plunkett RJ; Jacobowitz DM; Porrino L; di Porzio U; London WT; Kopin IJ; Oldfield EH. The effect of fetal mesencephalon implants on primate MPTP-induced parkinsonism. Histochemical and behavioral studies. *Journal of Neurosurgery*, 1990, **72**:231–44.

Barnes WM. Cloning and restriction map of the first part of the histidine operon of *Salmonella typhimurium*. *Journal of Bacteriology*, 1981, **147**:124–34.

Battini JL; Heard JM; Danos O. Receptor choice determinants in the envelope glycoprotein of amphotropic, xenotropic, and polytropic murine leukemia viruses. *Journal of Virology*, 1992, **66**:1468–75.

Bock E; Yavin Z; Jorgensen OS; Yavin E. Nervous system-specific proteins in developing rat cerebral cells in culture. *Journal of Neurochemistry*, 1980, **35**:1297–302.

Boris-Lawrie KA; Temin HM. Recent advances in retrovirus vector technology. *Current Opinion in Genetics and Development*, 1993, **3**:102–9.

Boris-Lawrie K; Temin HM. The retroviral vector. Replication cycle and safety considerations for retrovirus-mediated gene therapy. *Annals of the New York Academy of Sciences*, 1994, **16**:59–70.

Boviatsis EJ; Chase M; Wei MX; Tamiya T; Hurford RK Jr; Kowall NW; Tepper RI; Breakefield XO; Chiocca EA. Gene transfer into experimental brain tumors mediated by adenovirus, herpes simplex virus, and retrovirus vectors. *Human Gene Therapy*, 1994, **5**:183–91.

Caillaud C; Akli S; Vigne E; Koulakoff A; Perricaudet M; Poenaru L; Kahn A; Berwald-Netter Y. Adenoviral vectors as a gene delivery system into cultured rat neuronal and glial cells. *European Journal of Neuroscience*, 1993, **5**:1287–91.

Cepko C. Retrovirus vectors and their applications to neurobiology. *Neuron*, 1988, **1**:345–53.

Cepko CL; Ryder EF; Austin CP; Walsh C; Fekete DM. Lineage analysis using retrovirus vectors. *Methods in Enzymology*, 1993, **225**:933–60.

Chen LS; Ray J; Fisher LJ; Kawaja MD; Schinstine M; Kang UJ; Gage FH. Cellular replacement therapy for neurologic disorders: potential of genetically engineered cells. *Journal of Cellular Biochemistry*, 1991, **45**:252–7.

Chen SH; Shine HD; Goodman JC; Grossman RG; Woo SL. Gene therapy for brain tumors: regression of experimental gliomas by adenovirus-mediated gene transfer *in vivo*. *Proceedings of the National Academy of Sciences of the United States of America*, 1994, **91**:3054–7.

Chiocca EA; Choi BB; Cai WZ; DeLuca NA; Schaffer PA; DiFiglia M; Breakefield XO; Tuza RL. Transfer and expression of the *lacZ* gene in rat brain neurons mediated by herpes simplex virus mutants. *New Biologist*, 1990, **2**:739–46.

Clowes MM; Lynch CM; Miller AD; Miller DG; Osborne WR; Clowes AW. Long-term biological response of injured rat carotid artery seeded with smooth muscle cells expressing retrovirally introduce human genes. *Journal of Clinical Investigation*, 1994, **93**:644–51.

Cone RD; Mulligan RC. High-efficiency gene transfer into mammalian cells: generation of helper-free recombinant retrovirus with broad mammalian host range. *Proceedings of the National Academy of Sciences of the United States of America*, 1984, **81**:6349–53.

Cone RD; Mulligan RC. High-efficiency gene transfer into mammalian cells: Generation of helper-free recombinant retrovirus with broad mammalian host range. *Biotechnology*, 1992, **24**:420–4.

Cornetta K; Nguyen N; Morgan RA; Muenchau DD; Hartley JW; Laese RM; Anderson WF. Infection of human cells with murine amphotropic replication-competent retroviruses. *Human Gene Therapy*, 1993, **4**:579–88.

Cornetta K; Morgan RA; Gillio A; Sturm S; Baltrucki L; O'Reilly R; Anderson WF. No retroviremia or pathology in long-term follow-up of monkeys exposed to a murine amphotropic retrovirus. *Human Gene Therapy*, 1991, **2**:215–19.

Crystal RG; McElvaney NG; Rosenfeld MA; Dhu CS; et al. Administration of an adenovirus containing the human CFTR cDNA to the respiratory tract of individual with cystic fibrosis. *Nature Genetics*, 1994, **8**:42–51.

Culver KW; Van Gilder J; Link CJ; Carlstrom T; Buroker T; Yuh W; Koch K; Schabold K; Doornbas S; Wetjen B; et al. Gene therapy for the treatment of malignant brain tumors with *in vivo* tumor transduction with the herpes simplex thymidine kinase gene/ganciclovir system. *Human Gene Therapy*, 1994, **5**:343–79.

Dai Y; Roman M; Naviaux RK; Verma IM. Gene therapy via primary myoblasts: long-term expression of factor IX protein following transplantation *in vivo*. *Proceedings of the National Academy of Sciences of the United States of America*, 1992, **89**:10892–5.

Danos O; Mulligan RC. Safe and efficient generation of recombinant retroviruses with amphotropic and ecotropic host ranges. *Proceedings of the National Academy of Sciences of the United States of America*,

1988, **85** (17): 6460–4.

Davidson BL; Allen ED; Kozarsky KF; Wilson JM; Roessler BJ. A model system for *in vivo* gene transfer into the central nervous system using an adenoviral vector. *Nature Genetics*, 1993, **3**:219–23.

Dhawan J; Pan LC; Pavlath GK; Travis MA; Lanctot AM; Blau HM. Systemic delivery of human growth hormone by injection of genetically engineered myoblasts. *Science*, 1991, **254**:1509–12.

Donahue RE; Kessler SW; Bodine D; McDonagh K; Dunbar C; Goodman S; Agricola B; Byrne E; Raffeld M; Moen R; et al. Helper virus induced T cell lymphoma in non-human primate after retroviral mediated gene transfer. *Journal of Experimental Medicine*, 1992, **176**:1125–35.

Dornburg R; Temin HM. cDNA genes formed after infection with retroviral vector particles lack the hallmarks of natural processed pseudogenes. *Molecular and Cellular Biology*, 1990, **10**:68–74.

Dunnett SB. Transplantation of embryonic dopamine neurons: what we know from rats. *Journal of Neurology*, 1991a, **238**:65–74.

Dunnett SB. Towards a neural transplantation therapy for Parkinson's disease: experimental principles from animal studies. *Acta Neurochirurgica Supplementum*, 1991b, **52**:35–8.

Eglitis MA. Positive selectable markers for use with mammalian cells in culture. *Human Gene Therapy*, 1991, **2**:195–201.

Emi N; Friedmann T; Yee JK. Pseudotype formation of murine leukemia virus with the G protein of vesicular stomatitis virus. *Journal of Virology*, 1991, **65**:1202–7.

Emmerman M; Temin HM. Quantitative analysis of gene suppression in integrated retrovirus vectors. *Molecular and Cellular Biology*, 1986, **6**:792–800.

Engelhardt JF; Ye X; Doranz B; Wilson JM. Ablation of E2A in recombinant adenoviruses improves transgene persistence and decreases inflammatory response in mouse liver. *Proceedings of the National Academy of Sciences of the United States of America*, 1994, **91**:6196–200.

Ezzeddine ZD; Martuza RL; Platika D; Short MP; Malick A; Hoi B; Breakefield XO. Selective killing of glioma cells in culture and *in vivo* by retrovirus transfer of the herpes simplex virus thymidine kinase gene. *New Biologist*, 1991, **3**:608–14.

Faustinella F; Kwon H; Serrano F; Belmont JW; Caskey CT; Aguilar-Cordova E. A new family of murine retroviral vectors with extended multiple cloning sites for gene insertion. *Human Gene Therapy*, 1994, **5**:307–12.

Fink DJ; Sternberg LR; Weber PC; Mata M; Goins WF; Glorioso FC. *In vivo* expression of beta-galactosidase in hippocampal neurons by HSV-mediated gene transfer. *Human Gene Therapy*, 1992, **3**:11–19.

Fisher LJ; Gage FH. Grafting in the mammalian central nervous system. *Physiological Reviews*, 1993, **73**:583–616.

Fisher LJ; Schinstine M; Salvaterra P; Dekker AJ; Thal L; Gage FH. *In vivo* production and release of acetylcholine from primary fibroblasts genetically modified to express choline acetyltransferase. *Journal of Neurochemistry*, 1993a, **61**:1323–32.

Fisher LJ; Raymon HK; Gage FH. Cells engineered to produce acetylcholine: therapeutic potential for Alzheimer's disease. *Annals of the New York Academy of Sciences*, 1993b, **695**:278–84.

Fisher LJ; Young SJ; Tepper JM; Groves PM; Gage FH. Electrophysiological characteristics of cells within mesencephalon suspension grafts. *Neuroscience*, 1991, **40**:109–22.

Fisher LJ; Young SJ; Groves PM; Gage FH. Extracellular properties of cells within mesencephalon suspension grafts in rat striatum. *Progress in Brain Research*, 1990, **82**:473–9.

Flamant F; Aubert D; Legrand C; Cosset FL; Samarut J. Importance of 3′ non-coding sequences for efficient retrovirus-mediated gene transfer in avian cells revealed by self-inactivating vectors. *Journal of General Virology*, 1993, **74**:39–46.

Freed CR; Breeae RE; Tosenberf NL; Schneck SA; Kriek E et al. Survival of implanted fetal dopamine cells and neurologic improvement 12 to 46 months after transplantation for Parkinson's disease. *New England Journal of Medicine*, 1992, **327**:1549–55.

Freese A; Geller AI; Neve R. HSV-1 vector mediated neuronal gene delivery. Strategies for molecular neuroscience and neurology. *Biochemical Pharmacology*, 1990, **40**:2189–99.

Friedrich G; Soriano P. Promoter traps in embryonic stem cells: a genetic screen to identify and mutate developmental genes in mice. *Genes and Development*, 1991, **5**:1513–23.

Gage FH; Chen KS. Neural transplants: prospects for Alzheimer's disease. *Current Opinion in Neurology and Neurosurgery*, 1992, **5**:94–9.

Gage FH; Fisher LJ. Intracerebral grafting: a tool for the neurobiologist. *Neuron*, 1991, **6**:1–12.

Gage FH; Rosenberg MB; Tuszynski MH; Yoshida K; Armstrong DM; Hayes RC; Friedmann T. Gene therapy in the CNS: intracerebral grafting of genetically modified cells. *Progress in Brain Research*, 1990a, **86**:205–17.

Gage FH; Fisher LJ; Jinnah HA; Rosenberg MB; Tuszynski MH; Friedmann T. Grafting genetically modified cells to the brain: conceptual and technical issues. *Progress in Brain Research*, 1990b, **82**:1–10.

Gelinas R; Novak U. Retroviral vectors for the beta-globin gene that demonstrate improved titer and expression. *Annals of the New York Academy of Sciences*, 1990, **612**:427–41.

Geller AI. Influence of the helper virus on expression of beta-galactosidase from a defective HSV-1 vector, pHSVlac. *Journal of Virological Methods*, 1991a, **31**:229–38.

Geller AI. A system, using neural cell lines, to characterize HSV-1 vectors containing genes which affect neuronal physiology, or neuronal promoters. *Journal of Neuroscience Methods*, 1991b, **36**:91–103.

Geller AI; Keyomarsi K; Bryan J; Pardee AB. An efficient deletion mutant packaging system of effective herpes simplex virus vectors: potential applications to human gene therapy and neuronal physiology. *Proceedings of the National Academy of Sciences of the United States of America*, 1990, **87**:8950–4.

Ghattas IR; Sanes JR; Majors JE. The encephalomyocarditis virus internal ribosome entry site allows efficient coexpression of two genes from a recombinant retrovirus in cultured cells and in embryos. *Molecular and Cellular Biology*, 1991, **11**:5848–59.

Gilboa E; Mitra SW; Goff S; Baltimore D. A detailed model of reverse transcription and tests of crucial aspects. *Cell*, 1979, **18**:93–100.

Gritz L; Davies J. Plasmid-encoded hugromycin B resistance: the sequence of hygromycin B phosphotransferase gene and its expression in *Escherichia coli* and *Saccharomyces cerevisiae*. *Gene*, 1983, **25**:179–88.

Glorioso JC; Goins WF; Meaney CA; Fink DJ; DeLuca NA. Gene transfer to brain using herpes simplex virus vectors. *Annals of Neurology*, 1994, **35**:S28–34.

Haber DA; Heverly SM; Kiely ML; Schimke RT. Properties of an altered dihydrofolate reductase encoded by amplified genes in cultured mouse fibroblasts. *Journal of Biological Chemistry*, 1981, **256**:9501–10.

Hansson E; Ronnback L; Persson LI; Lowenthal A; Noppe M; Alling C; Karlsson B. Cellular composition of primary cultures from cerebral cortex, striatum, hippocampus, brainstem and cerebellum. *Brain Research*, 1984, **300**:9–18.

Hantzopoulous PA; Sullenger BA; Ungers G; Gilboa E. Improved gene expression upon transfer of the adenosine deaminase minigene outside the transcriptional unit of a retroviral vector. *Proceedings of the National Academy of Sciences of the United States of America*, 1989, **86**:3519–23.

Hatzoglou M; Hodgson CP; Mularo F; Hanson RW. Efficient packaging of a specific VL30 retroelement by psi 2 cells which produce MoMLV recombinant retroviruses. *Human Gene Therapy*, 1990, **1**:385–97.

Hawley TS; Sabourin LA; Hawley RG. Comparative analysis of retroviral vector expression in mouse embryonal carcinoma cells. *Plasmid*, 1989, **22**:120–31.

Ho DY; Mocarski ES; Sapolsky RM. Altering central nervous system physiology with a defective herpes simplex virus vector expressing the glucose transporter gene. *Proceedings of the National Academy of Sciences of the United States of America*, 1993, **90**:3655–9.

Hock RA; Miller AD; Osborne WR. Expression of human adenosine deaminase from various strong promoters after gene transfer into human hematopoietic cell lines. *Blood*, 1989, 74(2): 876–81.

Horellou P; Lundberg C; Le Bourdelles B; Wictorin K; Brundi J; Kalen P; Bjorklund A; Mallet J. Behavioural effects of genetically engineered cell releasing dopa and dopamine after intracerebral grafting in a rat model of Parkinson's disease. *Journal de Physiologie*, 1991, **85**:158–70.

Hu WS; Temin HM. Genetic consequences of packaging two RNA genomes on retroviral particle: pseudodiploidy and high rate of genetic recombination. *Proceedings of the National Academy of Sciences of the United States of America*, 1990a, **87**:1556–60.

Hu WS; Temin HM. Retroviral recombination and reverse transcription. *Science*, 1990b, **250**:1227–33.

Isobe T; Ichimura T; Okuyama T. Chemistry and cell biology of neuron- and glia-specific proteins. *Archives of Histology and Cytology*, 1989, **52**:25–32.

Iwanaga T; Takahashi Y; Fujita T. Immunohistochemistry of neuron-specific and glia-specific proteins. *Archives of Histology and Cytology*, 1989, **52**:13–24.

Jaffee EM; Dranoff G; Cohen LK; Hauda KM; Clift S; Marshal F; Mulligan RC; Pardoll DM. High efficiency gene transfer into primary human tumor explants without cell selection. *Cancer Research*, 1993, **53**:2221–6.

Jiao S; Wolff JA. Long-term survival of autologous muscle grafts in rat brain. *Neuroscience Letters*, 1992, **137**:207–10.

Jiao S; Gurevich V; Wolff JA. Long-term correction of rat model of Parkinson's disease gene therapy. *Nature*, 1993, **362**:450–3.

Johnson PA; Miyanohara A; Levine F; Cahill T; Friedmann T. Cytotoxicity of a replication-defective mutant of herpes simplex virus type 1. *Journal of Virology*, 1992, **66**:2952–65.

Jolly DJ; Warner JF. Retroviral vectors as vaccines and immunotherapeutics. *Seminars in Immunology*, 1990, **2**:329–39.

Kaleko M; Garcia JV; Miller AD. Persistent gene expression after retroviral gene transfer into liver cells *in vivo*. *Human Gene Therapy*, 1991, **2**:27–32.

Kang UJ; Fisher LJ; Joh TH; O'Malley KL; Gage FH. Regulation of dopamine production by genetically modified primary fibroblasts. *Journal of Neuroscience*, 1993, **13**:5203–11.

Kaplitt MG et al. Long-term gene expression and phenotypic correction using adeno-associated virus vectors in the mammalian brain. *Nature Genetics*, 1994, **8**:148–53.

Kavanaugh MP; Miller DG; Zhang W; Law W; Kozak SL; Kabat D; Miller AD. Cell-surface receptors for gibbon ape leukemia virus and amphotropic murine retrovirus are inducible sodium-dependent phosphate symporters. *Proceedings of the National Academy of Sciences of the United States of America*, 1994, **91**:7071–5.

Kawaja MD; Gage FH. Morphological and neurochemical features of cultured primary skin fibroblasts of Fischer 344 rats following striatal implantation. *Journal of Comparative Neurology*, 1992, **317**:102–16.

Kawaja MD; Fagan AM; Firestein BL; Gage FH. Intracerebral grafting of cultured autologous skin fibroblasts into the rat striatum: an assessment of graft size and ultrastructure. *Journal of Comparative Neurology*, 1991, **307**:695–706.

Kilpatrick TJ; Bartlett PF. Cloning and growth of multipotential neural precursors: requirements for proliferation and differentiation. *Neuron*, 1993, **10**:255–65.

Kim JW; Closs EI; Albritton LM; Cunningham JM. Transport of cationic amino acids by the mouse ecotropic retrovirus receptor. *Nature*, 1991, **352**:725–8.

Kozak M. Point mutations define a sequence flanking the AU initiator codon that modulates translation by eukaryotic ribosomes. *Cell*, 1986, **44**:283–92.

Kozak M. At least six nucleotides preceding the AUG initiator codon enhance translation in mammalian cells. *Journal of Molecular Biology*, 1987, **196**:947–50.

Kozak M. Structural features in eukaryotic mRNAs that modulate the initiation of translation. *Journal of Biological Chemistry*, 1991, **266**:19867–70.

Kozak M. Regulation of translation in eukaryotic systems. *Annual Review of Cell Biology*, 1992, **8**:197–225.

Kozarsky KF; Wilson JM. Gene therapy: adenovirus vectors. *Current Opinion in Genetics and Development*, 1993, **3**:499–503.

Le Gal La Salle G; Robert JJ; Berrard S; Ridoux V; Stratford-Perricaudet LD; Perricaudet M; Mallet J. An adenovirus vector for gene transfer into neurons and glia in the brain. *Science*, 1993, **259**:988–90.

Levison SW; Chuang C; Abramson BJ; Goldman JE. The migrational patterns and developmental fates of glia recursors in the rat subventricular zone are temporally regulated. *Development*, 1993, **119**:611–22.

Levison SW; Goldman JE. Both oligodendrocytes and astrocytes develop from progenitors in the subventricular zone of postnatal rat forebrain. *Neuron*, 1993, **10**:201–12.

Louis JC; Muir D; Varon S. Autocrine inhibition of mitotic activity in cultured oligodendrocyte-type-2 astrocyte (O-2A) precursor cells. *Glia*, 1992, **6**:30–8.

Luskin MB. Restricted proliferation and migration of postnatally generated neurons derived from the forebrain subventricular zone. *Neuron*, 1993, **11**:173–89.

Luskin MB. Neuronal cell lineage in the vertebrate central nervous system. *Faseb Journal*, 1994, **8**:722–30.

Lynch CM; Clowes MM; Osborne WR; Clowes AW; Miller AD. Long-term expression of human adenosine deaminase in vascular smooth muscle cells of rats: a model for gene therapy. *Proceedings of the National Academy of Sciences of the United States of America*, 1992, **89**:1138–42.

Lynch CM; Israel DI; Kaufman RJ; Miller AD. Sequences in the coding region of clotting factor VIII act as dominant inhibitors of RNA accumulation and protein production. *Human Gene Therapy*, 1993, **4**:259–72.

Mann R; Mulligan RC; Baltimore D. Construction of a retrovirus packaging mutant and its use to produce helper-free defective retrovirus. *Cell*, 1983, **33**:153–9.

Marty L; Roux P; Royer M; Piechaczyk M. MoMuLV-derived self-inactivating retroviral vectors possessing multiple cloning sites and expressing the resistance to either G418 or hygromycin B. *Biochimie*, 1990, **72**:885–7.

Mayer E; Dunnett SB; Fawcett JW. Mitogenic effect of basic fibroblast growth factor on embryonic ventral mesencephalic dopaminergic neurone precursors. *Brain Research: Developmental Brain Research*, 1993a, **72**:253–8.

Mayer E; Dunnett SB; Pellitteri R; Fawcett JW. Basic fibroblast growth factor promotes the survival of embryonic ventral mesencephalic dopaminergic neurons–I. Effects *in vitro*. *Neuroscience*, 1993b, **56**:379–88.

McIvor RS. Deletion in a recombinant retroviral vector resulting from a cryptic splice donor signal in the Moloney leukemia virus envelope gene. *Virology*, 1990, **176**:652–5.

McLachlin JR; Mittereder N; Daucher MB; Kadan M; Eglitis MA. Factors affecting retroviral vector function and structural integrity. *Virology*, 1993, **195**:1–5.

Miller AD. Retrovirus packaging cells. *Human Gene Therapy*, 1990, **1**:5–14.

Miller AD. Human gene therapy comes of age. *Nature*, 1992, **357**:455–60.

Miller AD; Buttimore C. Redesign of retrovirus packaging cell lines to avoid recombination leading to helper virus production. *Molecular and Cellular Biology*, 1986, **6**:2895–6.

Miller AD; Rosman GJ. Improved retroviral vectors for gene transfer: an expression. *Biotechniques*, 1989, **7**:980–2, 984–6, 989–90.

Miller AD; Law MF; Verma IM. Generation of helper-free amphotropic retroviruses that transduce a dominant-acting, methotrexate-resistant dihydrofolate reductase gene. *Molecular and Cellular Biology*, 1985, **5**:431–7.

Miller AD; Palmer TD; Hock RA. Transfer of genes into human somatic cells using retrovirus vectors. *Cold Spring Harbor Symposia on Quantitative Biology*, 1986, **51**:1013–19.

Miller AD; Miller DG; Garcia JV; Lynch CM. Use of retroviral vectors for gene transfer and expression. *Methods in Enzymology*, 1993, **217**:581–99.

Miller DG; Adam MA; Miller AD. Gene transfer by retrovirus vectors occurs only in cells that are actively replicating at the time of infection. *Molecular and Cellular Biology*, 1990, **10**:4239–42.

Miller DG; Edwards RH; Miller AD. Cloning of the cellular receptor for amphotropic murine retroviruses reveals homology to that for gibbon ape leukemia virus. *Proceedings of the National Academy of Sciences of the United States of America*, 1994, **91**:78–82.

Moolten FL; Wells JM. Curability of tumors bearing herpes thymidine kinase genes transferred by retroviral vectors. *Journal of the National Cancer Institute*, 1990, **82**:297–300.

Moolten FS; Wells JM; Mroz PJ. Multiple transduction as a means of preserving ganciclovir chemosensitivity in sarcoma cells carrying retrovirally transduced herpes thymidine kinase genes. *Cancer Letters*, 1992, **64**:257–63.

Moolten FL. Tumor chemosensitivity conferred by inserted herpes thymidine kinase genes: paradigm for a prospective cancer control strategy. *Cancer Research*, 1986, **46**:5276–81.

Morgan RA; Couture L; Elroy-Stein O; Ragheb J; Moss B; Anderson WF. Retroviral vectors containing putative internal ribosome entry sites: development of a polycistronic gene transfer system and applications to human gene therapy. *Nucleic Acids Research*, 1992, **20**:1293–9.

Morgenstern JP; Land H. Advanced mammalian gene transfer: high titre retroviral vectors with multiple drug selection markers and a complementary helper-free packaging cell line. *Nucleic Acids Research*, 1990, **18**:3587–3596.

Muenchau DD; Freeman SM; Cornetta K; Zwiebel JA; Anderson WF. Analysis of retroviral packaging lines for generation of replication-competent virus. *Virology*, 1990, **176**:262–5.

Mulligan RC. The basic science of gene therapy. *Science*, 1993, **260**:926–32.

Muzyczka N. Use of adeno-associated virus as a general transduction vector for mammalian cells. *Current Topics in Microbiology and Immunology*, 1992, **158**:97–129.

Nakajima K; Ikenaka K; Nakahira K; Morita N; Mikoshiba K. An improved retroviral vector for assaying promoter activity. Analysis of promoter interference in pIP211 vector. *FEBS Letters*, 1993, **315**:129–33.

Noble M; Barnett SC; Bogler O; Land H; Wolswijk G; Wren D. Control of division and differentiation in oligodendrocyte-type-2 astrocyte progenitor cells. *Ciba Foundation Symposium*, 1990, **150**:227–43.

Noble M; Wolswijk G. Development and regeneration in the O-2A lineage: studies *in vitro* and *in vivo*. *Journal of Neuroimmunology*, 1992, **40**:287–93.

Olson P; Temin HM; Dornburg R. Unusually high frequency of reconstitution of long terminal repeats in U3-minus retrovirus vectors by DNA recombination or gene conversion. *Journal of Virology*, 1992, **66**:1336–43.

Otto E; Jones-Trower A; Vanin EF; Stambaugh K; Mueller SN; Anderson WF; McGarrity GJ. Characterization of a replication-competent retrovirus resulting from recombination of packaging and vector sequences. *Human Gene Therapy*, 1994, **5**:567–75.

Palmer TD; Hock RA; Osborne WRA; Miller AD. Efficient retrovirus-mediated transfer and expression of a human adenosine deaminase gene in diploid skin fibroblasts from an adenosine deaminase-deficient human. *Proceedings of the National Academy of Sciences of the United States of America*, 1987, **84**:1055–9.

Palmer TD; Rosman GJ; Osborne WR; Miller AD. Genetically modified skin fibroblasts persist long after transplantation but gradually inactivate introduced genes. *Proceedings of the National Academy of Sciences of the United States of America*, 1991, **88**:1330–4.

Palmer TD; Thompson AR; Miller AD. Production of human factor IX in animals by genetically modified skin fibroblasts: potential therapy for hemophilia B. Blood, 1989, **73**:438–45.

Paludan K; Duch M; Jorgensen P; Kjeldgaard NO; et al. Graduated resistance to G418 leads to differential selection of cultured mammalian cells expressing the *neo* gene. *Gene*, 1989, **85**:421–6.

Perraud F; Labourdette G; Eclancher F; Sensenbrenner M. Primary cultures of astrocytes from different brain areas of newborn rats and effects of basic fibroblast growth factor. *Developmental Neuroscience*, 1990, **12**:11–21.

Pulsinelli GA; Temin HM. Characterization of large deletions occurring during a single round of retrovirus vector replication: novel deletion mechanism involving errors in strand transfer. *Journal of Virology*, 1991, **65**:4786–97.

Ram Z; Walbridge S; Shawker T; Culver KW; Blaese RM; Oldfield EH. The effect of thymidine kinase transduction and ganciclovir therapy on tumor vasculature and growth of 9L gliomas in rats. *Journal of Neurosurgery*, 1994, **81**:256–60.

Ramesh N; Lau S; Palmer TD; Storb R; Osborne WR. High-level human adenosine deaminase expression in dog skin fibroblasts is not sustained following transplantation. *Human Gene Therapy*, 1993, **4**:3–7.

Ray J; Peterson DA; Schinstine M; Gage FH. Proliferation, differentiation, and long-term culture of primary hippocampal neurons. *Proceedings of the National Academy of Sciences of the United States of America*, 1993, **90**:3602–6.

Ray J; Gage FH, Gene transfer into established and primary fibroblast cell lines: comparison of transfection methods and promoters. *Biotechniques*, 1992, **13**:598–603.

Ray J; Gage FH. Spinal cord neuroblasts proliferate in response to basic fibroblast growth factor. *Journal of Neuroscience*, 1994, **14**:3548–64.

Redmond DE Jr; Roth RH; Spencer DD; Naftolin F; Leranth C; Robbins RJ; Marek KL; Elsworth JD; Taylor JR; Sass KJ; et al. Neural transplantation for neurodegenerative diseases: past, present, and future. *Annals of the New York Academy of Sciences*, 1993, **695**:258–66.

Reynolds BA; Weiss S. Generation of neurons and astrocytes from isolated cells of the adult mammalian central nervous system. *Science*, 1992, **255**:1707–10.

Reynolds BA; Tetzlaff W; Weiss S. A multipotent EGF-responsive striatal embryonic progenitor cell produces neurons and astrocytes. *Journal of Neuroscience*, 1992, **12**:4565–74.

Ridoux V; Robert JJ; Zhang X; Perricaudet M; Mallet J; La Salle G. The use of adenovirus vectors for intracerebral grafting of transfected nervous cells. *Neuroreport*, 1994, **5**:801–4.

Roe T; Reynolds TC; Yu G; Brown PO. Integration of murine leukemia virus DNA depends on mitosis. *EMBO Journal*, 1993, **12**:2099–108.

Roman M; Axelrod JH; Dai Y; Naviaux RK; Friedmann T; Verma IM. Circulating human or canine factor IX from retrovirally transduced primary myoblasts and established myoblast cell lines grafted into murine skeletal muscle. *Somatic Cell and Molecular Genetics*, 1992, **18**:247–58.

Russell DW; Miller AD; Alexander IE. Adeno-associated virus vectors preferentially transduce cells in S phase. *Proceedings of the National Academy of Sciences of the United States of America*, 1994, **91**:8915–19.

Ryder EF; Cepko CL. Migration patterns of clonally related granule cells and heir progenitors in the developing chick cerebellum. *Neuron*, 1994, **12**:1011–28.

Sambrook J; Fritch EF; Maniatis T. Molecular cloning: a laboratory manual. 1989. Cold Spring Harbor Laboratory Press. Cold Spring Harbor, New York.

Samulski RJ. Adeno-associated virus: integration at a specific chromosomal locus. *Current Opinion in Genetics and Development*, 1993, **3**:74–80.

Scharfmann R; Axelrod JH; Verma IM. Long-term *In vivo* expression of retrovirus-mediated gene transfer in mouse fibroblast implants. *Proceedings of the National Academy of Sciences of the United States of America*, 1991, **88**:4626–30.

Schinstine M; Kawaja MD; Gage FH. Intracerebral delivery of growth factors: potential application of genetically modified fibroblasts. *Progress in Growth Factor Research*, 1991, **3**:57–66.

Schinstine M; Gage FH. Factors affecting proviral expression in primary cells grafted into the CNS. *Research Publications—Association for Research in Nervous and Mental Disease*, 1993, **71**:311–23.

Sensenbrenner M; Deloulme JC; Gensburger C. Proliferation of neuronal precursor cells from the central nervous system in culture. *Reviews in the Neurosciences*, 1994, **5**:43–53.

Shahar A; de Vellis J; Vernakakis A; Haber B eds. *A dissection and tissue culture manual of the nervous system*. Wiley-Liss, New York, 1993.

Shimohama S; Fisher LJ; Gage FH. Intracerebral grafting of genetically modified cells. Applications to a rat model of Parkinson's disease. *Advances in Neurology*, 1993, **60**:744–8.

Simon RH; Engelhardt JF; Yang Y; Zepeda M; Weber-Pendlet K; Grossman M; Wilson JM. Adenovirus-mediated transfer of the CFTR gene to lung of non-human primates: toxicity study. *Human Gene Therapy*, 1993, **4**:771–80.

Soriano P; Friedrich G; Lawinger P. Promoter interactions in retrovirus vectors introduced into fibroblasts and embryonic stem cells. *Journal of Virology*, 1991, **65**:2314–9.

Spencer DD; Robbins RJ; Naftolin F; Marek KL; Vollmer T et al., Unilateral transplantation of human fetal mesencephalic tissue in the caudate nucleus of patients with Parkinson's disease. *New England Journal of Medicine*, 1992, **327**:1541–8.

Stockschlaeder MA; Storb R; Osborne WR; Miller AD. L-histidinol provides effective selection of retrovirus-vector-transduced keratinocytes without impairing their proliferative potential. *Human Gene Therapy*, 1991, **2**:33–9.

Stromberg I; Wetmore CJ; Ebendal T; Ernfors P; Persson H; Olson L. Rescue of basal forebrain cholinergic neurons after implantation of genetically modified cells producing recombinant NGF. *Journal of*

Neuroscience Research, 1990, **25**:405–11.

Suhr ST; Gage FH. Gene therapy for neurologic disease. *Archives of Neurology*, 1993, **50**:1252–68.

Sullenger BA; Lee TC; Smith CA; Ungers GE; Gilboa E. Expression of chimeric tRNA-driven antisense transcripts renders NIH 3T3 cells highly resistant to Moloney murine leukemia virus replication. *Molecular and Cellular Biology*, 1990a, **10**:6512–23.

Sullenger BA; Gallardo HF; Ungers GE; Gilboa E. Overexpression of TAR sequences renders cells resistant to human immunodeficiency virus replication. *Cell*, 1990b, **63**:601–8.

Takayama H; Ray J; Raymon HK; Baird A; Hogg J; Fisher LJ; Gage FH. Basic fibroblast growth factor increases dopaminergic graft survival and function in a rat model of Parkinson's disease. *Nature Medicine* 1995, **1**:53–8.

Taketo M; Tanaka M. A cellular enhancer of retrovirus gene expression in embryonal carcinoma cells. *Proceedings of the National Academy of Sciences of the United States of America*, 1987, **84**:3748–52.

Taylor JR; Elsworth JD; Roth RH; Sladek JR Jr; Collier TJ; Redmond DE Jr. Grafting of fetal substantia nigra to striatum reverses behavioral deficits induced by MPTP in primates: a comparison with other types of grafts as controls. *Experimental Brain Research*, 1991, **85**:335–48.

Temin HM. Retrovirus variation and reverse transcription: abnormal strand transfers result in retrovirus genetic variation. *Proceedings of the National Academy of Sciences of the United States of America*, 1993, **90**:6900–3.

Torrent C; Gabus C; Darlix JL. A small and efficient dimerization/packaging signal of rat VL30 RNA and its use in murine leukemia virus-VL30-derived vectors for gene transfer. *Journal of Virology*, 1994, **68**:661–7.

Tuszynski MH; Peterson DA; Ray J; Baird A; Nakahara Y; Gage FH. Fibroblasts genetically modified to produce nerve growth factor induce robust neuritic ingrowth after grafting to the spinal cord. *Experimental Neurology*, 1994, **126**:1–14.

Tuszynski MH; Buzsaki G; Gage FH. Nerve growth factor infusions combined with fetal hippocampal grafts enhance reconstruction of the lesioned septohippocampal projection. *Neuroscience*, 1990, **36**:33–44.

Uchida K; Takamatsu K; Kaneda N; Toya S; Tsukada Y; Kurosawa Y; Fujita K; Nagatsu T; Kohsaka S. Synthesis of L-3,4-dihydroxyphenylalanine by tyrosine hydroxylase cDNA-transfected C6 cells: application for intracerebral grafting. *Journal of Neurochemistry*, 1989, **53**:728–32.

Walker AG; Chapman J; Bruce CB; Rumsby MG. Immunocytochemical characterisation of cell cultures grown from dissociated 1–2-day post-natal rat cerebral tissue. A developmental study. *Journal of Neuroimmunology*, 1984, **7**:1–20.

Walsh C; Cepko CL. Clonal dispersion in proliferative layers of developing cerebral cortex. *Nature*, 1993, **15**, **362**:632–5.

Wang H; Kavanaugh MP; North RA; Kabat D. Cell-surface receptor for ecotropic murine retroviruses is a basic amino-acid transporter. *Nature*, 1991, **352**:729–31.

Weiss R; Teich N; Varmus H; Coffin J. (eds.) *RNA Tumor Viruses*, New York, Cold Spring Harbor Laboratory, 1985.

Welsh R; Cooper NR, Jensen FC; Oldstone MB. Human serum lyses RNA tumor viruses. *Nature*, 1975, **257**:612–14.

Welsh RM; Jensen FC; Cooper NR; Oldstone MB. Inactivation of lysis of coronaviruses by human serum. *Virology*, 1976, **74**:432–40.

Whitcomb JM; Hughes SH. Retroviral reverse transcription and integration: progress and problems. *Annual Review of Cell Biology*, 1992, **8**:275–306.

Widner H; Tetrud J; Rehncrona S; Snow BJ; Brundin P; Bjorklund A; Lindvall O; Langston JW. Fifteen months' follow-up on bilateral embryonic mesencephalic grafts in two cases of severe MPTP-induced parkinsonism. *Advances in Neurology*, 1993, **60**:729–33.

Widner H; Tetrud J; Rehncrona S; Snow B; Brundin P; Gustavii B; Bjorklund A; Lindvall O; Langston JW. Bilateral fetal mesencephalic grafting in two patients with parkinsonism induced by 1-methyl-4-phenyl-1,2,3,6-tetrahydropyridine (MPTP). *New England Journal of Medicine*, 1992, **327**:1556–63.

Wolff JA; Fisher LJ; Xu L; Jinnah HA; Langlais PJ et al. Grafting fibroblasts genetically modified to produce L-dopa in a rat model of Parkinson disease. *Proceedings of the National Academy of Sciences of the United States of America*, 1989, **86**: 9011–14.

Wren D; Wolswijk G; Noble M. *in vitro*analysis of the origin and maintenance of O-2A adult progenitor cells. *Journal of Cell Biology*, 1992, **116**:167–76.

Yang HY; Lieska N; Shao D; Kriho V; Pappas GD. Proteins of the intermediate filament cytoskeleton as markers for astrocytes and human astrocytomas. *Molecular and Chemical Neuropathology*, 1994a, **21**:155–76.

Yang Y; Nunes FA; Berencsi K; Furth EE; Gonczol E; Wilson JM. Cellular immunity to viral antigens limits E1-deleted adenoviruses for gene therapy. *Proceedings of the National Academy of Sciences of the United States of America*, 1994b, **91**:4407–11.

Zhang J; Temin HM. Retrovirus recombination depends on the length of sequence identity and is not error prone. *Journal of Virology*, 1994, **68**:2409–14.

Zhang J; Temin HM. Rate and mechanism of non-homologous recombination during a single cycle of retroviral replication. *Science*, 1993, **259**:234–8.

CHAPTER 20

Murine Mucopolysaccharidosis Type VII: A Model System for Somatic Gene Therapy of the Central Nervous System

JOHN H. WOLFE AND MARK S. SANDS

Department of Pathobiology, School of Veterinary Medicine, University of Pennsylvania, 3800 Spruce St, Philadelphia, PA 19104-6051, USA. Tel: 215 898 2324; Fax: 215 573 2162; Email: jhwolfe@pobox.upenn.edu

1 INTRODUCTION

The mucopolysaccharidosis type VII (MPS VII) mouse carries a null mutation for β-glucuronidase (GUSB), a lysosomal acid hydrolase that is normally expressed in all tissues including the brain. The MPS VII mouse brain expresses no background GUSB activity, so even low amounts of transferred GUSB can be detected. The transferred normal GUSB activity can be both quantitated and localized, providing a powerful experimental system for following the fate of the transferred gene. The biochemical and histochemical protocols, and the optimal methods for evaluating changes in pathology, used in our laboratory are described in this chapter. A detailed description of the various viral and non-viral vectors that can be used to deliver genes into the brain are outlined elsewhere. Any of the currently used vector systems can be used for GUSB transfer since the coding sequence is less than 2 kb. Used in combination, the MPS VII mouse and various vectors expressing β-glucuronidase constitute an *in vivo* reporter gene system with defined lesions as an endpoint for disease correction.

1.1 The MPS VII Mouse Model

The enzyme β-glucuronidase is necessary for the normal degradation of glycosaminoglycans and its deficiency results in the lysosomal storage disease commonly referred to as Sly disease or MPS VII (Sly et al., 1973). The disease has been studied in detail in the dog (Haskins et al., 1984) and mouse (Birkenmeier et al., 1989) and has been diagnosed in the cat (Fyfe et al., unpublished data). The affected animals are true homologs of human patients, having mutations in the orthologous gene causing the biochemical and metabolic defects which produce essentially the same disease. Although MPS VII is rare in humans, collectively the lysosomal storage disorders occur with a frequency of approximately 1 in 1500 live births (Neufeld and Meunzer, 1995), more frequently than cystic fibrosis. Murine MPS VII is an effective model for gene therapy for most of the lysosomal storage disorders because the therapeutic strategy is similar for most of them.

MPS VII is a progressive degenerative disease resulting from the accumulation of undegraded glycosaminoglycans in the lysosomes of many types of cells. The disease affects the cornea, retina,

Protocols for Gene Transfer in Neuroscience: Towards Gene Therapy of Neurological Disorders
Edited by P.R. Lowenstein and L.W. Enquist

heart, trachea, skeletal system, liver, spleen and brain. The average life span of MPS VII mice is 5–6 months, and all die before 1 year of age (Birkenmeier et al., 1989). Gross skeletal deformities and corneal clouding are visible at maturity, and the animals become progressively weak and lame until they are nearly immobile. Histopathologically, lysosomal distension becomes apparent in most tissues of the body, including the brain, by 3 weeks of age. The meninges, neurons and glial cells are severely affected and distended lysosomes can readily be seen microscopically in all three cell types in young adult mice (Birkenmeier et al., 1989; Vogler et al., 1990; Snyder et al., 1995). However, lysosomal distension is present and accumulation of glycosaminoglycans can be detected biochemically in brain cells at birth (Vogler et al., 1990; Taylor and Wolfe, unpublished data).

β-Glucuronidase is one of the most thoroughly studied enzymes and genetic loci (*gus*) in the mouse (Paigen, 1989). The gene has been cloned from mice and humans (D'Amore et al., 1988; Miller et al., 1990), and GUSB cDNAs have been cloned from the mouse (Funkenstein et al., 1988; Gallagher et al., 1988), rat (Nishimura et al., 1986; Powell et al., 1988), human (Oshima et al., 1987) and dog (Bouvet et al., unpublished data). The cDNAs share 75–89% nucleic acid homology, thus both species-specific and common PCR primers can be synthesized to detect the presence of transferred genes by PCR (Wolfe et al., 1992a; Barker et al., 1993). The defect in the murine GUSB gene causing MPS VII is a single base deletion which results in a null mutant with profoundly reduced mRNA (< 1/200 of normal) and no detectable enzymatic activity in the CNS or other organs (Birkenmeier et al., 1989; Sands and Birkenmeier, 1993). The mouse mutation can be conveniently identified using the simple PCR-based assay described in Protocol #109.

1.2 Biochemical and Cellular Basis of Treatment

The basis of treatment for MPS VII, and most other lysosomal storage disorders, is cross-correction (Neufeld and Fratantoni 1970). This process involves the uptake of exogenous normal enzyme by mutant cells, either by mannose-6-phosphate receptor-mediated endocytosis (Sando and Neufeld, 1977) or by direct cell transfer (Olsen et al., 1981). Thus MPS VII cells may be corrected by supplying normal GUSB from transplanted heterologous cells (Haskins et al., 1991; Birkenmeier et al., 1991; Sands et al., 1993; Snyder et al., 1995), from injected preparations of purified GUSB protein (Vogler et al., 1993; Sands et al., 1994) or from genetically corrected mutant cells (Wolfe et al., 1990, 1992a, 1992b, 1995; Smith et al., 1990; Moullier et al., 1993; Marechal et al., 1993). In addition, GUSB from different species is processed and properly sorted to the acidified lysosomal compartment in MPS VII cells (Wolfe et al., 1990; Stramm et al., 1990), can cross-correct mutant cells (Hall et al., 1973; Lagunoff et al., 1973; Brot et al., 1974; Taylor and Wolfe, 1994) and can reverse the disease pathology *in vivo* (Kyle et al., 1990; Wolfe et al., 1992a; Moullier et al., 1993; Marechal et al., 1993; Snyder et al., 1995).

Secondary to the lack of GUSB activity in the MPS VII mouse is an increase in other lysosomal enzymes such as α-galactosidase and β-hexosaminidase (Birkenmeier et al., 1989). These enzymes are measured as control normal lysosomal enzymes and a decrease in the secondary elevations may be associated with a decrease in distended lysosomes and serve as indicator of therapeutic effectiveness, but the levels do not return to normal even in completely corrected tissues (Birkenmeier et al., 1991; Wolfe et al., 1992a; Sands et al., 1993, 1994).

1.3 Gene Transfer Experience in MPS VII Mice

Murine MPS VII is a powerful model for developing and testing various gene transfer strategies. Expression of the full-length human GUSB gene in a transgenic mouse with homozygous mutant *gus* loci resulted levels of enzyme 10–20 times higher than normal and completely eliminated the disease phenotype (Kyle et al., 1990). These experiments also show that over-expression of GUSB is not deleterious to cells or tissues because the mice are phenotypically normal by all criteria assessed. Similarly, 5–10 fold over-expression of GUSB from retroviral vectors *in vitro* has no apparent adverse affects on cells (Wolfe et al., 1995).

Retroviral vector-mediated gene transfer of the rat or human GUSB cDNA into hematopoietic stem cells from an MPS VII donor mouse reverses disease in the liver and spleen of recipient animals (Wolfe et al., 1992a; Marechal et al., 1993). Only 2% of normal activity can completely reverse fully established pathology in the liver and spleen (Wolfe et al., 1992a). Implantation of artificial organoids containing MPS VII fibroblasts transduced with a retrovirus containing the human GUSB cDNA also produced sufficient enzyme to decrease lysosomal distension in liver and spleen (Moullier et al., 1993). Although these experiments were successful in reversing pathology in visceral organs, they did not transfer GUSB into the brain.

Transplantation experiments in the brain with multipotent neuronal progenitor cells (Snyder et al., 1992) demonstrated increased GUSB activity throughout the MPS VII brain and decreased lysosomal storage with no apparent adverse effects (Snyder et al., 1995). This is analogous to bone marrow transplantation for the skeletal and visceral diseases. Intravenous injection of large amounts of biochemically purified GUSB at birth causes some GUSB to enter the brain and prevents lysosomal storage early in life in some neurons (Vogler et al., 1993; Sands et al., 1994). These experiments indicate that if enough enzyme can be expressed in the CNS on a sustained basis, it should be possible to correct the metabolic defect. Direct gene transfer of GUSB into the MPS VII brain has been shown using a herpesvirus vector encoding the rat GUSB cDNA driven by the LAT promoter, which is expressed during latency (Wolfe et al., 1992b). Although too few cells were corrected to alter the pathology this experiment illustrates the sensitivity of the histochemical stain by identifying single positive cells in whole sections.

1.4 Technical Advantages of the Murine MPS VII Model

The murine MPS VII model is well suited for gene transfer studies to the brain because of the availability of cDNAs from several species, sensitive biochemical and histochemical assays, readily detectable pathology in many areas of the brain and the lack of endogenous GUSB activity. Expression from most reporter gene systems can either be quantitated (e.g. chloramphenicol acetyl transferase, CAT) or localized (e.g. β-galactosidase) but not both. GUSB activity, however, can be quantitated using a sensitive fluorometric assay (Glaser and Sly, 1973; Kyle et al., 1992) and localized using naphthol-AS-BI β-D-glucuronide (Wolfe et al., 1990; Kyle et al., 1992) or 5-bromo-4-chloro-3-indolyl β-D-glucuronic acid (X-gluc) (Naleway, 1992; Kyle et al., 1992) as a substrate.

A further important advantage of the MPS VII system is that GUSB is extremely stable. It can survive fixation and retains 80% of its activity for days or weeks in culture medium at 37°C (Taylor and Wolfe, 1994). The stability in fixatives allows enzyme activity to be quantitated using the fluorometric assay or localized with histochemical stains. Morphology can be maintained sufficiently to observe distended lysosomes in samples prepared for electron microscopy. These characteristics make murine MPS VII an ideal system for studying new methods of delivering genes to the brain and for testing various CNS-specific promoters linked to GUSB cDNAs.

2 MATERIALS AND EQUIPMENT

2.1 Fluorometric Enzyme Activity Assays

(1) 0.1 M sodium acetate (pH 4.8).
(2) 0.2 M citrate-phosphate buffer (pH 4.8) (504 ml 0.2 M citric acid, 496 ml 0.2 M Na_2HPO_4).
(3) 10 mM 4-methylumbelliferyl β-D-glucuronide in 0.1 M sodium acetate buffer.
(4) 10 mM 4-methylumbelliferyl α-D-galactoside in 0.2 M citrate–phosphate buffer.
(5) 0.2 M sodium carbonate, 0.32 M glycine (pH 10.5) (stop buffer).
(6) 2 mM 4-methylumbelliferone in 100% ethanol.
(7) 0.2% Triton X-100, 0.9% NaCl.

2.2 Histochemical Localization of GUSB Activity

(1) 0.05 M sodium acetate buffer (pH 4.5).
(2) 0.05 M sodium acetate buffer (pH 5.2).
(3) 0.25 mM naphthol AS-BI β-D-glucuronic acid in 0.05 M sodium acetate buffer (pH 4.5).
(4) 0.25 mM naphthol AS-BI β-D-glucuronic acid in 0.05 M sodium acetate buffer (pH 5.2).

(5) 4% pararosaniline chloride in 2 N HCl (stable 1 week at 4°C), 6.4% sodium nitrite in distilled water (stable 1 week at 4°C).
(6) 1% chloral hydrate in 20% v/v neutral buffered formalin in distilled water (chloral hydrate–formalin fixative).
(7) Chloral-formal-acetone fixative (70 ml acetone, 30 ml solution prepared in Step 6).
(8) OCT embedding compound.
(9) 1% aqueous methyl green (extracted 3–4X with $CHCl_3$).

2.3 Genotyping by PCR

(1) Intron primer: 5′-CCTGTGTCATTTGCATGTG-3′.
(2) Mismatch primer: 5′-GATAACATCCACGTACCGG-3′.
(3) PCR buffer: 10 mM Tris (pH 8.8), 50 mM KCl, 2.5 mM $MgCl_2$, 0.01% gelatin.
(4) NuSieve agarose (FMC Corp., Rockland, ME).

2.4 Special equipment

(1) Fluorometer (365 nm excitation, 450 nm emission).
(2) Cryostat.
(3) Microscope with differential interference contrast (Nomarski), fluorescent capability and photomicroscopy attachment.

3 THE PROTOCOLS

Protocol #109: PCR Reaction for Genotyping B6.C-*H*-2^{bm1}/ByBir-*gus*^{mps}/+ Mice

(1) Prepare the PCR reaction: 2 μl intron primer (50 μM), 2 μl mismatched primer (50 μM), 1–10 μl DNA, 2.5 μl dNTPs (10 mM each of dGTP, dATP, dTTP, dCTP), 10 μl 10 × PCR buffer, 0.5 μl Taq polymerase (2.5 u), 72–82 μl distilled water.
(2) The thermocycler program is as follows: 95°C 5 min, then 32 cycles of the following steps: 94°C 1.5 min, 52°C 1.5 min, 72°C 1.5 min.

Protocol #110: Preparation of Homogenates or Supernatants for Quantitative Lysosomal Enzyme Assays

Media

(1) Harvest media from cultured cells and centrifuge (1000 rpm × 10 min, ≅900 × *g*) to remove cells.
(2) Pass the media through a 0.22 μm filter and freeze at −20°C until ready to assay.

Cells

(1) Rinse cells in culture with phosphate-buffered saline (PBS) to remove proteins, trypsinize, then neutralize with medium containing serum.
(2) Wash the cells 2–3 times by centrifugation (1000 rpm × 10 min, ≅900 × *g*) with 0.9% NaCl or PBS.
(3) Add 10 μl lysis buffer per milligram cell pellet.
(4) Freeze–thaw twice in a CO_2–ethanol bath.
(5) Collect supernatant and freeze at −20°C until ready to assay.

Tissue Sections

(1) Homogenize issue sections (25–100 mg) in lysis buffer (approximately the same weight to volume ratio as described for cells in culture) at 4°C with 5–10 strokes.

(2) Pellet cellular debris in a microcentrifuge (13 000 rpm 30–60 s).
(3) Freeze homogenates at −20°C until ready for assay.

Protocol #111: 4-MU Assay

Standard Curve

(1) Prepare 2 mM 4 methylumbelliferone (4-MU) solution: 19.8 mg 4-MU in 250 ml absolute ethanol, then add 50 ml sodium acetate buffer and heat at 50°C until 4-MU is completely in solution.
(2) Prepare 0.2 mM 4-MU solution (dilute 1 ml of 2 mM in 9 ml buffer). Store at 4°C.
(3) Make standards as follows: 10 ml (0.2 mM) in 90 ml distilled water (2 nmol 4-MU); 5 ml (2 mM) in 95 ml distilled water (10 nmol 4-MU); 10 ml (2 mM) in 90 ml distilled water (20 nmol 4-MU); 25 ml (2 mM) in 75 ml distilled water (50 nmol 4-MU).
(4) Prepare a blank with 100 μl distilled water.
(5) Add 100 μl 10 mM 4-MU glucuronide substrate to each dilution and blank and incubate at 37°C for 1–4 h.
(6) Add 1.8 ml stop buffer and read absorbance at 365 nm excitation, 450 nm emission.

Assay

(1) Perform assay in duplicate in glass tubes or disposable 4.5 ml four-sided methacrylate cuvettes.
(2) Add 10–100 μl of sample to tubes. Bring to 100 μl with distilled water.
(3) Add 100 μl distilled water to blanks.
(4) Add 100 μl of the appropriate 4-MU substrate to each tube.
(5) Incubate immediately in a water bath (37°C) for 1–4 h.
(6) Stop reaction with 1.8 ml stop buffer.
(7) Zero fluorometer with water blank.
(8) Read samples as in step (6) above.
(9) Calculate activity from standard curve.
(10) Assay α-galactosidase as a control using the same protocol (including the standard curve) except that the dilution buffer is 0.2 M citrate–phosphate.

Protocol #112: Localization of β-glucuronidase Activity; Naphthol-AS-BI β-D-Glucuronide Histochemical Staining

(1) Excise tissue samples (fixed or unfixed) and submerse in OCT embedding compound.
(2) Alternatively, slice the fixed brain into coronal sections to maintain orientation, lay flat on the bottom of a plastic cup and cover with OCT.
(3) Freeze sample in isopentane in a liquid nitrogen bath and store blocks at −70°C.
(4) Section blocks on a cryostat at 10–100 μm and place on polylysine coated slides.
(5) Store sections at −20°C until ready to stain.
(6) Thaw the slides and form a well around the section with a hydrophobic slide marker (e.g. PAP pen, Kiyota Intl, Inc.).
(7) Cover the section with chloral-formal-acetone fixative.
(8) Incubate 30 min at 4°C.
(9) Wash the slide with 3–5 changes of 0.05 M sodium acetate buffer (pH 4.5).
(10) Add 0.25 mM naphthol-AS-BI β-D-glucuronide (pH 4.5) and incubate 2–4 h at 4°C.
(11) Remove the substrate by aspiration.
(12) Mix equal volumes of 4% sodium nitrite and 4% pararosaniline chloride 10–30 min before staining. Add the pararosaniline to the sodium nitrite to minimize precipitation.
(13) Add 1/500 volume of hexazonium pararosaniline (prepared in Step 12) to 0.25 mM naphthol-AS-BI β-D-glucuronide (pH 5.2), pass through 0.45 μm filter and cover the sections.
(14) Stain sections for 2–16 h at 37°C in the substrate solution from step (13) in a humidified incubator.

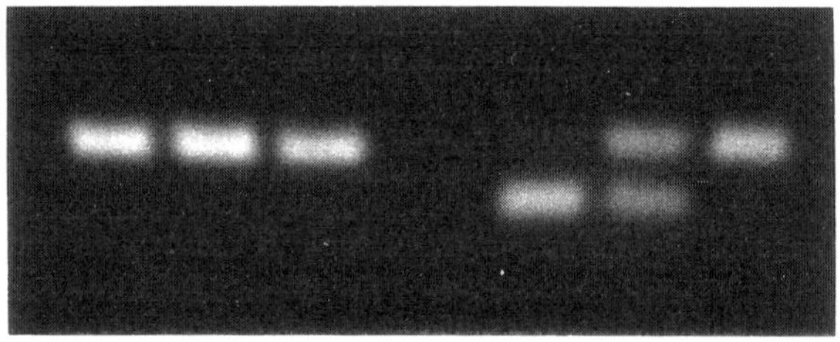

Figure 20.1 PCR-based assay for genotyping normal (+/+), carrier (+/−) and gus^{mps}/gus^{mps} (−/−) mice (15 μl on 3% NuSieve agarose gel, stained with ethidium bromide). Uncut PCR products of 95 base pairs from tissues of each genotype are shown in the three left-hand lanes. The lane labeled H_2O contains an equal volume of water blank. The three lanes on the right contain restriction fragments generated from digestion of the PCR products in the three left lanes. The mismatched nucleotide in the +/+ DNA creates an *Nci*I site and generates a 77 bp fragment, whereas the PCR from the mutant DNA remains uncut. PCR products from heterozygous DNA contain both alleles

(15) Stop reaction by rinsing in distilled water or 0.05 M sodium acetate.
(16) (Optional) Counterstain the slides with 1% methyl green for 1–10 min.

4 NOTES AND TROUBLESHOOTING

4.1 Genotyping, Husbandry and General Methods

Grossly, MPS VII mice are indistinguishable from normal animals at birth but the phenotype becomes apparent by 3–4 weeks of age. Adult MPS VII mice have a distinctive phenotype—flattened facies, shortened tail, corneal clouding, dull coat and impaired mobility—which makes them easily distinguishable from normal or heterozygous mice (Birkenmeier et al., 1989). Normal mice and heterozygous carriers are phenotypically indistinguishable.

These mice can be purchased from Dr E.H. Birkenmeier at the Jackson Laboratory (600 Main St, Bar Harbor, Maine 04609). However, the limited supply of mutant mice makes purchasing animals for large studies impracticable, and the investigator should consider maintaining a breeding colony. This is time-consuming and expensive, but the following methods will optimize the production of mutants.

The colony must be maintained by mating carriers; homozygous mutant mice will not breed. The animals should be maintained on a high-quality diet for optimum reproductive performance (Birkenmeier et al., 1989). Most litters will contain at least one affected pup but the overall yield of mutants by weaning is less than 20% of the total pups born. Identifying carriers for production can be problematic because they are phenotypically indistinguishable from normal mice. The specific activity of GUSB can be used to distinguish heterozygotes from normal mice, but activities in the two groups often overlap.

The most efficient method of identifying carriers is direct genotyping to detect the single base pair deletion in exon 10 (Sands and Birkenmeier, 1993). We have developed a simple PCR-based assay to distinguish the mutant from the normal allele (Protocol #109). A primer with a mismatched nucleotide creates a restriction site in the normal allele and none in the mutant allele. Following cleavage with *Nci*I or *Scr*FI the 77 bp restriction fragment present in the normal allele is easily distinguished on a 3% NuSieve agarose gel from the uncleaved 95 bp PCR product from the mutant allele (Fig. 20.1). DNA, usually obtained from a tail biopsy, can be isolated by a variety of methods but we routinely use the proteinase K–SDS method described by Sambrook et al., 1989.

For studies involving early application of a gene transfer technique it is crucial to distinguish mutants as early as possible. The fluorometric assay (Protocol #111) is sensitive enough to detect GUSB activity in a small (10 mm^3) tissue sample and can distinguish the mutant pups from carriers and normals. At birth a toe is removed from one of the hind limbs with a fine pair of dissecting scissors. The tissue sample is placed directly in buffer containing 4-methylumbelliferyl β-D-glucuronide substrate, crushed with a pipette tip, incubated at 37°C for 1 h, and the reaction stopped with sodium carbonate-glycine buffer. MPS VII mice will have a fluorometric reading similar to background whereas heterozygotes and normals will produce a clearly positive signal. The animals can be numbered by removing a different toe from each pup, and thereby distinguished throughout their lives. Newborn mutants can be identified within several hours of birth and can be ready for experimentation the same day.

! NEVER REMOVE THE INSIDE TOE: MICE REQUIRE THAT DIGIT FOR FULL MOBILITY !

4.2 On Protocol #109: PCR Reaction for Genotyping B6.C-*H*-2^{bm1}/ByBir-gus^{mps}/+ Mice

A total of 10–15 μl PCR product is usually sufficient to analyse for the mutation and can be accommodated on a mini-agarose gel. The PCR buffer is similar to the buffers required for *Nci*I or *Scr*FI digestion, with the exception of the $MgCl_2$ concentration. Therefore the restriction enzyme may be added directly to the PCR reaction mix after the appropriate amount of 10 × restriction enzyme buffer, containing no NaCl, has been added. Owing to the presence of mismatched nucleotide in one of the primers, the reaction is very sensitive to temperature and $MgCl_2$ concentrations.

4.3 Notes on Anesthesia, Transplantation, Infection and Neurosurgery of MPS VII Mice

The affected mice are very sensitive to anesthesia, requiring only half the dose of a normal animal to attain the same level of anesthesia and analgesia. We use Avertin (tribromoethanol, 20 mg/ml) which is very safe in normal animals. Normals should be anesthetized intraperitoneally with 0.4–0.5 ml, mutants should be given 0.2 ml to begin with and 0.05 ml increments until full anesthesia is reached. The animals will remain anesthetized for 30–45 min, which is sufficient time to place the animal in a stereotaxic frame, clip and clean the skin, incise the skin, drill the skull, inject the cells or virus, and suture the skin (typically 15–20 min).

The skulls of adult MPS VII mice are markedly thickened, which makes drilling more difficult than in normal skulls. The bone malformation also causes the shape of the MPS VII skull to be slightly different, so if precise placement of the injection is required coordinates for the MPS VII mouse should be established. Another consideration is that many MPS VII mice have dilated ventricles, which can distort neuroanatomical landmarks. The presence and size of ventricular dilation varies considerably among individual animals, but tends to be more pronounced in older animals.

Newborn mice may be treated by transilluminating the head with a cold fiberoptic light. Cells or virus can be injected into the brain or into the ventricles using a vital dye to guide the injection via a 30 G or thinner needle or a pulled glass pipette (Snyder et al., 1995). The mice are cryoanesthetized by placing them on wet ice for a few minutes before injection. After injection, the pups are warmed. All the pups of one litter should be treated together, and should be taken from and returned to the dam as a group. This will minimize the risk of the dam rejecting or killing individual pups.

Vectors or modified cells may also be injected intravenously in newborns through the superficial temporal vein (Sands et al., 1993; Vogler et al., 1993). This vein is located on the side of the face and travels from just below the eye towards the ear. A needle 30 G or smaller must be used because the vein is very small. Injection is best accomplished with two people: one to immobilize the mouse and hold the head so that the vein is facing up and the skin is taut, the second to perform the injection. If the skin is too loose the needle will not penetrate easily, and if the skin is too taut the vein is constricted and cannot be seen. The needle is inserted bevel up just under the skin next to the vein, positioned over the vein and advanced until the bevel is in the vessel and surrounded by blood (care is needed at this stage; the vein lies very superficial) and the solution injected slowly. Neonatal mice will tolerate up to 100 μl of solution with no apparent adverse effects. If the needle is not positioned in the vein, build up of subcutaneous fluid makes this immediately apparent. It is not usually possible to reinject if a vein is missed; the other side of the head should be used instead. The procedure can be facilitated by using an illuminated magnifying lens or a surgical microscope with a magnification of 1.5–6 ×. This route of administration is best attempted with pups 1–4 days old because the skin becomes pigmented after this and the position of the vein changes, making it difficult to inject.

4.4 On Protocol #110: Preparation of Homogenates or Supernatants for Quantitative Lysosomal Enzyme Assays

One of the advantages of the MPS VII mouse model is the availability of sensitive biochemical and histochemical assays for GUSB. In addition, the MPS VII mouse has no detectable GUSB activity in the brain, eliminating the problem of background activity. The activity of the gene product can be quantitated in tissue homogenates and active GUSB can be precisely localized in individual cells. Quantitation of the lysosomal enzyme activities measures the liberation and subsequent fluorescence of 4-MU from the appropriate substrate (Glaser and Sly, 1973). The substrate for GUSB is a glucuronic acid linked to 4-MU through a beta linkage. β-glucuronidase and α-galactosidase activities (as a control) can be determined from cell culture medium, from cultured cells or from tissue homogenates. Both enzyme activities can be determined on homogenates prepared by the same method and the relative scale for both enzymes is similar.

Protein should be measured and the enzymatic activity expressed as nanomoles of substrate cleaved per hour per milligram protein. Reference values should be established because considerable variation can occur although the relative relationships between normal, carrier and mutant cells should be similar. The values for experimental tissues or cells are thus often expressed as a percentage of normals for a specific tissue (Birkenmeier et al., 1991; Wolfe et al., 1992a).

4.5 On Protocol #111: 4-MU Assay

One unit of activity = 1 nmol 4-MU liberated per mg protein per hour. Fluorometer settings: excitation 365 nm; emission 450 nm. If readings are out of the linear range, dilute the reactions 1 to 10 in stop buffer and read again. It is critical to store the stopped reactions in the dark. The readings are stable for at least 24 h.

4.6 On Protocol #112: Localization of β-Glucuronidase Activity; Naphthol-AS-BI β-D-Glucuronide Histochemical Staining

Active GUSB can be localized in frozen sections of 10–100 mm^2 by two methods, using either naphthol-AS-BI β-D-glucuronide or X-gluc as substrates. We routinely use the former because it appears to be more sensitive and does not diffuse as readily throughout the sample. A detailed description of the protocol for X-gluc staining has been published by Kyle et al. (1992). Using naphthol-AS-BI β-D-glucuronide as a substrate, a single cell expressing GUSB can be identified (see Wolfe et al., 1992b). Active enzyme cleaves the substrate and in the presence of hexazonium pararosaniline a red precipitate is formed (Fishman et al., 1967). Although the assay is not quantitative, relative intensities correlate well with the values obtained from the fluorometric assay (Wolfe et al., 1990; Taylor and Wolfe, 1994). The enzyme is stable in the chloral-hydrate-formalin fixative and we routinely perfuse anesthetized mice through the left ventricle. By doing this adjacent sections of brain can be processed for histochemistry, plastic embedding and fluorometric assay.

Cells in suspension may be allowed to settle on a slide, the solution aspirated and the cells air-dried. Adherent cells can be stained in the culture dish. Positive control slides should always be run with the experimental samples. Control slides can be made from cultured GUSB-positive cells dried to slides and stored at −20°C.

The duration of the preincubation (Step 10) and staining (Step 14) is empirical but approximations can be made as follows: (1) transfected cells (high expressing) 2 h preincubation, 2 h stain; (2) transfected cells (low expressing) 2 h preincubation, 4–16 h stain; (3) liver, spleen, kidney sections 2 h preincubation, 2 h stain; (4) brain sections 4 h preincubation, 4–16 h stain. For very low levels of enzyme activity both the preincubation and the stain times may be increased to 16 h (Wolfe et al., 1992b). For tissue sections with very high levels of activity the preincubation step may be omitted and the staining step shortened to as little as 15 min (Vogler et al., 1993).

If few positive cells are present they can be visualized better without counterstaining, which can mask positive reactions. The sections should be viewed under a good quality microscope using Nomarski optics and an 80 A to D blue photographic filter, which enhances the appearance of the red stain. The color should be a bright cherry red (Fig. 20.2; see Plate VIII). Some tissues that are not positive (e.g. some muscle fibers or fibroblasts in brain grafts) may appear reddish brown after staining, but these cells are clearly distinguishable from positive cells. Mutant and normal controls should always be processed and used for comparison.

4.7 Notes on Identification of Engrafted Donor Cells

Various methods of identifying donor cells in the brain are described elsewhere in this volume. Frozen sections can be assayed with an immunofluorescent antibody (IFA) reaction and stained for GUSB activity to colocalize cells and enzyme. However, the test sections should be prepared and photographed for IFA first because the AS-BI reaction for GUSB causes the whole section to fluoresce non-specifically. The GUSB will remain stable at 4°C for at least 1–2 days. If DNA from tissue sections is to be Southern blotted or used for PCR, tissues should not be stained for GUSB activity because the reaction appears to degrade DNA. Adjacent sections should be used instead.

4.8 Notes on Evaluation of Changes in Pathology

One characteristic that makes the MPS VII model attractive is the prominent phenotype of the intact animal (Birkenmeier et al., 1989; Sands et al., 1993) and the abnormal morphology at the cellular level (Vogler et al., 1990). Improvements in the characteristic gross phenotype of the whole animal are observed only when the therapy is initiated at or before birth (Kyle et al., 1990; Sands et al., 1993, 1994). However, when therapy is initiated in adults with well established disease a reduction in size and number of distended lysosomes in cells from various tissues can be observed (Birkenmeier et al., 1991; Wolfe et al., 1992a; Moullier et al., 1993; Marechal et al., 1993), including the brain (Taylor and Wolfe, unpublished data). The reduction in lysosomal storage is one of the most stringent tests of how effective an experimental therapy can be. Cells of the meninges, neurons and glial cells in adult animals have distended lysosomes (Vogler et al., 1990; Sands et al., 1994; Snyder et al., 1995).

Samples for light and electron microscopy are best prepared in a pathology laboratory. To preserve the morphology in the CNS the anesthetized animal should be perfused with a fixative through the left ventricle of the heart. Chloral hydrate-formalin fixative should be used to obtain sections for both enzyme activity and histology. The best preservation of morphology is achieved by perfusing with 2% glutaraldehyde and 4% paraformaldehyde in PBS; however, enzymatic activity is diminished with this fixative.

To evaluate changes in lysosomal storage the samples should be fixed and embedded in plastic sections as for electron microscopy (the GUSB histochemical assay does not work on tissues processed in this way). Sections 0.5–1 μm thick should be cut and stained with toluidine blue to detect relatively large distended lysosomes by light microscopy. The best visualization is obtained when the staining reaction progresses to a dark blue color. This type of analysis is sufficient for most applications but if the therapy appears to be effective and no distended lysosomes are seen, thin sections may be cut for electron microscopy.

Electron micrographs must be very carefully compared with MPS VII and normal controls because, even in advanced disease, many neurons and glial cells in the MPS VII brain do not contain distended lysosomes. Therefore, comparisons must be made in regions where storage is prevalent and large numbers of cells from the region must be examined. Morphometric analysis can be performed (Haskins et al., 1992), but is difficult and the assistance of an expert should be sought.

4.9 Notes on Analysis of Changes in Substrate Metabolism

Undegraded glycosaminoglycan substrates can be quantitated from MPS VII cells or tissues. In cells this is done by metabolic labeling with $^{35}SO_4$, precipitation by cetylpyridinium chloride, resolution on cellulose acetate gel, autoradiography and quantitation by density scanning (Stramm et al., 1990). In tissues glycosaminoglycans are precipitated by cetylpyridinium chloride, resuspended and stained with Alcian Blue 8GN, and quantitated spectrophotometrically at 625 nm (Schuchman et al., 1989).

ACKNOWLEDGMENTS

Many colleagues have contributed to the development of methods and the animal models described, including G. Aguirre, J. Barker, E. Birkenmeier, N. Fraser, M. Haskins, J. Kyle, D. Patterson, W. Sly, E. Snyder and R. Taylor. This work was supported by NIH grants DK-42707, DK-46637 and NS-29390. MSS was supported in part by a fellowships from the National MPS Society and the Kleberg Foundation.

REFERENCES

Barker, J.E., Wolfe, J.H., Rowe, L.B. and Birkenmeier, E.H. (1993) Advantages of gradient vs 5-fluoro-uracil enrichment of stem cells for retroviral-mediated gene transfer. *Exp Hematol* **21**:47–54.

Birkenmeier, E.H., Davisson, M.T., Beamer, W.G., Ganschow, R.E., Vogler, C.A., Gwynn, B., Lyford, K.A., Maltais, L.M. and Wawrzyniak, C.J. (1989) Murine mucopolysaccharidosis type VII: Characterization of a mouse with β-glucuronidase deficiency. *J Clin Invest* **83**:1258–1266.

Birkenmeier, E.H., Barker, J., Vogler, C.A., Kyle, J.W., Sly, W.S., Gwynn, B., Levy, B. and Pegors, C. (1991) Increased lifespan and correction of metabolic defects in murine mucopolysaccharidosis type VII after syngeneic bone marrow transplantation. *Blood* **78**:3081–3092.

Brot, F.E., Glaser, J.H., Roozen, K.J., Sly, W.S. and Stahl, P.D. (1974) In vitro correction of human fibroblasts by beta-glucuronidase from different human sources. *Biochem Biophys Res Commun* **57**:1–8.

D'Amore, M.A., Gallagher, P.M. Korfhagen, T.R. and Ganschow, R.E. (1988) Complete sequence and organization of the murine beta-glucuronidase gene. *Biochemistry* **27**:7131–7140.

Fishman, W.H., Goldman, S.S. and DeLellis, R. (1967) Dual localization of beta-glucuronidase in endoplasmic reticulum and in lysosomes. *Nature* **213**:457–460.

Funkenstein, B., Leary, S.L., Stein, J.C. and Catterall, J.F. (1988) Genomic organization and sequence of the Gus-sa allele of the murine β-glucuronidase gene. *Mol Cell Biol* **8**:1160–1168.

Gallagher, P.M., D'Amore, M.A., Lund, S.D. and Ganschow, R.E. (1988) The complete nucleotide sequence of murine beta-glucuronidase mRNA and its deduced polypeptide. *Genomics* **2**:215–219.

Glaser, J.H. and Sly, W.S. (1973) β-glucuronidase deficiency mucopolysaccharidosis: methods for enzymatic diagnosis. *J Lab Clin Med* **82**:969–977.

Hall, C.W., Cantz, M. and Neufeld, E.F. (1973) A beta-glucuronidase deficient mucopolysaccharidosis: Studies in cultured fibroblasts. *Arch Biochem Biophys* **155**:32–38.

Haskins, M.E., Desnick, R.J., DiFerrante, N., Jezyk, P.F. and Patterson, D.F. (1984) Beta-glucuronidase deficiency in a dog: A model of mucopolysaccharidosis VII. *Pediatr Res* **18**:980–984.

Haskins, M.E., Baker, H.J., Birkenmeier, E., Hoogerbrugge, P.M., Poorthuis, B.J.H.M., Sakiyama, T., Shull, R.M., Taylor, R.M., Thrall, M.A. and Walkley, S.U. (1991) Transplantation in animal model systems. In: *Treatment of Genetic Diseases*. R.J. Desnick (ed). Churchill Livingstone: New York, pp.183–202.

Haskins, M.E., Otis, E.J., Hayden, J.E., Jezyk, P.F. and Stramm, L.E. (1992) Hepatic storage of glycosaminoglycans in feline and canine models of mucopolysaccharidosis I, VI, and VII. *Vet Pathol* **29**:112–119.

Kyle, J.W., Birkenmeier, E.H., Gwynn, B., Vogler, C., Hoppe, P.C., Hoffmann, J.W. and Sly, W.S. (1990) Correction of murine mucopolysaccharidosis VII by a human β-glucuronidase transgene. *Proc Natl Acad Sci USA* **87**:3914–3918.

Kyle, J.W., Grubb, J.H., Galvin, N. and Vogler, C. (1992) β-glucuronidase (GUS) assay in animal tissue. In: *GUS Protocols*. S.R. Gallagher (ed). Academic Press: San Diego, pp.189–203.

Lagunoff, D., Nicol, D.M. and Pritzl, P. (1973) Uptake of β-glucuronidase by deficient human fibroblasts. *Lab Invest* **29**:449–453.

Marechal, V., Naffakh, N., Danos, O. and Heard, J.-M. (1993) Disappearance of lysosomal storage in spleen and liver of mucopolysaccharidosis VII mice after transplantation of genetically-modified bone marrow cells. *Blood* **82:**1358–1365.

Miller, R.D., Hoffman, J.W., Powell, P.P., Kyle, J.W., Shipley, J.M., Bachinsky, D.R. and Sly, W.S. (1990) Cloning and characterization of the human β-glucuronidase gene. *Genomics* **7:**280–283.

Moullier, P., Bohl, D., Heard, J.-M. and Danos, O. (1993) Correction of lysosomal storage in the liver and spleen of MPS VII mice by implantation of genetically modified skin fibroblasts. *Nature Genet* **4:**154–159.

Naleway, J.J. (1992) Histochemical, spectrophotometric, and fluorometric GUS substrates. In: *GUS Protocols.* S.R. Gallagher (ed). Academic Press: San Diego, pp.61–76.

Neufeld, E.F. and Fratantoni, J.C. (1970) Inborn errors of mucopolysaccharide metabolism. *Science* **169:**141–146.

Neufeld, E.F. and Muenzer, J. (1995) The mucopolysaccharidoses. In: *Metabolic Basis of Inherited Disease* 7th ed. C.R. Scriver, A.L. Beaudet, W.S. Sly, D. Valle (eds). McGraw-Hill: New York, pp.2465–2494.

Nishimura, Y., Rosenfeld, M.G., Kreibich, G., Gubler, U., Sabatini, D.D., Adesnik, M. and Andy, R. (1986) Nucleotide sequence of rat preputial gland β-glucuronidase cDNA and *in vitro* insertion of its encoded polypeptide into microsomal membranes. *Proc Natl Acad Sci USA* **83:**7292–7296.

Olsen, I., Dean, M.F., Harris, G. and Muir, H. (1981) Direct transfer of a lysosomal enzyme from lymphoid cells to deficient fibroblasts. *Nature* **291:**244–247.

Oshima, A., Kyle, J.W., Miller, R.D., Hoffman, J.W., Powell, P.P., Grubb, J.H., Sly, W.S., Tropak, M., Guise, K.S. and Gravel, R.A. (1987) Cloning, sequencing and expression of cDNA for human β-glucuronidase. *Proc Natl Acad Sci USA* **84:**685–689.

Paigen, K. (1989) Mammalian beta-glucuronidase: Genetics, molecular biology, and cell biology. *Prog Nucl Acid Res Mol Biol* **37:**155–205.

Powell, P.P., Kyle, J.W., Miller, R.D., Pantano, J., Grubb, J.H. and Sly, W.S. (1988) Rat liver beta-glucuronidase. cDNA cloning, sequence comparisons and expression of a chimeric protein in COS cells. *Biochem J* **250:**547–555.

Sambrook, J., Fritsch, E.F. and Maniatis, T. (1989) *Molecular Cloning, a Laboratory Manual*, 2nd ed. Cold Spring Harbor Laboratory Press: Cold Spring Harbor, NY.

Sando, G.N. and Neufeld, E.F. (1977) Recognition and receptor-mediated uptake of a lysosomal enzyme, alpha-L-iduronidase, by cultured human fibroblasts. *Cell* **12:**619–627.

Sands, M. and Birkenmeier, E. (1993) A single-base-pair deletion in the β-glucuronidase gene accounts for the phenotype of murine mucopolysaccharidosis type VII. *Proc Natl Acad Sci USA* **90:**6567–6571.

Sands, M.S., Barker, J.E., Vogler, C., Levy, B., Gwynn, B., Galvin, N., Sly, W.S. and Birkenmeier, E. (1993) Treatment of murine mucopolysaccharidosis type VII by syngeneic bone marrow transplantation in neonates. *Lab Invest* **68:**676–686.

Sands, M.S., Vogler, C., Kyle, J.W., Grubb, J.H., Levy, B., Galvin, N., Sly, W.S. and Birkenmeier, E.H. (1994) Enzyme replacement therapy for murine mucopolysaccharidosis type VII. *J Clin Invest* **93:**2324–2331.

Schuchman, E.H., Toroyan, T.K., Haskins, M.E. and Desnick, R.J. (1989) Characterization of the defective B-glucuronidase activity in canine mucopolysaccharidosis type VII. *Enzyme* **42:**174–180.

Sly, W.S., Quinton, B.A., McAlister, W.H. and Rimoin, D.L. (1973) Beta-glucuronidase deficiency: Report of clinical, radiographic, and biochemical features of a new mucopolysaccharidosis. *J Pediatr* **82:**249–257.

Smith, B.F., Hoffman, R.K., Giger, U. and Wolfe, J.H. (1990) Genes transferred by retroviral vectors into normal and mutant myotubes in primary cultures are expressed in myotubes. *Mol Cell Biol* **10:**3268–3271.

Snyder, E.Y., Deitcher, D.L., Walsh, C., Arnold-Aldea, S., Hartwieg, E.A. and Cepko, C.L. (1992) Multipotent neural cell lines can engraft and participate in development of mouse cerebellum. *Cell* **68:**1–20.

Snyder, E.Y., Taylor, R.M. and Wolfe, J.H. (1995) Neural progenitor cell engraftment corrects lysosomal storage throughout the MPS VII mouse brain. *Nature* **374**: 367–370.

Stramm, L., Wolfe, J., Schuchman, E., Haskins, M., Patterson, D. and Aguirre, G. (1990) B-glucuronidase mediated pathway essential for retinal pigment epithelial degradation of glycosaminoglycans. *Exp Eye Res* **50:**521–532.

Taylor, R.M. and Wolfe, J.H. (1994) Cross-correction of β-glucuronidase deficiency by retroviral vector-mediated gene transfer. *Exp Cell Res* **214**: 606–613.

Vogler, C., Birkenmeier, E.H., Sly, W.S., Levy, B., Pegors, C., Kyle, J.W. and Beamer, W.G. (1990) A murine models of mucopolysaccharidosis VII: Gross and microscopic findings in beta-glucuronidase-deficient mice. *Am J Pathol* **136:**207–217.

Vogler, C., Sands, M.S., Higgins, A., Levy, B., Grubb, J., Birkenmeier, E.H. and Sly, W.S. (1993) Enzyme replacement with recombinant β-glucuronidase in the newborn mucopolysaccharidosis type VII mouse. *Pediatr Res* **34:**837–840.

Wolfe, J.H., Schuchman, E.H., Stramm, L.E., Concaugh, E.A., Haskins, M.E., Aguirre, G.D., Patterson, D.F., Desnick, R.J. and Gilboa, E. (1990) Restoration of normal lysosomal function in mucopolysaccharidosis type VII cells by gene transfer. *Proc Natl Acad Sci USA* **87:**2877–2881.

Wolfe, J.H., Sands, M.S., Barker, J.E., Rowe, L.B., Gwynn, B., Vogler, C.A. and Birkenmeier, E.H. (1992a) Reversal of pathology in murine mucopolysaccharidosis type VII by somatic cell gene transfer. *Nature* **360**:749–753.

Wolfe, J.H., Deshmane, S.L. and Fraser, N.W. (1992b) Herpesvirus vector gene transfer and expression of β-glucuronidase in the CNS of MPS VII mice. *Nature Genet* **1**:379–384.

Wolfe, J.H., Kyle, J.W., Sands, M.S., Sly, W.S., Markowitz, D.G. and Parente, M.J. (1995) Over-expression of β-Glucuronidase from a double-copy retroviral vector in MPS VII cells. *Gene Ther* **2**:70–78.

CHAPTER 21

Targeting Gene Products to the Brain and Neurons using Bone Marrow Transplantation: A Cell-mediated Delivery System for Therapy of Inherited Metabolic Human Disease

S.U. WALKLEY, M.A. THRALL* AND K. DOBRENIS

Sidney Weisner Laboratory of Genetic Neurological Disease, Department of Neuroscience, Rose F. Kennedy Center for Research in Mental Retardation and Human Development, Albert Einstein College of Medicine, Bronx, NY 10461, USA. Tel: 718 430 4025; Fax: 718 430 8821; Email: walkley@aecom.yu.edu

**Department of Pathology, College of Veterinary Medicine and Biomedical Sciences, Colorado State University, Fort Collins, CO 80523, USA. Tel: 970 491 7508; Fax: 970 491 0603; Email: mthrall@vines.colostate.edu*

1 INTRODUCTION

Bone marrow transplantation (BMT) has been used in attempts to treat a number of genetic neurological diseases in children that otherwise would progress to severe brain damage and death. These include lysosomal hydrolase deficiencies (e.g. Hurler and Gaucher diseases), peroxisomal disorders (e.g. adrenoleukodystrophy) and other rare enzyme deficiencies (e.g. Lesch–Nyhan disease) (Parkman, 1986; Pyeritz, 1984). Exactly how this therapy might correct a genetic metabolic defect is largely theoretical. A variety of possible mechanisms have been proposed (Whitley et al., 1986) and in terms of brain disease these can be summarized as follows (see Fig. 21.1). (1) Direct cell replacement: if the primary gene defect has major impact on bone marrow-derived cells in brain (as is believed to occur in Krabbe disease, for example) BMT would lead to replacement of these diseased cells with normal cells (Tsai et al., 1992). (2) Direct or indirect gene product transfer: normal donor bone marrow-derived cells located within the vasculature, perivascular spaces or brain parenchyma would transfer the missing gene product to diseased neurons and glia. An example would be a neuronal storage disease in which a lysosomal hydrolase is missing, e.g. α-mannosidosis (Walkley et al., 1994a). (3) "Metabolic filtration": correction of a metabolic defect would occur without the newly available gene product directly entering diseased cells. Rather, toxic metabolites in extracellular locations would be removed by normal, bone marrow-derived cells and thereby generate a gradient for further depletion of these products from diseased cells (see Barranger, 1984).

Protocols for Gene Transfer in Neuroscience: Towards Gene Therapy of Neurological Disorders
Edited by P.R. Lowenstein and L.W. Enquist

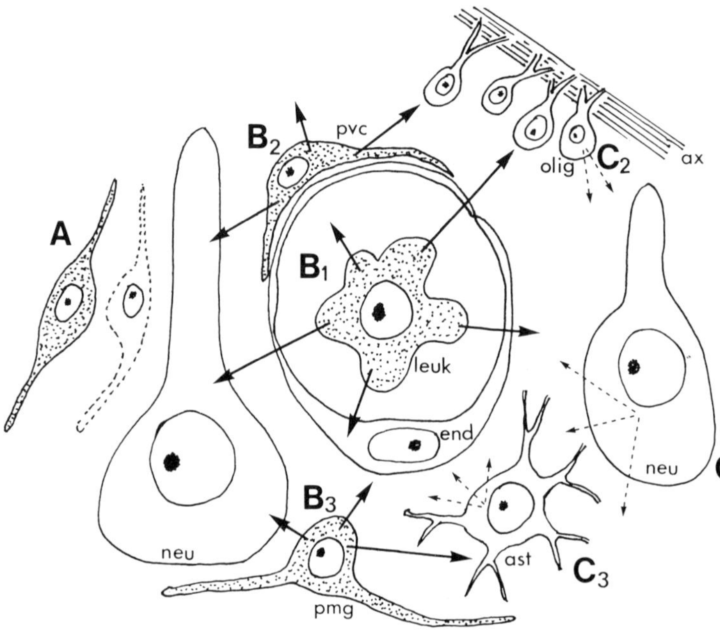

Figure 21.1 Mechanisms proposed to underlie possible metabolic correction in the CNS following BMT. (A) Direct cell replacement: normal donor bone marrow-derived cells may enter the CNS and slowly replace mesodermally derived cells of host origin. Cell in dotted lines indicates cell death. (B) Gene product release: gene products such as acid glycosidases may be released from donor bone marrow-derived cells and cross-correct metabolic defect in diseased cells. Possible locations of these cells include the vasculature (B_1), adjacent to blood vessels in brain (B_2), or within brain parenchyma (B_3). Straight arrows indicate release of gene product. (C) The metabolic filtration hypothesis: a gradient of substrate release may occur in which neurons (C_1), oligodendroglia (C_2) and astrocytes (C_3) eliminate abnormally accumulating products for metabolic processing in donor cells located elsewhere. Broken arrow indicates movement of substrate. Abbreviations: neu, neuron; leuk, blood leukocyte; end, endothelial cell; pvc, bone marrow-derived perivascular cell; pmg, parenchymal microglial cell; ast, astrocyte; olig, oligodendroglia; ax, axon

1.1 BMT for Treatment of Human Metabolic Brain Disease

Treatment of human genetic disease by BMT began in the late 1960s with attempts to correct severe combined immunodeficiency disease (Gatti et al., 1968). The first brain disease subjected to this therapy was mucopolysaccharidosis (MPS) type I, also known as Hurler disease (Hobbs et al., 1981). Over 150 children with a variety of inborn errors of metabolism affecting the brain have undergone BMT (Cowan, 1991; Krivit and Shapiro, 1991, 1994; Ozand and Gascon, 1992). Generally, three categories of genetic brain disease have been subject to BMT (see Table 21.1): (1) those with primary involvement of neurons due to deficiency of specific lysosomal hydrolases ("neuronal storage diseases"); (2) lysosomal hydrolase deficiencies with major involvement of glial cells, some of which manifest as leukodystrophies; (3) other types of brain diseases in which lysosomal hydrolases are not primarily involved.

1.2 Neuronal Storage Disorders

Long-term follow-up data (up to 10 years) of children with Hurler disease, a mucopolysaccharidosis resulting from deficiency of α-L-iduronidase, treated by BMT have recently become available (Hopwood et al., 1993; Krivit and Shapiro, 1991; Whitley et al., 1993). Successful engraftment led to normal or near-normal levels of plasma α-L-iduronidase activity and to reduced visceral

Table 21.1 Inherited brain diseases of humans treated by BMT

Category 1: Lysosomal enzyme deficiencies characterized by significant intraneuronal storage
Hurler disease (mucopolysaccharidosis type I)
Hunter disease (mucopolysaccharidosis type II)
Sanfilippo disease (mucopolysaccharidosis type III)
Niemann–Pick disease type A (sphingomyelin-cholesterol lipidosis type 1)
GM1 gangliosidosis
α-Mannosidosis
Pompe disease (Glycogenosis type II)
Category 2: Lysosomal enzyme deficiencies characterized by major glial cell involvement
Gaucher disease (glucosylceramide lipidosis)
Krabbe disease (globoid cell leukodystrophy)
Metachromatic leukodystrophy
Category 3: Other metabolic diseases of the nervous system
Adrenoleukodystrophy
Batten disease
Lesch–Nyhan disease

disease. Urinary glycosaminoglycan excretion was significantly lowered and splenomegaly and hepatomegaly reduced, with concomitant lowering of hepatic glycosaminoglycan content. Incidence of pneumonia, sleep apnea and heart failure were also reduced. Dysostosis multiplex, a severe skeletal change characteristic of this disease and some other mucopolysaccharidoses, remained unchanged but facial dysmorphology was reported to disappear. Analysis of CNS changes have been more difficult to evaluate fully. Reduced cerebrospinal fluid pressure has been documented, and may be of major benefit because pressure hydrocephalus is believed to contribute to brain dysfunction. Cognitive assessment provided equivocal results: although a few individuals were believed to improve following the transplant (Whitley et al., 1993), more commonly deterioration continued, though perhaps more slowly than in untreated patients. A key problem in evaluating the efficacy of BMT has been the wide clinical heterogeneity displayed by α-L-iduronidase deficiencies in children, ranging from severe forms of Hurler disease, to the considerably milder Scheie disease, and to intermediate variants referred to as Hurler–Scheie (Roubicek et al., 1985). It is impossible to predict the exact rate of disease progression and intellectual decline in patients exhibiting α-L-iduronidase deficiency, with the possible exception of the recently classified $W_{402}X$ homozygotes with severe Hurler disease (see Hopwood et al., 1993). Thus it is not known whether intraneuronal accumulation of glycosaminoglycans, gangliosides and other metabolic products in brain is actually reduced following BMT in Hurler children. Clinical studies have provided little insight into these issues and data on CNS changes in individuals dying at some stage following BMT are not available.

Other forms of MPS that exhibit direct or indirect CNS involvement, including type II (Hunter), type III (Sanfilippo), type IV (Morquio) and type VI (Maroteaux–Lamy), have also been treated with BMT. The pattern of findings mirrors that of Hurler disease: circulating levels of the missing enzyme increase after successful engraftment and visceral, cutaneous and other non-CNS effects, with the exception of some skeletal abnormalities, are largely ameliorated (Krivit and Shapiro, 1991, 1994; Krivit et al., 1984; McGovern et al., 1986; Vellodi et al., 1992). In forms of MPS characterized by intraneuronal storage in the CNS (types II and III) cognitive deterioration in a manner similar to Hurler disease has often been documented.

Several forms of sphingomyelin lipidosis, characterized by intraneuronal accumulation of sphingomyelin, gangliosides, cholesterol and related metabolic products, have also been subject to BMT. As a group these disorders exhibit substantial CNS involvement and variable visceral and skeletal affects. Results of BMT have been uniformly discouraging: two children with Niemann–Pick disease type A, a sphingomyelin lipidosis caused by lysosomal sphingomyelinase deficiency, exhibited no evidence of metabolic correction in viscera or brain (Bayever et al., 1992); one child with GM1 gangliosidosis, a lysosomal β-galactosidase deficiency with massive accumulation of ganglioside in neurons, exhibited no improvement after transplant (Shaw et al., 1986).

A 7-year-old patient with α-mannosidosis was treated with BMT but died 18 weeks after successful engraftment. Autopsy findings indicated that levels of α-mannosidase activity in liver and spleen had increased to near normal levels but activity in the brain was only marginally increased. The ultrastructure of liver and spleen revealed no lysosomal storage but CNS neurons remained heavily vacuolated. It was concluded that BMT reversed the disease in viscera but had no benefit in brain tissue (Will et al., 1987).

Type IIa glycogen storage disease (Pompe disease) in a 5-month-old child has been treated with BMT (Harris et al., 1986). This disorder is caused by lysosomal α-glucosidase deficiency which results in increased glycogen in most tissues, including the brain. The child died 5 months after successful engraftment and no evidence of metabolic correction was found. Glycogen storage persisted in all cells, including CNS neurons; only cells of the bone marrow and circulating lymphocytes were free of glycogen storage. It was speculated that the transplant was too late to be of benefit or that bone marrow-derived cells are incapable of transferring the needed enzyme to host cells.

1.3 Other Lysosomal Hydrolase Disorders

Other lysosomal disorders also exhibit CNS changes associated primarily with storage in macrophage-like cells in brain (Table 21.1, category 2) and BMT has been used to treat them. Examples include Gaucher disease, Krabbe disease and metachromatic leukodystrophy.

Gaucher disease is caused by deficiency of glucocerebrosidase and results in accumulation of glucosylceramide primarily in reticuloendothelial cells. Two of the three forms of Gaucher disease involve the CNS: acute (type 2) and chronic (type 3). In both, the CNS exhibits widespread distribution of lipid-laden macrophage-like cells known as Gaucher cells. Some degree of neuronal storage may also occur in type 2 disease, but a more prominent finding is death of neurons in select brain regions. A toxic effect of accumulating glucosylsphingosine has been proposed, but the pathogenic mechanisms are poorly understood.

BMT has been performed on several children with the neuronopathic forms of Gaucher disease (Rappeport et al., 1986; Tsai et al., 1992). Results indicate that Gaucher cells in brain and other tissues are replaced, albeit slowly, by normal donor bone marrow-derived cells and that neurological decline can be halted. Plasma glucosylceramide levels were normalized after transplant, and enzymic reconstitution was demonstrated in visceral tissue. However, little or no increase in brain levels of glucocerebrosidase was detected after transplant. Indeed, as this is a membrane-associated lysosomal hydrolase (Grabowski and Horowitz, 1990), direct cross-correction of diseased cells would not be anticipated.

Krabbe disease is caused by deficiency of lysosomal galactosylceramidase (galactocerebroside β-galactosidase) and exhibits several clinical phenotypes with different ages of onset. Swollen reticuloendothelial cells ("globoid cells"), which are similar to Gaucher cells, are abundant in brain white matter and contain large amounts of undigested galactocerebroside. Myelin loss is severe and appears secondary to death of oligodendroglia. These cells may die as a result of accumulation of a toxic compound, psychosine, which is normally metabolized by galactosylceramidase (Igisu and Suzuki, 1984). Astrocytosis is common; neurons are largely spared in terms of metabolic disease. Changes in white matter are believed to account for most of the neurological features of the disease.

Krabbe disease was thought to be a good candidate for BMT as globoid cells are probably mesodermal in origin (Suzuki and Suzuki, 1989). Both infantile and juvenile forms have been treated and have shown very different results. BMT had no apparent benefit on infantile Krabbe disease, possibly because of its rapid onset and progression (disease duration is 1 year or less). In contrast, BMT in juvenile Krabbe actually improved cognitive and motor skills in the first year after transplant (Shapiro et al., 1991).

Metachromatic leukodystrophy (MLD) is another lysosomal disease with substantial white matter involvement that has been treated with BMT (Krivit and Shapiro, 1994). This disorder is caused by a deficiency of arylsulfatase A and is characterized by accumulation of cerebroside sulfate primarily in white matter of the CNS. A variety of clinical forms are recognized, based on age of onset. Metachromatic granules accumulate in macrophages in brain, in oligodendroglia and some neurons. Several children with MLD have been subjected to BMT (Bayever et al., 1985; Krivit and Shapiro, 1994). Like Krabbe disease, BMT appears to have most benefit in late-onset, slowly developing clinical phenotypes (e.g. juvenile MLD) whereas disease in patients with late infantile MLD steadily progresses despite normalization of circulating enzyme levels.

1.4 Other Neurological Disorders

Adrenoleukodystrophy is an X-linked peroxisomal disorder that exhibits accumulation of very long chain fatty acids (VLCFA). As the name implies, this is primarily a white matter disease and is accompanied by adrenal insufficiency. Nutritional therapy has been shown to reduce VLCFA to normal levels and to be of some benefit in this disease. BMT has been reported to improve cognitive skills in some patients in whom disease was not advanced at the time of transplant (Krivit and Shapiro, 1994). Batten disease is characterized in part by lysosomal accumulation of subunit c of mitochondrial ATP synthase (Palmer et al., 1992) but exhibits no known defect in lysosomal enzymes. BMT in one patient was reported to have been of no value (Lake et al., 1995). Lesch–Nyhan disease is an X-linked disorder of purine metabolism in which the activity of hypoxanthine guanine phosphoribosyltransferase (HPRT) is defective. Affected individuals exhibit mental retardation, athetoid cerebral palsy and compulsive self-mutilation. Brains of Lesch–Nyhan patients show no overt cellular changes and the pathophysiology of this disease is poorly understood. BMT was of no benefit to a 22-year-old man with this disease (Nyhan et al., 1986).

1.5 BMT in Animal Models of Metabolic Brain Disease

The use of experimental animal models provides advantages in evaluating the efficacy of BMT. As most of these diseases are autosomal recessive conditions, heterozygotes can be identified and used to produce affected and unaffected offspring, the latter being ideal donors for BMT. The availability of affected animals with similar (or identical) genetic backgrounds reduces clinical variability and minimizes one of the major obstacles limiting evaluation of BMT in human disease. Colony-rearing of genetic models of brain disease also provides sufficient numbers of affected animals to evaluate disease pathogenesis in considerable detail. Animal models of lysosomal enzyme deficiencies have been particularly useful in this regard (Siegel and Walkley, 1994; Walkley, 1988; Walkley et al., 1991). Induced models of storage diseases using specific enzyme inhibitors have supplied important information on pathogenesis of brain dysfunction and on reversibility of disease-induced changes in brain tissue (Walkley et al., 1987; Walkley, 1988). The age of transplant can be systematically varied to determine its effects, and tissues can be collected at multiple time points. The ability to rapidly collect tissues for freezing or optimal fixation is a major advantage in terms of evaluating the tissue changes resulting from a transplant procedure. A variety of animal models of neurological diseases have been subject to BMT (Table 21.2), and include the human brain disease categories given in Table 21.1 (Haskins et al., 1991).

1.5.1 Category 1 Diseases

One of the most extensively studied animal models has been fucosidosis (α-L-fucosidase deficiency) as it occurs in English Springer Spaniels (Kelly et al., 1983). Disease begins at 4–8 months with mild hypermetria and behavioral abnormalities and progresses steadily to severe mental and motor system disease and death at 24–30 months. Onset and progression of intraneuronal storage occurs at a rate commensurate with clinical progression. Fifteen dogs have been successfully engrafted at various ages and detailed analyses summarized (Taylor et al., 1992). Generally, BMT increased levels of fucosidase activity in a variety of tissues and this was coupled with evidence for significant amelioration of the metabolic defect. Fucosidase activity in brain reached 10% of normal by 6 months after transplant and neurons exhibited reduced intracellular storage. Transplants in the early postnatal period gave the best results; BMT performed later did

Table 21.2 Inherited brain diseases in animals that have been treated by BMT

Disease	*Category*	*Species*	*Reference*
Fucosidosis	1	Dog	Taylor et al., 1992
α-Mannosidosis	1	Cat	Walkley et al., 1994a
MPSI (Hurler–Scheie)	1	Dog	Shull et al., 1988
MPSVI (Maroteaux–Lamy)	1	Cat	Gasper et al., 1984
MPSVII (Sly)	1	Mouse	Birkenmeier et al., 1991
GM1 Gangliosidosis	1	Cat	Baker and Walkley (unpublished data)
GM2 Gangliosidosis	1	Cat	Walkley et al. (unpublished data)
Krabbe	2	Mouse	Hoogerbrugge et al., 1988a,b
Niemann–Pick type C	3	Mouse	Sakiyama et al., 1983
		Cat	Brown et al., 1994
Batten	3	Dog	Deeg et al., 1990

not reverse the established clinical disease. This study provided the first clear evidence that BMT could significantly affect events within neurons in a genetic metabolic disease. Unfortunately the specific mechanism (see Fig. 21.1) responsible for the correction could not be identified.

A similar disease in cats, α-mannosidosis, has also been studied. Lysosomal α-mannosidase deficiency in Persian-cross cats manifests as a progressive neurological disease with onset just after weaning (6 weeks of age) and death generally by 6 months (Vandevelde et al., 1982). Storage of mannose-rich oligosaccharides is widespread in brain and viscera. BMT at 8–12 weeks of age not only prevented further disease progression but also reversed intraneuronal storage at the time of transplant (Walkley et al., 1994a) (Fig. 21.2). Lysosomal α-mannosidase activity in brain after treatment was 10–15% of normal. Histochemical studies demonstrated activity of this enzyme specifically within neurons and glia in the CNS and thus established for the first time that BMT could elevate levels of a given gene product in diseased cells (Figs 21.3 and 21.4; see Plates VII and VIII). Recent studies indicate that the probable explanation for this is that microglia from donor bone marrow are present in brain and secrete substantial amounts of acidic α-mannosidase which is internalized by diseased neurons (Dobrenis et al., 1994). Studies of bovine α-mannosidosis have provided additional evidence that normal blood-derived cells can cross-correct diseased neurons *in vivo*. In this case partial reduction in intraneuronal storage was observed in a chimeric calf with α-mannosidosis whose twin was normal (Jolly et al., 1976).

Animal models of mucopolysaccharidosis have also been subject to BMT. The clinical condition of several dogs with MPS type I (Hurler–Scheie form) transplanted at 5 months improved and the animals showed evidence of reduced glycosaminoglycan storage in a variety of tissues, including brain (Shull et al., 1987, 1988). Activity of α-L-iduronidase in liver reached 45% of normal and was accompanied by markedly reduced glycosaminoglycan storage in hepatocytes. Levels of iduronidase in brain were considerably lower (less than 10% of normal) but there was evidence of significantly reduced storage in vascular endothelial cells and smaller decreases in intraneuronal storage.

Maroteaux–Lamy disease (MPS VI) is caused by deficiency of arylsulfatase B and exhibits pathological changes in visceral and skeletal tissues (Spranger et al., 1970). Brain tissue generally is spared, at least in terms of neurons. However, the feline model of this disease has been found to exhibit significant intracellular storage in occasional neurons in the cerebral cortex (Walkley and Thrall, unpublished data). The storage material appeared floccular and membranous and resembled cytoplasmic inclusions typical of other mucopolysaccharidoses. Extensive studies have clearly established that BMT corrects metabolism in visceral tissues and reduces severity of skeletal changes (Gasper et al., 1984; Wenger et al., 1986). Preliminary studies of brain tissue from BMT-treated MPS VI cats suggest only partial reduction in intracellular storage (Walkley and Thrall, unpublished data).

A murine model of MPS VII has also been studied. Mice with this disorder exhibit significant visceral, skeletal and CNS disease (Vogler et al., 1990). BMT in neonatal and adult animals has significantly reduced storage of glycosaminoglycans and increased life span. The greatest improvements occurred in animals treated early. The most significant reduction of storage in

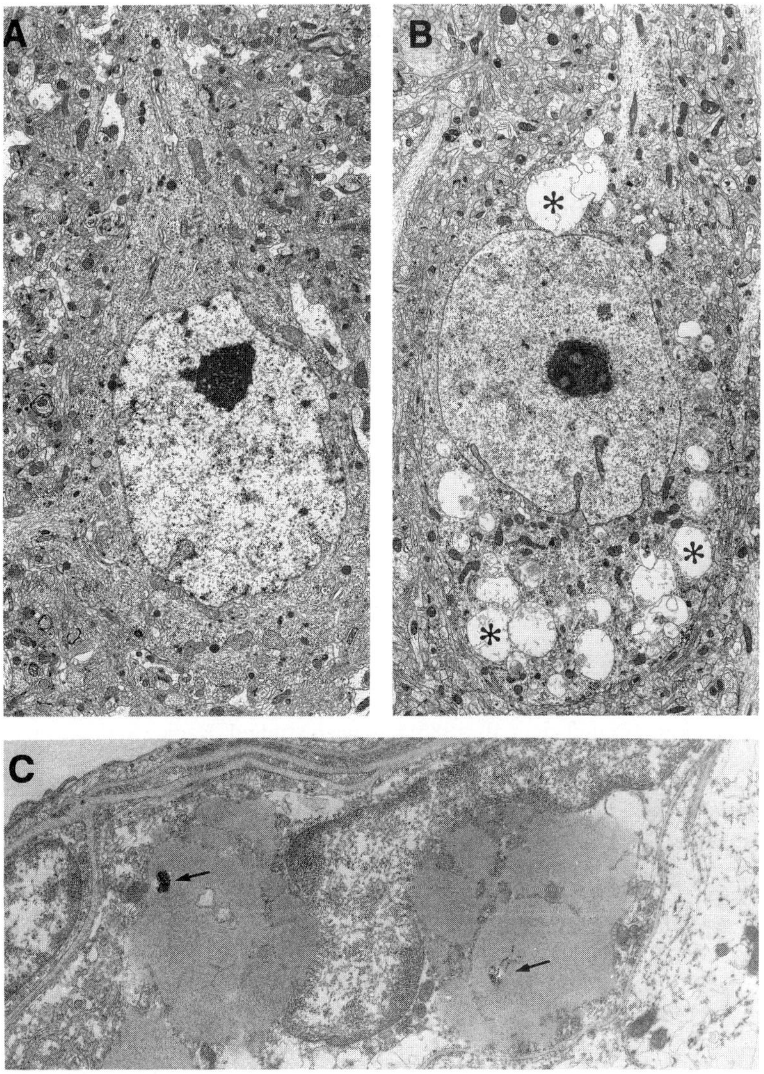

Figure 21.2 Electron micrographs of CNS cells in cats with α-mannosidosis with and without BMT. (A) Cortical pyramidal neuron (× 5280), showing lack of intracellular storage 2 years after receiving BMT at 2 months of age. (B) Cortical pyramidal neuron (× 7720) in a 2-month-old affected, untreated cat. Typical storage vacuoles are indicated by asterisks. (C) Perivascular microglia-like cell in the cat shown in A (× 14 040), exhibiting histochemical evidence of acidic α-mannosidase (arrows). Light micrographs of cell type shown in C are given in Fig. 21.4 (Plate VIII)

brain occurred in leptomeningeal cells rather than neurons, and histochemical studies revealed that β-glucuronidase activity was limited to perivascular cells (Birkenmeier et al., 1991; Sands et al., 1993).

Animal models of ganglioside storage diseases also appear considerably less amenable to BMT than other types of storage disorders. A Portuguese water dog with GM1 gangliosidosis (Saunders et al., 1988) was transplanted at 12 weeks and plasma β-galactosidase levels normalized following successful engraftment (O'Brien et al., 1990). However, neurological disease progressed in a manner similar to untreated controls and autopsy at 7 months revealed accumulation of GM1 ganglioside in brain. In contrast, cytoplasmic vacuolation in liver disappeared with treatment. BMT in 5- and 7-month-old cats with GM1 gangliosidosis produced similar results in terms of reversing CNS disease, but clinical progression did appear slower (Baker and Walkley, unpublished data). Although storage in CNS neurons was severe at death, neurons in dorsal root ganglia were free of storage. In a 7-week-old kitten with GM2 gangliosidosis neurological deterioration progressed in a manner identical to that of an untreated control and morphological study revealed massive accumulation of ganglioside in CNS neurons. In contrast, levels of β-hexosaminidase in the cerebral cortex were high—30% of normal activity was detected. Subsequent histochemical studies using an indigogenic substrate for β-hexosaminidase revealed that the enzyme was confined to microglial cells (Walkley et al., 1994b).

1.5.2 Category 2 Diseases

A murine model of galactosylceramidase deficiency known as "twitcher" is analogous to human globoid cell leukodystrophy (Krabbe disease) (Duchen et al., 1980) and has been used in BMT studies (Hoogerbrugge et al., 1988a, 1988b; Yeager et al., 1984). Twitcher mice are neurologically impaired, have a shortened life span, and exhibit white matter disease very similar to the human disorder. BMT has been found to result in migration of donor bone marrow-derived cells into brain and the slow disappearance of globoid cells, followed by remyelination and improved clinical condition.

1.5.3 Category 3 Diseases

Neuronal storage diseases not caused by lysosomal hydrolase defects have also been studied. The efficacy of BMT for Niemann–Pick disease type C, a lipidosis associated with a defect in cholesterol trafficking (Pentchev et al., 1985) has been studied in mice and cats. Clinical disease progresses secondary to accumulation of cholesterol, gangliosides and related metabolic products in lysosomes in cells of many tissues. The mouse model designated *spm/spm* showed reduced accumulation of sphingomyelin and cholesterol in liver but no improvement in neurological features, despite evidence of donor bone marrow-derived cells in brain (Sakiyama et al., 1983, 1992). Similar results were found in the feline model (Brown et al., 1993). A second murine model in Balb/c mice was subject to a reverse transplant—diseased marrow was transplanted into a normal host. Bone marrow-derived cells remained abnormal and slight increases in sphingomyelin and cholesterol were noted in visceral tissues (Boothe et al., 1984). Treatment has also been attempted in a canine model of Batten disease but the disease process appeared unaltered (Deeg et al., 1990).

1.6 Bone Marrow-derived Cells in the CNS

Experience with BMT as a treatment for lysosomal storage diseases indicates that macromolecules normally excluded by the blood–brain barrier (BBB) can be delivered to the CNS from the periphery. This delivery can be substantial and result in therapeutic efficacy. For those diseases in which BMT proved successful, the most common explanation has been cellular invasion of the CNS by bone marrow-derived cells, with subsequent secretion of relevant macromolecules. There are two possible explanations for the presence of bone marrow-derived cells in brain: first, extravasation of blood cells can accompany pathological change in brain as in other tissues; secondly, even the normal CNS is populated by cells of hematopoietic lineage—that is, in addition to neurons and macroglia (astrocytes and oligodendroglia), the vertebrate CNS contains another abundant class of cells, microglia, some or all of which may be bone marrow-derived. Estimates of microglial numbers in the adult reach 20% of the total glial population and microglia are present in all major regions of the CNS (Lawson et al., 1990; Perry and Gordon, 1991). The origin of these cells has been debated since the turn of the century. Some of the argument can today be linked in part to the realization that the cells in question may constitute both a fundamentally heterogeneous and a highly mutable population. In examining the evidence for bone marrow-derived cells in the normal CNS it is therefore useful to first consider some general categories of microglia and brain macrophages.

1.6.1 *Types of Microglia and Brain Macrophages*

The developing CNS contains cells with characteristic macrophage-like properties referred to as "ameboid" microglia. Generally, these phagocytes are evident initially in the fetus, become most abundant in the perinatal period, and decline in number over a period of days or weeks. The precise timing varies with species and CNS region (Rio-Hortega, 1932; Choi, 1981; Ling, 1981; Murabe and Sano, 1982; Innocenti et al., 1983; Perry et al., 1985; Cuadros, 1992; Hutchins et al., 1992). Relatively few appear to be present in adult parenchyma but similar cells can be found in the circumventricular organs (areas lacking a BBB) and the choroid plexus (Perry and Gordon, 1991). In contrast, cells characteristic of normal adult CNS are the "ramified", "quiescent", or "parenchymal" microglia (terms dependent on circumstance or investigator, but essentially interchangeable). These cells typically have limited perikaryal cytoplasm and variably display several fine processes with numerous short branches and spiny projections. Parenchymal microglia are common in both white and gray matter where they appear free-standing or as "perineuronal" cells (Rio-Hortega, 1932; Lawson et al., 1990; Peters et al., 1991; Perry and Gordon, 1991) . Some also reside near blood vessels but lie within the parenchyma proper and may contribute to the glia limitans (Lassmann et al., 1991). It has been argued that these are the only perivascular cells that should be considered "microglia" and are distinct from the **perivascular** cells that reside between the glia limitans and the endothelial layer (Graeber and Streit, 1990; Streit and Graeber, 1991). The latter population of cells is not ramified and resembles ameboid microglia or macrophage-like cells (Honda et al., 1990; Graeber et al., 1992; Hickey et al., 1992; Graeber, 1993; Perry et al., 1994). Within the perivascular space, cells have also been identified as macrophages, pericytes and lipid phagocytes (Jordan and Thomas, 1988; Kida et al., 1993). Finally, it should be noted that macrophage-like cells are also present within the ventricular system of the CNS, the subarachnoid spaces and the leptomeninges (Perry and Gordon, 1991; Perry et al., 1994).

1.6.2 *Origin and Turnover of Microglia and Brain Macrophages*

Current opinion strongly favors a myelomonocytic origin for the ameboid microglia prominent during brain development. This is largely based on cellular and molecular similarities, including numerous antigenic/histochemical markers shared with other tissue macrophages. Apparent transitions from round monocyte-like cells to ameboid cells have been frequently described (Ling, 1981; Jordan and Thomas, 1988; Perry and Gordon, 1991; Thomas, 1992; Ling and Wong, 1993). Furthermore, in tracer studies, monocytes labeled with carbon particles *ex vivo* are found as carbon-positive ameboid microglia following reinjection into neonatal rats (Ling et al., 1980). The timing of appearance of ameboid cells in brain correlates with vascularization of the CNS, supporting the notion of a blood-borne origin. They are also abundant in brain at the time of normal cell death, and this finding has led to the concept that invasion of monocytes from the vasculature is stimulated by cellular degeneration (Innocenti et al., 1983; Perry et al., 1985; Matsumoto and Ikuta, 1985; Ashwell, 1990, 1991). This view appears reasonable in light of similar infiltration that can occur in pathologic states in the adult CNS. The dynamics of proliferation and fate/turnover of these microglia are poorly understood.

There is considerable evidence to show that the non-parenchymal, perivascular cells of the adult CNS are derived from bone marrow. These cells, like ameboid microglia, have macrophage-like characteristics and express monocyte–macrophage lineage markers. They can also express major histocompatibility complex molecules and present antigen (Hickey and Kimura, 1988; Streit et al., 1989; Hickey et al., 1992; Graeber et al., 1992; Graeber, 1993; Flaris et al., 1993; Perry et al., 1994). Numerous BMT studies using specific antigenic or genetic markers to identify donor-derived cells have confirmed that this perivascular population is of bone marrow origin. These experiments have been performed both on young and adult recipients of a variety of species, including humans, and suggest that substantial turnover of this population may occur throughout life (Hickey and Kimura, 1988; De Groot et al., 1992; Hickey et al., 1992; Unger et al., 1993; Walkley et al., 1994a; Krall et al., 1994). For example, detailed studies with adult rats estimate a 20–40% turnover of perivascular cells of monocyte–microglial lineage in 2–3 months (Hickey et al., 1992). Similar putative donor-derived perivascular cells were prominent in brains of cats with α-mannosidosis that received BMT and demonstrated replacement of gene product in CNS neurons (Walkley et al., 1994a). The extent to which procedures associated with BMT, such as irradiation, may influence the turnover of bone marrow-derived perivascular cells is unclear: some studies with adult rats suggest that the BMT protocol has no significant effect on the size of the perivascular population (Hickey et al., 1992; Lassmann et al., 1993). Given the procedural and species variability, particularly when young animals are used, further study would be appropriate (Sands et al., 1993).

Although most studies also support a monocytic origin for the adult parenchymal microglial cell some debate remains. Over the course of development the appearance of ramified microglia overlaps the disappearance of ameboid microglia. Numerous studies have suggested that ameboid cells transform into ramified microglia after passing through transitional stages (e.g. Rio-Hortega, 1932; Perry et al., 1985; Cuadros et al., 1992; Wu et al., 1992, 1994) but other studies have failed to find these transitional cells (Schelper and Adrian, 1986; De Groot et al., 1992), have suggested the simultaneous appearance of ameboid and ramified cells (Chugani et al., 1991), or have claimed transitional forms between neuroepithelium-derived cells and microglia (Kitamura et al., 1984). Ramified microglia also lack many antigenic and molecular markers of monocyte–macrophage lineage. For some this has served as an argument against a monocytic origin (Oehmichen et al., 1979; Miyake et al., 1984; Matsumoto and Ikuta, 1985); however, it is now recognized that the adult parenchymal cells can be viewed as normally "quiescent" but can respond to CNS injury by expressing these otherwise absent markers (Graeber et al., 1990b; Thomas, 1992; Gerhmann and Kreutzberg, 1993). On the other hand, evidence of antigenic markers for ramified microglia that are absent from other monocyte–macrophage lineage cells and present on neuroepithelium lineage cells is lacking (McKanna, 1993; Fedoroff and McKanna, 1994; Wolswijk, 1994).

Tagging prospective progenitor populations by a variety of techniques has done little to clarify the origin of ramified microglia. However, studies involving BMT in mice, rats and humans have made it clear that if these microglia are derived from hematopoietic cells, immigration into the adult CNS is minimal. Replacement of resident with donor-derived cells has been estimated as 1% or less of total parenchymal microglia even several months after transplantation (Matsumoto and Fujiwara, 1987; Hickey et al., 1992; Krall et al., 1994). A study combining [^{3}H]thymidine labeling with F4/80 immunohistochemistry, a reliable marker for mouse microglia, has suggested that the adult ramified microglial population is turned over once in the life of the animal, half through local division of resident cells and half through replacement from circulating monocytes (Lawson et al., 1992). The use of transfection with viral constructs bearing the *E. coli* β-galactosidase gene, as applied to the investigation of neuronal and macroglial lineage *in vivo*, has revealed no evidence of colineage between CNS cell types and microglia (Grove et al., 1993; Levinson et al., 1993; Luskin et al., 1993). In cell culture studies, ameboid microglia isolated from fetal or neonatal brain can remain apparently unchanged for extended periods but under some conditions can acquire characteristics of ramified microglia (Giulian and Baker, 1986; Suzumura et al., 1991; Liu et al., 1994). A recent study has shown that blood monocytes and spleen macrophages can develop into ramified microglia-like cells when cultured with astrocytes (Sievers et al., 1994). The strongest evidence of a neuroepithelial origin for microglia has come from a series of cell culture studies by Fedoroff and colleagues (Richardson et al., 1994), suggesting that microglial cells develop in CNS cultures of C_3H/HeJ mice from progenitor cells that (1) lack monocyte–macrophage lineage characteristics (Hao et al., 1991), (2) are positive for lipocortin-1, also present in primitive neuroepithelium (Fedoroff and McKanna, 1994; McKanna, 1993), and (3) may also give rise to astrocytes (Hao et al., 1991; Novak and Federoff, 1994). Furthermore, microglia were found to develop in cultures prepared from neural tube of 9-day embryos, before vascularization and when mesodermal, hematopoietic progenitor cells are probably absent (Hao et al., 1991).

Other cells of bone marrow origin associated with the normal CNS are lymphocytes and macrophages found in meninges, ventricles and choroid plexus. Turnover of these macrophages appears rapid in the adult (Hickey et al., 1992, De Groot et al., 1992; Lawson et al., 1993). In BMT studies in rats 50–70% of meningeal macrophages were replaced by donor cells in 2–3 months (Hickey et al., 1992). Although the number of lymphocytes in the adult CNS is normally exceedingly low, activated T lymphocytes appear to cycle through the brain parenchyma even in the absence of CNS disease (Hickey et al., 1991, 1992).

In the context of therapy for neurologic diseases it is worth reiterating that pathologic states may themselves increase the influx of bone marrow-derived cells into the CNS. The extent to which this occurs and the cell types involved may vary widely from one condition to another. Inflammation can occur in the CNS as in other tissues, and macrophages are a major and often sustained element in both immunologic and non-immunologic conditions (Oehmichen, 1983). Several human neurologic disorders marked by demyelination, such as multiple sclerosis, involve infiltration of lymphocytes as well as the presence of phagocytes (Compston, 1993; Couraud, 1994). However, genetic deficiency of galactocerebrosidase (Krabbe disease) leads to demyelination and infiltration of macrophages without lymphocytic involvement (Matsushima et al., 1994, Hoogerbrugge et al., 1988b; Suzuki and Suzuki, 1989). A prominent blood-borne macrophage invasion with no significant immune component occurs when the BBB is compromised following mechanical or cryogenic injury and severe ischemia (Schelper and Adrian, 1986; Streit et al., 1988; Perry and Gordon, 1991; Flaris et al., 1993; Fernaud-Espinosa et al., 1993; Raivich et al., 1993; Myers and Cremer, 1994).

Macrophage-like cells are also apparent in pathologic conditions that do not overtly compromise the BBB or involve an immunologic process. Resident parenchymal microglia can become "activated" to proliferate and in some cases become phagocytic, thereby potentially contributing to "macrophage" populations in CNS pathology. This has been best documented using models of retrograde neuronal degeneration where contribution of macrophages from the vasculature in the region of dying neuronal cell bodies has been largely excluded (Graeber et al., 1988a, b; Streit and Kreutzberg, 1988; Streit et al., 1988; Rieske et al., 1989; Graeber et al., 1990a; Thanos et al., 1992; Streit and Graeber, 1993). Evidence for activated, and in some cases phagocytic, cells originating from local parenchymal microglia has been found in a wide variety of disorders affecting the CNS, including Alzheimer's, Parkinson's, and Huntington's diseases and amyotrophic lateral sclerosis (McGeer et al. 1988a, b; McGeer et al., 1993, Dickson et al., 1993). Experimental studies to model processes that may occur in some neurodegenerative diseases (Choi, 1988) suggest that a microglial reaction can occur in response to excitotoxic neuronal death as well as leukocyte invasion (Akiyama et al., 1988; Perry and Andersson, 1992; Fernaud-Espinosa et al., 1993; Topper et al., 1993). Similarly, phagocytic populations following penetrating injuries and ischemia may derive, to some extent, from local microglial populations (Brierley and Brown, 1982; Perry and Gordon, 1991; Fernaud-Espinosa et al., 1993; Gehrmann and Kreutzberg, 1993; Korematsu et al., 1994). Changes in bone marrow-derived perivascular cell populations can also occur (Streit and Graeber, 1993). Examples are studies suggesting entry of perivascular cells into the parenchyma in Alzheimer's disease (Wisniewski and Weigel, 1993) and following retrograde neuronal degeneration (Streit et al., 1989). The rate of turnover of perivascular cells can be enhanced, as demonstrated in bone marrow chimeras with experimental autoimmune encephalomyelitis, a model of immune-mediated demyelinating disease (Lassmann et al., 1993).

1.6.3 Secretory Capacity of Microglia

In considering the potential for microglial populations to act as agents of gene product delivery to the brain the question of their capacity for secretion is paramount. Microglia have been shown to release significant amounts of a wide variety of molecules, including cytokines, growth factors, neurotoxins, proteases, nitric oxide and lysosomal glycosidases (Giulian and Baker, 1985; Vaca and Wendt, 1992; Nakajima et al., 1992a, 1992b; Banati et al., 1993; Chao et al., 1993; Fischer et al., 1993; Giulian et al., 1993; Mallat and Chamak, 1994; Gebicke-Haerter et al., 1994; Dobrenis et al., 1994). The investigation of secretion has been facilitated by the availability of virtually pure cultures of microglial cells, usually ameboid or macrophage-like. These are typically prepared by generating high-density cultures of mixed glial populations from the CNS of newborn animals, removing the microglia preferentially by a "shaking" procedure and further enriching them by differential adhesion. Microglia have been isolated from many species including rats, mice, rabbits, goats and cats (Giulian and Baker, 1986; Suzumura et al., 1987; Dow et al., 1990; Hassan et al., 1991b, 1991c; Roque and Caldwell, 1993; Baszler et al., 1994; Dobrenis et al., 1994) and from CNS of fetal and adult humans (Hassan et al., 1991a; Lee et al., 1992; Williams et al., 1992; Norenberg et al., 1994). Microglial cell lines have been recently obtained by immortalization (Hosaka et al., 1992; Sacerdote et al., 1993; Briers et al., 1994).

Studies on the ability of microglia to secrete acid glycosidases may provide important insights into BMT treatment of lysosomal hydrolase deficiencies in humans and other experimental models. The extracellular release of several lysosomal glycosidases has been evaluated using purified microglial cultures from cat neocortex. Acid-optimum α-mannosidase activity rapidly accumulated in culture medium, reaching levels equivalent to intracellular levels within 3 days. The apparent relative "secretion" of all other enzymes assessed was substantially less or undetectable by enzyme activity. Of those detectable, β-D-*N*-acetylhexosaminidase and β-D-galactosidase were lowest. The high α-mannosidase and low hexosaminidase and galactosidase secretion findings closely correlate with CNS findings following BMT in the feline neuronal storage diseases described in Section 1.5.1.

2 MATERIALS AND EQUIPMENT

2.1 Major Equipment and Miscellaneous Supplies for BMT in Cats and Dogs

(1) Sterile laminar flow unit.
(2) Sterile tissue sieve.
(3) Osgood or Rosenthal 18-gauge bone marrow biopsy needles.
(4) Linear accelerator (6 MeV).
(5) Spinal needle, 30 cm.
(6) Sterile plastic syringes (12 and 20 ml).
(7) Isoflurane gas for anesthesia.
(8) Refrigerated centrifuge, Beckman model TJ6.
(9) Tissue culture plate, 96-well.
(10) Hemocytometer.

2.2 Drugs, Chemicals, Buffers

(1) Antibiotics: cyclosporin, enrofloxacin, ampicillin, cefoxitin.
(2) Prednisone.
(3) Recombinant canine G-CSF.
(4) Erythropoietin.
(5) Preservative-free heparin.
(6) Hanks buffered salt solution (HBSS).
(7) Potassium chloride, 0.075 M.
(8) Tris buffer.
(9) Lactated Ringer's solution for injection.
(10) RPMI culture medium (Gibco/BRL).
(11) Colchicine (Gibco).
(12) Penicillin/streptomycin solution in normal saline (10 000 U penicillin, 10 μg streptomycin per ml).

3 THE PROTOCOLS

The technique of allogeneic BMT consists of donor selection, recipient conditioning, donor cell preparation and infusion (bone marrow transplant) and evaluation of engraftment and medical management following BMT (Gasper et al., 1989, 1992a, b).

Protocol #113: Allogeneic Bone Marrow Transplant in the Cat—Donor Selection

(1) Select normal healthy full siblings, usually littermates, as marrow donors.
(2) To determine the degree of chimerism established, sex mismatch donors and recipients if possible (SEE SECTION 4.5, PAGE 289).
(3) Mixed leukocyte reactions (Protocol #114) may be performed to aid donor selection (Gasper et al., 1984), but this method is labor intensive and of minimal value so is seldom used.

Protocol #114: Allogeneic Bone Marrow Transplant in the Cat—Mixed Leukocyte Reaction

(1) Separate leukocytes from siblings using ficoll–metrizoate gradients.
(2) Assay for one and two-way mixed leukocyte reactivity against similarly separated lymphocytes of the recipient according to Peck and Bach (1973).
(3) Mix lymphocytes (2×10^5) in 96-well plates with either 2×10^5 leukocytes treated with mitomycin C (2 μg mitomycin C per 10 lymphocytes, 45 min incubation at 37°C) or with 2×10^5 untreated leukocytes.
(4) Incubate at 37°C in a humidified, 5% CO_2 atmosphere for 7 days.
(5) Eighteen hours before collection, add 0.5 μCi [^{3}H]-thymidine to each well.
(6) Select the animal with the lowest stimulation index as bone marrow donor.

Protocol #115: Allogeneic Bone Marrow Transplant in the Cat—Recipient Preparation and Conditioning

(1) Perform complete blood count and biochemical profile.
(2) Administer 2.5 mg/kg oral enrofloxacin twice daily from 7 days before BMT to 4 days after BMT to selectively decontaminate the gut and prevent bacterial infections.
(3) Deliver total body irradiation (TBI) (9.0 or 10.0 Gy given in six fractions of 1.5 or 1.67 Gy), twice daily 6 hours apart on days −2, −1, and 0 with a 6 MeV linear accelerator to ablate marrow.
(4) Prepare cyclosporin (24 mg/ml) for oral use by mixing 180 mg cyclosporin with 7 ml olive oil and 0.5 ml cod liver oil in a beaker. Introduce a magnetic stir bar, and heat the mixture with stirring at approximately 80°C. Do not exceed 100°C. Mix for 30 min, dispense the solution into sterile 20 ml bottles and seal. Mixture is stable for about 5 days.
(5) Administer cyclosporin (15 mg/kg orally) on days −1, 0, and +1 and then from the time of hematologic engraftment (neutrophil count = 1000/μl) until day 100 after BMT.
(6) Obtain marrow from an anesthetized donor by aspiration of long bones (proximal femur, humerus, tibia) and iliac crests using an 18-gauge marrow biopsy needle.
(7) Collect the marrow into sterile heparinized (preservative-free heparin) 20 ml syringes.
(8) Move to a laminar flow hood, where all of the following procedures should be performed.
(9) Place a volume of HBSS equivalent to the volume of marrow collected in a sterile 250 ml beaker at room temperature.
(10) Following stringent aseptic procedures add marrow to the beaker of HBSS and filter through a sterile tissue sieve with a fine metal screen or through six layers of sterile gauze into a second sterile beaker.
(11) Aliquot samples into sterile 15 ml conical centrifuge tubes with caps.
(12) Centrifuge at 1000*g* (2225 r.p.m.) for 10 min at 4°C to remove fat.
(13) Aspirate buffy coat (at the plasma/red cell interface) with a sterile 12 ml syringe and a 30 cm spinal needle.
(14) Dilute 0.2 ml of sample with 1.8 ml of 0.83% NH_4Cl/0.01M Tris buffer.
(15) Allow to stand 5 min to lyse erythrocytes.
(16) Dilute 0.1 ml of cell suspension with 0.1 ml new methylene blue in one well of a 96-well plate.
(17) Store the rest of the sample at 2–8°C until ready to transplant.
(18) Count nucleated cells in the four outside squares and center square of the red cell/platelet area of a hemocytometer. Multiply cell number by 10 to correct for dilution factor, thus giving the number of cells/ml $\times 10^5$. Multiply this by volume (ml) of marrow to be transfused

to obtain the total number of cells to be transplanted. Divide the total number of cells by the weight of the cat (kg) to determine the total number of cells/kg administered.

(19) Give recipients as many marrow cells as possible intravenously, immediately after the sixth dose of TBI.

(20) Inject cells as a bolus over a period of approximately 5 min.

(21) Give a second injection of donor marrow cells on day 5. Again, give as many cells as possible.

Protocol #116: Allogeneic Bone Marrow Transplant in the Cat—Engraftment and Medical Management

(1) House the recipient in a laminar flow unit for approximately 4 weeks after BMT. If the recipient is still nursing, also house the queen and littermates in the unit.

(2) Provide food and water *ad libitum.*

(3) Evaluate the recipient by taking body temperature and determining state of hydration 3–4 times daily, weigh daily, and provide nutritional support, intravenous or subcutaneous fluids and antibiotics as needed.

(4) If fevers of 39.2°C or above are present, take cultures of blood and stools and treat with ampicillin and cefoxitin intramuscularly, pending culture results.

(5) Perform complete blood counts weekly, or as needed if the animal appears ill.

Protocol #117: Allogeneic Bone Marrow Transplant in the Cat—Karyotypic Analysis to Determine the Degree of Hematologic Chimerism

(1) Collect 1 ml bone marrow aspirate or 2 ml peripheral blood in a 12 ml heparinized syringe. Use preservation-free heparin, 1000 U/ml.

(2) Add 8 ml RPMI with 25 mM HEPES, 1 ml heat-inactivated fetal bovine serum, 30 μl L-glutamine, 30 μl heparin, 50 μl gentamicin sulfate (10 mg/ml) and 200 μl penicillin/streptomycin solution, to a sterile 125 ml bottle with screw cap.

(3) Add 0.5 ml whole blood or bone marrow.

(4) Incubate at 37°C, 5% CO_2 for 72 h.

(5) Add 200 μl colchicine. Incubate at 37°C for 30–60 min.

(6) Pellet cells as follows: Place sample into 15 ml conical tube and centrifuge for 10 min at 200 g. Aspirate supernatant and add 8 ml hypotonic (0.075 M KCl to sediment, vortex, and allow to stand for 30 min at 37°C.

(7) Centrifuge and repeat step (6). Add 2 ml fixative (1 : 3 dilution of acetic acid : methanol) and allow to stand for 5 min, then centrifuge for 10 min at 200 *g*.

(8) Aspirate supernatant down to 2 ml. Add 3 ml fixative, mix, and allow to stand for 30 min.

(9) Centrifuge for 10 min at 200 *g*, then decant all supernatant. Add 5 ml of fixative, re-suspend and let stand overnight in refrigerator.

(10) Drop the final cell suspension on clean glass slides, dry at room temperature and stain with 2% Giemsa stain for 6–8 min.

(11) Examine metaphase chromosomes at × 1000.

4 NOTES AND TROUBLESHOOTING

4.1 On Protocol #113: Donor Selection

Although cats have the usual components of the histocompatibility complex (Pollack et al., 1982), MLR stimulation indices are almost always low, even in unrelated cats, and cats have a lower incidence of graft-versus host disease than dogs and humans (Gasper et al., 1992a). Because it is labor-intensive and of apparent minimal value in the donor selection process, MLR is usually considered unnecessary for BMT studies involving cats.

4.2 On Protocol #115: Recipient Preparation and Conditioning

General health should be as good as possible. Cats with common disorders such as upper respiratory infections and dermatophytosis often die when immunosuppressed. Routine vaccinations are given, but killed, rather than modified live virus, vaccines are used. Age does not appear to be a significant factor in the success of the procedure; however, recently weaned kittens usually do not do well, presumably because of the added stress of weaning. Nursing kittens are most tolerant to BMT, as they usually continue to nurse, unlike older kittens which may need to be force fed.

4.2.1 Irradiation-induced Bone Marrow Ablation

The marrow is ablated to eliminate defective cells, to provide space for donor cell hematopoiesis and to blunt host immunologic resistance to donor cells.

The 9.0 Gy dose is used in kittens less than 6 weeks of age. The dosage schedule described appears to be optimal; cats given 7.0 Gy as a single dose developed as hematopoietic chimeras and cats given 12.0 Gy in 6 fractions developed severe vomiting and diarrhea and died, despite intensive fluid therapy.

4.2.2 Drug-induced Bone Marrow Ablation

Because linear accelerators are not widely available and a cobalt source for TBI has not been successful in cats, marrow ablation has also been attempted using a myelotoxin (busulphan, 16–20 mg/kg) and an immunosuppressive agent (cyclophosphamide, 120–180 mg/kg). Ablation was not achieved using 16 mg/kg busulphan and 120 mg/kg cyclophosphamide (marrow autologously recovered); using 20 mg/kg busulphan, 50% of cats had autologous recovery. Cyclophosphamide at 180 mg/kg induced acute renal failure and death. In summary, effective and toxic doses of busulphan and cyclophosphamide are similar; TBI alone is much more effective in the cat.

4.3 Notes on Donor Cell Collection, Preparation and Infusion

The quantity of marrow that can be obtained from each site depends on the size of the donor.

On the first infusion, we have given an average of 12.4×10^8 donor-origin nucleated marrow cells per kilogram body weight.

On the second infusion, we have given a mean of 5.6×10^8 cells on day 5, for a total mean of 18×10^8 cells/kg.

Giving as many cells as possible, and a second infusion of cells, appears to hasten engraftment.

4.4 On Protocol #116: Engraftment and Medical Management

Growth factors (erythropoietin and recombinant G-CSF) have been given to some recipients. Both normal cats (Fulton et al., 1991) and cats receiving BMT have slightly higher neutrophil counts following administration of G-CSF. Benefits have not been fully evaluated but there is some evidence that the use of recombinant human (rh) G-CSF may result in a delayed neutropenia, presumably because antibodies formed against the growth factor. This has not been observed with recombinant canine G-CSF.

4.5 Notes on Karyotypic Analysis to Determine the Degree of Hematologic Chimerism

Following TBI, white blood cells and platelets are depleted but subsequently increase by days 12–18 after irradiation. If graft rejection occurs, autologous recovery of the marrow is usually seen but hematologic evidence of engraftment is usually not seen until days 20–30. Karyotypic analysis showed that most recipients have approximately 98% donor engraftment. In cats receiving only 7 Gy as a single dose, donor engraftment was only approximately 60%.

We are currently using DNA fingerprinting to determine the degree of chimerism. Briefly, DNA is digested with the restriction enzymes *Msp*I or *Pst*I and Southern analysis is performed on 1% agarose gels with transfer to nylon membranes (Southern, 1975). Probes used for hybridization are feline origin VNTR mini-satellite probes, digoxigenin-labeled and detected using the Genius (Boehringer Mannheim) non-radioactive DNA labeling and detection kit. Fingerprints are evaluated to assess engraftment and chimerism (Blazar and Orr, 1985; Knowlton and Brown, 1985; Yam et al., 1987; Neitzel, 1991).

4.6 Modifications used to Perform BMT in Dog, Mouse and Human

4.6.1 Dog

Most bone marrow transplant techniques were developed and tested in dogs, and the dog continues to be evaluated as a model for humans (Bean et al., 1994; de Revel et al., 1994; Raff et al., 1993a, 1993b; Storb et al., 1993, 1994). Methods for BMT in dogs with lysosomal storage diseases are similar to those used in the cat (Haskins, personal communication; Shull et al., 1987; Taylor et al., 1986).

Current methodology for donor selection and conditioning in experiments involving MPS VII dogs is as follows (Haskins, personal communication). Normal healthy siblings serve as donors and are selected using mixed lymphocyte reactivity. Marrow is ablated by 7.0 Gy in a single dose using a linear accelerator. Nucleated marrow cells (3–4 × 10^8) are infused intravenously following TBI. Cyclosporin (25 mg/kg orally once daily) is given from time of engraftment until day 100, gradually decreasing the dose towards the end of treatment. Oral L-glutamine, an amino acid which is enterocyte protective, is given orally (1 ml 200 mM solution twice daily) from a few days before TBI to 2 weeks after.

In another conditioning regimen which has been used, dogs with MPS I (Shull et al., 1987) were given 7.5–8.5 Gy in a single dose (0.20 Gy per minute) from a cobalt 60 source, and 2.20–4.03 × 10^8 cells were infused. Methotrexate was given on days 1, 3, 6, 11, and weekly until day 102 to help prevent GVHD. Total lymphoid irradiation has been used as a conditioning regimen in fucosidosis-affected dogs receiving BMT (Taylor et al., 1986). It was claimed to enable engraftment across major histocompatibility barriers without the development of GVHD and it carries no risk of marrow failure if the graft fails. This was delivered at 18 Gy over 4–6 weeks in 1 Gy fractions to intermediate width, mantle and abdominal fields with lung, kidney and rectal shielding. Skull and distal limbs were outside the fields of irradiation, and engraftment was successful without development of GVHD.

Medical management of dogs includes housing in HEPA-filtered rooms, administering fluids and antibiotics as necessary and controlling GVHD with cyclosporin and corticosteroids. The most significant complication immediately after TBI is gastrointestinal damage with subsequent diarrhea and fluid loss (Haskins, personal communication).

4.6.2 Mouse

The mouse is commonly used as a model for BMT in humans. In MPS VII affected mice, optimal engraftment occurred with 8–10 Gy TBI followed by BMT giving 6 × 10^6 nucleated marrow cells (Birkenmeier et al., 1991). Hematopoietic chimerism was achieved with lower doses. As the mice are syngeneic, failure to engraft and development of GVHD are not significant problems. To perform successful BMT in Twitcher mice, a model for human Krabbe disease, 9 Gy TBI was given, followed by infusion of 3–5 × 10^7 donor marrow cells (Hoogerbrugge et al., 1988a,b).

4.6.3 Humans

In humans TBI is associated with acute effects including fluid shifts, diarrhea and fever, and long-term effects including cataracts, interstitial pneumonitis and increased incidence of radiation-induced malignancy (Pearson, 1986). Most of the children with lysosomal storage diseases are conditioned with busulphan (14 mg/kg) and cyclophosphamide (200 mg/kg) (Barrett and Gordon, 1993). Recombinant hematopoietic growth factors such as G-CSF and granulocyte macrophage colony stimulating factor (GM-CSF) have been shown to lessen morbidity of BMT in humans by enhancing neutrophil recovery and function.

New approaches are constantly being developed in the areas of conditioning (including use of cytokines), medical management and treatment of GVHD (Armitage, 1994; Fowler et al., 1994; Pepe et al., 1993; Rowe et al., 1994; Xenocostas et al., 1994). The most significant complication in man is still GVHD; other significant complications are infections and hepatic veno-occlusive disease as a complication of high-dose chemotherapy (Rowe et al., 1994).

4.7 General Complications of BMT

Although BMT is technically simple, medical management of recipients is complex and often difficult. Using fractionated TBI we have observed no complications in cats related to radiation other than stunted growth. Male and female cats treated by the above protocols have been successfully bred. Mice irradiated at early ages as part of BMT studies later exhibited cerebellar and retinal defects in addition to skeletal changes (Sands et al., 1993). Pathological changes in blood vessels of the CNS have been reported in rats after brain irradiation (Reinhold et al., 1990), but the intensity of exposure used in these experiments (20–25 Gy given in singe doses) exceeded that given in the BMT studies reported here.

The most serious complications related to BMT in cats include graft failure with either death or autologous recovery, infections secondary to immunosuppression and GVHD. Incidence of graft failure is very low in the cat (< 10%) if the appropriate dose of TBI is used and adequate numbers of cells are infused. In cats which failed to engraft and then autologously recovered, a second BMT months later was also unsuccessful.

Thrombocytopenia-related bleeding may occur in the first 2 weeks after BMT. Corticosteroids (prednisone) appear to decrease the severity of bleeding in these cats. Fresh whole blood transfusions, preferably from the donor, may be required. Cats are susceptible to bacterial infections during the period of neutropenia, and remain immunosuppressed for at least 200 days after BMT. The percentage of T lymphocytes and the ratio of T-helper to T-cytotoxic lymphocytes decreases immediately after transplantation but returns to normal by day 200. Immune function, as evaluated by lymphoblast transformation assay and serum immunoglobulin levels, is also impaired up to 105 days after BMT. Complications associated with immunosuppression include septicemia, pneumonia, diarrhea and severe dermatophytosis. Organisms most commonly cultured at necropsy include *Enterobacter cloacae*, non-hemolytic streptococcus, *E. coli* and *Streptococcus faecium* (Fulton et al., 1990).

4.8 Graft Versus Host Disease

Graft versus host disease remains one of the major complications of BMT, particularly in humans. It occurs in up to 80% of patients receiving HLA-matched sibling BMT, and is responsible for up to 20% mortality (Barrett and Gordon, 1993). Immunologically competent donor origin cells target antigens on the cells of the recipient; GVHD manifests primarily by signs associated with the skin, gastrointestinal system, biliary tree of the liver, and exocrine glands. The most life-threatening component of the disorder is the accompanying immune suppression (Armitage, 1994). Graft versus host disease may occur as two distinct entities: acute disease, occurring in the first 1–2 months, and chronic disease, developing at least 2–3 months following transplantation. The acute disease does not necessarily precede chronic GVHD.

In acute GVHD skin disorders usually occur first, often followed by involvement of the mucosa of the gastrointestinal tract and biliary epithelium of the liver. The major feature which characterizes chronic GVHD is collagen deposition with development of sclerosis; lungs, exocrine glands and musculoskeletal system are often also involved. Patients undergoing BMT commonly receive prophylactic treatment for GVHD. The most common methods of prophylaxis in humans are administration of cyclosporin (with or without methotrexate), corticosteroids, and removal of T cells from the graft. Treatment includes corticosteroids, antithymocyte globulin, thalidomide and monoclonal antibodies (Armitage, 1994). Although T-cell depletion of marrow often helps to prevent GVHD, it is associated with increased incidence of failure to engraft (Barrett and Gordon, 1993).

Graft versus host disease is not as significant in cats as it is in dogs and humans. Although 19%

of cats develop some form of the disease, only about 5% die. In cats acute GVHD first manifests as erythema of the skin, particularly the ears (thickening of the ears is one of the first manifestations in the dog). Gastrointestinal GVHD is seen in cats and dogs, manifesting as diarrhea and malabsorption. Exocrine pancreatic insufficiency has also been observed in dogs receiving BMT. Liver GVHD is a less significant problem in dogs and cats than in humans. Cyclosporin is usually used as prophylaxis in both dogs and cats, although methotrexate has been used in dogs (Shull et al., 1987). Treatment of GVHD consists of cyclosporin and high-dose corticosteroids such as prednisone. Gene therapy using autologous marrow is particularly attractive because GVHD remains a serious problem in patients receiving allogeneic BMT.

4.9 Notes on the Assessments and Future Directions

4.9.1 BMT as a Cell-mediated Delivery System

The repopulation of widespread body tissues with nucleated donor cells following BMT offers considerable potential for direct and/or indirect correction of many metabolic processes in genetically abnormal cells. That cells of bone marrow origin are capable of releasing a variety of biological products, ranging from cytokines to lysosomal enzymes, suggests they may be useful for delivering missing gene products in a variety of disease states. The extent to which this delivery system will be successful appears to depend on factors ranging from intrinsic events such as the nature of the primary metabolic defect (and disease-related processes) to the age at which BMT is carried out. For diseases of the brain in particular, current findings argue that these factors exert substantial influence over the final outcome.

Considerable evidence supports the view that microglial and macrophage populations of the CNS originate from monocytes derived from bone marrow. This is particularly well established for the ameboid microglia present during development of the CNS, for a population of perivascular cells and for macrophage populations found in the meninges, ventricles and choroid plexus. Turnover from the bone marrow continues in the adult CNS at different rates for the various cell types, being slowest for parenchymal microglia. In pathologic conditions monocytic and, in some cases, lymphocytic infiltration can increase. Thus BMT can serve to deliver cells (carrying therapeutic molecules) to the CNS. The efficiency of cell delivery may be expected to be higher in younger recipients, before CNS maturation, and may be improved in some diseases in which leukocyte infiltration is heightened. However, while macrophage-like cells may be evident within the CNS in a particular disease, some of these cells may be derived from the resident microglial population. Therefore it is important for the investigator to identify the source of these cells.

Studies to date suggest that BMT is effective for some lysosomal hydrolase deficiencies. It leads to significant correction of the metabolic defect in CNS neurons in α-mannosidosis and fucosidosis and possible partial correction in the mucopolysaccharidoses. No correction appears to occur in the gangliosidoses. Leukodystrophies secondary to lysosomal enzyme defects also benefit from BMT, and replacement of diseased macrophages in the brain (e.g. in white matter) with normal cells appears to be the key event underlying efficacy. For neuronal storage diseases such as α-mannosidosis evidence suggests that enzyme transfer from normal donor-derived cells within the brain is important for treatment. Studies that have confirmed the presence of acidic α-mannosidase in host cells following BMT, have provided evidence suggesting the presence of donor-derived perivascular cells in brain, and have indicated that high levels of α-mannosidase are secreted by normal microglia. The presence of donor bone marrow-derived cells in brain in feline GM2 gangliosidosis, coupled with an absence of correction of neuronal storage, portrays a more ominous picture: getting donor cells into the brain may be only the first step in correcting the metabolic defect. Release of enzyme by donor-derived cells may be a major limiting factor. However, genetic manipulation leading to gene product overexpression, coupled with normal secretory pathways employed by microglia/CNS macrophages, might be a means of overcoming this limitation (Ioannou et al., 1992). Determining the exact mechanisms responsible for successful therapy in diseases like α-mannosidosis may provide crucial insight into exactly what combination of factors is necessary for successful therapy in other types of neurological diseases.

4.9.2 *In utero Stem Cell Transplantation*

Because many of the problems associated with bone marrow transplantation are related to the immunologic status of the donor and recipient, and because potentially devastating effects of neurological diseases can occur during fetal life, performing transplants *in utero* before immunocompetence is established could circumvent difficulties associated with BMT (Diukman and Mitchell, 1992; Flake et al., 1991; Simpson and Golbus, 1985). During its first trimester the mammalian fetus is immunotolerant and *in utero* transplantation can be performed without tissue matching, marrow ablation, immunosuppressive drugs or GVHD. Fetal bone marrow at this time is relatively empty, awaiting the migration of hematopoietic stem cells from the fetal liver. Furthermore, ameboid microglia arising from monocytic infiltration first appear in fetal development. Investigations employing mouse (Pallavicini et al., 1992), sheep (Flake et al., 1991; Srour et al., 1992; Zanjani al., 1991) and monkey (Harrison et al., 1989; Zanjani, et al., 1991) models have shown that *in utero* allogeneic and even xenogeneic stem cell transplantation, when both donor and recipient are immunologically tolerant, will result in long-term stable hematopoietic chimerism of lymphoid, erythroid and myeloid cells of donor origin. Clinical trials involving human fetal transplants are beginning and at least three have been partially successful (Flake et al., 1991; Raudrant et al., 1992; Touraine 1991, 1992; Touraine et al., 1991, 1992). The procedure appears relatively safe for both mother and fetus (Slavin et al., 1990).

Although *in utero* stem cell transplants have resulted in hematopoietic chimeras with relatively low levels of donor cell expression, these levels could be sufficient to prevent some metabolic diseases. Donor cell expression in the successful human *in utero* stem cell transplant was 10% at 1 month and 26% at 1 year (Touraine, 1991, 1992; Touraine et al., 1991, 1992). Donor cell expression in mouse, sheep, and monkey models was 5–10% (Pallavicini et al., 1992), 10–12% (Zanjani et al., 1991; Srour et al., 1992), and 5–15% (Harrison et al., 1989; Zanjani et al., 1991), respectively. Importantly, there is evidence that enzyme production may be upregulated by donor cells in enzyme-deficient tissues, which could compensate for low numbers of donor cell expression. This may be important as, even with current advances in stem cell purification, enrichment and expansion using cytokines (Miller, 1993), donor cell expression may remain relatively low following stem cell transplantation *in utero* because the fetal recipient's own stem cells are not ablated before the procedure.

Fetal liver is an excellent source of hematopoietic cells (Champlin et al., 1987; Lasky, 1991), and contains at least a third of the number of stem cells in bone marrow (Simpson and Golbus, 1985). Ultimately, hematopoietic stem cell transplantation *in utero* may be combined with gene therapy to treat patients with inherited metabolic disorders.

4.9.3 *Gene Therapy using Autologous BMT*

Although BMT can prevent manifestations of some neuronal storage disorders, allogeneic BMT carries a high risk of morbidity and mortality. Perhaps more importantly, it is difficult or impossible to identify an HLA (human leukocyte or histocompatibility antigen)-identical donor; failure to engraft and GVHD are common complications. With the development of replication-defective retroviral vectors capable of efficient transfer and expression of genes in a variety of mammalian cells, somatic gene therapy for genetic disorders has become feasible (Desnick and Schuchman, 1991; Friedmann, 1989; Miller et al., 1991; Wolfe et al., 1992). Gene transfer into pluripotent stem cells followed by autologous BMT (allotransplantation) would be expected to allow long-term correction of enzyme deficiency. The benefits of this therapy for lysosomal storage disorders should be similar to that of allogeneic bone marrow transplantation, but risks should be lower because the recipient also serves as donor. This has been studied using the MPS VII mouse model. Following retroviral mediated gene transfer of the β-glucuronidase gene to marrow stem cells, the genetically modified cells were transplanted into the recipient's marrow. Long-term low levels of β-glucuronidase were produced in recipient tissues and storage in liver and spleen was reduced (Wolfe et al., 1992). Krall and colleagues (1994) have shown in mice that cells expressing human glucocerebrosidase from a retroviral vector repopulate a variety of tissues, including brain. Although stable expression of gene products in hematopoietic cells has been reported in the murine system (Correll et al., 1989; Sly, 1993; Wolfe et al., 1992), long-term expression has been less successful in larger animals like dogs and monkeys (Kantoff et al., 1987; Stead et al., 1988). More encouragingly, in a study in cats Lothrop et al. (1991) transduced the neomycin-resistance gene (gene for neomycin phosphotransferase) using a retrovirus vector. The marker gene was retained in some of the cats for more than 200 days.

ACKNOWLEDGMENTS

We wish to thank our many collaborators: Doctors H. Baker, D. Brown, S. Dial, P. Gasper, R. Fulton, M. Haskins, P. March and M. Rattazzi. We are grateful to the NIH and to the Dr Louis Sklarow Memorial Fund for support.

REFERENCES

Akiyama, H., S. Itagaki, and P.L. McGeer. 1988. Major histocompatibility complex antigen expression on rat microglia following epidural kainic acid lesions. *J. Neurosci. Res.* **20**:147–157.

Armitage, J.O. 1994. Bone marrow transplantation. *N. Engl J. Med.* **330**:827–838.

Ashwell, K. 1990. Microglia and cell death in the developing mouse cerebellum. *Dev. Brain Res.* **55**:219–230.

Ashwell, K. 1991. The distribution of microglia and cell death in the fetal rat forebrain. *Dev. Brain Res.* **58**:1–12.

Banati, R.B., J. Gehrmann, P. Schubert, and G.W. Kreutzberg. 1993. Cytotoxicity of microglia. *Glia* **7**:111–118.

Barranger, J.A. 1984. Marrow transplantation in genetic disease. *N. Engl J. Med.* **311**:1629–1631.

Barrett, A.J., and M.Y. Gordon. 1993. In: *Bone Marrow Disorders—The Biological Basis of Treatment.* Baszler, T.V., W.G. Harwood, K.L. Lester, W.C. Davis, and D.P. Knowles. 1994. Characterization of caprine microglial cells and *in vitro* infection with caprine arthritis-encephalitis lentivirus. *Lab. Invest.* **70**:933–943.

Blackwell Scientific Publications, Oxford, p.190.

Bayever, E., N. Kamani, C.S. August, Ferreira, D.A. Wenger, and W. Krivit. 1992. Allogeneic BMT for Niemann–Pick type Ia disease. *Bone Marrow Transplant.* **10**:85–86.

Bayever, E., Ladisch, M. Philippart, N. Brill, M. Nuwer, R.S. Sparkes, and S.A. Feig. 1985. Bone-marrow transplantation for metachromatic leucodystrophy. *Lancet* **ii**:471–473.

Bean, M.A., T. Graham, F.R. Applebaum, J.H. Deeg, F. Schuening, F.E. Sale, and R. Storb. 1994. Gamma-irradiation of pretransplant blood transfusions from unrelated donors prevents sensitization to minor histocompatibility antigens on dog leukocyte antigen-identical canine marrow grafts. *Transplantation* **57**:423–426.

Birkenmeier, E.H., J.E. Barker, C.A. Vogler, J.W. Kyle, W.S. Sly, B. Gwynn, B. Levy, and C. Pegors. 1991. Increased life span and correction of metabolic defects in murine mucopolysaccharidosis type VII after syngeneic bone marrow transplantation. *Blood* **78**:3081–3092.

Blazar, B.R., and H.T. Orr. 1985. Restriction fragment length polymorphisms as markers of engraftment in allogeneic marrow transplantation. *Blood* **66**:1436–1444.

Boothe, A.D., H. Weintroub, P.G. Pentchev, J. Jones, J. Butler, J.E. Barry, B. Neumeyer, J.A. Stivers, and R.O. Brady. 1984. A lysosomal storage disorder in the Balb/c mouse: bone marrow transplantation. *Vet. Pathol.* **21**:432–441.

Brierley, J.B., and A.W. Brown. 1982. The origin of lipid phagocytes in the central nervous system: I. The intrinsic microglia. *J. Comp. Neurol.* **211**:397–406.

Briers, T.W., C. Desmaretz, and E. Vanmechelen. 1994. Generation and characterization of mouse microglial cell lines. *J. Neuroimmunol.* **52**:153–164.

Brown, D.E., M.A. Thrall, D.A. Wenger, T. Mitchell, S.U. Walkley, and M. Smith. 1993. Bone marrow transplantation in feline Niemann–Pick disease type C. *Vet. Pathol.* **30**: 428.

Brown, D.E., M.A. Thrall, S.U. Walkley, D.A. Wenger, T. Mitchell, M. Smith, K. Royals, P. March, and R. Allison. 1994. Animal model of human disease: Feline Niemann–Pick disease type C. *Am. J. Pathol.* **144**:1412–1415.

Champlin, R.E., G. Cain, K. Stitzel, and R.P. Gale. 1987. Sustained recovery of hematopoiesis and immunity following transplantation of fetal liver cells in dogs. *Thymus* **10**:13–18.

Chao, C.C., T.W. Molitor, and S. Hu. 1993. Neuroprotective role of IL-4 against activated microglia. *J. Immunol.* **151**:1473–1481.

Choi, B.H. 1981. Hematogenous cells in the central nervous system of developing human embryos and fetuses. *J. Comp. Neurol.* **196**:683–694.

Choi, D.W. 1988. Glutamate neurotoxicity and disease of the nervous system. *Neuron* **1**:623–634.

Chugani, D.C., N.L. Kedersha, and L.H. Rome. 1991. Vault immunofluorescence in the brain: New insights regarding the origin of microglia. *J. Neurosci.* **11**:256–268.

Compston, A. 1993. Inflammation and the brain. *Mol. Chem. Neuropathol.* **19**:47–64.

Correll, P.H., J.K. Fink, R.O. Brady, L.K. Perry, and S. Karlsson. 1989. Production of human glucocerebrosidase in mice after retroviral gene transfer into multipotential hematopoietic progenitor cells. *Proc. Natl Acad. Sci. USA* **86**:8912–8916.

Couraud, P.O. 1994. Interactions between lymphocytes, macrophages, and central nervous system cells. *J. Leukoc. Biol.* **56**:407–415.

Cowan, M.J. 1991. Bone marrow transplantation for the treatment of genetic diseases. *Clin. Biochem.* **24**:375–381.

Cuadros, M., A. Moujahid, G. Martin-Partido, and J. Navascues. 1992. Microglia in the mature and developing quail brain as revealed by a monoclonal antibody recognizing hemopoietic cells. *Neurosci. Lett.* **148**:11–14.

Deeg, H.J., H.M. Shulman, D. Albrechtsen, T.C. Graham, R. Storb, and N. Koppang. 1990. Batten's disease: Failure of allogeneic bone marrow transplantation to arrest disease progression in a canine model. *Clin. Genet.* **37**:264–270.

De Groot, C.J.A., W. Huppes, T. Sminia, G. Kraal, and C. Dijkstra. 1992. Determination of the origin and nature of brain macrophages and microglial cells in mouse central nervous system, using non-radioactive in situ hybridization and immunoperoxidase techniques. *Glia* **6**:301–309.

de Revel, T., F.R. Applebaum, R. Storb, F. Scheuning, R. Nash, J. Deeg, I. McNiece, R. Andrews, and T. Graham. 1994. Effects of granulocyte colony stimulating factor and stem cell factor, alone and in combination on the mobilization of peripheral blood cells that engraft lethally irradiated dogs. *Blood* **83**:3795–3799.

Desnick, R.J., and E.H. Schuchman. 1991. Human gene therapy: Strategies and prospects for inborn errors of metabolism. In: *Treatment of Genetic Diseases.* R.J. Desnick, editor. Churchill Livingstone, NY. pp.239–259.

Dickson, D.W., S.C. Lee, L.A. Mattiace, S.C. Yen, and C. Brosnan. 1993. Microglia and cytokines in neurological disease, with special reference to AIDS and Alzheimer's disease. *Glia* **7**:75–83.

Diukman, R., and S.G. Mitchell. 1992. *In utero* stem cell therapy. *J. Reprod. Med.* **37**:515–520.

Dobrenis, K., D.A. Wenger, and S.U. Walkley. 1994. Extracellular release of lysosomal glycosidases in cultures of cat microglia. *Mol. Biol. Cell* **5**:113a.

Dow, S.W., M.L. Poss, and E.A. Hoover. 1990. Feline immunodeficiency virus: A neurotropic lentivirus. *J. Acq. Immuno. Def.* **3**:658–668.

Duchen, L.W., E.M. Eicher, J.M. Jacobs, F. Scarvilli, and F. Teixeira. 1980. Hereditary leucodystrophy in the mouse: The new mutant twitcher. *Brain* **103**:695–710.

Fedoroff, S., and J.A. McKanna. 1994. Lipocortin-1 is expressed in micgrolia and their progenitor cells in cultures. *Mol. Biol. Cell* **5**:228a.

Fernaud-Espinosa, I., M. Nieto-Sampedro, and P. Bovolenta. 1993. Differential activation of microglia and astrocytes in aniso- and isomorphic gliotic tissue. *Glia* **8**:277–291.

Fischer, H.G., A.K. Bielinsky, B. Nitzgen, W. Dubener, and U. Hadding. 1993. Functional dichotomy of mouse microglia developed *in vitro*: Differential effects of macrophage and granulocyte/macrophage colony-stimulating factor on cytokine secretion and antitoxoplasmic activity. *J. Neuroimmunol.* **45**:193–202.

Flake, A.W., M.R. Harrison, and E.D. Zanjani. 1991. *In utero* stem cell transplantation. *Exp. Hematol.* **19**:1061–1064.

Flaris, N.A., T.L. Densmore, M.C. Molleston, and W.F. Hickey. 1993. Characterization of microglia and macrophages in the central nervous system of rats: Definition of the differential expression of molecules using standard and novel monoclonal antibodies in normal CNS and in four models of parenchymal reaction. *Glia* **7**:34–40.

Fowler, D.H., K. Kurasawa, R. Smith, M.A. Eckhaus, and R.E. Gress. 1994. Donor CD4-enriched cells of the cytokine phenotype regulate graft-versus-host disease without impairing allogeneic engraftment in sublethally irradiated mice. *Blood* **84**:3540–3549.

Friedmann, T. 1989. Progress toward human gene therapy. *Science* **244**:1275–1281.

Fulton, R., W. Gasper, G.K. Ogilvie, T.C. Boone, and R.E. Dornsife. 1991. Effect of recombinant human granulocyte colony-stimulating factor on hematopoiesis in normal cats. *Exp. Hematol.* **19**:759–767.

Fulton, R., P.W. Gasper, M.A. Thrall, R.W. Norrdin, J.B. Rose, C.A. Macy, S.M. Dial, and S.P. Colgan. 1990. Complications associated with bone marrow transplantation in the cat. *Vet. Clin. Path.* **19**:5.

Gasper, P.W. 1989. Bone marrow transplantation. In: *Current Veterinary Therapy XI.* R.W. Kirk editor. W.B. Saunders, Philadelphia. p.115.

Gasper, P.W., R. Fulton, and M.A. Thrall. 1992a. Bone marrow transplantation: update and current considerations. In: *Current Veterinary Therapy XI*. R.W. Kirk editor. W.B. Saunders, Philadelphia. pp.493–496.

Gasper, P.W., M.A. Thrall, R. Fulton, B.J. Rose, and T.N. Thomas. 1992b. Allogeneic bone marrow transplantation in cats. *J. Cell. Biochem.* suppl. 16a, 213.

Gasper, P.W., M.A. Thrall, D.A. Wenger, D.W. Macy, L. Ham, R.E. Dornsife, S.L. Quackenbush, M.L. Kesel, E.L. Gillette, and E.A. Hoover. 1984. Correction of feline arylsulfatase B deficiency (mucopolysaccharidosis VI) by bone marrow transplantation. *Nature* **312**:467–469.

Gatti, R.A., H.D. Allen, H.J. Meuwissen, R. Hong, and R. Good. 1968. Immunological reconstitution of sex-linked lymphopenic immunological deficiency. *Lancet* **ii**:1366–1369.

Gebicke-Haerter, P.J., K. Appel, G.D. Taylor, A. Schobert, I.N. Rich, H. Northoff, and M. Berger. 1994. Rat microglial interleukin-3. *J. Neuroimmunol.* **50**:203–214.

Gehrmann, J., and G.W. Kreutzberg. 1993. Monoclonal antibodies against macrophages/microglia: Immunocytochemical studies of early microglia activation in experimental neuropathology. *Clin. Neuropathol.* **12**:301–306.

Ginns, E.I., D.B. Caplan, J.M. Rappeport, and J.A. Barranger. 1984. Bone marrow transplantation in severe Gaucher's disease: Rapid correction of enzyme deficiency accompanied by continued long term survival of storage cells. In: *Molecular Basis of Lysosomal Storage Disorders*. J.A. Barranger and R.O. Brady editors. Academic Press, NY, pp.429–440.

Giulian, D., and T.J. Baker. 1985. Peptides released by ameboid microglia regulate astroglial proliferation. *J. Cell Biol.* **101**:2411–2415.

Giulian, D., and T.J. Baker. 1986. Characterization of ameboid microglia isolated from developing mammalian brain. *J. Neurosci.* **6**:2163–2178.

Giulian, D., K. Vaca, and M. Corpuz. 1993. Brain glia release factors with opposing actions upon neuronal survival. *J. Neurosci.* **13**:29–37.

Grabowski, G.A., and G.S. Horowitz. 1990. Acid β-glucosidase: enzymology and molecular biology of Gaucher disease. *Crit. Rev. Biochem. Mol. Biol.* **25**:385.

Graeber, M.B. 1993. Microglia, macrophages and the blood-brain barrier. Clin. *Neuropathol.* **12**:296–297.

Graeber, M.B., and W.J. Streit. 1990. Perivascular microglia defined. *Trends Neurosci.* **13**:366.

Graeber, M.B., W.J. Streit, D. Buringer, D.L. Sparks, and G.W. Kreutzberg. 1992. Ultrastructural location of major histocompatibility complex (MHC) class II positive perivascular cells in histologically normal human brain. *J. Neuropathol. Exp. Neurol.* **51**:303–311.

Graeber, M.B., W.J. Streit, R. Kiefer, S.W. Schoen, and G.W. Kreutzberg. 1990a. New expression of myelomonocytic antigens by microglia and perivascular cells following lethal motor neuron injury. *J. Neuroimmunol.* **27**:121–132.

Graeber, M.B., W.J. Streit, and G.W. Kreutzberg. 1988a. Axotomy of the rat facial nerve leads to increased CR3 complement receptor expression by activated microglial cells. *J. Neurosci. Res.* **21**:18–24.

Graeber, M.B., W.J. Streit, and G.W. Kreutzberg. 1990b. The third glial cell type, the microglia: cellular markers of activation in situ. *Acta Histochem Suppl.* **38**: S157–S160.

Graeber, M.B., W. Tetzlaff, W.J. Streit, and G.W. Kreutzberg. 1988b. Microglial cells but not astrocytes undergo mitosis following rat facial nerve anatomy. *Neurosci. Lett.* **85**:317–321.

Grove, E.A., B.P. Williams, L. Da-Qing, M. Hajihosseini, A. Friedrich, and J. Price. 1993. Multiple restricted lineages in the embryonic rat cerebral cortex. *Development* **117**:553–561.

Hao, C., A. Richardson, and S. Fedoroff. 1991. Macrophage-like cells originate from neuroepithelium in culture: Characterization and properties of the macrophage-like cells. *Int. J. Dev. Neurosci.* **9**:1–14.

Harris, R.E., D. Hannon, C. Vogler, and G. Hug. 1986. Bone marrow transplantation in type IIa glycogen storage disease. In: *Bone Marrow Transplantation for Treatment of Lysosomal Storage Diseases*. W. Krivit, and N.W. Paul editors. Alan R. Liss, NY. pp.119–132.

Harrison, M.R., R.N. Slotnick, T.M. Crombleholme, M.S. Golbus, A.F. Tarantal, and E.D. Zanjan. 1989. *In utero* transplantation of fetal liver haemopoietic stem cells on monkeys. *Lancet* **ii**:1425.

Haskins, M., H.J. Baker, E. Birkenmeier, P.M. Hoogerbrugge, B.J.H.M. Poorthuis, T. Sakiyama, R.M. Shull, R.M. Taylor, M.A. Thrall, and S.U. Walkley. 1991. Transplantation in animal model systems. In: *Treatment of Genetic Diseases*. R.J. Desnick editor. Churchill Livingstone, NY. pp. 183–201.

Hassan, N.F., D.E. Campbell, S. Rifat, and S.D. Douglas. 1991a. Isolation and characterization of human fetal brain-derived microglia in *in vitro* culture. *Neuroscience* **41**:149–158.

Hassan, N.F., K. Prakash, J. Chehimi, L.J. McCawley, and S.D. Douglas. 1991b. Isolation and characterization of newborn rabbit brain derived microglia. *Clin. Immunol. Immunopathol.* **59**:426–435.

Hassan, N.F., S. Rifat, D.E. Campbell, L.J. McCawley, and S.D. Douglas. 1991c. Isolation and flow cytometric characterization of newborn mouse brain-derived microglia maintained *in vitro*. *J. Leukoc. Biol.* **50**:86–92.

Hickey, W.F., and H. Kimura. 1988. Perivascular microglial cells of the CNS are bone marrow-derived and present antigen *in vivo*. *Science* **239**:290–292.

Hickey, W.F., B.L. Hsu, and H. Kimura. 1991. T-lymphocyte entry into the central nervous system. *J. Neurosci. Res.* **28**:254–260.

Hickey, W.F., K. Vass, and H. Lassmann. 1992. Bone marrow-derived elements in the central nervous system: An immunohistochemical and ultrastructural survey of rat chimeras. *J. Neuropathol. Exp. Neurol.* **51**:246–256.

Hobbs, J.R., K. Hugh-Jones, A.J. Barrett, N. Byrom, D. Chambers, K. Henry, D.C.O. James, C.F. Lucas, P.F. Benson, L.R. Tansley, A.D. Partick, J. Mossman, and E.P. Young. 1981. Reversal of clinical features of Hurler's disease and biochemical improvement after treatment by bone-marrow transplantation. *Lancet* **ii**:709–712.

Honda, H., H. Kimura, W.K. Silvers, and A. Rostami. 1990. Perivascular location and phenotypic heterogeneity of microglial cells in the rat brain. *J. Neuroimmunol.* **29**:183–191.

Hoogerbrugge, P.M., B.J.H.M. Poorthuis, A.E. Romme, J.J.P. Van de Kamp, G. Wagemaker, and D.W. van Bekkum. 1988a. Effect of bone marrow transplantation on enzyme levels and clinical course in the neurologically affected twitcher mouse. *J. Clin. Invest.* **81**:1790–1794.

Hoogerbrugge, P.M., K. Suzuki, K. Suzuki, B.J.H.M. Poorthuis, T. Kobayashi, G. Wagemaker, and D.W. van Bekkum. 1988b. Donor-derived cells in the central nervous system of twitcher mice after bone marrow transplantation. *Science* **239**:1035–1038.

Hopwood, J.J., A. Vellodi, H.S. Scott, C.P. Morris, T. Litjens, P.R. Clements, D.A. Brooks, A. Cooper, and J.E. Wraith. 1993. Long-term clinical progress in bone marrow transplanted mucopolysaccharidosis type I patients with a defined genotype. *J. Inherit. Metab. Dis.* **16**:1024–1033.

Hosaka, Y., A. Kitamoto, M. Shimojo, K. Nakajima, Y. Imai, H. Handa, and S. Kohsaka. 1992. Generation of microglial cell lines by transfection with simian virus 40 large T gene. *Neurosci. Lett.* **141**:139–142.

Hutchins, K.D., D.W. Dickson, W.K. Rashbaum, and W.D. Lyman. 1992. Localization of microglia in the human fetal cervical spinal cord. *Dev. Brain Res.* **66**:270–273.

Igisu, H., and K. Suzuki. 1984. Progressive accumulation of toxic metabolite in a genetic leukodystrophy. *Science* **224**:753–755.

Innocenti, G.M., S. Clarke, and H. Koppel. 1983. Transitory macrophages in the white matter of the developing visual cortex II. Development and relations with axonal pathways. *Dev. Brain Res.* **11**:55–66.

Ioannou, Y.A., D.F. Bishop, and R.J. Desnick. 1992. Overexpression of human α-galactosidase A results in its intracellular aggregation, crystallization in lysosomes, and selective secretion. *J. Cell Biol.* **119**:1137–1150.

Jolly, R.D., K.G. Thompson, C.E. Murphy, B.W. Manktelow, A.N. Bruere, and B.G. Winchester. 1976. Enzyme replacement therapy—an experiment of nature in a chimeric mannosidosis calf. *Pediatr. Res.* **10**:219–224.

Jordan, F.L., and W.E. Thomas. 1988. Brain macrophages: questions of origin and interrelationship. *Brain Res. Rev.* **13**:165–178.

Kantoff, P.W., A.P. Gillio, J.R. Lachlin, C. Bordignon, M.A. Eglitis, N.A. Kernan, R.C. Moen, D.B. Kohn, S-F. Yu, E. Karson, S. Karlsson, J.A. Zwiebel, E. Gilboa, R.M. Blaese, A. Nienhuis, R.J. O'Reilly, and W.F. Anderson. 1987. Expression of human adenosine deaminase in nonhuman primates after retrovirus-mediated gene transfer. *J. Exp. Med.* **166**:219–234.

Kelly, W.R., A.E. Clague, R.J. Barns, M.J. Bate, and B.M. MacKay. 1983. Canine α-L-Fucosidosis: A storage disease of springer spaniels. *Acta Neuropathol.* **60**:9–13.

Kida, S., P.V. Steart, E. Zhang, and R.O. Weller. 1993. Perivascular cells act as scavengers in the cerebral perivascular spaces and remain distinct from pericytes, microglia and macrophages. *Acta Neuropathol.* **85**:646–652.

Kitamura, T., T. Miyake, and S. Fujita. 1984. Genesis of resting microglia in the gray matter of mouse hippocampus. *J. Comp. Neurol.* **226**:421–433.

Knowlton, R.G., and V.A. Brown. 1985. Use of highly polymorphic DNA probes for genotype analysis following bone marrow transplantation. *Blood* **68**:378–385.

Korematsu, K., S. Goto, S. Nagahiro, and Y. Ushio. 1994. Microglial response to transient focal cerebral ischemia: an immunocytochemical study on the rat cerebral cortex using anti-phosphotyrosine antibody. *J. Cereb Blood Flow Metab.* **14**:825–830.

Krall, W.J., P.M. Challita, L.S. Perimutter, D.C. Skelton, and D.B. Kohn. 1994. Cells expressing human glucocerebrosidase from a retroviral vector repopulate macrophages and central nervous system microglia after murine bone marrow transplantation. *Blood* **9**:2737–2748.

Krivit, W., and E.G. Shapiro. 1991. Bone marrow transplantation for storage diseases. In: *Treatment of Genetic Diseases*. R.J. Desnick editor. Churchill Livingstone, London, pp.203–221.

Krivit, W., and E.G. Shapiro. 1994. Marrow transplantation for storage diseases: The plan and need for a control study. In: *Bone Marrow Transplantation*. S. Forman, E.D. Thomas, and K. Blume editors.

Blackwell Scientific, London. pp.883–894.

Krivit, W., M.E. Pierpont, K. Ayaz, M. Tsai, N.K.C. Ramsay, J. Kersey, S. Weisdorf, R. Sibley, D. Snover, M.M. McGovern, M.F. Schwartz, and R J. Desnick. 1984. Bone-marrow transplantation in the Maroteauz-Lamy syndrome (mucopolysaccharidosis type VI) biochemical and clinical status 24 months after transplantation. *N. Engl J. Med.* **311**:1606–1611.

Lake, B.D., D.C. Henderson, A. Oakhill, and A. Vellodi. 1995. Bone marrow transplantation in Batten disease (neuronal ceroid-lipofuscinosis). Will it work? Fifth International Symposium on Neuronal Ceroid Lipofuscinosis. *Am. J. Med. Genet.* **57**:369–373.

Lasky, L.C. 1991. The role of laboratory in marrow manipulation. *Arch. Pathol. Lab. Med.* **115**:293–298.

Lassmann, H., M. Schmied, K. Vass, and W.F. Hickey. 1993. Bone marrow derived elements and resident microglia in brain inflammation. *Glia* **7**:19–24.

Lassmann, H., F. Zimprich, K. Vass, and W.F. Hickey. 1991. Microglial cells are a component of the perivascular glia limitans. *J. Neurosci. Res.* **28**:236–243.

Lawson, L.J., M.K. Matyszak, and V.H. Perry. 1993. Lessons from microglia in special sites. *Clin. Neuropathol.* **12**:310–315.

Lawson, L.J., V.H. Perry, and S. Gordon. 1992. Turnover of resident microglia in the normal adult mouse brain. *Neuroscience* **48**:405–415.

Lawson, L.J., V.H. Perry, P. Dri, and S. Gordon. 1990. Heterogeneity in the distribution and morphology of microglia in the normal adult mouse brain. *Neuroscience* **39**:151–170.

Lee, S.C., W. Liu, C.F. Brosnan, and D.W. Dickson. 1992. Characterization of primary human fetal dissociated central nervous system cultures with an emphasis on microglia. *Lab. Invest.* **67**:465–476.

Levinson, S.W., C. Chuang, B.J. Abramson, and J.E. Goldman. 1993. The migrational patterns and developmental fates of glial precursors in the rat subventricular zone are temporally regulated. *Development* **119**:611–622.

Ling, E.A. 1981. The origin and nature of microglia. *Adv. Cell. Neurobiol.* **2**:33–82.

Ling, E.A., D. Penney, and C.P. LeBlond. 1980. Use of carbon labeling to demonstrate the role of blood monocytes as precursors of the 'ameboid cells' present in the corpus callosum of postnatal rats. *J. Comp. Neurol.* **193**:631–657.

Ling, E., and W. Wong. 1993. The origin and nature of ramified and ameboid microglia: A historical review and current concepts. *Glia* **7**:9–18.

Liu, W., C.F. Brosnan, D.W. Dickson, and S.C. Lee. 1994. Macrophage colony-stimulating factor mediates astrocyte-induced microglial ramification in human fetal central nervous system culture. *Am. J. Pathol.* **145**:48–53.

Lothrop, C.D., Z.S. Al-lebban, G.P. Niemeyer, J.B. Jones, M.G. Peterson, J.R. Smith, H.J. Baker, R.A. Morgan, M.A. Eglitis, and W.F. Anderson. 1991. Expression of a foreign gene in cats reconstituted with retroviral vector infected autologous bone marrow. *Blood* **78**:237–245.

Luskin, M.B., J.G. Parnavelas, and J.A. Barfield. 1993. Neurons, astrocytes, and oligodendrocytes of the rat cerebral cortex originate from separate progenitor cells: An ultrastructural analysis of clonally related cells. *J. Neurosci.* **13**:1730–1750.

Mallat, M., and B. Chamak. 1994. Brain macrophages: neurotoxic or neurotrophic effector cells? *J. Leukoc. Biol.* **56**:416–422.

Matsumoto, Y., and M. Fujiwara. 1987. Absence of donor-type major histocompatibility complex class I antigen-bearing microglia in the rat central nervous system of radiation bone marrow chimeras. *J. Neuroimmunol.* **17**:71–82.

Matsumoto, Y., and F. Ikuta. 1985. Appearance and distribution of fetal brain macrophages in mice. *Cell Tissue. Res.* **239**:271–278.

Matsushima, G.K., M. Taniike, L.H. Glimcher, M.J. Grusby, J.A. Frelinger, K. Suzuki, and J.P.-Y. Ting. 1994. Absence of MHC class II molecules reduces CNS demyelination, microglial/macrophage infiltration, and twitching in murine globoid cell leukodystrophy. *Cell* **78**:645–656.

McGeer, P.L., S. Itagaki, B.E. Boyes, and E.G. McGeer. 1988a. Reactive microglia are positive for HLA-DR in the substantia nigra of parkinson's and alzheimer's disease brains. *Neurology* **38**:1285–1291.

McGeer, P.L., S. Itagaki, and P.L. McGeer. 1988b. Expression of the histocompatibility glycoprotein HLA-DR in neurological disease. *Acta Neuropathol.* **76**:550–557.

McGeer, P.L., T. Kawamata, D.G. Walker, H. Akiyama, I, Tooyama, and E. McGeer. 1993. Microglia in degenerative neurological disease. *Glia* **7**:84–92.

McGovern, M.M., M. Ludman, M.P. Short, L. Steinfeld, M. Kattan, E.L. Raab, W. Krivit, and R. Desnick. 1986. Bone marrow transplantation in Maroteaux–Lamy syndrome (MPS type 6): Status 40 months after BMT. In: *Bone Marrow Transplantation for Treatment of Lysosomal Storage Diseases.* W. Krivit and N.W. Paul editors. Alan R. Liss, NY. pp.41–53.

McKanna, J.A. 1993. Lipocortin I immunoreactivity identifies microglia in adult rat brain. *J. Neurosci. Res.*

36:491–500.

Miller, A.D., J.V. Garcia, N. von-Suhr, C.M. Lynch, C. Wilson, and M.V. Eiden. 1991. Construction and properties of retrovirus packaging cells based on gibbon ape leukemia virus. *J. Virol.* **65:**2220–2224.

Miller, A.M. 1993. Hematopoietic growth factors in autologous bone marrow transplantation. *Semin. Oncol.* **20:**88–95.

Miyake, T., Y. Tsuchihashi, T. Kitamura, and S. Fujita. 1984. Immunohistochemical studies of blood monocytes infiltrating into the neonatal rat brain. *Acta Neuropathol.* **62:**291–297.

Murabe, Y., and Y. Sano. 1982. Morphological studies on neuroglia. *Cell. Tissue Res.* **225:**469–485.

Myers, R., and J. Cremer. 1994. Imaging inflammation in the CNS. *Neuropathol. Appl. Neurobiol.* **20:**213–215.

Nakajima, K., M. Shimojo, M. Hammanoue, S. Ishiura, H. Sugita, and S. Kohsaka. 1992a. Identification of elastase as a secretory protease from cultured rat microglia. *J. Neurochem.* **58:**1401–1408.

Nakajima, K., N. Takemoto, and S. Kohsaka. 1992b. Retinoic acid enhances the secretion of plasminogen from cultured rat microglia. *FEBS Lett.* **314:**167–170.

Neitzel, H. 1991. Routine applications of DNA fingerprinting with the oligonucleotide probe (CAC)/(GTG). *Clin. Genet.* **39:**97–103.

Norenberg, W., P. Illes, and P.J. Gebicke-Haerter. 1994. Sodium channel in isolated human brain macrophages (microglia). *Glia* **10:**165–172.

Novak, J.P., and S. Federoff. 1994. A mathematical model to test hypotheses about the development of microglia in cultures. *Mol. Biol. Cell* **5:**228a.

Nyhan, W.L., T. Page, H.E. Gruber, and R. Parkman. 1986. Bone Marrow transplantation in Lesch–Nyhan disease. In: *Bone Marrow Transplantation for Treatment of Lysosomal Storage Diseases.* W. Krivit and N.W. Paul editors. Alan R. Liss, NY. pp.113–117.

O'Brien, J.S., R. Storb, R.F. Raff, J. Harding, F. Appelbaum, S. Morimoto, Y. Kishimoto, T. Graham, A. Ahern-Rindell, and S.L. O'Brien. 1990. Bone marrow transplantation in canine Gm1 gangliosidosis. *Clin. Genet.* **38:**274–280.

Oehmichen, M. 1983. Inflammatory cells in the central nervous system: an integrating concept based on recent research in pathology, immunology, and forensic medicine. *Progr. Neuropathol.* **5:**277–335.

Oehmichen, M., H. Wietholter, and M.F. Greaves. 1979. Immunological analysis of human microglia: Lack of monocytic and lymphoid membrane differentiation antigens. *J. Neuropathol. Exp. Neurol.* **38:**99–103.

Ozand, P.T., and G.G. Gascon. 1992. Treatment of inherited neurometabolic diseases: the future. *J. Child Neurol.* **7:**S132–S140.

Pallavicini, M.G., A.W. Flake, D. Madden, C. Bethel, B. Duncan, M.L. Gonzalgo, S. Haendel, T. Montoys, and L. Roberts. 1992. Hemopoietic chimerism in rodents transplanted *in utero* with fetal human hemopoietic cells. *Transplant Proc.* **24:**542–543.

Palmer, D.N., I.M. Fearly, J.E. Walker, N.A. Hall, B.D. Lake, L.S. Wolfe, M. Haltia, R.D. Martinus, and R.D. Jolly. 1992. Mitochondrial ATP synthase subunit c storage in the ceroid lipofuscinoses (Batten disease). *Am. J. Med. Genet.* **42:**551–567.

Parkman, R. 1986. The application of bone marrow transplantation to the treatment of genetic diseases. *Science* **232:**1373–1378.

Pearson, A.D.J. 1986. Survey of preparative regimens and complications of bone marrow transplantation in patients with lysosomal storage disease. In: *Bone Marrow Transplantation for Treatment of Lysosomal Storage Disease.* W. Krivit and N.W. Paul editors. Alan R. Liss, New York. pp.153–162.

Peck, A.B., and F.H. Bach. 1973. A miniaturized mouse mixed leukocyte culture in serum-free and mouse serum supplemented media. *J. Immunol. Meth.* **3:**147–150.

Pentchev, P.G., M.E. Comly, H.S. Kruth, M.T. Vanier, D.A. Wenger, S. Patel, and R.O. Brady. 1985. A defect in cholesterol esterification in Niemann–Pick disease (type C) patients. *Proc. Natl Acad. Sci. USA* **82:**8247.

Pepe, M.S., G. Longton, M. Pettinger, M. Mori, L.D. Fisher, and R. Storb. 1993. Summarizing data on survival, relapse, and chronic graft-versus-host disease after bone marrow transplantation: motivation for and description of new methods. *Br. J. Haematol.* **83:**602–607.

Perry, V.H., and P.B. Andersson. 1992. The inflammatory response in the CNS. *Neuropathol. Appl. Neurobiol.* **18:**454–459.

Perry, V.H., and S. Gordon. 1991. Macrophages and the nervous system. *Int. Rev. Cytol.* **125:**203–244.

Perry, V.H., D.A. Hume, and S. Gordon. 1985. Immunohistochemical localization of macrophages and microglia in the adult and developing mouse brain. *Neuroscience* **18:**313–326.

Perry, V.H., L.J. Lawson, and D.M. Reid. 1994. Biology of the mononuclear phagocyte system of the central nervous system and HIV infection. *J. Leukoc. Biol.* **56:**399–406.

Peters, A., S.L. Palay, and H. deF. Webster. 1991. *The Fine Structure of the Nervous System.* Oxford University Press, NY.

Pollack, M., F. Mastrota, J. Chin-Loui, S. Mooney, and A. Hayes. 1982. Preliminary studies of the feline histocompatibility system. *Immunogenetics* **16:**339–347.

Pyeritz, R.E. 1984. Treatment of inborn errors of metabolism by transplantation. *Nature* **312:**405–406.

Raff, R.F., E.M. Severns, R. Storb, T.C. Graham, G. Sale, F.G. Schuening, and F.R. Applebaum. 1993a. Studies of the use of L-leucyl-L-leucine methyl ester in canine allogeneic marrow transplantation. *Transplantation* **55:**1244–1249.

Raff, R.F., R. Storb, T. Graham, H.J. Deeg, M. Pepe, R. Schaffer, G.E. Sale, F. Schuening, and F.R. Applebaum. 1993b. What role for 15-deoxyspergualin in enhancing engraftment of unrelated histocompatible canine marrow grafts and preventing graft-versus-host disease? *Transplantation* **55:**684–688.

Rappeport, J.M., J.A. Barranger, and E.I. Ginns. 1986. Bone marrow transplantation in Gaucher disease. In: *Bone Marrow Transplantation for Treatment of Lysosomal Storage Diseases.* W. Krivit and N.W. Paul editors. Alan R. Liss, NY. pp.101–109.

Raudrant, D., J.L. Touraine, and A. Rebaud. 1992. In utero transplantation of stem cells in humans: technical aspects and clinical experience during pregnancy. *Bone Marrow Transplant.* **9:**98.

Raivich, G., J. Gehrmann, M. Moreno-Floros, and G.W. Kreutzberg. 1993. Microglia: growth factor and mitogen receptors. *Clin. Neuropathol.* **5:**293–295.

Reinhold, H.S., W. Calvo, J.W. Hopewell, and A.P. van der Berg. 1990. Development of blood vessel-related radiation damage in the fimbria of the central nervous system. *Int. J. Radiat. Oncol. Biol. Phys.* **18:**37–42.

Richardson, A., J. Neuhaus, and S. Fedoroff. 1994. Microglia progenitor cells and development of microglia. *Neuropathol. Appl. Neurobiol.* **20:**183–185.

Rieske, E., M.B. Graeber, W. Tetzlaff, A. Czlonkowska, W.J. Streit, and G.W. Kreutzberg. 1989. Microglia and microglia-derived brain macrophages in culture: generation from axotomized rat facial nuclei, identification and characterization *in vitro. Brain Res.* **492:**1–14.

Rio-Hortega, P.D. 1932. Microglia. In: *Cytology & Cellular Pathology of the Nervous System.* W. Penfield editor. Hafner Publishing Co., NY. pp.483–534.

Roque, R.S., and R.B. Caldwell. 1993. Isolation and culture of retinal microglia. *Curr. Eye Res.* **12:**285–290.

Roubicek, M., J. Gehler, and J. Spranger. 1985. The clinical spectrum of α-L-iduronidase deficiency. *Am. J. Med. Genet.* **20:**471–481.

Rowe, J.M., N. Ciobanu, J. Ascensao, E.A. Stadtmauer, R.S. Weiner, D.P. Schenkein, P. McGlave, and H.M. Lazarus. 1994. Recommended guidelines for the management of autologous and allogeneic bone marrow transplantation. *Ann. Intern. Med.* **120:**143–158.

Sacerdote, P., S. Dennis-donini, P. Paglia, F. Granucci, A.E. Paneral and P. Ricciardi-Castagnoli. 1993. Cloned microglial cells but not macrophages synthesize β-Endorphin in response to CRH activation. *Glia* **9:**305–310.

Sakiyama, T., M. Tsuda, K. Horinouchi, A. Akatsuka, S. Miyawaki, M. Tadokoro, T. Kunieda, and T. Kitagawa. 1992. Study of bone marrow transplantation for Niemann-Pick mice using sry and zfy genes. *J. Inherit. Metab. Dis.* **15:**821–826.

Sakiyama, T., M. Tauda, M. Owada, K. Joh, S. Miyawaki, and T. Kitagawa. 1983. Bone marrow transplantation for Niemann–Pick mice. *Biochem. Biophys. Res. Commun.* **113:**605–610.

Sands, M.S., J.E. Barker, C. Vogler, V. Levy, B. Gwynn, N. Galvin, W.S. Sly, and E. Birkenmeier. 1993. Treatment of murine mucopolysaccharidosis type VII by syngeneic bone marrow transplantation in neonates. *Lab. Invest.* **68:**676–686.

Saunders, G.K., P.A. Wood, R.K. Myers, L.G. Shell, and R. Carithers. 1988. G_{M1} gangliosidosis in Portuguese water dogs: pathologic and biochemical findings. *Vet. Pathol.* **25:**265–269.

Schelper, R.L., and E.K. Adrian Jr. 1986. Monocytes become macrophages; they do not become microglia: A light and electron microscopic autoradiographic study using 125–Iododeoxyuridine. *J. Neuropathol. Exp. Neurol.* **45:**1–19.

Shapiro, E.G., L. Lockman, W. Kennedy, D. Zimmerman, E.H. Kolodny, S. Raghavan, G. Wiederschain, D.A. Wenger, J. Sung, C.G. Summers, and W. Krivit. 1991. Bone marrow transplantation as treatment for globoid cell leukodystrophy. In: *Treatment of Genetic Diseases.* R.J. Desnick Editor. Churchill Livingstone, London, pp.223–238.

Shaw, P., K. Hugh-Jones, J. Hobbs, A. Cooper, and G. Lealman. 1986. GM1 gangliosidosis: failure to halt regression by bone marrow transplantation. *Bone Marrow Transplant.* **1:**339.

Shull, R.M., M.A. Breider, and G.C. Constantopoulos. 1988. Long-term neurological effects of bone marrow transplantation in a canine lysosomal storage disease. *Pediatr. Res.* **23:**347–352.

Shull, R.M., N.E. Hastings, R.R. Selcer, J.B. Jones, J.R. Smith, W.C. Cullen, and G. Constantopoulos. 1987. Bone marrow transplantation in canine mucopolysaccharidosis I. *J. Clin. Invest.* **79:**435–443.

Siegel, D.A., and S.U. Walkley. 1994. Growth of ectopic dendrites on cortical pyramidal neurons in neuronal storage diseases correlates with abnormal accumulation of GM2 ganglioside. *J. Neurochem.* **62:**1852–1862.

Sievers, J., J. Schmidtmayer, and R. Parwaresch. 1994. Blood monocytes and spleen macrophages differentiate into microglia-like cells when cultured on astrocytes. *Ann. Anat.* **176:**45–51.

Simpson, T.J., and M.S. Golbus. 1985. *In utero* fetal hematopoietic stem cell transplantation. *Semin. Perinatol.* **9:**68–73.

Slavin, S., E. Neparstek, M. Ziegler, G. Bach, J.G. Schenker, and A. Lewin. 1990. Intrauterine bone marrow transplantation for correction of genetic disorders in man. *Exp. Hematol.* **18**:658.

Sly, W.S. 1993. Gene therapy on the Sly. *Nature Genet.* **4**:105–106.

Southern, E.M. 1975. Detection of specific sequences among DNA fragments separated by gel electrophoresis. *J. Molec. Biol.* **98**:503–517.

Spranger, J.W., F. Koch, V.A. McKusick, J. Natzschka, H.R. Wiedemann, and H. Zellweger. 1970. Mucopolysaccharidosis VI (Maroteaux–Lamy's disease). *Helv. Paediatr. Acta* **25**:337–362.

Srour, E.F., E.D. Zanjani, J.E. Brandt, T. Leemhuis, R.A. Briddell, N.A. Heerema, and R. Hoffman. 1992. Sustained human hematopoiesis in sheep transplanted in utero during early gestation with fractionated adult human bone marrow cells. *Blood* **79**:1404–1412.

Stead, R.B., W.W. Kwok, R. Storb, and A.D. Miller. 1988. Canine model for gene therapy: Inefficient genc expression in dogs reconstituted with autologous marrow infected with retroviral vectors. *Blood* **71**:742–747.

Storb, R., R.F. Raff, F.R. Applebaum, H.J. Deeg, W. Fitzsimmons, T.C. Graham, M. Pepe, M. Pettinger, G. Sale, R. van der Jagt, and R.G. Schuening. 1993. FK-506 and methotrexate prevent graft-versus-host disease in dogs given 9.2 Gy total body irradiation and marrow grafts from unrelated dog leukocyte antigen-nonidentical donors. *Transplantation* **56**:800–807.

Storb, R., R.F. Raff, F.R. Applebaum, J.H. Deeg, T.C. Graham, F.G. Schuening, G. Sale, E. Bryant, and K. Seidel. 1994. Fractionated versus single-dose total body irradiation at low and high dose rates to condition canine littermates for DLA-identical marrow grafts. *Blood* **83**:3384–3389.

Streit, W.J., and M.B. Graeber. 1991. Perivascular location and phenotypic heterogeneity of microglial cells in the rat brain. *J. Neuroimmunol.* **33**:87.

Streit, W.J., and M.B. Graeber. 1993. Heterogeneity of microglial and perivascular cell populations: Insights gained from the facial nucleus paradigm. *Glia* **7**:68–74.

Streit, W.J., M.B. Graeber, and G.W. Kreutzberg. 1988. Functional plasticity of microglia: A review. *Glia* **1**:301–307.

Streit, W.J., M.B. Graeber, and G.W. Kreutzberg. 1989. Expression of Ia antigen on perivascular and microglial cells after sublethal and lethal motor neuron injury. *Exp. Neurol.* **105**:115–126.

Streit, W.J., and G.W. Kreutzberg. 1988. Response of endogenous glial cells to motor neuron degeneration induced by toxic ricin. *J. Comp. Neurol.* **268**:248–263.

Suzuki, K., and Y. Suzuki. 1989. Galactyosylceramide lipidosis: Globoid-cell leukodystrophy (Krabbe disease). In: *The Metabolic Basis of Inherited Disease.* C.R. Scriver, A.L. Beaudet, W.S. Sly, and D. Valle editors. McGraw-Hill, NY. pp.1699–1720.

Suzumura, A., S.G.E. Mezitis, N.K. Gonatas, and D.H. Silverberg. 1987. MHC antigen expression on bulk isolated macrophage-microglia from newborn mouse brain: induction of Ia antigen expression by γ-interferon. *J. Neuroimmunol.* **15**:263–278.

Suzumura, A., T. Marunouchi, and H. Yamamoto. 1991. Morphological transformation of microglia *in vitro*. *Brain Res.* **45**:301–306.

Taylor, R.M., B.R.H. Farrow, G.J. Stewart, and P.J. Healy. 1986. Enzyme replacement in nervous tissue after allogeneic bone-marrow transplantation for fucosidosis in dogs. *Lancet* **ii**:772–774.

Taylor, R.M., B.R.H. Farrow, and G.J. Stewart. 1992. Amelioration of clinical disease following bone marrow transplantation in fucosidase-deficient dogs. *Am. J. Med. Genet.* **42**:628–632.

Thanos, S., C. Pavlidis, J. Mey, and H. Thiel. 1992. Specific transcellular staining of microglia in the adult rat after traumatic degeneration of carbocyanine-filled retinal ganglion cells. *Eye Res.* **55**:101–117.

Thomas, W.E. 1992. Brain macrophages: evaluation of microglia and their functions. *Brain Res. Rev.* **17**:61–74.

Topper, R., J. Gehrmann, M. Schwarz, F. Block, J. Noth, and G.W. Kreutzberg. 1993. Remote microglial activation in the quinolinic acid model of Huntington's disease. *Exp. Neurol.* **123**:271–283.

Touraine, J.L. 1991. Stem cell transplantation in primary immunodeficiency with special reference to the first prenatal, in utero transplants. *Allergol. Immunopathol.* **19**:49–51.

Touraine, J.L., D. Raudrant, C. Royo, A. Rebaud, F. Barbier, M.G. Roncarolo, F. Touraine, S. Laplace, L. Gebuhrer, H. Betuel, D. Frappaz, F. Freycon, and C. Vullo. 1991. In utero transplantation of hemopoietic stem cells in humans. *Transplant Proc.* **23**:1706–1708.

Touraine, J.L. 1992. In-utero transplantation of fetal liver stem cells into human fetuses. *Hum. Reprod.* **7**:44–48.

Touraine, J.L., D. Raudrant, A. Rebaud, M.G. Roncarolo, S. Laplace, L. Gebuhhrer, H. Betuel, D. Frappaz, F. Freycon, M.T. Zabot, F. Touraine, G. Souillet, N. Phillipe, and C. Vullo. 1992. *In utero* transplantation of stem cells in humans: immunological aspects and clinical follow-up of patients. *Bone Marrow Transplant.* **9**:121.

Tsai, P., J.M. Lipton, I. Sahdev, V. Najfeld, L.R. Rankin, A.H. Slyper, M. Ludman, and G.A. Grabowski. 1992. Allogenic bone marrow transplantation in severe Gaucher disease. *Pediatr. Res.* **31**:503–507.

Unger, E.R., J.H. Sung, J.C. Manivel, M.L. Chenggis, B.R. Blazar, and W. Krivit. 1993. Male donor-derived cells in the brains of female sex-mismatched bone marrow transplant recipients: A Y-chromosome specific in situ hybridization study. *J. Neuropathol. Exp. Neurol.* **52:**460–470.

Vaca, K., and E. Wendt. 1992. Divergent effects of astroglial and microglial secretions on neuron growth and survival. *Exp. Neurol.* **118:**62–72.

Vandevelde, M., R. Frankhauser, P. Bischel, U. Weismann, and N. Hershkowitz. 1982. Hereditary neurovisceral mannosidosis associated with α-mannosidase deficiency in a family of persian cats. *Acta Neuropathol.* **58:**64–68.

Vellodi, A., E. Young, M. New, C. Pot-Mees, and K. Hugh-Jones. 1992. Bone marrow transplantation for Sanfilippo disease type b. *J. Inherit. Metab.* **15:**911–918.

Vogler, C., E.H. Birkenmeier, W.S. Sly, B. Levy, C. Pegors, J.W. Kyle, and W.G. Beamert. 1990. Murine model of mucopolysaccharidosis VII. Gross and microscopic findings in β-glucuronidase-deficient mice. *Am. J. Pathol.* **136:**207–217.

Walkley, S.U. 1988. Pathobiology of neuronal storage disease. *Int. Rev. Neurobiol.* **29:**191–244.

Walkley, S.U., H.J. Baker, M.C. Rattazzi, M.E. Haskins, and J.-Y. Wu. 1991. Neuroaxonal dystrophy in neuronal storage disorders: Evidence for major GABAergic neuron involvement. *J. Neurol. Sci.* **104:**1–8.

Walkley, S.U., M.A. Thrall, K. Dobrenis, M. Huang, P.A. March, D.A. Siegel, and S. Wurzelmann. 1994a. Bone marrow transplantation corrects the enzyme defect in neurons of the central nervous system in a lysosomal storage disease. *Proc. Natl Acad. Sci. USA* **91:**2970–2974.

Walkley, S., M. Thall, K. Dobrenis, P. March, and S. Wurzelmann. 1994b. Bone marrow transplantation in neuronal storage diseases. *Brain Pathol.* **4:**376.

Walkley, S.U., S. Wurzelmann, and D.A. Siegel. 1987. Ectopic axon hillock-associated neurite growth is maintained in metabolically-reversed swainsonine-induced neuronal storage disease. *Brain Res.* **410:**89–96.

Wenger, D.A., P.W. Gasper., M.A. Thrall, S.M. Dial, R.A. LeCouteur, and E.A. Hoover. 1986. Bone marrow transplantation in the feline model of arylsulfatase B deficiency. In: *Bone Marrow Transplantation for Treatment of Lysosomal Storage Diseases.* W. Krivit and N.W. Paul editors. Alan R. Liss, NY. pp.177–186.

Whitley, C.B., K.G. Belani, P. Chang, C.G. Summers, B.R. Blazer, M.Y. Tsai, R.E. Latchaw, N.K.C. Ramsay, and J.H. Kersey. 1993. Long-term outcome of hurler syndrome following bone marrow transplantation. *Am. J. Med. Genet.* **46:**209–218.

Whitley, C.B., N.K.C. Ramsay, J.H. Kersey, and W. Krivit. 1986. Bone marrow transplantation for Hurler syndrome: Assessment of metabolic correction. In: *Bone Marrow Transplantation for Treatment of Lysosomal Storage Diseases.* W Krivit and N.W. Paul editors. Alan R. Liss, NY. pp.7–24.

Will, A., A. Cooper, C. Hatton, I.B. Sardharwalla, D.I.K. Evans, and R.F. Stevens. 1987. Bone marrow transplantation in the treatment of α-mannosidosis. *Arch. Dis. Child.* **62:**1044–1049.

Williams, K., A. Bar-Or, E. Ulvestad, A. Olivier, J.P. Antel, and V.W. Yong. 1992. Biology of adult human microglia in culture: Comparisons with peripheral blood monocytes and astrocytes. *J. Neuropathol. Exp. Neurol.* **51:**538–549.

Wisniewski, H.M., and J. Weigel. 1993. Migration of perivascular cells into the neurophil and their involvement in β-amyloid plaque formation. *Acta Neuropathol.* **85:**586–595.

Wolfe, J.H., M.S. Sands, J.E. Barker, B. Gwynn, L.B. Rowe, C.A. Volger, and E.H. Birkenmeier. 1992. Reversal of pathology in murine mucopolysaccharidosis type VII by somatic cell gene transfer. *Nature* **360:**749–753.

Wolswijk, G. 1994. G_{D3}+ cells in the adult rat optic nerve are ramified microglia rather than O-$2A^{adult}$ progenitor cells. *Glia* **10:**244–249.

Wu, C.H., C.Y. Wen, J.Y. Shieh, and E.A. Ling. 1992. A quantitative and morphometric study of the transformation of ameboid microglia into ramified microglia in the developing corpus callosum in rats. *J. Anat.* **181:**423–430.

Wu, C.H., C.Y. Wen, J.Y. Shieh, and E.A. Ling. 1994. Down-regulation of membrane glycoprotein in ameboid microglia transforming into ramified microglia in postnatal rat brain. *J. Neurocytol.* **23:**258–269.

Xenocostas, A., T. Ghayur, J.-C. Setrakian, W.S. Lapp, and D.G. Osmond. 1994. A donor-derived asialo-GM1 cell induces depression of B-cell genesis during systemic graft-versus-host disease. *Blood* **84:**3965–3973.

Yeager, A.M., S. Brennab, and C. Tiffany. 1984. Prolonged survival and remyelination after hematopoietic cell transplantation in the twitcher mouse. *Science* **225:**1052.

Yam, P.Y., Petz, L.D., Knowlton, R.G., and Wallace, R.B. 1987. Use of DNA restriction fragment length polymorphisms to document marrow engraftment and mixed hematopoietic chimerism following bone marrow transplantation. *Transplantation* **43:**99–140.

Yeager, A.M., H.W. Moser, P.J. Tutschka, R. Saral, A.E. Moser, A.A.J. Kumar, and G.W. Santos, 1986. Allogeneic bone marrow transplantation in adrenoleukodystrophy: clinical, pathologic, and biochemical studies. In: *Bone Marrow Transplantation for Treatment of Lysosomal Storage Diseases.* W. Krivit and N.W. Paul editors. Alan R. Liss, NY. pp.79–100.

Zanjani, E.D., F.R. Mackintosh, and M.R. Harrison. 1991. Hematopoietic chimerism in sheep and nonhuman primates by in utero transplantation of fetal hematopoietic stem cells. *Blood Cells* **17:**349–363.

SECTION 6

Protocols for *in vivo* Application of Gene Transfer Methods

CHAPTER 22

Replication-competent Viral Therapy of Tumors in the Central Nervous System

William D. Hunter, Takahito Yazaki, Samuel D. Rabkin and Robert L. Martuza

Molecular Neurosurgery Laboratory and Georgetown Brain Tumor Center, Department of Neurosurgery, Georgetown University Medical Center, 3800 Reservoir Road NW, Washington DC 20007, USA. Tel: 202 687 4972; Fax: 202 687 3744; Email: whunte02@gumedlib.dml.georgetown.edu

1 INTRODUCTION

The prognosis for a patient with glioblastoma multiforme has not changed dramatically over the past few years despite advances in surgical techniques, chemotherapy, and radiation treatment (Onoyama et al., 1976; Salazar et al., 1979; Walker et al., 1980; Daumas-Duport et al., 1988; Mahaley et al., 1989; Shapiro et al., 1989; Kim et al., 1991). The 5-year survival is less than 5.5% (Walker et al., 1980; Mahaley et al., 1989). Clearly, new approaches are required for brain tumor therapy.

Viruses have been used over the past few years as an alternative anti-tumor therapy (Moore, 1960; Austin and Boone, 1979; Lobayashi, 1979); they are the most efficient means for getting foreign genes into cells. Some of the problems from early studies have been overcome by genetic engineering techniques which allow directed mutations of viruses to be made and tested.

A number of viral vectors are currently being examined for tumor therapy. These include herpes simplex virus (HSV-1)(Martuza et al., 1991; Markert et al., 1992, 1993; Boviatsis et al., 1994a, b; Jia et al., 1994; Kaplitt et al., 1994; Mineta et al., 1994), adenovirus (Le Gal La Salle et al., 1993; Boviatsis et al., 1994a; Chen et al., 1994) and retroviral vectors (Short et al., 1990; Ezzeddine et al., 1991; Culver et al., 1992; Takamiya et al., 1992; Yamada et al., 1992; Oldfield et al., 1993; Ram et al., 1993). In the latter two, essential genes are deleted (*gag*, *pol*, *env*-deleted retrovirus, or *E1*-deleted adenovirus), and therefore these viral vectors derive from replication-incompetent viruses, and are classified as replication-incompetent viral vectors. The retroviral vector is genetically modified to the point that it is incapable of producing active viral particles in infected host cells (Boris-Lawrie and Temin, 1993). Each particle of the retrovirus can integrate and express only the gene to be delivered in a single dividing cell and cannot spread to other dividing cells. Adenovirus will infect most cells, not just proliferating cells. Its advantages over the retrovirus are the higher titers that can be obtained, useful in treating tumors, and the fact that larger DNA constructs can be placed into recombinant adenovirus vectors (Boviatsis et al., 1994a). However, the virus itself is not specifically targeted to tumor cells and at high titers adenovirus vectors can be toxic to cells. A problem with the replication-incompetent vectors is that they do not spread.

Protocols for Gene Transfer in Neuroscience: Towards Gene Therapy of Neurological Disorders
Edited by P.R. Lowenstein and L.W. Enquist

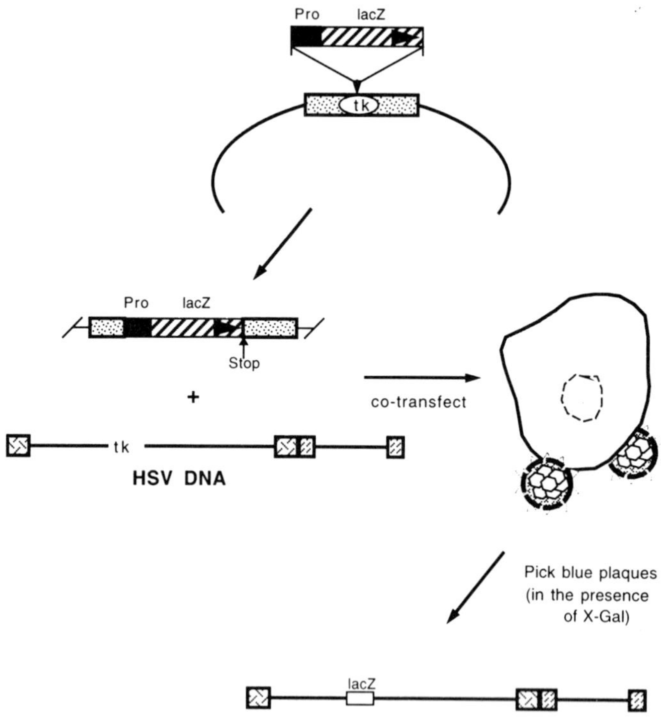

Figure 22.1 Generation of *tk*D:*lacZ* insertion recombinant HSV-1. The gene of interest is inserted with promotor (e.g. Pro *lacZ*) into the thymidine kinase (tk) sequence, leaving sufficient flanking HSV-1 sequences for homologous recombination and the recombinant plasmid DNA cotransfected with HSV-1 DNA. Recombinant viruses will contain the gene insert into the *tk* gene. Recombinant HSV-1 (containing the *lacZ* gene) can be identified using X-gal to stain positive plaques. Blue plaques may then be isolated

Our current strategy utilizes replication-competent vectors derived from HSV-1 for tumor therapy (Fig. 22.1). HSV-1 mutants may be constructed which are attenuated for growth in non-dividing cells but replication-competent within the tumor. This allows the virus to enter one tumor cell, make multiple copies, kill the cell and spread to other tumor cells. The surrounding normal brain cells are non-dividing and therefore unable to support replication of these vectors.

HSV-1 has several advantages over other possible vectors: the HSV-1 genome has been sequenced; the DNA is linear, double stranded and 152 kilobase pairs in length; its large genome allows insertion of reasonably large constructs into recombinant vectors; the viral genome does not integrate into the host genome and mutants with decreased neurovirulence have been isolated; HSV-1 is also known to infect tumor cells with high efficiency.

A concern regarding the use of HSV-1 in the treatment of brain gliomas is the potential for killing surrounding normal brain, mostly composed of non-dividing neurons and slowly dividing glia. However, clinical studies indicate that even wild-type HSV-1 generally does not spread far from the site of initial infection or cause serious systemic disease in immunocompetent individuals (Sacks et al., 1989).

Malignant glioma cells are a dividing tumor cell population. We have hypothesized that HSV-1 mutants would replicate in gliomas while sparing normal brain tissue. The ability of HSV-1 mutants to kill glioma cells can be easily determined in cell culture, where infections at low multiplicity of infection (MOI) of 0.1 or 0.01 should lead to a spreading infection that destroys the entire monolayer of tumor cells. When injected into animals that contain tumors originated from these cell lines (subcutaneous, subrenal or intracranial) these HSV-1 mutants are associated with tumor death or growth inhibition (Martuza et al., 1991). Similar results have been shown with other nervous system tumors (Market et al., 1992).

Great care should be taken in planning viral constructs. These are replication-competent viruses and the possible impact on the human environment if such a recombinant were to spread outside the laboratory must be considered. For example, the hazard of constructing a replication-competent virus mutant expressing an oncogene or with new tropism needs to be carefully evaluated before constructing one.

2 MATERIALS AND EQUIPMENT

2.1 Instruments

(1) Adson dissecting forceps.
(2) Autoclip applier 9 mm.
(3) Autoclip (9 mm).
(4) Zeiss stereomicroscope with ocular micrometer accurate to 0.1 mm and 60 × magnification.
(5) Clinical centrifuge.
(6) Polypropylene conical tubes: 6 ml, 15 ml, 50 ml.
(7) Hemacytometer, Bright-Line.
(8) Disposable No. 11 blade scalpel.
(9) Deaver straight, sharp–sharp scissors.
(10) Foredom burr, cutting, 2 mm in diameter.
(11) Foredom burr hand drill.
(12) Halsted mosquito hemostatic forceps.
(13) Hamilton needle, microliter.
(14) Kopf stereotactic frame with microinjection adaptor for mice.
(15) Micro friedman bone Rongeur.
(16) Automatic pipettes (1000 μl, 200 μl, 20 μl).
(17) Tissue culture flasks: 75 cm^2, 150 cm^2.
(18) Dressing sponges 4 × 30″.
(19) Ultrasonic bath.
(20) Winged infusion set 25 gauge × 0.75″.
(21) Insulin syringes, 1 ml.

2.2 Mice

(1) Balb/c, nu/nu (National Cancer Institute, Bethesda, MD).
(2) C57B1/6 (Charles Rivers Company, Boston, MA).

2.3 Reagents

(1) Sterile Dulbecco's Modified Eagle Medium 1 × (DMEM), containing 584 mg/l L-glutamine, 4.5 g/l D-glucose, 0.11 g/l sodium pyruvate.
(2) Sterile Dulbecco's phosphate-buffered saline 1 × (PBS), containing 1.0 g/l glucose.
(3) Fixative solution: 2% paraformaldehyde, 5 mM EGTA, 2 mM $MgCl_2$ in 0.1 M piperazine-*N*-*N*′-bis(2-ethanesulfonic acid) (Pipes) (pH 7.3).
(4) Formaldehyde (36.5%).
(5) Inactivated fetal calf serum (IFCS); heat inactivated at 56°C for 30 min.
(6) Methanol, absolute.

(7) PBS/IFCS; PBS containing glucose and 1% IFCS.
(8) Sodium pentobarbital solution: 3 ml sodium pentobarbital (50 mg/ml), 2 ml absolute ethanol, 25 ml bacteriostatic saline.
(9) Substrate solution (X-gal stain): 1 mg/ml X-gal (5-bromo-4-chloro-3-indolyl-β-D-galactoside), 5 mM potassium ferricyanide, 5 mM potassium ferrocyanide, 2 mM $MgCl_2$, 0.01% sodium deoxycholate, 0.02% Nonidet P-40 detergent.
(10) Trypan blue solution (0.4%).
(11) Sterile trypsin–EDTA solution: 0.5 g/l trypsin, 0.2 g/l EDTA.
(12) Versene 1:5000 (0.2 g EDTA·4Na/l in PBS).
(13) Virus buffer: 150 mM NaCl, 20 mM Tris (pH 7.5), sterilized by autoclaving.
(14) Virucide: e.g. LpHse One-step Germicidal Detergent (Calgon Vestal labs, St Louis, MO).
(15) X-gal stain in PBS: 1 mg/ml X-gal, 5 mM potassium ferricyanide, 5 mM potassium ferrocyanide, 2 mM $MgCl_2$.

3 THE PROTOCOLS

Protocol #118: Purification of HSV-1

For growing and titering HSV-1, consult the Protocols in Chapters 14–17. All steps of virus purification should be carried out at 4°C.

(1) Harvest infected cells when cytopathic effect is maximal.
(2) Collect infected cells by centrifugation at 500 g for 7 min at 4°C.
(3) Remove supernatant (which contains released virus) without disturbing infected cell pellet. Save the supernatant.
(4) Centrifuge supernatant again at 970 g for 7 min at 4°C. Save the supernatant for Step 8.
(5) Resuspend the infected cell pellets with a small volume of virus buffer.
(6) Release the intracellular virus by sonicating the infected cells for 30 s in an ultrasonic cup sonicator. Place on ice for 30 s. Repeat this procedure six times (total sonication time: 3 min). Sonication releases virus from cells and cell debris.
(7) Separate virus from cell debris by centrifugation at 1600 r.p.m. for 7 min.
(8) The supernatant that contains free virus from Steps 3 and 4 can be pooled with the released virus and concentrated by centrifugation at 20 000*g* for 2 h at 4°C.
(9) Resuspend the virus pellet in a small volume (usually about one-tenth of the starting volume) of virus buffer.

Protocol #119: Tumor Preparation

For one T150 flask of tumor cells.

(1) Grow tumor cells to confluence.
(2) Remove the medium by aspiration.
(3) Wash cells twice with 10 ml Versene and remove washes by aspiration.
(4) Trypsinize cells by adding 5–6 ml of trypsin–EDTA.
(5) Incubate at room temperature or 37°C until cells come off the surface.
(6) Add 8 ml DMEM/10% IFCS to inactivate the trypsin.
(7) Move cells up and down in pipette to disperse and transfer to 15 ml polypropylene tube. Centrifuge at 500*g* for 7 min.
(8) Remove supernatant by aspiration.
(9) Resuspend cell pellet in 10 ml DMEM/10% IFCS; pipette up and down to resuspend thoroughly.

(10) Count the number of viable cells: remove 20 μl of cells (well resuspended), add 20 μl trypan blue and count immediately. Using hemocytometer (this must be thoroughly cleaned before use), count five different quadrants. Viable cells stay round and refractile, dead cells take up dye, becoming large and blue. To obtain the number of viable cells per ml, multiply the number counted by 2 (cells are diluted by half with trypan blue), divide by 5 (five quadrants counted), multiply by 10^4 (conversion of 0.1 mm^3 counting volume to ml), and multiply by 10 to obtain the total number cells in the 10 ml suspension.
(11) Cells prepared in this way are suitable for the subcutaneous or intracranial tumor models (see below). For the subcutaneous model, cells should be at 5×10^6 cells/10μl. For the intracranial model, cells should be at 2×10^5 cells/2μl.

Protocol #120: Subcutaneous Tumor Model

Implantation of Tumor

(1) Using cells prepared in Protocol #119, inject 5×10^6 cells/10μl subcutaneously into an anesthetized mouse. Allow several weeks for tumor to grow.
(2) Kill the animal by injecting 0.5 ml 0.25% sodium pentobarbital solution intraperitoneally. Allow 5 min for the anesthesia to take effect.
(3) Remove the tumor by making an incision and circumferentially freeing tumor from the subcutaneous tissue.
(4) Be sure to discard the instruments used above and continue with fresh instruments. Split fragments of tumor into pieces of 2 mm using disposable scalpel.
(5) Inject 0.25 ml of 0.25% sodium pentobarbital solution intraperitoneally into a mouse for tumor implantation. Allow 5 min for the anesthesia to take effect then swab skin with alcohol.
(6) Make a 1.0 cm incision at flank (above hind leg).
(7) Open a subcutaneous pocket with a hemostat.
(8) Place the tumor fragment into the space, keeping away from the incision site.
(9) Place auto clip at incision site to close wound.
(10) Wrap mouse with cotton 4″ × 3″ sheet to keep warm and allow the animal to come out of the anesthesia. If animal stays cold, cover it with your own hands—the cold could kill the animal. Alternatively, place a lamp above the cage for warmth. Monitor the animal closely at this stage.
(11) Allow a few weeks for the implanted tumor to grow until it reaches 5 mm diameter.

Experimental Treatment of Tumor with Virus

(1) Inject 0.25 ml of 0.25% sodium pentobarbital solution intraperitoneally into a tumor-bearing mouse. Allow 5 min for the anesthesia to become effective.
(2) Slowly inject the desired HSV-1 mutant into the subcutaneous tumor using a microsyringe. Typically, our experiments use 5×10^6 p.f.u./40 μl.
(3) Wrap mouse with cotton sheet to keep warm and allow the animal to come out of the anesthesia as in Step 10 above.
(4) Measure the tumor volume at regular intervals with external callipers (see Fig. 22.2). Plot tumor growth directly as an increase in volume or as a growth ratio (length (l) × width (w) × height (h)/l × w × h (day 0)).

Protocol #121: Subrenal Capsule Tumor Model

(1) Take a fragment of the tumor obtained in Protocol #120, Steps 1–3 and dissect into pieces of appropriate size (usually about 1 mm) using a disposable scalpel.
(2) Inject 0.25 ml of 0.25% sodium pentobarbital solution intraperitoneally into mouse. Allow 5 min for the anesthesia to take effect.
(3) Swab peritoneum with alcohol.
(4) Make a 1.5 cm retroperitoneal skin incision and expose the peritoneum, incise the peritoneum and expose the kidney (Fig. 22.3a).

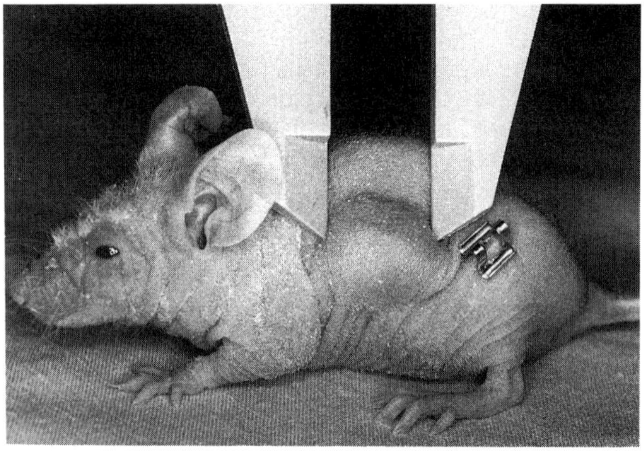

Figure 22.2 A subcutaneous tumor in a nude mouse. The calliper used to measure tumor size is illustrated. Note the surgical clip distant from the subcutaneous tumor

(5) View the surgical field through a stereomicroscope (with an ocular micrometer accurate to 0.1 mm and × 60 amplification), lift the kidney capsule with microforceps and place outside the body.
(6) Cut the renal membrane using a crushed flat aluminum needle (19 gauge), and place a tumor fragment into the subrenal space. Advance the tumor so that it is at least 5 mm from the cut membrane. Apply cotton swab to the cut renal membrane to stop bleeding (Fig. 22.3b).
(7) Place two auto clips at the incision site to close both peritoneum and skin.
(8) Wrap mouse with cotton sheet to keep warm and allow to come out of the anesthesia.
(9) Ten days later open the wound and expose the kidney using the same method as above to examine tumor growth. Measure the tumor size with an ocular micrometer within the stereomicroscope. Inject the tumor with 1 μl of virus (10^5 or 10^6 p.f.u.) or control media (or mock extract) (Fig. 22.3c).
(10) Repeat this measurement technique two further times to observe tumor growth and produce a growth curve. Also observe and chart the neovascularization of the tumor by visualization (Lee et al., 1990).

Protocol #122: Intracranial Tumor Model

(1) Prepare a tumor cell suspension at 2 × 10^5 cells/2μl (Protocol #119).
(2) Inject 0.25 ml of 0.25% sodium pentobarbital solution intraperitoneally into a mouse. Allow 5 min for the anesthesia to take effect.
(3) Set up stereotactic frame, placing sterile towels in the area.
(4) Place anesthetized animal in the stereotactic frame, making sure that all joints of the frame are placed at zero (you will reinject the animal with virus at exactly the same site at a later date).
(5) Clean the head with ethanol.
(6) Allow to air dry.
(7) Make a midline incision in the skin about 4 mm in size, using cotton swabs for assistance.
(8) Identify the coronal and sagittal sutures.
(9) With the hand drill, place a small burr hole 2 mm off midline and 1 mm in front of the coronal suture.
(10) Load 2 μl tumor cells into a Hamilton syringe.
(11) Place needle into the stereotactic frame and align the tip just above the brain surface.
(12) Slowly introduce the tip of the syringe through the neocortex, 3 mm in the ventral direction.

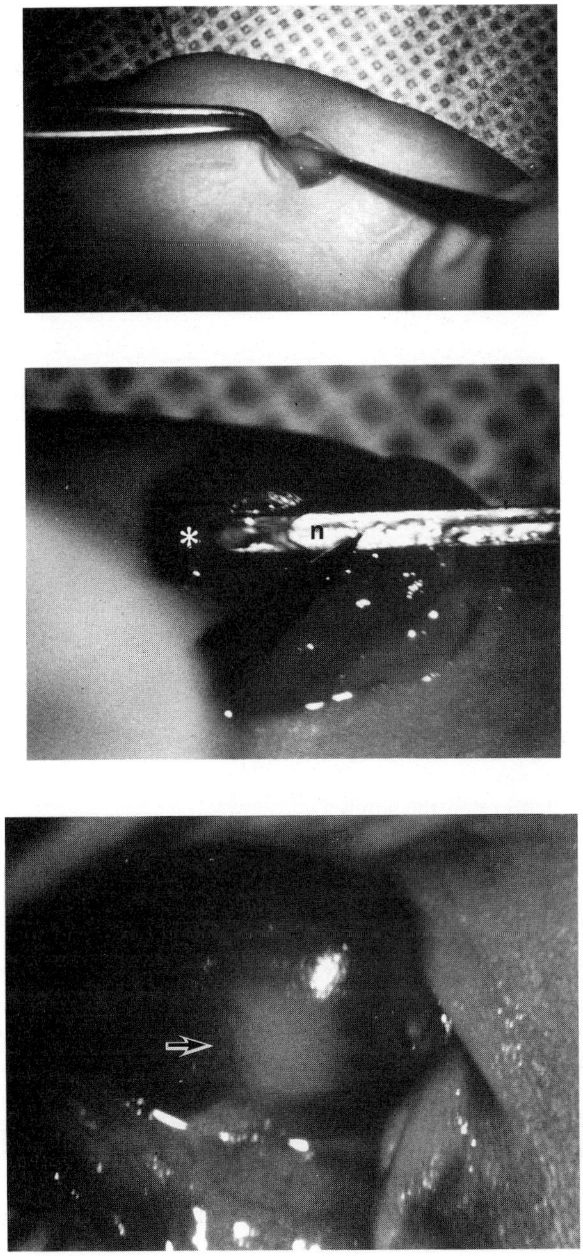

Figure 22.3 Subrenal capsule model. (a) A 1.5 cm retroperitoneal skin incision is made and the peritoneum is incised, exposing the kidney. (b) A flattened 19 gauge needle (n) is inserted under the translucent renal membrane. The needle is advanced at least 5 mm from the incised membrane (*) and the tumor fragment placed into the subrenal space. (c) Ten days after placement of tumor fragment, the kidney is again exposed. Tumor size and vascularity can be measured and/or virus (or mock) can be inoculated into the tumor. The arrow points to the region representing the growing tumor

(13) Retract the needle 1 mm so that the needle depth is only 2 mm.
(14) Inject the tumor cells very slowly, avoiding any fluid leakage.
(15) Wait 1 min, then place a small clip at the site of incision and close the wound.
(16) Wrap mouse with cotton and keep it warm until it comes out of the anesthesia.
(17) Allow the tumor to grow for 10 days.
(18) Anesthetize the animal and place in the stereotaxic frame.
(19) Reopen the wound and expose the brain surface.
(20) Inoculate the tumor location with 10^5–10^6 p.f.u./2 μl of virus or media (mock extract) using the technique used for tumor injection (Steps 10–14).
(21) Closely monitor the animal's condition and survival. To evaluate the brain using histochemical techniques the animal should be killed and cardiac perfusion performed as in Protocol #123.

Protocol #123: Intracardiac Perfusion

(1) Inject 0.25 ml of 0.25% sodium pentobarbital solution intraperitoneally into a mouse. Allow 5 min for the anesthesia to take effect.
(2) Spray ethanol on animal's abdomen.
(3) Make a skin incision, and then incise the peritoneum to expose the intestines.
(4) Expose the diaphragm and open it to produce bilateral pneumothoraces.
(5) Cut through ribs with scissors; stay off midline, avoiding the internal thoracic artery.
(6) Expose the heart and place a butterfly needle into the left ventricle.
(7) Incise the right atrium and allow to bleed.
(8) Infuse 20 ml PBS over 10 min.
(9) Infuse 20 ml fixative solution over 10 min.
(10) After all of the fixative has been infused, turn the animal over and incise the skin over the skull midline (about 1 cm).
(11) Use the Rongeur to open the sinuses.
(12) Expose the olfactory bulbs bilaterally.
(13) Expose the frontal lobes.
(14) Remove the temporal bone to allow adequate exposure of the brain.
(15) Visualize the region of the brain that was implanted with tumor cells and injected.
(16) Remove the whole brain and place into fixative solution for 1 h.
(17) Place into PBS at 4°C overnight. Note: if the brain is to be sectioned, it should be cryoprotected in cold PBS (4°C) containing 30% sucrose rather than PBS. Cryoprotection is complete when the brain sinks to the bottom of the sucrose solution. Histochemical or immunocytochemical procedures may now be undertaken.

Protocol #124: Staining with X-Gal

(1) After transcardiac perfusion remove brain into cold PBS and cut in half coronally (try not to cut into the frontal cortex with tumor).
(2) Replace the PBS with X-Gal substrate solution overnight at room temperature.
(3) Remove substrate solution and wash tissue with PBS.
(4) Place tissue in cold PBS containing 30% sucrose and 2mM $MgCl_2$ until the brain sinks.
(5) Remove the brain from the sucrose and freeze on dry ice.
(6) Section brains on cryostat or freezing microtome at 20–40 μm.
(7) Stain sections at this stage again with X-gal if staining was incomplete.
(8) Mount sections onto gelatin-coated glass slides and counterstain with carmalin or neutral red solution (Bolam, 1992).
(9) Dehydrate sections with increasing concentrations of ethanol (e.g. 80, 90, 95, 100%), treat with xylene for 5 min, then cover with coverslip and examine.

4 NOTES AND TROUBLESHOOTING

4.1 Sterile Technique and Safety

Always use sterile technique—develop this habit early, so that contamination does not become part of your results.

Some of the chemical solutions are potentially harmful so perform manipulations after careful planning and take precautions to avoid contact. Take special care when working with herpes simplex viruses. Avoid producing aerosols and avoid exposure of skin, cuts or abrasions and eyes to virus. It is appropriate to wear two pairs of gloves when handling virus. Use a BSL2 biological containment hood when working with virus solutions. Decontaminate all waste and exposed materials with diluted bleach or virucide. Protect yourself and your surgical area.

4.2 On Protocol #118: Purification of HSV-1

4.2.1 Growing Virus and Cells

Develop the habit of counting cells and determine viability, a decrease in viability is a sign that cell cultures are old or contaminated. Some viral strains yield higher titers after growth at 34°C. Repeated passage of stocks at high MOI will increase amounts of defective interfering particles and selects for reversion of slower growing mutants. When handling the virus keep solutions on ice: virus titer drops after prolonged exposure to room temperature, even in medium. Aliquot the virus in clearly labeled cryotubes containing 1 ml, 0.5 ml, 0.25 ml, 0.1 ml of virus, etc. Use the aliquot with the amount of virus needed for the experiments. The virus is sensitive to freezing and thawing so do not refreeze thawed virus repeatedly because this may decrease virus titer.

Always titer the virus used for intratumoral injection after completing an animal experiment to verify the viability and concentration of inoculum.

4.2.2 Virus Purification

This procedure should take approximately 3 h.

Once the primary stock solution has been titrated it is important to purify the virus and concentrate it for *in vivo* injections. Crude viral stock contains cellular debris that can be toxic to cells. Remove debris by low-speed centrifugation (2500*g*) for 7 min then proceed with virus purification. An important control is the virus-free mock extract. Prepare this from mock-infected cells using the same procedures used to make the virus.

4.3 On Protocol #119: Tumor Preparation

Once a virus has been constructed and shown to be effective against tumor cells *in vitro* it is appropriate to use animal tumor models. The different animal models have their advantages and disadvantages.

The subcutaneous tumor model is probably the simplest to use. Injection of tumor cells into a subcutaneous space should lead to proliferation and formation of a solid tumor. Tumor fragments can also be implanted subcutaneously. Subcutaneous tumors are easy to measure for growth and evaluation of tumor therapy. The subrenal cavity model often allows tumor growth for primary tumor fragments obtained from the operating room. This model enables the investigator to evaluate the tumor by measuring the tumor size *in situ* and the vascularity of the tumor. The most representative model for brain tumor therapy is intracranial implantation of malignant tumor cells into the cerebral cortex. The choice of animal species depends on the tumor cell line. For human tumors nude mice (or nude rats) are required. The use of an immunocompetent host requires a syngeneic tumor cell line (i.e. GL261 in a C57/B6 mouse). In constructing experiments with animal models it is critical to take into account the variability of tumor cell growth *in vivo*. Animals can die from complications due to anesthesia, surgery and complications arising after surgery. Each animal used should be clearly identified (e.g. ear tag) and accurate records kept—it is easy to confuse animals from different or even the same group. Tumor growth should be measured blind, without knowing the treatment regime.

4.3.1 Preparation of Tumor Cells for Implantation

This procedure should take approximately 1 h.

Primary cultured cells or a tumor fragment (from the operating room) may be difficult to initiate as subcutaneous tumors in animals. We use established tumor cell lines or passaged tumor fragments to obtain a subcutaneous tumor fragment.

It is important to obtain accurate cell counts so that equivalent numbers of cells are implanted in different experiments. The cells should be resuspended well, so that animals receive the same number of cells.

For mice an intracranial injection requires about 2×10^5 cells in a volume of 2 μl and a subcutaneous injection requires about 5×10^6 cells in 10 μl.

4.4 On Protocol #120: Subcutaneous Model

This protocol should take approximately 10 min per animal.

This model is particularly useful in evaluating tumor growth and is a straightforward procedure. It is easy to measure the tumor size of each animal (without anesthetic; see Fig. 22.2). The subcutaneous tumor is easily accessible for injection of the therapeutic herpes virus mutant under study. Each animal must be clearly identified and recorded.

It is important to make a big subcutaneous pocket before placing the tumor inside the animal. Wrapping the animal in cotton sheet will keep the animal warm and decrease complications due to anesthesia.

The size of the tumor must not be allowed to become a burden for the animal (it should not interfere with daily activities such as eating, drinking, or moving).

After implantation, tumor fragments may shrink for about one week before beginning to grow. Different tumors grow at different rates; these must be determined empirically. Treatment with virus injections can begin once the tumor has reached 5 mm in diameter.

Make sure the inoculum does not leak out of the tumor during injection. Depending upon the density and size of the tumor, even 40 μl may be too great a volume. We routinely inject into a number of sites in one tumor.

The mock infection is a useful control in which a group of animals receives virus-free medium prepared from mock-infected cells following the procedure used to prepare virus stock. Tumor-bearing animals should be randomly divided into treatment and control groups before injections.

4.5 On Protocol #121: Subrenal Capsule Model

This procedure should take approximately 15 min per animal.

The ocular microscope is invaluable when implanting into the subrenal cavity because the renal membrane is very thin and requires careful handling while implanting. It is important to prevent hemorrhage when cutting the renal membrane as this will invariably result in adhesions around the kidney that will make it difficult to re-expose and re-explore the implanted tumor several weeks later.

The subrenal space is excellent for initiating tumor growth. If attempting to implant a tumor directly from the operating room, the tumor must be placed into DMEM in the operating room and then implanted immediately into the subrenal space (see Fig. 22.3). Tumor material should be 1 mm in size. Begin implantation at Step 1 of Protocol #120.

4.6 On Protocol #122: Intracranial Model

This procedure should take approximately 30 min per animal.

This is the most representative procedure for the exploration of novel therapies for brain tumors. However, because it is not possible to re-explore the tumor on a living animal, you have the choice of evaluating the life expectancy of a single animal or of evaluating the tumor at a single time point.

The stereotactic frame is essential because the virus inoculum must be placed precisely where the tumor was placed. Once an animal is anesthetized, it must be positioned in the stereotactic frame properly, keeping all the joints of the frame on zero and checking the alignments carefully.

Once the skin incision has been made, locate the sagittal and coronal coordinates with precision. Do not rush this procedure: veins are located in the same region and you could make a serious mistake. **Slowly** inject 2 μl cells or virus. If you see solution leakage **stop**. It does the experiment no good if the cells or virus are leaking outside of the brain. Leakage indicates that either the injection was too fast or the track is not big enough. Either way, slow down the rate of injection (we routinely allow 5 min for each injection). You also may try inserting the needle to a depth of 4 mm into the brain and then moving back to 3 mm, making a larger track for the inoculum.

4.7 On Protocol #123: Intracardiac Perfusion

This procedure should take approximately 35 min per animal.

Intracardiac perfusion is required to wash blood from the brain vasculature and to fix the brain adequately for staining. If the brain is not fixed using this method it will be too soft for useful sectioning and staining and blood in the vasculature will compromise histological analyses.

It is important to make fresh fixative each time. As this solution can cause serious damage to skin and eyes, take appropriate precautions including the use of gloves and masks.

Stay off the midline when using the scissors to cut through the ribs because major vessels (e.g. the internal thoracic artery) are present along the midline. Once you have produced bilateral pneumothoraces, expose the heart and place a 25-gauge butterfly needle into the left ventricle. After incision of the right atrium, infuse PBS (20 ml) until you observe that the fluid emerging from the right atrium is lighter in color than blood. When the fixative is first infused, you may note two events: (1) the liver may turn pale, indicating that the fixative is infusing through the vasculature; (2) the animal may start to quiver, which is another sign that the fixative has infused properly.

Special care should be taken when starting to remove the brain. The rongeur is large and is good for violating the sinuses, but a small hemostat should be used to remove the skull. Take extra time when removing the brain because this tissue is the most important part of the whole experiment and a mistake may ruin several weeks of work.

ACKNOWLEDGMENTS

This work is supported by grants from the NIH (N532677), NF Inc., and the American Association of Neurological Surgeons.

REFERENCES

Austin, F.C. and Boone, C.W. (1979). Virus augmentation of the antigenicity of tumor cell extracts. *Adv. Cancer Res.* **30:** 301–345.

Bolam, J.P. (ed.) (1992). Preparation of central nervous system tissue for light and electron microscopy. In *Experimental Neuroanatomy: A practical approach*, pp.1–29. Oxford: Oxford University Press.

Boris-Lawrie, K.A. and Temin, H.M. (1993) Recent advances in retrovirus vector technology. *Curr. Opin. Genet. Dev.* **3:** 102–109.

Boviatsis, E.J., Chase, M., Wei, M.X., Tamiya, T., Hurford, R.K., Kowall, N.W., Tepper, R.I., Breakefield, X.O. and Chiocca, E.A. (1994a). Gene transfer into experimental Brain Tumors Mediated by Adenovirus, Herpes Simplex Virus, and Retrovirus. *Hum. Gene Ther.* **5:** 183–191.

Boviatsis, E.J., Scharf, J.M., Chase, M., Harrington, K., Knowall, N.W., Breakefield, X.O. and Chiocca, E.A. (1994b). Antitumor activity and reporter gene transfer into rat brain neoplasms inoculated with herpes simplex virus vectors defective in thymidine kinase or ribonucleotide reductase. *Gene Ther.* **1:** 323–331.

Chen, S.H., Shine, H.D., Goodman, J.C., Grossman, R.G. and Woo, S.L. (1994). Gene therapy for brain tumors: regression of experimental gliomas by adenovirus-mediated gene transfer *in vivo*. *Proc. Natl Acad. Sci. USA* **91(8):** 3054–3057.

Culver, K.W., Ram, Z., Wallbridge, S., Ishii, H., Oldfield, E.H. and Blaese, R.M. (1992). In vivo gene transfer with retroviral vector-producer cells for treatment of experimental brain tumors. *Science* **256:** 1550–1552.

Daumas-Duport, C., Scheithauer, B., O'Fallon, J. and Kelly, P. (1988). Grading of astrocytomas. A simple and reproducible method. *Cancer* **62:** 2152–2165.

Ezzeddine, Z.D., Martuza, R.L., Platika, D., Short, M.P., Malick, A., Choi, B. and Breakefield, X.O. (1991). Selective killing of glioma cells in culture and *in vivo* by retrovirus transfer of the herpes simplex virus thymidine kinase gene. *New Biologist* **3:** 608–614.

Jia, W.W-G., McDermott, M., Goldie, J., Cyander, M., Tan, J. and Tufaro, F. (1994). Selective destruction of gliomas in immunocompetent rats by thymidine kinase-defective Herpes Simplex Virus type I. *J. Natl Cancer Inst.* **86:** 1209–1215.

Kaplitt, M.G., Tjuvajev, J.G., Leib, D.A., Berk, J., Pettigrew, K.D., Posner, J.B., Pfaff, D.W., Rabkin, S.D. and Blasberg, R.G. (1994). Mutant herpes simplex virus induced regression of tumors growing in immunocompetent rats. *J. Neurooncol.* **19:** 137–147.

Kim, T.S., Halliday, A.L., Heldey-Whyte, E.T. and Convery, K. (1991). Correlates of survival and the Daumas-Duport grading system for astrocytomas. *J. Neurosurg.* **74:** 27–37.

Le Gal La Salle, G., Robert, J.J., Berrard, S., Ridoux, V., Stratford-Perricaudet, L.D., Pericaudet, M. and Mallet, J. (1993). An adenovirus vector for gene transfer into neurons and glia in the brain. *Science* **259:** 988–990.

Lee, J.K., Choi, B., Sobel, R.A., Chiocca, E.A. and Martuza, R.L. (1990). Inhibition of growth and angiogenesis of human neurofibrosarcoma by heparin and hydrocortisone. *J. Neurosurg.* **73:** 429–435.

Lobayashi, H. (1979). Viral xenogenization of intact tumor cells. *Adv. Cancer Res.* **30:** 279–299.

Mahaley, M.S., Jr., Mettlin, C., Natarajan, N., Laws, E.R., Jr. and Peace, B.B. (1989). National survey of patterns of care for brain-tumor patients. *J. Neurosurg.* **71:** 826–836.

Markert, J.M., Coen, D.M., Malick, A., Mineta, T. and Martuza, R.L. (1992). Expanded spectrum of viral therapy in the treatment of nervous system tumors. *J. Neurosurg.* **77:** 590–594.

Markert, J.M., Malick, A., Coen, D.M. and Martuza, R.L. (1993). Reduction and elimination of encephalitis in an experimental gliomas therapy model with attenuated herpes simplex mutants that retain susceptibility to acyclovir. *Neurosurgery* **32:** 597–603.

Martuza, R.L., Malick, A., Markert, J.M., Ruffner, K.L. and Coen, D.M. (1991). Experimental therapy of human glioma by means of a genetically engineered virus mutant. *Science* **252:** 854–856.

Mineta, T., Rabkin, S.D. and Martuza, R.L. (1994). Treatment of malignant gliomas using ganciclovir-hypersensitive, ribonucleotide reductase-deficient herpes simplex viral mutant. *Cancer Res.* **54:** 3963–3966.

Moore, A.E. (1960). The oncolytic viruses. *Prog. Exp. Tumor Res.* **1:** 411–439.

Oldfield, E.H., Ram, Z., Culver, K.W., Blaese, R.M., Devroom, H.L. and Anderson, W.F. (1993). Gene therapy for the treatment of brain tumors using intra-tumoral transduction with the thymidine kinase gene and intravenous ganciclovir. *Hum. Gene Ther.* **4:** 39–69.

Onoyama, Y., Abe, M., Yabumoto, E., Sakamoto, T. and Nishidai, T. (1976). Radiation therapy in the treatment of glioblastoma. *Am. J. Roentgenol.* **126:** 481–492.

Ram, Z., Culver, K.W., Walbridge, S., Blease, R. M. and Oldfield, E.H. (1993). In situ retroviral-mediated gene transfer for the treatment of brain tumors in rats. *Cancer Res.* **53:** 83–88.

Sacks, S.L., Wanklin, R.L., Reece, D.E., Hicks, K.A., Tyler, K.L. and Coen, D.M. (1989). Progressive esophagitis from acyclovir-resistant herpes simplex. Clinical roles for DNA polymerase mutants and viral heterogeneity? *Ann. Int. Med.* **111:** 893–899.

Salazar, O.M., Rubin, P., Feldstein, M.L. and Pizzutiello, R. (1979). High dose radiation therapy in the treatment of malignant gliomas: Final report. *Int. J. Radiat. Oncol. Biol. Phys.* **5:** 1733–1749.

Shapiro, W.R., Green, S.B., Burger, P.C., Mahaley, M.S., Jr., Selker, R.G., VanGilder, J.C., Robertson, J.T., Ransohoff, J., Mealey, J., Jr., Strike, T.A. and Pistenmaa, D.A. (1989). Randomized trial of three chemotherapy regimens and two radiotherapy regimens in postoperative treatment of malignant glioma. Brain Tumor Cooperative Group Trial 8001. *J. Neurosurg.* **71:** 1–9.

Short, M.P., Choi, B.C., Lee, J.K., Malick, A., Breakefield, X.O. and Martuza, R.L. (1990). Gene delivery to glioma cells in rat brain by grafting of a retrovirus packaging cell line. *J. Neurosci. Res.* **27:** 427–439.

Takamiya, Y., Short, M.P., Ezzeddine, Z.D., Moolten, F.L., Breakefield, X.O. and Martuza, R.L. (1992). Gene therapy of malignant brain tumors: A rat glioma line bearing the herpes simplex virus type-I thymidine kinase gene and wild type retrovirus kills other tumor cells. *J. Neurosci. Res.* **33:** 493–503.

Walker, M.D., Green, S.B., Byar, D.P., Alexander, E., Jr., Batzdorf, U., Brooks, W.H., Hunt, W.E., MacCarty, C.S., Mahaley, M.S., Mealey, J. Jr., Owens, G., Ransohoff, J., Robertson, J.T., Shapiro, W.R., Smith, K.R., Wilson, C.B. and Strike, T.A. (1980). Randomized comparisons of radiotherapy and nitroureas for the treatment of malignant glioma after surgery. *N. Engl. J. Med.* **303:** 1323–1329.

Yamada, M., Shimizu, K., Miyao, Y., Hayakawa, T., Ikenaka, K., Nakahira, K., Nakajima, K., Kagawa, T. and Mikoshiba, K. (1992). Retrovirus-mediated gene transfer targeted to malignant glioma cells in murine brain. *Jpn. J. Cancer Res.* **83:** 1244–1247.

CHAPTER 23

Osmotic Blood–brain Barrier Disruption Methodologies for Global Delivery of Genetic Vectors to the Brain

EDWARD A. NEUWELT AND LESLIE L. MULDOON*

*Department of Neurology, Division of Neurosurgery and Department of Biochemistry and Molecular Biology, and *Department of Cell and Developmental Biology, Oregon Health Sciences University, 3181 SW Sam Jackson Park Road, Portland OR 97201, USA. Tel: 503 494 5626; Fax: 503 494 5627; Email: neuwelte@ccmail.ohsu.edu; *Email: muldoonl@ohsu.edu*

1 INTRODUCTION

Gene therapy of the central nervous system (CNS) with recombinant viral vectors, whether it be replacement of faulty genes in neurons or transfer of toxic genes to tumor cells, is close to becoming a reality (Fleischman, 1991; Boviatsis et al., 1994; Davidson et al., 1994). A major impediment to both viral gene therapy of neurodegenerative diseases affecting the brain and virus-mediated treatment of brain tumors, however, will be the delivery of virus to the target cells in the CNS. Many diseases of the brain that may potentially be targets of gene therapy, such as Alzheimer's disease or the lysosomal storage disorders, are global disorders affecting either the whole brain or large regions of it (Fleischman, 1991; Neuwelt et al., 1995). Such disorders will require global therapy. Viral therapy of brain tumors will also require a mechanism to obtain delivery of vector to a large portion of the brain, in order to target those neoplastic cells distant from the main tumor mass that are most invasive and divide most rapidly (Markert et al., 1993; Chen et al., 1994). Thus it is important to develop methods to maximize the regional and global delivery of viral vectors to brain.

The most commonly used mechanism to deliver recombinant virus to the brain is focal intracerebral injection. Primary infection by this method is limited by diffusion of virus to 1–3 mm surrounding the injection site, as has been demonstrated by several laboratories using recombinant herpes virus type I (HSV-1) or adenovirus vectors expressing the bacterial *lac*Z gene for β-galactosidase (Breakefield and DeLuca, 1991; Wolfe et al., 1992; Akli et al., 1993; Davidson et al., 1993; Bajocchi et al., 1993). Delivery volumes of up to 1 ml have been obtained by combining intracerebral inoculation with convection-enhanced diffusion (Bobo et al., 1994; Laske et al., 1994; our unpublished observations). Although this is a large volume of distribution in a 1 g rat brain, it is a small volume in the 1100 g human brain. The restricted access of inoculated virus to most of the human brain indicates that this method of delivery is not suitable for treatment of global neurodegenerative diseases or disseminated tumors.

In the normal mammalian brain, passage of viral particles from the systemic circulation to the brain parenchyma is completely blocked by the blood–brain barrier (BBB). The BBB is a capillary barrier that results from a continuous layer of endothelial cells bound together with tight

Protocols for Gene Transfer in Neuroscience: Towards Gene Therapy of Neurological Disorders
Edited by P.R. Lowenstein and L.W. Enquist

junctions, or zonula occludens, that allow very little pericellular transport of blood-borne molecules (Rapoport, 1976; Neuwelt and Kroll, 1994; Brightman, 1989; Rapoport and Robinson, 1986). The BBB excludes molecules from the brain based on electric charge, lipid solubility, and molecular weight, normally excluding molecules of greater than 180 M_r (Brightman, 1989; Smith, 1989). This anatomical feature protects the brain from potentially noxious compounds in the blood, but also markedly reduces the delivery of therapeutic agents. A major area of emphasis of this laboratory has been to circumvent the BBB for delivery of various therapies to brain and brain tumors (Neuwelt et al., 1981a, 1991a,b, 1994a; Doran et al., 1995; Dahlborg et al., 1996).

Delivery of a variety of agents across the BBB can be accomplished by transiently modifying the BBB with a hypertonic solution. Perfusion of the cerebral vasculature with a hypertonic solution appears to cause cerebrovascular endothelial cell shrinkage and subsequent increased permeability of the tight junctions (Rapoport et al., 1980, 1986; Brightman, 1989). We refer to this process as BBB disruption. Although a number of hyperosmotic agents have been used for BBB disruption (See Section 4.3.11, Page 328), our laboratory most often employs hypertonic mannitol (25%), which is the only agent approved for this procedure in humans. Vascular permeability to small molecules such as amino-isobutyric acid, as well as relatively large molecules such as antibodies, is increased maximally at 15 min after infusion of hypertonic agent, after which it decreases rapidly and returns to preinfusion levels within 2 h (Rapoport et al., 1980; Neuwelt et al., 1994b; Barnett et al., 1995).

The BBB disruption technique may provide a mechanism for the global delivery of infectious virions to brain and intracerebral tumors. In an initial experiment we found that BBB disruption produced four times as much radiolabeled UV-inactivated herpesvirus in normal rat brain than in the contralateral non-disrupted hemisphere (Neuwelt et al., 1991b). We also performed a series of studies demonstrating that virus-sized monocrystalline iron oxide nanoparticles (MIONs) could be delivered to rat brain cells when administered with osmotic BBB disruption (Neuwelt et al., 1994a). MIONs provide a tool to follow virus delivery to brain, as they can be imaged non-invasively by magnetic resonance techniques and can be detected in brain sections with a sensitive histochemical stain. The distribution of MIONs in rat brain closely matches that of virus transgene expression, whether delivery is by focal intracerebral inoculation or by BBB disruption (Muldoon et al., 1995). We have demonstrated the delivery of recombinant adenovirus across the BBB in normal rat brain (Doran et al., 1995). Our most recent results have demonstrated delivery of both adenovirus and recombinant HSV-1 across the BBB in intracerebral tumor-bearing animals (unpublished observations).

Our previous preclinical studies of BBB disruption in an animal model of intracerebral metastatic carcinoma focused on delivery of anti-tumor antibodies (Neuwelt et al., 1993, 1994b), MIONs (Neuwelt et al., 1994a) and monoclonal antibody immunoconjugates (Remsen et al., 1995), with the goal of imaging, diagnosis and treatment of intracerebral tumors. BBB disruption to enhance delivery of chemotherapy to brain tumors is also used clinically and results in prolonged survival without cognitive loss (Neuwelt et al., 1991a; Dahlborg et al., 1996). Our current studies are directed towards applying this methodology to the treatment of CNS disease, including treatment of brain tumors in our nude rat intracerebral xenograft model (Neuwelt et al., 1985a, 1994a) and treatment of global neurodegenerative disease in a feline model of GM2 gangliosidosis (Neuwelt et al., 1985b; Muldoon et al., 1994; Kroll et al., 1995). Although clinical application of gene replacement therapy in the CNS will require development of safe and effective viral vectors, applying the BBB disruption technique with currently available viral vectors will allow us to investigate gene transfer therapy to neurons in diseased brain from a global perspective.

2 MATERIALS AND EQUIPMENT

2.1 Reagents

(1) Heparinized saline (10 units/ml heparin in 0.9% NaCl).
(2) Normal saline (0.9% NaCl).

(3) Phosphate-buffered saline (PBS): 0.9% NaCl, 50 mM Na_2HPO_4, 50 mM KH_2PO_4, pH 7.4.
(4) Lactated Ringer's solution.
(5) Mannitol: 25% (1.37 M), sterile filtered through 0.22 μm membrane.
(6) Evans Blue dye: 2% solution in PBS and sterile filtered through 0.22 μm membrane.
(7) Betadine scrub.
(8) Lidocaine: 2% solution without epinephrine (adrenaline).
(9) Isoflurane anesthetic.
(10) Pentobarbital sodium solution.

2.2 Specialized Equipment

(1) Anesthesia vaporizer.
(2) Rodent ventilator.
(3) Operating microscope.
(4) Infusion pump.
(5) Fluoroscope.

2.3 Surgical Instruments

If more than one of an item is needed, the number recommended is indicated in parentheses.

(1) Kelly hemostat, 5.5″, curved.
(2) Thumb forceps.
(3) Metzenbaum scissors, 7″, curved (Aesculap BC603).
(4) Micro-suturing needle holders (Aesculap FD231) (2).
(5) Biemer vessel clips (Aesculap FD562) (2).
(6) Clip applier, Biemer (Aesculap FD568).
(7) Micro suture tying forceps (Aesculap FD281) (2).
(8) Micro dissecting scissors.
(9) Needle retractors: Hooked needles, with suture attached, used as tissue retractors (3 or 4).
(10) Scalpel blades, #15.
(11) Battery-operated cauterization tool.

2.4 Miscellaneous Supplies

(1) Induction chamber.
(2) Heating pad, wrapped with a towel.
(3) Umbilical tape (1/8″ wide).
(4) Cellophane tape.
(5) 4-0 silk thread.
(6) PE-240 tubing, approximately 3 cm.
(7) Intravenous catheter, 14 gauge (2.25″, non-radio-opaque Teflon), needle stylet removed.
(8) Cotton-tipped applicator.
(9) Three-way stopcock (3).
(10) Luer stub adapter (23 gauge).
(11) Syringes, monoject luer tip, 1,3,6,12 and 20 ml.
(12) Needles, 22 and 27 gauge.
(13) Polyethylene (PE-50) arterial pressure tubing: 25 cm, 0.28 cm outer diameter, 0.17 cm inner diameter.
(14) Additional supplies for BBB disruption in dogs include catheters, extension set, 60 ml and 140 ml syringes.
(15) Sterile 0.22 μm filters.

3 THE PROTOCOLS

Protocol #125: BBB Disruption in Rats—Anesthesia and Ventilation

(1) Induce anesthesia using 5% isoflurane in room air, in a small purpose-built chamber.
(2) After anesthesia induction lay the animal on its back on a slant board and expose the larynx, using a speculum to depress the tongue.
(3) Apply lidocaine (lignocaine) to the larynx with a cotton-tipped applicator.
(4) Rapidly insert an endotracheal tube, with a paper clip as stylet, under external illumination.
(5) Ventilate the rat with 2–2.5% isoflurane in oxygen, to maintain a surgical plane of anesthesia.

Protocol #126: BBB Disruption in Rats—Preparation of the Animal

(1) Place the rat on its back on a heating pad wrapped in a towel.
(2) Secure the front and hind limbs toward the corners of the heating pad.
(3) Make sure the animal is immobilized in the correct position and a hind limb is available for injection of Evans Blue dye.
(4) Use umbilical tape for the restraining ties, and secure these to the work surface with cellophane tape.
(5) Secure the head by placing umbilical tape around the upper incisors and taping to the work surface.
(6) Shave the surgical sites and prepare them aseptically with Betadine scrub.

Protocol #127: BBB Disruption in Rats—Exposure of the Carotid Artery

(1) Make a skin incision about 4 cm in length directly along the ventral midline, starting from between the angles of the mandible at the point of the chin, and extending down to the top of the sternum (Fig. 23.1).
(2) Retract the skin laterally using two needle retractors. The incision will expose the muscles over the trachea (along the midline).
(3) Pull these muscles to the left with one needle retractor, and pull the large salivary gland to the right with the second needle retractor (Fig. 23.2).
(4) Use blunt dissection to expose the carotid artery at the level of the bifurcation (internal and external branches).
(5) Free the external carotid artery from connective tissue, starting at the bifurcation and extending up 4–5 mm. The occipital and superior thyroid arteries, which branch from the external carotid artery, must be ligated or cauterized before infusion. It is not necessary to occlude the pterygopalatine branch of the internal carotid artery.

Protocol #128: BBB Disruption in Rats—Catheterization of the Carotid Artery

(1) Use a dissecting or operating microscope to place the carotid catheter.
(2) Tie off the external carotid artery as far up from the bifurcation as possible, using a 15–20 cm piece of 4-0 silk thread. Apply traction to the artery by placing the suture into Kelly forceps and gently retract the suture towards the nose.
(3) Place a fine Biemer clip on the external carotid, just up from the bifurcation to seal off a section of the carotid artery approximately 1 cm in length, and to provide maximum exposure of the external carotid for cannula insertion.
(4) Apply another length of 4-0 silk around the artery, just rostral to the Biemer clip, and loosely tie a half of a square knot, to secure the catheter later (see Step 10).
(5) Prepare the cannula (approximately 25 cm of PE-50 tubing) by cutting a bevel at one end and connecting the other end of the tubing to a 23 gauge luer stub adapter attached to a three-way stopcock.
(6) Attach the stopcock to a 3 ml syringe containing warmed (37°C) heparinized saline, and fill the tubing.
(7) Make a small nick incision (arteriotomy) in the external carotid, approximately 4 mm up

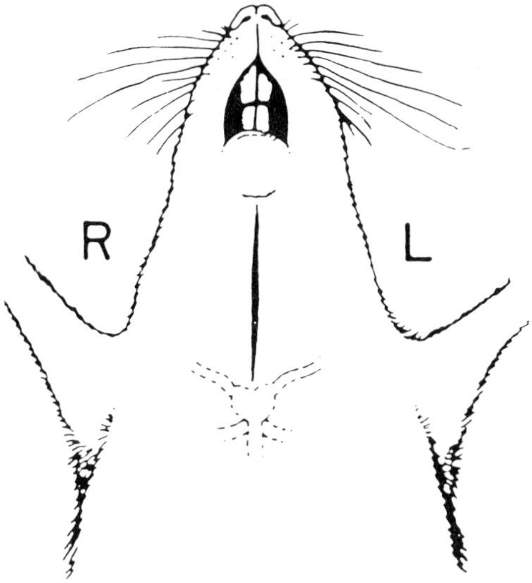

Figure 23.1 Site of incision in a rodent BBB disruption procedure. The anesthetized rat is secured to the heating pad. A 4-cm skin incision is made along the midline from between the angles of the mandible to the manubrium sternum

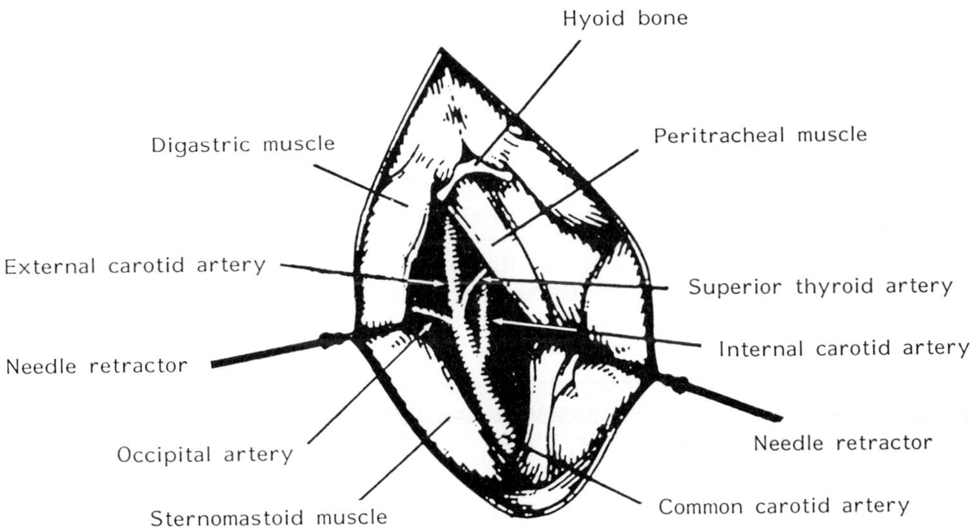

Figure 23.2 Exposure of the right carotid artery. The artery is revealed by blunt dissection of the overlying muscles and tissues. The common carotid artery bifurcates into the external and internal carotid arteries. The occipital and superior thyroid arteries, which branch from the external carotid artery, must be ligated or cauterized before infusion

from the bifurcation using micro dissecting scissors.

(8) Apply a few drops of lidocaine (lignocaine) (2%) to the arteriotomy site to cause vasodilatation and facilitate introduction of the catheter.

(9) Insert the catheter towards the bifurcation through the arteriotomy site, taking care that the beveled tip does not perforate the opposite side of the artery.

(10) Advance the catheter towards the Biemer clip and gently but firmly secure in place with the ligature of 4-0 silk thread (Step 4).

(11) Carefully remove the Biemer clip.
(12) Draw a small amount of blood into the syringe to clear the cannula of any air bubbles and then flush through the heparinized saline.
(13) Make sure the beveled tip of the catheter is located approximately 1 mm away from the bifurcation of the internal and external carotid arteries, as illustrated in Fig. 23.3.
(14) Following catheterization, inject the rat with Evans Blue through the femoral vein (SEE SECTION 4.1.2).

Protocol #129: BBB Disruption in Rats—Administration of Mannitol and Virus

(1) Induce osmotic BBB disruption by retrograde infusion of warm (37°C) sterile, filtered 25% mannitol (or another agent such as arabinose). In control animals (sham disrupted) infuse normal saline in place of the hyperosmotic agent.
(2) Place the syringe filled with mannitol into the Harvard infusion pump.
(3) Connect the syringe to the 3-way stopcock attached to the PE-50 cannula via the arterial pressure tubing.
(4) Infuse the osmotic agent at a constant rate of 0.09–0.12 ml/s for 30 s, depending on anesthetic agent and hemodynamic variables.
(5) Ventilate animals mechanically during the infusion.
(6) Keep the wound area irrigated with saline throughout the disruption and subsequent virus infusion.
(7) Administer the viral vector slowly through the same carotid catheter immediately after osmotic disruption: infuse 2 ml of HSV-1 vectors (5×10^8–5×10^9 p.f.u./ml) or adenovirus or adenovirus (5–50 $\times 10^{10}$ particles/ml of adenovirus, corresponding to 0.5–25 $\times 10^9$ p.f.u./ml, depending on the percentage of viral particles that are infectious) over a 20 min period (0.1 ml/min).

Protocol #130: BBB Disruption in Rats—Completion of Procedure

(1) Complete the procedure by reapplying the Biemer clip and withdrawing the cannula.
(2) Tie off the external carotid artery caudal to the arteriotomy site using the 4-0 silk suture already in place. Close the wound in a single layer by apposing the skin edges with skin staples or sutures.
(3) Administer 5–7 ml warm (37°C) lactated Ringer's solution by intraperitoneal inoculation.
(4) Allow the animal to recover in an incubator or other warmed environment.
(5) Maintain rats that received virus in a BL-2 containment facility and observe daily for any signs of neurotoxicity, such as seizures.

Protocol #131. BBB Disruption in Dogs—Preparation of the Animal

(1) Anesthetize adult, mongrel male dogs weighing 20–25 kg with diazepam (15 mg, intramuscular) and 20 mg/kg intravenous (i.v.) sodium pentothal.
(2) Intubate the dog with an endotracheal tube and ventilate with an animal respirator.
(3) Maintain anesthesia with supplemental i.v. pentothal (50 mg increments) as needed.
(4) Ventilate with 60% O_2, 40% N_2O.
(5) Monitor blood gases and maintain at a $p\text{CO}_2$ of 25–35 mmHg and a $p\text{O}_2$ of 80 mmHg.
(6) Maintain fluid balance with i.v. lactated Ringer's solution.
(7) Monitor urinary output by collecting urine with a catheter connected to an i.v. drip set and empty fluid bag placed below the dog.
(8) Keep fluid input up with urine output.

Protocol #132: BBB Disruption in Dogs—Catheterization of the Carotid Artery

(1) Shave the left side of the neck and prepare for surgery.
(2) Make a 10–12 cm incision using aseptic technique, starting at the ramus of the mandible and directed caudally to a point lateral to the end of the trachea.

(3) Expose the jugular vein and parotid and mandibular salivary glands by blunt dissection and retract.
(4) Isolate the left internal carotid artery infundibulum by gentle blunt dissection and expose the bifurcation of the carotid artery.
(5) Insert a 16 gauge catheter into the vessel approximately 3–4 mm in a rostral direction.
(6) Secure the catheter in the vessel using a rummel clamp and flush with heparinized saline.
(7) Give frusemide (0.5 mg/kg i.v.) to diurese the animal to compensate for the 1.5% increase in brain water anticipated from the mannitol infusion.
(8) Inject Evans Blue dye (2% dye, 3 ml/kg i.v.).

Protocol #133: BBB Disruption in Dogs—Administration of Mannitol and Virus

(1) Infuse warm, filtered 25% mannitol into the carotid catheter for a period of 30 s at a rate of 1.5 ml/s.
(2) Ventilate the dog mechanically during infusion.
(3) Infuse the viral vector immediately after mannitol, through the same catheter.

Protocol #134: BBB Disruption in Dogs—Completion of Procedure

(1) Remove the catheter and apply bulldog vascular clamps to the common and external carotid arteries to prevent hemorrhage.
(2) Repair the internal carotid artery with 6-0 Prolene (Ethicon Inc, Somersville, NJ).
(3) Close the incision in three layers—deep tissue, subcutaneous tissue, and skin.
(4) Allow the dog to wake up and constantly monitor during recovery.
(5) Administer supplemental diazepam (5–10 mg) i.v. or by intramuscular injection as needed to ease the recovery period.

4 NOTES AND TROUBLESHOOTING

4.1 General Comments

4.1.1 Materials and Equipment

Although osmotic BBB disruption has been reported for several animal models, including dogs (Neuwelt et al., 1985a), rabbits (Strasbaugh and Brinker, 1983) and primates (Rapoport, 1976; Neuwelt and Kroll, 1994), experimental procedures such as virus delivery to the CNS are performed predominantly in rodents. Therefore the protocols given in this chapter are devoted primarily to the materials and equipment required for rodent BBB disruptions. Specialized articles or reagents necessary for disruption in dogs or cats are indicated.

4.1.2 Reagents and Solutions

The following solutions will be needed at different stages: heparinized saline (to maintain catheter patency); sterile normal saline (for wound irrigation and sham disruptions); sterile PBS (for virus dilution); lactated Ringer's solution (administered after the procedure to rodents, and during the procedure to dogs and cats, to minimize dehydration due to the diuretic effects of mannitol); Evans Blue dye (marker of BBB disruption). All these solutions are sterilized by filtration through a 0.22 μm filter before use. Betadine scrub is used to aseptically prepare the surgical sites, lidocaine (lignocaine) is applied locally as an arterial dilator, isoflurane is used as the anesthesia in chronic studies in rodents and pentobarbital sodium solution is used for anesthesia in all BBB disruption studies in dogs and cats. It is also used as anesthesia for acute studies in rodents.

4.1.3 Specialized Equipment

An anesthesia vaporizer is used with isoflurane anesthesia, which is delivered through a mechanical ventilator. This is used together with a small animal volume-controlled ventilator to maintain anesthesia in rodents during the BBB disruptions, and should be specifically dedicated for virus work. The small animal ventilator can also be used for BBB disruption of dogs and cats. A Harvard Instruments infusion/withdrawal pump is useful to regulate the rate at which hypertonic mannitol and virus preparations are infused. For experiments involving the disruption of the vertebral artery in dogs and cats fluoroscopic guidance for correct placement of the catheter is required. We utilize hospital equipment and personnel for these procedures.

4.1.4 Miscellaneous Supplies

For rapidly anesthetizing rodents we converted a small plastic freezer box with a tightly fitting lid into an induction chamber by inserting two luer locks through one of the plastic sides. This allows for easily managed constant ventilation of a single rat. Polyethylene PE-240 tubing is used as a tracheostomy tube in acute studies during which anesthesia is maintained with pentobarbital sodium. It is inserted so as to control airway patency and provide ventilatory assistance. The endotracheal tube used in studies utilizing inhalation anesthetic consists of a 14-gauge intravenous catheter with needle stylet removed, which allows maintenance of the animal on a ventilator with 2% isoflurane.

4.2 Problems that May be Encountered

We recommend that several animals are used for short-term experiments to practice the procedure.

4.3 On Protocols #125–129: BBB Modification in the Rat

The technique requires catheter placement in the right external carotid artery for infusion of hyperosmotic agent into the internal carotid artery. This catheter is also used for administration of the virus. Our studies are usually performed on normal adult female rats, Long/Evans (obtained from Simonsen), Sprague Dawley (obtained from B & K Industries), or nude rats (available through the National Cancer Institute), weighing 220–250 g. The protocols are easily adapted for larger rats.

4.3.1 Anesthesia and Ventilation

For chronic studies the rat is anesthetized with and maintained on isoflurane. This allows rapid recovery from anesthesia as well as consistent successful disruptions. The intubation must be performed rapidly, as the animal will begin to recover from the anesthesia within 1 min.

4.3.2 Animal Dies during Anesthesia

If an animal dies, reduce the percentage of isoflurane anesthetic for other animals, so that cardiovascular parameters are not depressed. Check that the animal is intubated in the trachea, not the esophagus, by gently blowing into the tube and observing that the chest walls expand.

4.3.3 Difficulty in Finding the Carotid Artery

The carotid artery is located deep in the neck, midway between the trachea and the salivary gland, but is easy to recognize due to its pulse. Bluntly dissect more tissue until the relatively large vessel with the pulse is found. The jugular vein is also relatively large, but it is located under the salivary gland and does not pulse.

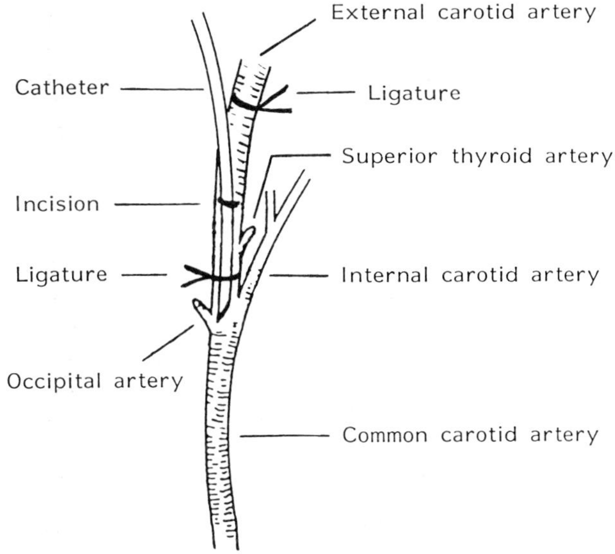

Figure 23.3 Correct placement of the catheter in the carotid artery of the rodent. The cannula is inserted into the external carotid artery such that the tip is within 1 mm of the bifurcation. Correct placement is essential for adequate infusion of mannitol into the internal carotid artery

4.3.4 Carotid Artery is Perforated

If the integrity of the carotid artery wall is in question it is probably not worthwhile going through the procedure. This could happen in a number of ways during the set up for catheterization; for example, during cauterization of the collateral arteries or insertion of the cannula.

4.3.5 Catheterization of the Carotid Artery

If the cannula is correctly placed blood from the common carotid artery and saline from the catheter should both flow through the internal carotid artery. Correct placement is essential for effective BBB disruption. The catheter may be gently advanced, if necessary, to achieve the position indicated in Fig. 23.3. It is important to remember that this is a one-time procedure in the rat because the external carotid is sacrificed.

4.3.6 Administration of Mannitol

Because the animals become apneic during administration of the osmotic agent, they **must** be mechanically ventilated during the infusion.

4.3.7 Administration of Virus

Dilution of virus in PBS appears to reduce toxicity compared to administration of the same amount as a concentrated aliquot. Herpesvirus stocks are titered on Vero African green monkey kidney cells (Wolfe et al., 1992; Boviatsis et al., 1994). The virus stocks can be stored indefinitely at −70°C, and we have found no apparent reduction in activity of thawed virus. We have found that adenovirus preparations are best used fresh, in contrast to HSV-1. Purified concentrated adenovirus in cesium chloride can be desalted by flowing through a G25 Sephadex column followed by detection of viral particles with spectroscopy at 260 nm.

4.3.8 Cannula Slips out During Infusion

If this happens, **stop**: it is not worth your while trying to reinsert the cannula. To avoid the problem, make sure that the cannula is firmly held in place by the silk ligature, yet not so firmly as to cut through the arterial wall.

4.3.9 Animal does not Recover from Procedure

If the animal does not begin breathing on its own (without ventilator assistance) within 30–60 min of finishing the procedure it will probably not recover. This is most likely to occur if the animal has been over-disrupted, but may also represent toxicity of the virus or a reaction to anesthesia.

4.3.10 Factors Influencing BBB Disruption

BBB disruption is a threshold event dependent on a number of factors including the osmolality, duration, rate and volume of infusate; the type of anesthetic used; and the cardiac output and $Pa\mathrm{CO_2}$ of the subject animal (Gumerlock and Neuwelt, 1990; Neuwelt and Kroll, 1994). Steroids decrease vascular permeability and also decrease the degree of disruption that can be obtained with hyperosmotic mannitol, both in tumor and normal brain (Neuwelt et al., 1993). A number of alterations to the basic BBB disruption procedure can be attempted that may increase the efficacy of the procedure in smaller or larger animal models.

4.3.11 Alternate Osmotic Agents

Hypertonic solutions that have been used to osmotically disrupt the BBB include mannitol, arabinose, sucrose, urea, dimethyl sulfoxide and several radiographic contrast agents (Studer et al., 1974; Rapoport, 1976; Rapoport et al., 1980; Bullard and Bigner, 1984; Rapoport and Robinson, 1986; Neuwelt and Barnett, 1989; Gumerlock and Neuwelt, 1990; Neuwelt and Kroll, 1994). The increased cerebral vascular permeability must be reversible to have any role in the delivery of therapeutic viral vectors to brain or intracerebral tumor. Therefore many of these osmotic agents are not recommended because they cause prolonged disruption or even permanent vascular damage. In our laboratory, and in the clinical setting, we use hypertonic mannitol (25%: 1.4 M). However, in some preclinical studies we occasionally use arabinose as the disrupting agent because of the higher concentration of sugar that can be obtained (1.6 M).

4.3.12 Anesthesia

We have previously performed a series of studies to examine the impact of various anesthetics on our ability to obtain consistently reproducible, high quality, survivable BBB disruptions in normal rats (Gumerlock and Neuwelt, 1990; Neuwelt and Kroll, 1994). Osmotic disruption is highly dependent on such physiological variables as cardiac output and vascular tone. Thus cardiovascular changes associated with different anesthetic agents can alter the environment to make BBB disruptions more difficult.

In rodents excellent BBB disruptions were obtained with pentobarbital or isoflurane anesthesia. In contrast, with methoxyflurane, ketamine–xylazine or fentanyl–droperidol, pharmacological manipulation to normalize the cardiac index was necessary before good BBB disruption could be obtained (Gumerlock and Neuwelt, 1990; Neuwelt and Kroll, 1994). Pentobarbital decreases blood pressure slightly, so disruption agent is infused at a slower rate than that used with isoflurane, in which blood pressure is maintained at a steady level. Pentobarbital is used for anesthesia in all BBB disruption studies in dogs and cats. Pentobarbital is also used in rodents for acute studies that do not require recovery, in contrast to the virus studies which require the animal to survive several days in order to assess viral infection and gene expression.

In addition to the mechanics of the BBB disruption itself, the survivability of the procedure becomes important in long-term studies of virus infection. Pentobarbital anesthesia requires several hours of intensive care before the animal recovers. We have found that isoflurane provides the best disruptions with minimal postoperative complications in chronic studies. If pentobarbital is used the animal must be ventilated during the BBB disruption procedure.

4.3.13 Additional Parameters that may be Altered

The rate of infusion must be determined empirically in larger or smaller animals than those specified here. Infusion rates that are too low or too high will result in sub-threshold levels of osmotic agent and failure to attain BBB disruption. The flow rate and/or the time of exposure to hyperosmotic agent can be increased incrementally. For example, begin rat experiments with a flow rate of 0.09 ml/s for 30 s. In successive rats, increase the flow rate to 0.10, 0.11 or 0.12 ml/s, or increase the time of infusion to 35 or 40 s. Excessive infusion rates may lead to intravascular hypertension, brain edema and irreversible damage (Johansson, 1989). For vertebral BBB disruption, in the event that blood flow through the rostral cerebral circulation dilutes the hyperosmotic agent too much for good BBB disruption, the carotid arteries can be briefly occluded with external pressure. Alternatively, as osmotic BBB leak is primarily in the post-capillary venule, temporary occlusion of one or both jugular veins may accentuate BBB opening.

4.3.14 Grading Osmotic Disruption

Approximately 15 minutes before administration of mannitol all animals receive Evans Blue dye as a marker of BBB disruption. The dye rapidly complexes with serum albumin to form a high molecular weight marker (68 kDa) that is excluded from the normal brain by the BBB. The dye should be administered only after the carotid artery has been catheterized, as it becomes very difficult to distinguish the artery from the dark blue adjacent tissues. After death, the brain is examined and the degree of disruption is graded on a scale of 0 (no disruption) to 3+ (excellent disruption), based on the intensity and distribution of the blue color (Neuwelt and Kroll, 1994; Roman-Goldstein et al., 1994). The dye : albumin complex remains as an extracellular compound and is largely washed out during tissue preparation. We have found that Evans Blue dye does not appear to compromise immunocytochemistry or X-gal histochemistry.

BBB disruption can be monitored in humans using computed tomography or magnetic resonance imaging (Roman-Goldstein et al., 1994). We have been able to image disruption in rodent brain using MIONs as the contrast agent (Neuwelt et al., 1994a).

4.4 On Protocols #131–134: BBB Disruption in Dogs

Dogs can also be osmotically disrupted via the vertebral artery to deliver virus to the cerebellum and brain stem (Neuwelt et al., 1981b). We have performed vertebral disruptions by surgically exposing the vertebral artery at the base of the neck and inserting a cannula as described for carotid infusions. However, this was a lengthy and technically difficult procedure; therefore we use percutaneous insertion of the catheter into the femoral artery and advancement to the vertebral artery under fluoroscopic guidance. Mannitol is infused at a rate of 2.08 ml/s for 30 s.

4.5 Notes on Osmotic BBB Disruption in Cats

Unlike that in rodents, canines and primates, the feline internal carotid artery separates into an anastomotic rete mirabile which allows dilution of the mannitol infusion below the threshold concentration necessary for disruption. Owing to this anatomic feature, we have been unable to perform reversible BBB disruption via the carotid artery without neurological sequelae. It is therefore not suitable for the long-term studies of viral infection.

The availability of steerable catheters and new angiographic techniques permits fluoroscopically guided transfemoral catheter placement in vessels with an inside diameter as small as 0.6 mm. With this system we are developing techniques for modification of the cat caudal fossa BBB via the vertebral circulation. In one experiment, infusion of a contrast agent at the rate of 2 ml/s resulted in reflux down the contralateral vertebral artery and complete filling of the rostral and caudal brain circulations, including the middle cerebral artery. Infusion of mannitol at the same rate resulted in patchy areas of blue staining, indicating a moderate degree of BBB disruption in focal areas. Canine BBB disruption following catheterization of the vertebral artery is successful in our laboratory (Neuwelt et al., 1981b). In our clinical studies human patients routinely undergo BBB disruption via the vertebral artery with no neurological sequelae (Neuwelt et al., 1991a). These data suggest that osmotic BBB disruption may also be successfully performed in the cat via this route.

ACKNOWLEDGMENTS

We would like to thank the personnel in the laboratory, including Dr Robert A. Kroll, Dr Laura G. Remsen, Mr Christopher I. McCormick and Mr Michael A. Pagel.

REFERENCES

Akli S., C. Caillaud, E. Vinge, L. D. Stratford-Perricaudet, L. Poenaru, M. Perricaudet, A. Kahn, and M. R. Peschanski. 1993. Transfer of a foreign gene into the brain using adenovirus vectors. *Nature Genet.* **3:**224–228.

Bajocchi G., S. H. Feldman, R. G. Crystal, and A. Mastrangeli. 1993. Direct *in vivo* gene transfer to ependymal cells in the central nervous system using recombinant adenovirus vectors. *Nature Genet.* **3:**229–234.

Barnett P. A., S. Roman-Goldstein, F. Ramsey, C. McCormick, E. M. Shannon, and E. A. Neuwelt. 1995. Differential Permeability and Quantitative MR Imaging of a Human Lung Carcinoma Brain Xenograft in the Nude Rat. *Am. J. Pathol.* **146:**436–449.

Bobo R. H., D. W. Laske, A. Akbasak, P. F. Morrison, R. L. Dedrick, and E. H. Oldfield. 1994. Convection-enhanced delivery of macromolecules in the brain. *Proc. Natl Acad. Sci. USA.* **91:**2076–2080.

Boviatsis E. J., J. S. Park, M. Sena-Esteves, C. M. Kramm, M. Chase, J. T. Efird, M. X. Wei, X. O. Breakefield, and E. A. Chiocca. 1994. Long-term survival of rats harboring brain neoplasms treated with ganciclovir and a herpes simplex virus vector that retains an intact thymidine kinase gene. Cancer Res. **54:**5745–5751.

Breakefield, X. O. and N. A. DeLuca. 1991. Herpes simplex virus for gene delivery to neurons. *New Biologist* **3:**203–218.

Brightman M. W. 1989. The anatomic basis of the blood–brain barrier. In *Implications of the Blood–Brain Barrier and Its Manipulation, Vol* 1 *Basic Science Aspects.* E. A. Neuwelt, editor. Plenum Publishing Co, New York, 53–83.

Bullard, D. E. and D. D. Bigner. 1984. Blood brain barrier disruption in immature Fischer 344 rats. *J. Neurosurg.* **60:**743–750.

Chen S.-H., H. D. Shine, J. C. Goodman, R. G. Grossman, and S. L. C. Woo. 1994. Gene therapy for brain tumors: regression of experimental gliomas by adenovirus-mediated gene transfer *in vivo. Proc. Natl Acad. Sci. USA* **91:**3054–3057.

Dahlborg, S.A., E.A. Neuwelt, W.D. Henner, J.R. Crossen, M. Tableman, and A. Petrillo. 1996. Non-AIDS primary CNS lymphoma: The first example of durable response in a primary brain tumor using enhanced chemotherapy delivery without cognitive loss and without radiotherapy. *Cancer J. Sci. Am.*, in press.

Davidson, B. L., E. D. Allen, K. F. Kozarsky, J. M. Wilson, and B. J. Roessler. 1993. A model system for *in vivo* gene transfer into the central nervous system using an adenoviral vector. *Nature Genet.* **3:**219–223.

Davidson B. L., S. E. Doran, E. S. Shewach, J. M. Latta, J. W. Hartman, and B. J. Roessler. 1994. Expression of *Escherichia coli* β-Galactosidase and rat HPRT in the CNS of *Macaca mulatta* following adenoviral mediated gene transfer. *Exp. Neurol.* **125:**258–267.

Doran S. E., X. D. Ren, A. L. Betz, M. A. Pagel, E. A. Neuwelt, B. J. Roessler, and B. L. Davidson. 1995. Gene Expression from Recombinant Viral Vectors in the CNS following Blood–Brain Barrier Disruption. *Neurosurgery* **36:**965–970.

Fleischman R. A. 1991. Southwestern internal medicine conference: human gene therapy. *Am. J. Med. Sci.* **301:**353–363.

Gumerlock, M. K. and E. A. Neuwelt. 1990. The effects of anesthesia on osmotic blood–brain barrier disruption. *Neurosurgery* **26:**268–277.

Johansson, B. B. 1989. Hypertension and the blood-brain barrier. In *Implications of the Blood–Brain Barrier and Its Manipulation, Vol 2 Clinical Aspects.* E. A. Neuwelt, editor. Plenum Publishing Co, New York, 389.

Kroll, R. A., M. A. Pagel, S. Roman-Goldstein, A. J. Barkovich, A. N. D'Agostino, and E. A. Neuwelt. 1995. White matter changes associated with feline GM2 Gangliosidosis (Sandhoff disease): correlation of MRI with the Pathological and Ultrastructural Abnormalities. *Am. J. Neuroradiol.* **16:**1219–1226.

Laske D. W., R. J. Youle, O. Ilercil, D. M. Lieberman, J. C. Reynolds, P. A. Stewart, C. Paik, D. Katz, H. L. DeVroom, and E. H. Oldfield. 1994. Clinical Experience with Convection Enhanced Drug Delivery in the Brain. *Neurosurgery* **35:**576.

Markert J. M., A. Malick, D. M. Coen, and R. L. Martuza. 1993. Reduction and elimination of encephalitis in an experimental glioma therapy model with attenuated herpes simplex mutants that retain susceptibility to acyclovir. *Neurosurgery* **32:**597–603.

Muldoon, L. L., G. Nilaver, R. A. Kroll, M. A. Pagel, X. O. Breakefield, E.A. Chiocca, B. L. Davidson, R. Weissleder, and E. A. Neuwelt. 1995. Comparison of intracerebral inoculation and osmotic blood–brain disruption for delivery of adenovirus, herpesvirus and iron oxide particles to normal rat brain. *Am. J. Pathol.* **147:**1840–1851.

Muldoon, L. L., M. A. Pagel, E. A. Neuwelt, and D. L. Weiss. 1994. Characterization of the molecular defect in a feline model for Type II GM2–gangliosidosis (Sandhoff disease). *Am. J. Pathol.* **144:**1109–1118.

Neuwelt E. A., J. A. Barranger, R. O. Brady, M. Pagel, F. S. Furbish, J. M. Quirk, G. E. Mook, and E. P. Frenkel. 1981a. Delivery of hexosaminidase-A to the cerebrum after osmotic modification of the blood-brain barrier. *Proc. Natl Acad. Sci. USA.* **78:**5838–5841.

Neuwelt E. A., M. Glasberg, J. Diehl, E. P. Frenkel, and P. Barnett. 1981b. Osmotic blood-brain barrier disruption in posterior fossa of the dog. *J. Neurosurg.* **55:**742–748.

Neuwelt E. A., E. P. Frenkel, A. N. D'Agostino, D. N. Carney, J. D. Minna, P. A. Barnett, and C. I. McCormick. 1985a. Growth of human lung tumor in the brain of the nude rat as a model to evaluate antitumor agent delivery across the blood-brain barrier. *Cancer Res.* **45:**2827–2833.

Neuwelt E. A., W. G. Johnson, N. K. Blank, M. A. Pagel, D. Maslen-McClure, M. J. McClure, and P. M. Wu. 1985b. Characterization of a new model of GM2–gangliosidosis (Sandhoff's disease) in Korat cats. *J. Clin. Invest.* **76:**482–490.

Neuwelt, E. A. and P. A. Barnett. Blood–brain barrier disruption in the treatment of brain tumors: Animal studies. 1989. In *Implications of the Blood–Brain Barrier and Its Manipulation, Vol 2 Clinical Aspects.* E. A. Neuwelt, editor. Plenum Publishing Co, New York, 107.

Neuwelt, E. A., D. L. Goldman, S. A. Dahlborg, J. Crossen, F. Ramsey, S. Roman-Goldstein, R. Braziel, and B. Dana. 1991a. Primary Central Nervous System Lymphoma Treated with Osmotic BBBD and Combination Chemotherapy: Prolonged Survival and Preservation of Cognitive Function. *J. Clin Oncol.* **9:**1580–1590.

Neuwelt E. A., M. A. Pagel, and R. D. Dix. 1991b. Delivery of UV-inactivated [35S]-Herpesvirus across the BBB after osmotic modification. *J. Neurosurg.* **74:**475–479.

Neuwelt, E. A., P. A. Barnett, F. L. Ransey, K. E. Hellstrom, and C. I. McCormick. 1993. Dexamethasone decreases the delivery of tumor-specific monoclonal antibody to both intracerebral and subcutaneous tumor xenografts. *Neurosurgery* **33:**478–484.

Neuwelt E. A., R. Weissleder, G. Nilaver, R. A. Kroll, S. Roman-Goldstein, J. Szumowski, M. A. Pagel, R. S. Jones, L. G. Remson, C. I. McCormick, E. M. Shannon, and L. L. Muldoon. 1994a. Delivery of virus sized iron oxide particles in rodent CNS neurons. *Neurosurgery* **34:**777–784.

Neuwelt, E. A., P. A. Barnett, K. E. Hellstrom, I. Hellstrom, C. I. McCormick, and F. L. Ramsey. 1994b. Effect of Blood–brain Barrier Disruption on Intact and Fragmented Monoclonal Antibody Localization in Intracerebral Human Carcinoma Xenografts. *J. Nucl. Med.* **35:**1831–1841.

Neuwelt, E. A. and R. A. Kroll. 1994. Osmotic blood-brain barrier modification: Increasing delivery of diagnostic and therapeutic agents to the brain. *Meth. Neurosci.* **21:**52–67.

Neuwelt E. A., M. A. Pagel, A. I. Geller, and L. L. Muldoon. 1995. Gene Replacement Therapy in the Central Nervous System: Viral vector mediated therapy of global neurodegenerative disease. *Behav. Brain Sci.* **18:**1–9.

Rapoport, S. I. 1976. *Blood–Brain Barrier in Physiology and Medicine.* Raven Press, New York.

Rapoport, S. I., W. R. Fredericks, K. Ohno, and K. D. Pettigrew. 1980. Quantitative aspects of reversible osmotic opening of the blood–brain barrier. *Am. J. Physiol.* **238:**R421–R431.

Rapoport, S. I. and P. J. Robinson. 1986. Tight-junctional modification as the basis of osmotic opening of the blood–brain barrier. *Ann. NY Acad. Sci.* **481:**250–267.

Remsen, L. G., C. I. McCormick, S. Roman-Goldstein, G. Nilaver, R. Weissleder, A. Bogdanov, K. E. Hellstrom, I. Hellstrom, R. A. Kroll, and E. A. Neuwelt. 1996. MR imaging of MION conjugated carcinoma specific monoclonal antibody in a rodent model of intracerebral human lung cancer: The potential for noninvasive diagnosis. *AJNR Am J. Neuroradiol.* **17:** March, 1996.

Roman-Goldstein, S., D. A. Clunie, J. Stevens, R. Hogan, J. Monard, F. Ramsey, and E. A. Neuwelt. 1994. Osmotic blood-brain barrier disruption: CT and radionuclide imaging. *Am. J. Neuroradiol.* **15:**581–590.

Smith, Q. R. 1989. Quantitation of Blood–Brain Barrier Permeability. In *Implications of the Blood–Brain Barrier and Its Manipulation, Vol 1 Basic Science Aspects.* E. A. Neuwelt, editor. Plenum Publishing Co, New York, 85–118.

Strausbaugh, L. J. and G. S. Brinker. 1983. Effect of osmotic blood-brain barrier disruption on gentamicin penetration into the cerebrospinal fluid and brains of normal rabbits. *Antimicrob. Agents Chemother.* **24:**147–150.

Studer, R. K., D. M. Welch, and B. A. Siegel. 1974. Transient alteration of the blood brain barrier: Effect of hypertonic solutions administered via carotid artery injection. *Exp. Neurol.* **44:**266–273.

Wolfe, J. H., S. L. Deshmane, and N. W. Fraser. 1992. Herpesvirus vector gene transfer and expression of beta-glucuronidase in the central nervous system of MPS VII mice. *Nature Genet.* **1:**379–384.

CHAPTER 24

Pseudorabies Virus: A Tool For Tracing Neuronal Connections

LYNN W. ENQUIST AND J. PATRICK CARD*

Department of Molecular Biology, Princeton University, Princeton, NJ 08544, USA. Tel: 609 258 2415; Fax: 609 258 1035; Email: lenquist@molbiol.princeton.edu

**Departments of Neuroscience and Psychiatry, 446 Crawford Hall, University of Pittsburgh, Pittsburgh, PA 15260, USA. Tel: 412 624 6995; Fax: 412 624 9198; Email: card@bns.pitt.edu*

1 INTRODUCTION

Neurotropic alpha herpesviruses invade and spread in the nervous system of their hosts. This attribute can be exploited to define populations of neurons that are functionally connected because these viruses invade and replicate within neurons in a predictable fashion and then pass transneuronally through synapses to infect neurons presynaptic to the infected cell (Dolivo, 1980; Kuypers and Ugolini, 1990). As the infection proceeds, virus passes through chains of synaptically linked neurons, and the organization of these circuits can be defined by immunohistochemical localization of virus antigen in fixed tissue (Strick and Card, 1992; Card and Enquist, 1994) (Figs 24.1 and 24.2). Although it is possible to use any neurotropic herpesvirus as a neural circuit tracer, numerous studies have used a swine alpha herpesvirus known as pseudorabies virus or PRV (see Enquist, 1994 for a recent review). An attenuated strain of this virus (PRV-Bartha; Bartha, 1961), originally developed as a vaccine, is particularly popular for circuit analysis because of its broad host range and reduced cytopathogenicity. Nevertheless, the availability of a number of well defined viral strains and isogenic mutants that differ in virulence (Bartha, 1961; Becker, 1967; Lomniczi et al., 1984; Wittmann and Rziha, 1989; Card et al., 1992; Kimman et al., 1992; Heffner et al., 1993; Kritas et al., 1994; Mettenleiter, 1994) also make PRV an attractive tool for analysis of viral pathogenesis in rodent models of neuroinvasiveness.

Dolivo and collaborators pioneered the use of PRV as a transneuronal tracer, demonstrating that the virus replicated within multisynaptic circuits in both the peripheral and the central nervous system (CNS) (Dolivo et al., 1978, 1979; Dolivo, 1980; Martin and Dolivo, 1983). Since then, PRV has been used extensively to define circuits that modulate the output of both the sympathetic (Marchand and Schwab, 1986; Rouiller et al., 1986, 1989; Strack et al., 1989a, b; Strack and Loewy, 1990; Jansen et al., 1992, 1993; Rotto-Percelay et al., 1992) and parasympathetic (Card et al., 1990; Nadelhaft et al., 1992; Barrett et al., 1994; Dobbins and Feldman, 1994; Standish et al., 1994) components of the autonomic nervous system. In contrast, use of PRV to characterize the synaptic organization of other circuits in the CNS has been restricted to a few systems. Babic and colleagues (1993) recently used PRV-Bartha to identify premotor neurons that

Protocols for Gene Transfer in Neuroscience: Towards Gene Therapy of Neurological Disorders
Edited by P.R. Lowenstein and L.W. Enquist

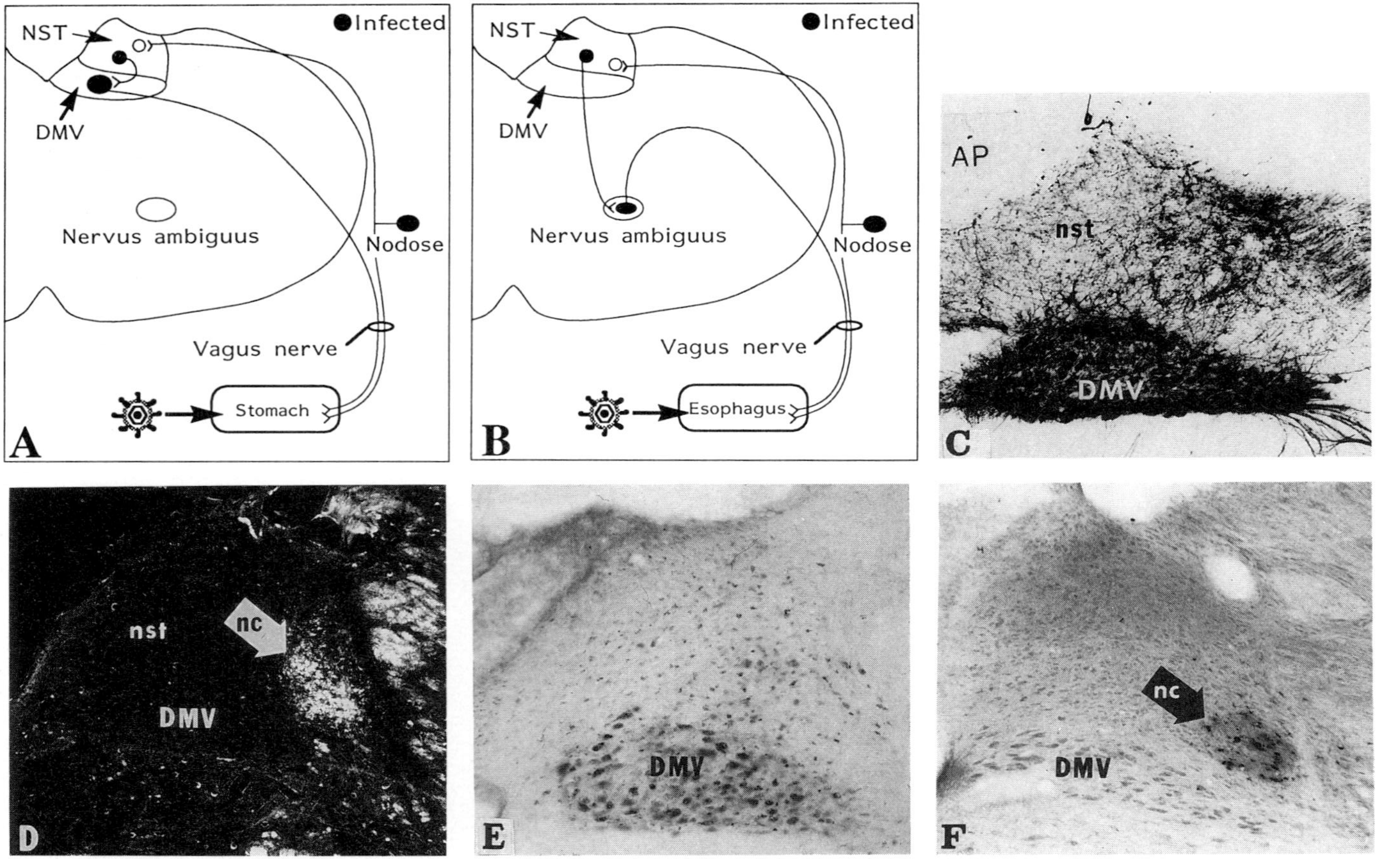

Figure 24.1 Retrograde transneuronal infection of brainstem neurons resulting from injection of PRV into the stomach or the subdiaphragmatic portion of the esophagus. The schematic diagrams in A and B illustrate the organization of the vagal circuitry innervating these organs as well as the distribution of infected neurons within each circuit. The motor and sensory innervation of both organs are susceptible to infection by PRV, but infection of brainstem neurons initially occurs by virtue of retrograde transport of virus to motor neurons. Infection of brainstem neurons through sensory circuits is delayed because the virus must replicate within neurons of nodose ganglion before anterograde transport to the nucleus of the solitary tract (nst). C and D illustrate labeled cells and processes in the dorsal brainstem resulting from injection of conventional tracer (the beta subunit of cholera toxin) into each organ. Note that injection of the stomach labels neurons in the dorsal motor nucleus of the vagus nerve (DMV) as well as sensory fibers in the nst. In contrast, after injection of esophagus, labeling in dorsal brainstem is confined to a dense group of fibers in the subnucleus centralis (nc; arrow) of the nst. The distribution of infected neurons following injection of PRV into the stomach or esophagus is shown in E and F. After stomach injection (D) virus replicates in DMV neurons and passes transneuronally to infect neurons in the overlying nst in a time frame that precedes transneuronal infection of nst neurons through sensory afferents. Similarly, early postinoculation intervals following esophagus injection are characterized by retrograde transneuronal infection of neurons in the nc that project to esophageal motor neurons in the nucleus ambiguus. AP, Area postrema.

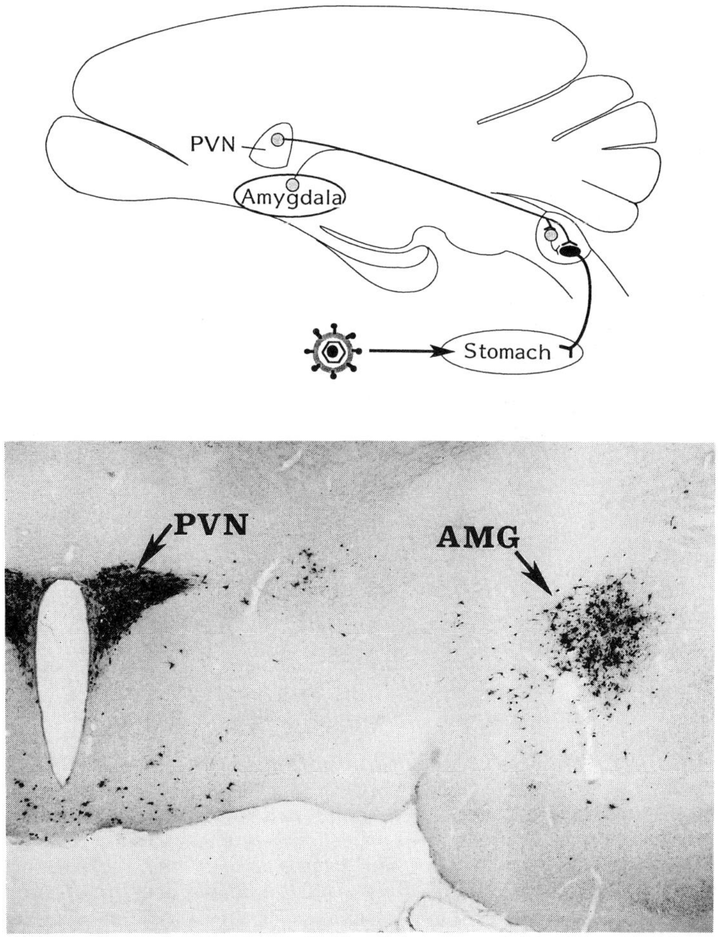

Figure 24.2 The same experimental paradigm that leads to infection of DMV neurons following injection of PRV into the stomach (see Fig. 24.1) ultimately infects forebrain neurons at longer postinoculation intervals. Two groups of forebrain neurons that become infected through their descending projections to the DMV/NST after stomach injection are shown here. Neurons in both the paraventricular nucleus of hypothalamus (PVN) and the central nucleus of the amygdala (AMG) exhibit dense viral immunoreactivity. Subsets of these neurons reproducibly become infected after injection of virus into other visceral organs indicating that there is a viscerotopic organization of forebrain neurons involved in this circuitry

influence the activity of hypoglossal motor neurons, and we have conducted an extensive analysis of visual circuitry with a number of genetically defined strains of PRV (Card et al., 1991, 1992; Whealy et al., 1993) (Fig. 24.3). Our studies of the visual system revealed a remarkable restricted tropism of PRV-Bartha for functionally distinct components of the central visual projections and we demonstrated that the restricted phenotype was due to deletion of two genes encoding viral envelope glycoproteins (Fig. 24.4). The demonstration that deletions in the viral genome can alter the invasiveness of PRV has proven fortuitous for analysis of components of the visual system involved in the photic modulation of circadian function. However, this observation has further emphasized the importance of critically evaluating circuit data produced with this method and of carefully documenting viral invasiveness by comparative analysis with conventional tract tracers.

A number of other factors relating to the virus or the host organism must be critically considered in using viruses for transneuronal tracing. Care must be taken when using PRV as

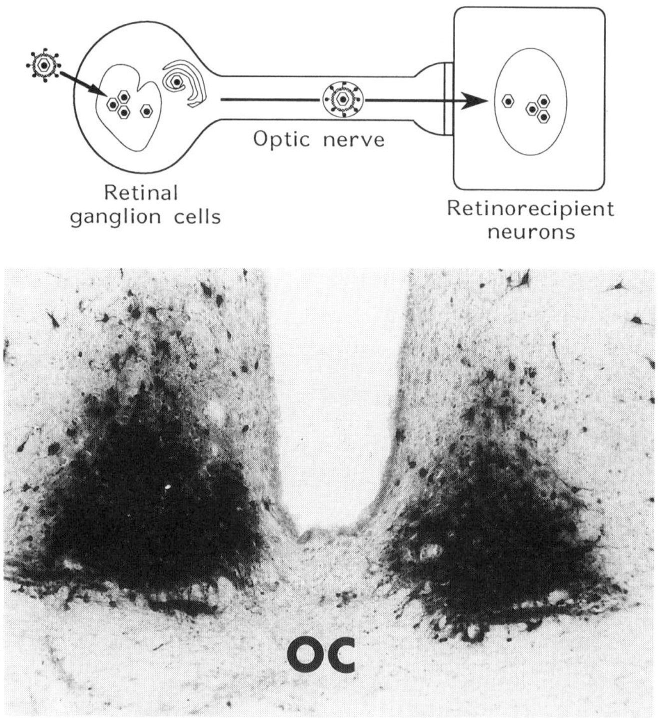

Figure 24.3 Anterograde transneuronal infection of neurons in the CNS occurs following injection of PRV into the vitreous body of the eye. In this experimental paradigm, illustrated in the schematic, virus infects and replicates within retinal ganglion cells and then is transported anterogradely through the axons of these neurons. Upon reaching axon terminals the virus passes transneuronally to infect retinorecipient neurons. The lower micrograph illustrates the presence of viral immunoreactivity in the suprachiasmatic nuclei of the hypothalamus four days after injection of PRV-Bartha into the vitreous body. Neurons in this nucleus are involved in timing of rhythmic phenomena and their circadian activity is entrained to the environmental light-dark cycle via a dense retinal projection through the optic chiasm (OC)

circuit tracers because all strains ultimately produce lethal infections in CNS neurons (McCracken et al., 1973; McCracken and Dow, 1973). As the infection proceeds, more virulent strains of virus will show signs of infecting non-neuronal cells in the vicinity of chronically infected neurons (Card et al., 1990, 1993; Rinaman et al., 1993). Thus, anyone using neurotropic viruses as tracers must be able to prove that viral spread through the CNS occurs in response to transsynaptic passage rather than non-specific release of virions following neuronal lysis and infection of glial cells. Fortunately, the brain responds to the viral infection by mounting a localized inflammatory response that effectively limits the non-neuronal spread of the virus. Our work has demonstrated a temporally organized mobilization of astrocytes, microglia and peripheral macrophages to the site of neuronal infection that effectively limits non-specific dissemination of PRV through the extracellular space. Spread of virus across synapses to afferents synapsing upon these cells is far more rapid than the non-neuronal response to isolate the infection, so the virus is transported to other areas of the nervous system even while a strong response is mounting to earlier infected cells (Card et al., 1990, 1993; Rinaman et al., 1993). Nevertheless, demonstration of specificity of viral transport through a circuit remains the pre-eminent concern in all studies employing this methodology and must be thoroughly documented in each circuit. This requires use of the proper virus (preferably attenuated strains), appropriate controls and, importantly, detailed temporal analysis of the route of invasiveness. In this chapter we review the basic technical considerations for use of PRV in immunohistochemical

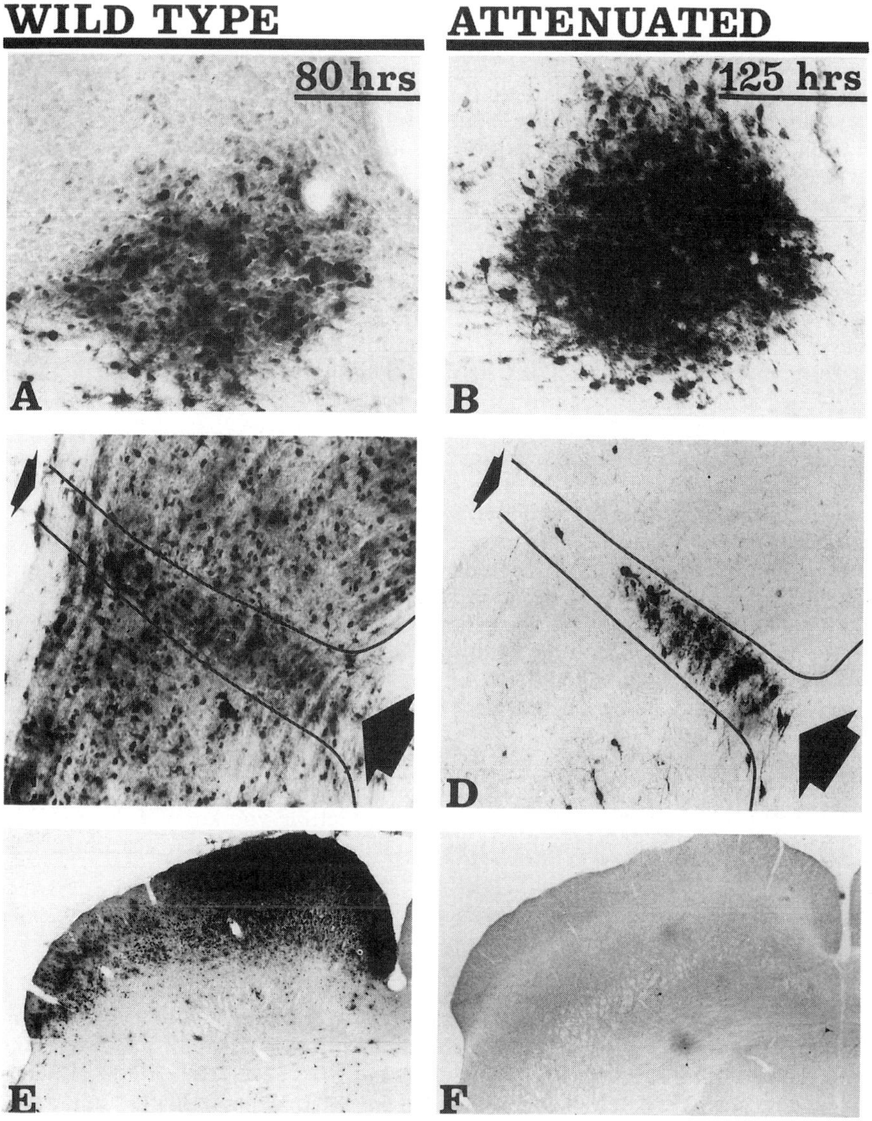

Figure 24.4 Some populations of CNS neurons are differentially sensitive to infection by different strains of PRV. This is particularly evident in comparing the patterns of central infection produced by injection of PRV-Becker (column labeled wild type; A, C and E) and PRV-Bartha (column labeled attenuated; B, D and F) into the vitreous body of the eye. PRV-Becker produces a productive infection in all retinorecipient neurons within 80 hours of inoculation whereas PRV-Bartha infects only a subset of these regions at survival times extending to 125 hours. A and B are of the suprachiasmatic nuclei, C and D illustrate the geniculate complex, and E and F pass through the superior colliculus. Note that viral immunoreactivity is largely restricted to the SCN and a distinct subdivision of the geniculate known as the intergeniculate leaflet (demarcated by arrows) after injection of PRV-Bartha

studies of multisynaptic circuits and detail the factors that must be considered in designing and interpreting experiments of this nature. Issues related to the use of human herpes simplex virus (HSV) are available in several publications (Ugolini et al., 1987, 1989; McLean et al., 1989; Glorioso et al., 1992; Ugolini, 1992).

2 MATERIALS AND EQUIPMENT

2.1 Tissue Culture and Virus Production

(1) Dulbecco's Modified Eagle's Medium (DMEM). Aliquot 100 ml and 500 ml quantities in screw-cap glass bottles. Before use, add penicillin/streptomycin (Pen/Strep) at 100 U/ml penicillin G and 100 μg/ml streptomycin, bicarbonate and the proper concentration of fetal bovine serum (FBS) as indicated in Step 6.
(2) Phosphate-buffered saline (PBS): 0.1 mM Na_2HPO_4, 2.7 mM KCl, 1.5 mM KH_2PO_4, 137 mM NaCl. Sterilize.
(3) Trypsin–EDTA: 0.5% trypsin, 5.3 mM EDTA. Freeze at −20°C in 2 ml aliquots. Stock solution obtained from Gibco/BRL (Life Technologies, Ltd., Grand Island, NY). To prepare final working concentration dilute in PBS to 0.1% trypsin and 1.06 mM EDTA.
(4) Penicillin–streptomycin (Pen/Strep): stock solution obtained from Gibco/BRL #15140–031 (10 000 U/ml penicillin G and 10 000 μg/ml streptomycin sulfate in 0.85% saline). Freeze at −20°C in 2.5 ml aliquots. Final working concentration: 100 U/ml penicillin G and 100 μg/ml streptomycin sulfate in DMEM.
(5) Fetal bovine serum (FBS). Use only qualified, performance tested, mycoplasma, virus and endotoxin tested serum. It is best to use the same lot number as much as possible. Heat-inactivate and freeze 50 ml aliquots at −20°C.
(6) Methocel (methyl cellulose). Prepare a 2% methocel solution as follows: weigh out 2% weight/volume solution of methocel in distilled water. Add a stirrer bar to the solution and shake to disperse. Autoclave 30 min using a liquid cycle; be sure to keep the stirrer still in the solution during autoclaving. Resuspend the autoclaved methocel by stirring overnight at 4°C. Prepare the final solution in a sterile bottle by adding equal volumes of 2 × DMEM and the methocel suspension. Add 2.5 ml Pen/Strep to 500 ml final solution. Be sure to add 5 ml of a 7.5% solution of sodium bicarbonate per 100 ml medium or the buffering capacity will not be optimal. Finally, add FBS to 2%.
(7) Cryoguard™ M-40 thermal exposure indicators. Indicators are green in cryoenvironments maintained continuously below −50°C, but turn irreversibly red when the temperature rises above −40°C. These indicators are invaluable for letting you know if there was a freezer failure and the viability of your virus stocks should be suspect. Order from Control Chemicals Inc. Phone: 313 769 5940.
(8) Humidified, 5% CO_2 incubator at 37°C.

2.2 Material for Stereotaxic Injection

(1) Stereotaxic apparatus, small animal frame.
(2) Microinjection unit.
(3) Hamilton microliter syringes; fixed needle, 1–10 μl.
(4) Appropriate anesthesia (e.g. ketamine 60 mg/kg or xylazine 7 mg/kg, administered by intramuscular injection).
(5) Heating pad to maintain animal body temperature during and after surgery.
(6) Fiberoptic light source.
(7) Binocular surgical microscope.
(8) Dremile drill or dental drill with finest drill tip.
(9) Stereotaxic rat atlases (Paxinos, 1986; Cooley and Vanderwolf, 1990).

3 THE PROTOCOLS

Protocol #135: Preparing Standard PRV Stocks

(1) The day before infection, prepare monolayers of PK15 cells in DMEM + 10% FBS on ten 100 mm plastic dishes. Split cells such that the monolayers will reach about 80% confluence the next day, when you will be ready to infect them.

(2) Remove medium from each dish by aspiration. Infect with PRV at a multiplicity of infection (MOI) of 0.01 (e.g. with 6×10^4 p.f.u./6×10^6 cells) in 1.0 ml DMEM + 2% FBS. The MOI may be varied to accommodate viral strain differences.
(3) Adsorb virus to cells for 1 h at 37°C, 5% CO_2 incubator. Tilt plates slowly twice every 15 min to moisten the cell surface and to keep liquid uniform over monolayer.
(4) Aspirate and discard liquid containing unabsorbed virus. Add 10 ml fresh, warm DMEM containing 2% FBS and Pen/Strep.
(5) Incubate at 37°C, 5% CO_2 for 2–3 days. Wait until complete cytopathic effect is visible (this depends on virus strain) and harvest cells and medium with a plastic scraper. Collect cells and medium in sterile 50 ml screw-cap polypropylene centrifuge tubes. If volume exceeds 50 ml, combine contents of all infected plates in a sterile glass bottle of appropriate size. Mix contents carefully and then aliquot into 50 ml plastic tubes with screw caps.
(6) Freeze each tube at −70°C until frozen solid. Stocks may be kept indefinitely at −70°C.
(7) Rapidly thaw virus samples by placing tubes in a water bath at 37°C, gently mixing every 5 min until ice just disappears. Place tubes on ice and sonicate one tube at a time in cup sonicator (10 pulses for a total of 10 s; amplitude at 80%) to disrupt aggregated virus and to release virus from debris. This allows you to keep the tubes tightly sealed during sonication to avoid creation of aerosols.
(8) Keeping plastic tubes on ice, mix contents by turning tubes upside down. Aliquot 1 ml volumes to sterile 1.7 ml centrifuge tubes or cryovials (use different colors of tubes for different virus strains).
(9) Determine the virus titer from one 1.7 ml centrifuge tube and freeze the remaining aliquots at −70°C as in Step 6.

Protocol #136: Preparing a "Neurostock" from Standard Virus Stocks

This preparation is necessary to remove cell debris from virus stocks.

(1) Thaw two 1 ml samples of stock (from Step 9 of Protocol #135) rapidly in a 37°C water bath and sonicate each sealed tube in a cup sonicator (Protocol #135, Step 7).
(2) Remove cell debris from each sample by centrifugation at 5000 r.p.m. (about 2000*g*) for 5 min.
(3) Remove the supernatant, carefully avoiding the cell debris that forms as a loose pellet.
(4) Aliquot the supernatant into 50–100 μl samples in small screw-cap freezer vials.
(5) Freeze vials rapidly on dry ice and then transfer to −70°C until ready for use.

Protocol #137: Titering PRV Stocks

PRV generally grows to titers of 10^8–10^9 p.f.u./ml.

(1) Prepare monolayers of PK15 cells in six-well dishes the day before titering by splitting a 100 mm dish of PK15 cells that has just reached confluence and plating onto three six-well dishes.
(2) Rapidly thaw the sample to be titered in a 37°C water bath.
(3) Standard stocks should be sonicated in cup sonicator to release virus from aggregates and cell debris prior to determining titer. Neurostocks do not need to be sonicated.
(4) Prepare a series of 10-fold dilutions. Prepare seven tubes with 0.9 ml DMEM containing 2% FBS and Pen/Strep. Add 0.1 ml of the stock to the first tube. Mix well and, with a fresh pipette, add 0.1 ml of this dilution to the next tube. Continue this process through all seven tubes, changing pipette tip each time. The final dilution will be 1×10^7 (indicated as a 10^{-7} dilution).
(5) Aspirate the medium from the monolayers in six-well dishes and wash with warm PBS.
(6) Add 0.2 ml of the desired dilution to appropriate wells containing the washed monolayers and return the plates to the incubator. Duplicate platings should be made of each dilution.
(7) Adsorb virus for 1 h at 37°C, 5% CO_2. Rock the plates every 15 min to keep monolayer evenly moist.
(8) Remove the inoculum and replace with 3 ml DMEM containing 1% methocel, sodium bicarbonate, 2% FBS and Pen/Strep. This semi-solid liquid facilitates the formation of plaques by physically blocking the diffusion of virus.

Table 24.1 Dilution values for primary antibodies

Final dilution PBS (μl)	Stock (μl)	Normal serum (μl)	Triton X-100 (μl)	
Using 1:10 stock				
1:100	100	10	30	860
1:500	20	10	30	940
1:1000	10	10	30	950
1:2000	5	10	30	955
1:5000	2	10	30	958
Using 1:100 stock				
1:1000	100	10	30	860
1:5000	20	10	30	940
1:10 000	10	10	30	950
1:15 000	6.67	10	30	954
1:20 000	5	10	30	955

The values in this table are based on the following: (i) Prepare the primary antibody stock in a final volume of 1 ml; (ii) use a 10 mM PBS solution (pH 7.6) for all dilutions and washes; (iii) normal serum is a 10% solution of serum that matches the species of the secondary (bridge) antibody; and (iv) use a 10% solution of Triton X-100 for dilutions such that the final concentration will be 0.3%

(9) Return the plates to the incubator and **do not disturb** for 2 days. **Do not** pick up the plates and look at them. You may have to wait 3 days to see plaques, depending on the virus strain and your experience.

(10) Count the plaques on the monolayers. These will appear as distinct and usually uniform holes in the monolayer with a halo of round cells. Multiply the number of plaques by the reciprocal of the dilution and then multiply by 5 to obtain the titer in p.f.u./ml. For example, if there are 12 plaques on the 10^{-7} dilution and 175 plaques on the 10^{-6} dilution, the average would be 147.5×10^6. After multiplication by 5, the titer of the stock would be 7.4×10^8 p.f.u./ml.

Protocol #138: Detecting PRV Antigens by Immunoperoxidase and Light Microscopy

(1) Immerse fixed sections of tissue in a solution containing primary antibody, 2% normal serum and 0.3% Triton X-100. The amount of standard stock reagents necessary to achieve a variety of dilutions are indicated in Table 24.1. We routinely use a 1:10 000 dilution to achieve robust and reproducible staining with rabbit polyclonal antisera generated against inactivated PRV. Incubate the tissue in primary antibody at 4°C for 24–48 h. Normal serum for blocking should be of the same species used to raise the secondary (bridge) antibody.

(2) Bring tissue to room temperature over a period of 30–60 min with agitation and wash in multiple changes of a 10 mM solution of PBS (pH 7.6) for 30 min. This is most effectively accomplished by immersing sections in a large excess of buffer (e.g. 100 ml) while agitating the solution on a rocker table.

(3) Place tissue sections in biotinylated secondary antibody raised in another species. For example, if the primary antiserum is generated in rabbit, an appropriate secondary would be biotinylated donkey anti-rabbit IgG. A 1:200 dilution is made as follows: 5 μl of secondary antibody, 20 μl normal serum, 30 μl 10% Triton X-100, 955 μl PBS. Incubate tissue for 60–90 min at room temperature.

(4) Prepare the avidin-biotin complex 60–90 min before use. Two aliquots, designated "A" and "B" are available in the Vectastain Elite kit sold by Vector Laboratories (Burlinghame, CA). Combine 5 μl of each of these reagents in the bottom of an Eppendorf tube and incubate at room temperature with slight agitation.

(5) Wash tissue in multiple changes of PBS for 30 min as described in Step 2.

(6) Mix the components of "A" and "B" from Step 4 with 960 μl PBS and 30 μl 10% Triton X-100. Incubate the tissue in this mixture for 60–90 min at room temperature with agitation.

(7) Repeat Step 5.

(8) Prepare a "saturated" solution of diaminobenzidine (DAB) in Tris buffer (pH 7.2) by placing

an excess of DAB in buffer and vigorously stirring it for 5 min. Filter the solution, and incubate the tissue for 10 min. Add 35 μl hydrogen peroxide and monitor the development of a brown reaction product visually with the aid of a light microscope. Terminate the reaction by repeatedly washing the tissue in multiple changes of PBS.

(9) Mount sections on gelatin-coated microscope slides and allow to air dry. After a period of 1–2 days dehydrate the sections with a graded ethanol series, clear in xylene and coverslip.

Protocol #139: Detecting PRV and other Antigens by Dual Immunoperoxidase Reactions

(1) It is sometimes desirable to localize more than one antigen in the same tissue section. For example, co-injection of PRV with a conventional tracer such as the beta fragment of cholera toxin (CT) permits one to definitively separate first- and second-order neurons since the CT is incapable of crossing synapses and only labels first-order connections. In these dual injection paradigms nickel intensification of DAB can be used to generate a blue-black reaction product that is distinct from the brown, unintensified, DAB precipitate. However, the nickel intensification should always be used to localize the first antigen in this procedure. Start by repeating Steps 1–7 of Protocol #138.

(2) Prepare the "saturated" solution of DAB in Tris buffer as described in Step 8 of Protocol #138. Immediately before tissue incubation add 0.3% NiCl, preincubate the tissue in this solution for 10 min and add 35 μl hydrogen peroxide. Monitor the development of the blue–black reaction product visually and terminate the reaction with repeated washes of PBS.

(3) Repeat Steps 1–8 of Protocol #138 using the second antibody. This will produce a brown reaction product that can be easily distinguished from the nickel intensified signal.

(4) Mount, clear and coverslip tissue as described in Step 9 of Protocol #138.

Protocol #140: Detecting PRV and other Antigens by Immunofluorescence

(1) Mount sections of tissue (10 μm cryostat sections) on gelatin coated slides and store at −20°C until antibody incubation.

(2) Tissue can be incubated sequentially or simultaneously. The optimal dilution for each antibody must be determined separately, but we suggest trying first in the range of 1 : 500. Use the antibody diluent described for the immunoperoxidase localizations. The tissue sections should be ringed with rubber cement, covered with primary antibody, and incubated overnight at room temperature in a humidified box.

(3) Wash tissue in several changes of PBS for 30 min.

(4) Incubate tissue in isotype-specific antibodies tagged with fluorescein isothiocyanate or tetramethylrhodamine isothiocyanate to label antigens green and red, respectively. Other combinations of fluorophors are also available.

(5) Rinse slides in several changes of buffer and coverslip. Examine tissue with a fluorescence microscope using the appropriate excitation filters. Fluorophors often fade quickly during examination, so it is best to photograph the material upon first examination.

Protocol #141: Stereotactic Injection of PRV into the CNS

(1) Use adult Sprague-Dawley rats weighing 280–310 g for stereotaxic injections. (This size animal of correlates with the coordinates defined by Paxinos, 1986.)

(2) Anesthetize the animal by intramuscular injection with ketamine (60 mg/kg) and xylazine (7 mg/kg) or other anesthesia. Shave the skull and swab the scalp with 70% ethanol. Place the animal on a heating pad during surgery.

(3) Place the earbars in the external auditory meatus of each ear and secure the head in the stereotaxic frame. Firmly secure the animal's head and center the animal using the scales on each ear bar. Place the front teeth over the tooth bar and secure the snout. Adjust the angle of the toothbar to the desired angle using the atlas as a guide (Paxinos, 1986; Cooley and Vanderwolf, 1990).

(4) Make a midline incision in the scalp and scrape the periosteum from the surface of the skull. Locate the desired coordinates and mark the skull.

(5) Drill a hole in the cranium at the desired coordinates and make an incision in the dura mater to expose the surface of the brain at the region of injection.
(6) Thaw frozen aliquots of virus immediately before injection and load the Hamilton microliter syringe. Swab the outside of the needle with PBS to remove any virus that could contaminate the needle track. Lower the needle to the desired coordinates and inject 10–100 nl virus at a controlled rate (approximately 10 nl/min). Leave the needle in place for 5 min after virus injection to help reduce reflux of the inoculum up the needle tract. Remove the needle, fill the hole in the cranium with bone wax and close the scalp with wound clips. Remove the animal from the stereotaxic frame and place on the heating pad until it recovers from the anesthetic. Return the animal to its cage in the biosafety housing unit.

4 NOTES AND TROUBLESHOOTING

4.1 Safety Precautions

Alpha herpesviruses are class II infectious agents by CDC/NIH standards and all experiments using these viruses must be conducted in a laboratory sanctioned for Biosafety Level 2 experiments. PRV is not a human pathogen (Card and Enquist, 1994), but appropriate precautions should be taken when handling the virus, infected animals and infectious waste. Specific regulations required for BSL-2 experiments are available in the Health and Human Services Publication #88–8395 *Biosafety in Microbiological and Biomedical Laboratories.* The pertinent regulations regarding the use of viruses for definition of neuronal circuits have been reviewed (Strick and Card, 1992; Card and Enquist, 1994). Every investigator must rigorously apply these standards.

4.2 Selection of Appropriate PRV Strain

There are many isolates of PRV available that vary in their ability to invade and replicate within the nervous system. However, PRV strains are not interchangeable. A number of mutants of well studied strains enable a variety of experimental paradigms to be employed, and knowledge of the strain and its history are therefore important in designing a study. Neuroinvasiveness, the ability to selectively infect some neural circuits and not others, and neurovirulence vary substantially among even closely related strains of PRV. We have shown that deletion of a single gene from the PRV-Becker strain blocks the mutant virus's ability to productively infect some functionally distinct subdivisions of visual circuitry. This gene is also missing in PRV-Bartha (Wittmann and Rziha, 1989; Card et al., 1992), the strain of PRV that has been used most extensively for transneuronal analysis. Thus it is important to apply rigorous standards in evaluating the extent of viral transport through any circuit to ensure that all of its constituent neurons are susceptible to infection. This can be most effectively accomplished by comparing the patterns of viral labeling to previous literature on the connections of a given region and by using the virus in combination with conventional tract tracers.

The Bartha strain is used in most tract tracing studies employing PRV because the reduced neuropathogenicity produced by this attenuated strain permits analysis of viral transport over a longer survival interval. Moreover, Bartha infection often labels the somata and dendrites of infected neurons in a "Golgi-like" fashion. Despite these features, it is important to realize that the Bartha strain contains several characterized and uncharacterized mutations that might affect neural circuit analysis. For example, the restricted neurotropism exhibited by the Bartha strain of PRV in the visual system has obvious advantages for those interested in studying neuronal circuitry involved in the regulation of circadian rhythmicity. However, it is also easy to envision circumstances when reduced neurotropism of a strain of virus could become a serious impediment to experimental analysis or could produce misleading data. All studies to date indicate that the Bartha strain is a very effective tool for delineating circuits influencing the activity of the autonomic nervous system (ANS). Loewy's group in particular has used PRV to characterize multisynaptic circuits extending from the forebrain to spinal cord that modulate the outflow of the ANS (Strack et al., 1989a, b; Strack and Loewy, 1990; Jansen et al., 1992, 1993; Rotto-Porcelay et al., 1992). However, their work has also shown that PRV is less efficient in infecting the somatic nervous system than it is in infecting the sympathetic neurons (Rotto-Porcelay et al., 1992). We stress that the pattern of neuronal infection resulting from viral inoculation is dependent upon properties of the virus (i.e. neuroinvasiveness) as well as the permissiveness of the host neuron. Each of these factors should be carefully considered in evaluating the results of these studies, and the patterns of infection should be compared with data acquired with conventional tract tracers to insure that the pattern of viral transport represents an accurate and complete picture of the circuit.

4.3 On Protocol #137: Titering PRV Stocks

4.3.1 Virus Titer and the Fragility of PRV

It is essential to know the titer of PRV used in each analysis since the concentration of infectious virus dramatically affects viral invasiveness. We measure viral titer in p.f.u./ml after plating dilutions of the stock on monolayers of PK15 cells. It is best to determine the lowest concentration of virus that will give an infection in 100% of infected animals. In general, for standard strains of PRV, at least 10^5 p.f.u. of virus is required to achieve high and reproducible rates of infection. Injection of less than this will reduce the percentage of animals that display productive infection. For example, we have found that less than 20% of animals showed infection of visual circuitry after injection of 10^4 p.f.u. into the vitreous body of the eye whereas 100% were infected with 10^5 p.f.u.

Herpesviruses in general are sensitive to damage by external agents such as heat, desiccation, ultraviolet light, detergents, bleach, alcohols. Because they have a lipid envelope, they are particularly sensitive to detergents, freeze/thaw cycles and ice formation. Therefore it is important to store virus in frozen aliquots at −70°C or below and to thaw virus immediately before inoculation. Storage at −20°C is guaranteed to reduce the virus titer substantially. Unused virus should never be refrozen as this will reduce the titer and introduce unnecessary variability. We routinely store our viral stocks in 50–100 μl aliquots at −70°C and use a single aliquot for each experiment. We make every effort to use the same stock of virus for each set of experiments to further standardize the infectivity and rate of transport of virus through a neuronal circuit.

Detergents and bleach are commonly used to clean syringes and surgical instruments but these agents also inactivate virus and can severely compromise virus titer. All instruments used in the surgery and inoculation need to be free of any of these reagents. Finally, viral stocks should be stored in the portion of the freezer that experiences the least variation in temperature (i.e. the bottom of a chest freezer) and the temperature of the freezer should be carefully monitored to identify variations in temperature. A rise in temperature to −40°C due to short-term freezer failure can reduce the titer of a viral stock and decrease neuronal infectivity. Since freezers have an annoying tendency to break down, spelling disaster for virus stocks, we divide our virus stocks among several freezers on separate electrical circuits to circumvent the problem.

4.4 On Protocol #138: Detecting PRV Antigens by Light Microscopic Immunoperoxidase

4.4.1 Tissue Fixation

We fix all tissue for immunohistochemical localizations with a modification of the paraformaldehyde–lysine–periodate (PLP) fixative developed by McLean and Nakane (1974). It consists of paraformaldehyde, lysine-HCl and sodium meta-periodate in 0.1 M PBS. We have found this fixative to be superior for preserving the antigenicity of virus as well as a variety of peptides and neurotransmitters and therefore routinely employ it in all of our immunohistochemical applications. It is prepared by heating 0.1 M PBS (pH 7.4) to approximately 80°C and adding 4 g of paraformaldehyde for each 100 ml buffer to create a final concentration of 4%. This solution is stirred vigorously until it clears and is then cooled to room temperature with ice. Immediately before use, lysine and sodium meta-periodate are added to a final concentration of 0.075 M and 0.01 M, respectively. Addition of these reagents reduces the pH of the solution to approximately 6.5, and it is not readjusted before use.

Tissue is fixed by transcardiac infusion of 200–400 ml of the fixative, preceded by 50–100 ml physiological saline to wash the blood from the vascular tree. All solutions are infused at a controlled pressure using a peristaltic pump. Aldehydes inactivate the virus, so we perfuse the entire animal rather than clamping the descending aorta as is often done when perfusion of the brain is the ultimate goal. Upon completion of the fixative infusion, the brain and other tissues to be included in the analysis are removed, post-fixed in the primary fixative, washed in 0.1 M PBS (pH 7.4) and placed in 20% phosphate-buffered sucrose for cryoprotection of the tissue. All of these steps are carried out at 4°C. The length of the post-fixation period varies with the application. If localization of virus is the sole objective of the analysis, tissue can be post-fixed overnight to further optimize structural preservation. However, if double labeling procedures are going to be used to localize virus along with a peptide or neurotransmitter it is best to restrict the post-fixation to 1 h. The buffer washes consist of two or more changes of the buffer over a period of 1 or 2 h, followed by cryoprotection in 20% phosphate-buffered sucrose. Cryoprotection of the tissue is judged adequate when it sinks to the bottom of the vial (24–48 h).

4.4.2 Preparation of Tissue

Tissue is sectioned by freezing it onto the chuck of a sliding microtome using dry ice or a commercially available freezing unit. Sections (35 μm) through the rostrocaudal extent of the neuraxis are then collected in consecutive bins of buffer and a single bin of tissue is immediately processed for immunohistochemical localization of virus to determine the extent of viral transport and evaluate the preservation of tissue morphology. The remaining bins can be used to analyse viral immunoreactivity in a more frequent series of sections, or to localize other antigens either alone or in combination with the virus. To obtain maximum information from the material we section tissue into multiple wells of buffer and transfer excess tissue to an ethylene glycol-based cryopreservant for long-term storage at −20°C with no evident loss of antigenicity or morphology (Watson et al., 1986). Any tissue that is not processed within the first 2 days following sectioning is transferred to cryoprotectant and stored at −20°C. The cryoprotectant is made by mixing 200 g sucrose and 10 g polyvinyl pyrrolidone-40 in a large beaker and then slowly stirring in 500 ml of 0.1 M PBS. Thereafter, another 100 g sucrose is added to the solution, followed by 300 ml ethylene glycol and enough distilled water to a final volume of 1000 ml. The solution is then stored in the freezer.

4.5 On Protocol #139: Detecting PRV and other Antigens by Dual Immunoperoxidase Reactions

4.5.1 Localization of Virus Antigen by Immunoperoxidase

Localization of virus with immunoperoxidase methods is straightforward and can be accomplished with polyclonal antisera generated against the entire virus, or with monospecific antisera generated against individual viral envelope glycoproteins. Polyclonal antisera are preferable because they are more readily available and produce a more robust signal. We use the avidin–biotin modification (Hsu et al., 1981) of the peroxidase antiperoxidase procedure (Sternberger, 1979). This procedure (Strick and Card, 1992; Card and Enquist, 1994) provides a sensitive means of detecting virus localization using the standard Vectastain kit (Vector Laboratories) and dilutions of rabbit polyclonal antisera in the range of 1:1000–1:2000. However, the recent introduction of more sensitive methods of detection now permits the use of dilutions of primary antisera extending to 1:30 000 with no apparent loss in either the intensity of staining or the extent of immunoreactivity. The procedure we now employ uses the Vectastain Elite modification of the avidin–biotin immunoperoxidase procedure.

4.6 On Protocol #140: Detecting PRV and other Antigens by Immunofluorescence

4.6.1 Localization of Virus Antigens by Immunofluorescence

Several different color fluorophors are available that can be effectively applied for localization of antigens in the same tissue section, and this methodology has been successfully applied to localize PRV in combination with a variety of antigens (Strack et al., 1989a, b; Strack and Loewy, 1990;

Rinaman et al., 1993). In addition, this method can be effectively applied to localizing PRV in combination with other tracers such as the beta subunit of cholera toxin. Other fluorescent tracers such as Fluorogold (Schmued and Fallon, 1986) have been shown to interfere with HSV infection in the trigeminal ganglion (Carter et al., 1992). Negative data on the colocalization of PRV with tract tracers should be viewed conservatively. In addition, the pathological changes that PRV causes in neurons may affect peptide or neurotransmitter content. The best approach is to apply the method early in the course of neuronal infection to minimize any adverse effects that viral infection may have upon host cell synthesis. Colchicine should be used to increase intracellular levels of peptides or neurotransmitters with caution because it could interfere with the transneuronal passage of virus and compromise the health of the animal.

4.6.2 Interpretation of Results

The parameters used to evaluate the transport of conventional tracers through the nervous system are also relevant to the analysis of viral transport. The most obvious variables influencing the interpretation of labeling include the route of administration, the volume of the inoculum, and the spread of virus from the site of injection. However, the postinjection survival interval and the cytopathogenicity of the virus are also extremely important in evaluating studies of this nature. The best results are achieved when the same stock of an attenuated strain of virus is used throughout a single set of experiments. This reduces any variability that might result from injection of differing concentrations of virus, particularly with respect to standardizing the extent of viral transport in different animals with similar postinoculation survival intervals.

PRV does not diffuse significant distances after either peripheral or central inoculation (Card et al., 1990; Luc Jasmin, personal communication). Following direct injection of PRV into the rat cortex virus does not appear to spread from the injection site (Card et al., 1996). It is likely that the high affinity of the virus for neurons and glia effectively limits the spread of virus from the injection site and contributes to its effectiveness as a neuronal track tracer. Nevertheless, it is important to clearly document the extent of viral dissemination by examining representative sections throughout the extent of the injection site and/or by injecting conventional tracers in combination with the virus. The extent of diffusion of a conventional tracer should be used only as a relative index of the diffusion of virus from the injection site as it is inappropriate to assume that they exhibit identical rates of spread. The most reliable determinant of the extent of viral spread is immunohistochemical localization of virus in closely spaced sections through the injection site.

The volume of virus injected will also contribute to the extent of diffusion from the injection site. As a general rule it is best to inject small volumes. When injecting the vitreous body of the eye in rats we inject 1–2 μl of virus syringe and leave the needle in the globe of the eye for a minimum of 5 min to reduce leakage of virus into the orbit. Successful injections of the viscera also employ small volumes of virus (1–5 μl) injected into multiple sites in the organ of interest using a microliter syringe and a surgical microscope. The needle is left in place for a short time to reduce reflux along the needle tract, and the surface of the injection site is washed with saline-soaked cotton swabs to prevent dissemination of virus through the peritoneal cavity. When injecting the virus directly into the CNS, a small cannula is placed in the desired area using a stereotaxic apparatus and virus (10–100 nl) is injected at a controlled rate of approximately 10 nl/min. Upon completion of the injection the cannula is left in place for a minimum of 5 min. These parametrics have produced specific transport of virus through multisynaptic pathways subserving visual, visceral and cortical function, but are only provided as general reference points for designing a study. Independent parametrics should be rigorously characterized in each experimental application.

It is important to do a temporal analysis of virus spread through a particular circuit. A significant feature of the viral life cycle relevant to interpreting the transport of virus through a multisynaptic circuit is that, upon infecting a neuron, the virus must reproduce before it can pass to the next neuron. Replication of virus in a neuron is a complex process involving transport of a capsid containing viral DNA to the cell nucleus, replication of viral DNA and assembly of new virions, and intracellular transport of newly replicated virions to sites of afferent synaptic contact. This process requires time, and the length of time necessary varies substantially in different neurons. For example, viral replication and transneuronal passage occurs more quickly in interneurons than in projection neurons due to the shorter length of the axon. Consider the transport of virus through central circuits following injection of virus into the viscera. Following injection of virus into the stomach we noted that viral antigens could be detected by immunohistochemical techniques in preganglionic parasympathetic neurons of the DMV as early as 30 h after inoculation, with robust viral immunoreactivity apparent at 45–50 h (Card et al., 1990). In contrast, short axon second-order neurons in the overlying nucleus of the solitary tract (NST) and nearby brainstem tegmentum displayed viral immunoreactivity 50–55 h after injection. In subsequent studies of longer survival intervals, infected neurons were observed in areas of the forebrain known to give rise to descending projections to the DMV/NST complex (Miselis et al., 1996). However, although neurons in the DMV and NST exhibited pathological changes consistent with neuronal death, the distribution of infected forebrain neurons was highly reproducible in different animals and always became infected in a predictable temporal sequence. All available evidence indicates that virus begins to cross synapses shortly after replication, within a time frame preceding the appearance of any overt neuropathology in the infected neuron.

ACKNOWLEDGMENTS

We thank Paul Husak, Anita Knapp-Rysek and Marlies Eldrige for careful reading and testing the protocols. L.W.E. is supported by National Institutes of Health grant NINDS R01 33506. J.P.C. is supported by National Institutes of Health grant ROI MH 53574.

REFERENCES

Babic, N., T. C. Mettenleiter, A. Flamand, and G. Ugolini. 1993. Role of essential glycoproteins gII and gp50 in transneuronal transfer of pseudorabies virus from the hypoglossal nerve of mice. *J Virol* **67**:4421–4426.

Barrett, R. T., X. Bao, R. R. Miselis, and S. M. Altschuler. 1994. Brain stem localization of rodent esophageal premotor neurons revealed by transneuronal passage of pseudorabies virus. *Gastroenterology* **107**:728–737.

Bartha, A. 1961. Experimental reduction of virulence of Aujeszky's disease virus. *Magy Allatorv Lapja* **16**: 42.

Becker, C. H. 1967. Zur primären Schädigung vegetativer Ganglien nach Infektion mit dem Herpes Suis Virus bei verschiedenen Tierarten. *Experientia* **23**: 209–217.

Card, J. P. and L. W. Enquist. 1994. The use of pseudorabies virus for definition of synaptically linked populations of neurons. In *Methods in Molecular Genetics* (K. W. Adolph, ed.), 363–382. Academic Press Inc., Orlando Florida.

Card, J. P., L. Rinaman, J. S. Schwaber, R. R. Miselis, M. E. Whealy, A. K. Robbins, and L. W. Enquist. 1990. Neurotropic properties of pseudorabies virus: uptake and transneuronal passage in the rat central nervous system. *J Neurosci* **10**:1974–1994.

Card, J. P., L. Rinaman, R. B. Lynn, B. H. Lee, R. P. Meade, R. R. Miselis, and L. W. Enquist. 1993. Pseudorabies virus infection of the rat central nervous system: ultrastructural characterization of viral replication, transport and pathogenesis. *J Neurosci* **13**:2515–2539.

Card, J. P., L. W. Enquist, and P. Levitt. 1996. Differential invasiveness of two strains of pseudorabies virus injected into rat prefrontal cortex. In preparation.

Card, J. P., M. E. Whealy, A. K. Robbins, and L. W. Enquist. 1992. Pseudorabies virus envelope glycoprotein gI influences both neurotropism and virulence during infection of the rat visual system. *J Virol* **66**:3032–3041.

Card, J. P., M. E. Whealy, A. K. Robbins, R. Y. Moore, and L. W. Enquist. 1991. Two α-herpesvirus strains are transported differentially in the rodent visual system. *Neuron* **6**:957–969.

Carter, S. R., L. Pereira, P. Paz, and J. H. LaVail. 1992. A quantitative assay of retrograde transported HSV in the trigeminal ganglion. *Invest Opthal Vis Sci* **33**:1934–1939.

Cooley, R. K. and A. J. Vanderwolf. 1990. *Stereotaxic Surgery In The Rat: A Photographic Series.* A.J. Kirby Co., Ontario.

Dobbins, E. G. and J. L. Feldman. 1994. Brainstem network controlling descending drive to phrenic motoneurons in rat. *J Comp Neurol* **347**:64–86.

Dolivo, M. 1980. A neurobiological approach to neurotropic viruses. *Trends Neurosci* **3**:149–152.

Dolivo, M., E. Beretta, Y. Bonifas, and C. Foroglou. 1978. Ultrastructure and function in sympathetic ganglia isolated from rats infected with pseudorabies virus. *Brain Res* **140**:111–123.

Dolivo, M., P. Honegger, C. George, M. Kiraly, and W. Bommeli. 1979. In *Progress in Brain Research*, vol 51 (M. Cuenod, G. W. Kreutzberg and F. E. Bloom, eds), 51. Elsevier/North Holland, Amsterdam.

Enquist, L. W. 1994. Infection of the mammalian nervous system by pseudorabies virus (PRV). *Semin Virol* **5**:221–231.

Glorioso, J. C., W. F. Goins, and D. J. Fink. 1992. Herpes simplex virus-based vectors. *Semin Virol* **3**:265–276.

Heffner, S., F. Kovacks, B. Klupp, and T. C. Mettenleiter. 1993. Glycoprotein gp50-negative pseudorabies virus: a novel approach toward a nonspreading live herpesvirus vaccine. *J Virol* **67**:1529–1537.

Hsu, S. M., L. Raine, and H. Fanger. 1981. The use of avidin-biotin-peroxidase complex (ABC) in immunoperoxidase techniques: A comparison between ABC and unlabeled antibody (PAP) procedures. *J Histochem Cytochem* **29**:577–580.

Jansen, A. S. P., D. G. Farwell, and A. D. Loewy. 1993. Specificity of pseudorabies virus as a retrograde marker of sympathetic preganglionic neurons: implications for transneuronal labeling studies. *Brain Res* **617**:103–112.

Jansen, A. S. P., G. J. Ter Horst, T. C. Mettenleiter, and A. D. Loewy. 1992. CNS cell groups projecting to the submandibular parasympathetic preganglionic neurons in the rat: a retrograde transneuronal viral cell body labeling study. *Brain Res* **572**:253–260.

Kimman, T. G., N. De Wind, N. Oei-Lie, J. M. A. Pol, A. J. M. Berns and A. J. J. Gielkens. 1992. Contribution of single genes within the unique short region of Aujeszky's disease virus (suid herpesvirus type 1) to virulence, pathogenesis and immunogenicity. *J Gen Virol* **73**:243–251.

Kritas, S. K., M. B. Pensaert, and T. C. Mettenleiter. 1994. Role of envelope glycoproteins gI, gp63 and gIII in the invasion and spread of Aujesky's disease virus in the olfactory nervous pathway of the pig. *J Gen Virol* **75**:2319–2327.

Kuypers, H. G. J. M. and G. Ugolini. 1990. Viruses as transneuronal tracers. *Trends Neurosci* **13**:71–75.

Lomniczi, B., S. Watanabe, T. Ben-Porat and A. S. Kaplan. 1984. Genetic basis of the neurovirulence of pseudorabies virus. *J Virol* **61**:796–801.

Marchand, C. F. and M. Schwab. 1986. Binding, uptake and retrograde axonal transport of herpes virus suis in sympathetic neurons. *Brain Res* **383**:262–270.

Martin, X and M. Dolivo. 1983. Neuronal and transneuronal tracing in the trigeminal system of the rat using herpes virus suis. *Brain Res* **273**:253–276.

McCracken, R. M. and C. Dow. 1973. An electron microscope study of Aujeszky's disease. *Acta Neuropathol (Berl.)* **25**: 207.

McCracken, R. M., J. B. McFerran, and C. Dow. 1973. The neural spread of pseudorabies virus in calves. *J Gen Virol* **20**:17–28.

McLean, I. W. and P. K. Nakane. 1974. Periodate-lysine-paraformaldehyde fixative. A new fixative for immunoelectron microscopy. *J Histochem Cytochem* **22**:1077–1083.

McLean, J. H., M. T. Shipley, and D. I. Bernstein. 1989. Golgi-like, transneuronal retrograde labeling with CNS injections of herpes simplex virus type 1. *Brain Res Bull* **22**:867–881.

Mettenleiter, T. C. 1994. Review: Pseudorabies (Aujeszky's Disease) virus: state of the art, August 1993. *Acta Vet Hung* **42**:153–177.

Miselis, R. R., M. Yang, B. H. Lee, J. P. Card, and L. W. Enquist. 1996. Visceral neuraxis defined by transneuronal passage of neurotropic viruses from structures of the alimentary canal. In preparation.

Nadelhaft, I., P. L. Vera, J. P. Card, and R. R. Miselis. 1992. Central nervous system neurons labeled following the injection of pseudorabies virus into the rat urinary bladder. *Neurosci Lett* **143**:271–274.

Paxinos, G. 1986. *The Rat Brain In Stereotaxic Coordinates*, 2nd Edition. Academic Press/Harcourt Brace, San Diego.

Rinaman, L., J. P. Card, and L. W. Enquist. 1993. Spatiotemporal responses of astrocytes, ramified microglia and brain macrophages to central neuronal infection with pseudorabies virus. *J Neurosci* **13**:685–702.

Rotto-Percelay, D. M., J. G. Wheeler, F. A. Osorio, K. B. Platt, and A. D. Loewy. 1992. Transneuronal labeling of spinal interneurons and sympathetic preganglionic neurons after pseudorabies virus injections in the rat medial gastrocnemius muscle. *Brain Res* **574**:291–306.

Rouiller, E. M., M. Capt, M. Dolivo, and F. DeRibaupierre. 1986. Tensor tympani reflex pathways studied with retrograde horseradish peroxidase and transneuronal viral tracing techniques. *Neurosci Lett* **72**:247–252.

Rouiller, E. M., M. Capt, M. Dolivo, and F. DeRibaupierre. 1989. Neuronal organization of the stapedius reflex pathways in the rat: a retrograde HRP and viral transneuronal tracing study. *Brain Res* **476**:21–28.

Schmued, L. C. and J. H. Fallon. 1986. Fluoro-Gold: A new fluorescent retrograde axonal tracer with numerous unique properties. *Brain Res* **377**:147–154.

Standish, A., L. W. Enquist, and J. S. Schwaber. 1994. Innervation of the heart and its central medullary origin defined by viral tracing. *Science* **263**:232–234.

Sternberger, L. A. 1979. The unlabeled antibody peroxidase-antiperoxidase (PAP) method. In *Immunocytochemistry* (L. A. Sternberger, ed.), 104. Wiley, New York.

Strack, A. M. and A. D. Loewy. 1990. Pseudorabies virus: a highly specific transneuronal cell body marker in the sympathetic nervous system. *J Neurosci* **10:**2139–2147.

Strack, A. M., W. B. Sawyer, J. H. Hughes, K. B. Platt, and A. D. Loewy. 1989a. A general pattern of CNS innervation of the sympathetic outflow demonstrated by transneuronal pseudorabies viral infections. *Brain Res* **491:**156–162.

Strack, A. M., W. B. Sawyer, K. B. Platt, and A. D. Loewy. 1989b. CNS cell groups regulating the sympathetic outflow of the adrenal gland as revealed by transneuronal cell body labeling with pseudorabies virus. *Brain Res* **491:**274–296.

Strick, P. L. and J. P. Card. 1992. Transneuronal mapping of neuronal circuits with alpha-herpesviruses. In *Experimental Neuroanatomy. A Practical Approach* (J. P. Bolam, ed.), p. 81. IRL Press, Oxford.

Ugolini, G. 1992. Transneuronal transfer of herpes simplex virus type 1 (HSV 1) from mixed limb nerves to the CNS. I. Sequence of transfer from sensory, motor and sympathetic nerve fibers to the spinal cord. *J Comp Neurol* **326:**527–548.

Ugolini, G., H. G. M. J. M. Kuypers, and A. Simmons. 1987. Retrograde transneuronal transfer of herpes simplex virus type 1 (HSV-1) from motoneurones. *Brain Res* **422:**242–256.

Ugolini, G., H. G. M. J. M. Kuypers, and P. L. Strick. 1989. Transneuronal transfer of herpes virus from peripheral nerves to cortex and brainstem. *Science* **243:**89–92.

Watson, R. E., S. T. Wiegand, R. W. Clough, and G. E. Hoffman. 1986. Use of cryoprotectant to maintain long-term peptide immunoreactivity and tissue morphology. *Peptides* **7:** 155–159.

Whealy, M. E., J. P. Card, A. K. Robbins, J. R. Dubin, H. J. Rziha, and L. W. Enquist. 1993. Specific pseudorabies virus infection of the rat visual system requires both gI and gp63 glycoproteins. *J Virol* **67:**3786–3797.

Wittmann, G. and H. J. Rziha. 1989. Aujeszky's disease (pseudorabies) in pigs. In *Herpesvirus diseases of cattle, horses and pigs* (G. Wittmann, ed.), 230–325. Kluwer, Boston.

CHAPTER 25

Tracing Connected Neurons with Herpes Simplex Virus Type 1

GABRIELLA UGOLINI

Laboratoire de Génétique des Virus, CNRS, F-91198 Gif-sur-Yvette, France.
Tel: 33 1 69 82 37 69; Fax: 33 1 69 82 43 08

1 INTRODUCTION

Considerable efforts have been made to develop transneuronal tracers, markers that can be used to trace a whole chain of serially connected neurons that supply a given organ or a specific CNS cell group. To be an effective transneuronal tracer a marker should be able to produce intense labeling of all groups of connected neurons that are part of a given circuit. Alpha-herpesviruses have these features: they propagate very efficiently through transneuronal transfer and function as a self-amplifying marker by replicating in recipient neurons (Kuypers and Ugolini, 1990; Strick and Card, 1992; Ugolini, 1995). Because of viral replication, transneuronal labeling with alpha-herpesviruses is as intense as the labeling of first-order neurons (Fig. 25.1) and can involve all groups of second-order neurons and higher-order neurons (Kuypers and Ugolini, 1990; Strick and Card, 1992; Ugolini, 1995). Viral transneuronal labeling can be easily detected immunohistochemically in tissue sections.

The two alpha-herpesviruses used as tracers are Herpes simplex virus type 1 (HSV-1) and Pseudorabies virus (PRV, Suid Herpesvirus 1) (reviewed in Kuypers and Ugolini, 1990; Strick and Card, 1992; Ugolini, 1995 and Chapter 24). Tracing studies on PRV were initiated by Martin and Dolivo in 1983 and the first demonstration that HSV-1 is an effective retrograde transneuronal tracer was provided by Ugolini and collaborators in 1987. The transneuronal transfer of another alpha-herpesvirus (B virus; herpesvirus simiae), has also been reported (Gosztonyi et al., 1992), but this virus should not be used because it is fatal for humans. In contrast, both HSV-1 and PRV may be safely manipulated if simple protection measures are adopted (SEE SECTION 4.1.2, PAGE 355).

HSV and PRV differ in host range: only HSV-1 is able to produce transneuronal labeling in primates, although both viruses are transferred transneuronally in rodents (see Strick and Card, 1992; Ugolini, 1995; SEE ALSO SECTION 4.2, PAGE 356). The choice between HSV-1 or PRV may be determined by local biosafety regulations: for example, PRV has been eradicated in the UK and its use is not authorized there.

The properties of HSV-1 and PRV as transneuronal tracers are very similar: the extent and specificity of transfer of the two viruses depend on several experimental parameters related both to the virus (virus strain and dose) and to the host (species, strain and age) (SEE SECTIONS 4.2–4.4 PAGE 356). If these parameters are optimized and kept constant, transneuronal transfer of HSV-1 and PRV is very efficient, bidirectional and strictly time-dependent. As serially connected neurons are labeled at sequential intervals, it is very important to study the propagation of the virus at

Protocols for Gene Transfer in Neuroscience: Towards Gene Therapy of Neurological Disorders
Edited by P.R. Lowenstein and L.W. Enquist

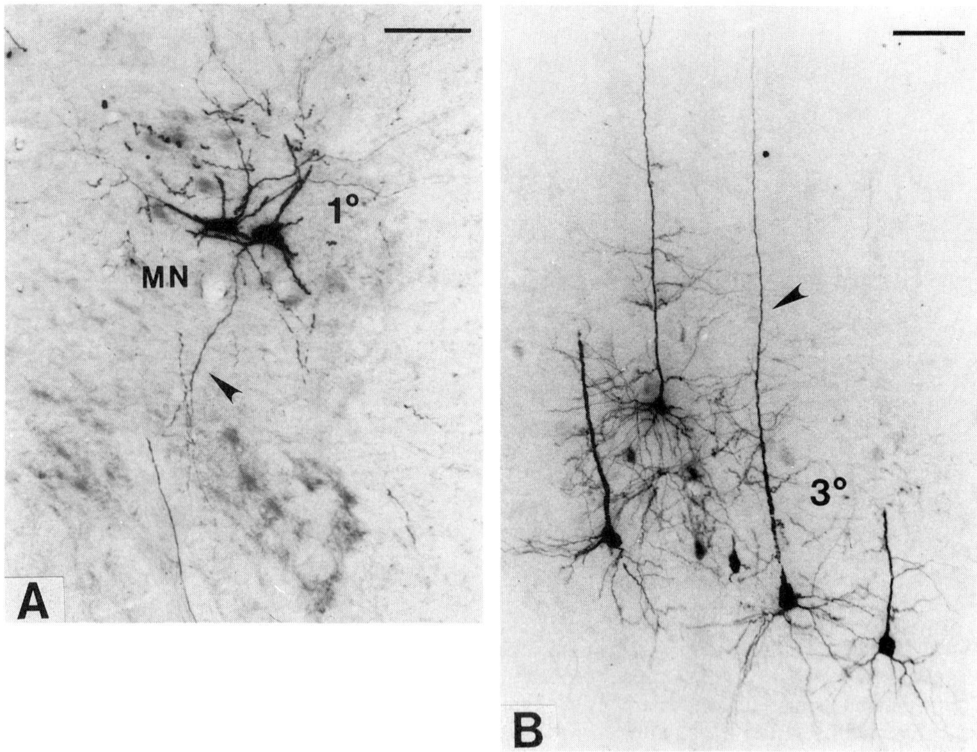

Figure 25.1 Similarity in labeling intensity of first-order neurons (A) and third-order neurons (B) with HSV-1. The virus was injected unilaterally into forelimb nerves (ulnar and median) of rats (Ugolini et al., 1989; Ugolini, 1992). (A) First-order neurons (1°): retrograde labeling of forelimb motoneurons (MN) in spinal segment C8 (28 h after inoculation; see Fig. 25.2). Labeling comprises the cell bodies, dendrites and axons (arrowhead) of the motoneurons. At early times of infection, labeled MN show normal size and morphology. Glial cells are not labeled. Bar: 100 μm. Taken with permission from Ugolini (1992). (B) Retrograde transneuronal labeling of third-order neurons (3°) with HSV-1: corticospinal neurons in layer V in forelimb area of the contralateral sensorimotor cortex infected by transneuronal transfer of HSV-1 from forelimb nerves (Ugolini et al., 1989). Intense labeling of neuronal cell bodies, basal dendrites and long apical dendrites (arrowhead). Bar: 180 μm. Immunoperoxidase detection of HSV-1 (peroxidase-antiperoxidase method) in frozen sections using a rabbit polyclonal antiserum generated against the entire virus

different times after inoculation, to distinguish first, second and third-order neurons on the basis of their sequential appearance. However, the analysis may be complicated by the fact that labeling of different groups of second-order neurons may also occur at different times (Fig. 25.2; SEE ALSO SECTION 4.9.4, PAGE 361).

All strains of alpha-herpesviruses that can function as transneuronal tracers have some disadvantages: they induce neuronal degeneration and may also produce a small amount of spurious labeling due to local virus spread from degenerating neuronal cell bodies and axons to nearby cells. However, local (non-specific) spread of virus is much less efficient than transneuronal (specific) transfer and may be minimized with careful control of dose and time after inoculation (SEE SECTION 4.9.3, PAGE 361).

If used correctly, transneuronal tracing with alpha-herpesviruses is a very powerful technique, which can be exploited to clarify important aspects of neuronal connectivity that could never be studied with conventional tracing methods. This chapter will focus on the methodology for

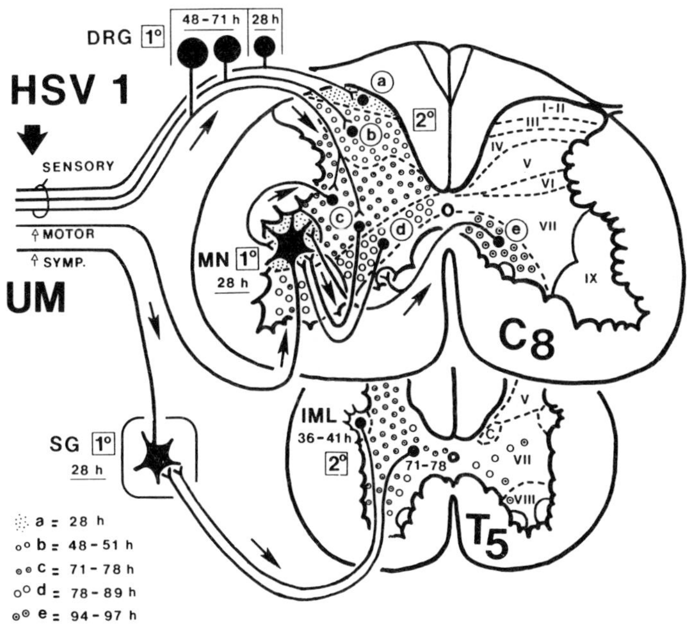

Figure 25.2 Asynchronous transneuronal transfer of HSV-1 from sensory, motor and sympathetic axons of mixed forelimb nerves (ulnar and median, UM) to connected spinal neurons. Left: different symbols indicate the increase in spinal distribution at different times after inoculation (a–e). Right: boundaries of laminae I–IX. HSV-1 infects all groups of first-order neurons (1°): sensory neurons in dorsal root ganglia (DRG), motoneurons (MN), sympathetic neurons in stellate ganglion (SG). However, retrograde transneuronal transfer from the SG to second-order (2°) sympathetic neurons in intermediolateral cell group (IML) occurs by 36–41 h, whereas the first labeling consistent with retrograde transneuronal transfer from motoneurons occurs much later (c–e). Similarly, anterograde transneuronal transfer from small primary sensory afferents to laminae I–II occurs at 28 h (a), whereas transfer from sensory afferents of intermediate and large diameter to deeper spinal laminae is obtained later (b, c). This sequence indicates that transneuronal transfer from axons of small diameter (small cutaneous afferents and sympathetic axons, largely unmyelinated) precedes transfer from axons of large diameter (myelinated sensory afferents and motor axons). Asynchronous labeling of second-order neurons also occurs during transfer from the same population of first-order neurons (e.g. sympathetic neurons in SG): at 36 h, labeling involves only the preganglionic cell groups that provide the strongest input to the SG (e.g. IML at T5); cell groups that have only a few connections with the SG (e.g. medial sympathetic preganglionic cell groups at T5) are labeled later (e.g. 71 h). Adapted with permission from Ugolini (1992). (Copyright 1992 of Wiley-Liss, a division of Wiley & Sons, Inc.)

transneuronal tracing with HSV-1. Some data on PRV will be also discussed, to exemplify the similarities in the behavior of the two viruses.

2 MATERIALS AND EQUIPMENT

Experimental manipulation of HSV-1 requires straightforward safety precautions (SEE SECTION 4.1.2, PAGE 355). Transneuronal tracing with HSV-1 does not require anything more than the standard equipment used in any neuroscience laboratory for the administration and detection of classical tracers: conventional materials and equipment for surgery and microinjection of tracers, perfusion-fixation, dissection, tissue sectioning, and histological processing. The main items are listed below. Additional items are required for virus culture. The protocols for culture and titration of HSV-1 are described in other protocols in this book.

2.1 Injection of HSV-1 into Peripheral Nerves

(1) Microsurgery microscope.
(2) Anesthetic agents such as sodium pentobarbital.
(3) Instruments for microsurgery: fine forceps, scissors, needle holders, scalpels, etc.
(4) Glass micropipettes for inoculating the virus. We make our own micropipettes with long taper length and tip diameter 50–60 μm.
(5) A microinjection unit for pressure delivery of tracers. A number of units are available. We use a modified infusion–withdrawal pump that is connected with a home-made timer. This unit guides a 5–10 μl microsyringe with fixed needle (e.g. Hamilton 701 or Dynatech A-100), connected by fine tubing to the glass micropipette used to inject the virus. The system is filled with paraffin oil before filling the micropipette with the virus.
(6) Suture material: e.g. Ethicon W502 (3/0) for skin sutures, W6594 (7/0) or W1708 (10/0) for nerve ligatures.
(7) Absorbable gelatine sponge.
(8) Heat pad for animals.

2.2 Stereotactic Injection of HSV-1 into the Brain

Items 1–8 above, plus:

(1) A small-animal stereotaxic frame.
(2) A dental drill with a fine tip.
(3) Bone wax.
(4) A stereotaxic atlas of the rat brain (Paxinos and Watson, 1986).

2.3 Perfusion-fixation of Infected Animals

(1) Surgical instruments.
(2) Infusion pump.
(3) Microsurgery microscope for dissection.
(4) Phosphate-buffered saline, 0.9%, pH 7.4 (PBS; standard buffer solution).
(5) Fixative: 4% paraformaldehyde in 0.1 M phosphate buffer, pH 7.4. For 1 liter: heat 500 ml distilled water to 70–80°C, add 40 g of paraformaldehyde and continue heating until it is dissolved. Add a few drops of 1 N NaOH until the solution becomes clear. Cool. Add 500 ml 0.2 M phosphate buffer. Filter and adjust the pH to 7.4.
(6) Fixative-sucrose solution: add 15% sucrose to the fixative solution (Step 5) and adjust the pH to 7.4.
(7) Solution for cryoprotecting the tissue before histological processing: 20% sucrose in 0.1 M phosphate buffer (pH 7.4–7.5).

2.4 Equipment for Histological Processing

(1) Freezing microtome or cryostat.
(2) Standard agitator.

2.5 Solutions for Immunoperoxidase Staining

(1) Buffer for diluting antibodies and washes: many standard buffers can be used, for example 0.1 M Tris buffer or PBS, provided that the pH is adjusted to 7.4.
(2) Diaminobenzidine (DAB) substrate solutions. Because DAB is carcinogenic, it is important to avoid exposure to the powder. As a substrate for HSV-1 immunoperoxidase staining, we make a solution of 0.05% DAB in PBS, pH 7.4. To enhance the staining, a solution of 0.03% DAB and 0.04–2.5% $NiSO_4$ in PBS (or Tris buffer) may be used. Good results can be also obtained with the metal-enhanced DAB substrate kit from Pierce (N. 34065).

2.6 Antibodies for HSV-1 Immunoperoxidase Detection (Ugolini, 1992)

(1) Primary antibody: rabbit polyclonal antibodies to HSV-1, followed by immunoperoxidase labeling with the peroxidase anti-peroxidase (PAP) method (Steps 2 and 3) or immunoperoxidase labeling with the Avidin-biotin method (ABC), using the Vectastain Elite ABC Kit, rabbit (Vector Labs, USA).
(2) Secondary antibody: swine anti-rabbit IgG.
(3) Rabbit peroxidase anti-peroxidase (PAP) complex, Z113 Dako Ltd.

3 THE PROTOCOLS

Protocol #142: Inoculation of HSV-1 into Peripheral Nerves

(1) Inoculate HSV-1 into peripheral nerves using glass micropipettes with long taper length (tip diameter 50–60 μm) (Ugolini et al., 1987; Ugolini, 1992).
(2) Lightly crush the nerve to maximize viral contact with nerve fibers just before introducing the taper of the micropipette into the nerve.
(3) Using surgical silk (size 10/0) make a ligature around the nerve proximal to the point where the micropipette has penetrated, to prevent any leakage of virus from the nerve. Keep the ligature in tension while inoculating with virus. After inoculation, withdraw the micropipette while further tightening the ligature, and wipe the area around the nerve with gelatine sponge. This procedure avoids leakage of virus from the nerve during or after the injection (Ugolini et al., 1987, 1989; Ugolini, 1992).

Protocol #143: Terminal Anesthesia, Transcardiac Perfusion, Tissue Fixation and Sectioning for Immunohistochemical Detection of HSV-1

(1) Anesthetize rats deeply, and wait for total absence of response to painful stimuli.
(2) Open abdomen and enlarge the incision to expose the diaphragm. Grasp the sternum with hemostat and cut a wide incision into the diaphragm. Cut sides of the rib cage to expose the thoracic cavity. Introduce a trocar into the left ventricle, taking care not to puncture the interventricular wall or the aorta.
(3) Perfuse with 60 ml PBS, pH 7.4, to wash out the blood (atrial effluent becomes clear). At the start of perfusion cut an incision into the right atrium.
(4) Continue the perfusion with 120 ml fixative.
(5) Complete the perfusion with 120 ml of fixative containing 15% sucrose.
(6) Dissect out brain, spinal cord or any other tissue of interest.
(7) Post-fix tissue in fixative solution containing 15% sucrose for 3–4 h at room temperature.
(8) Transfer tissue to ice-cold 20% sucrose in 0.1 M phosphate buffer (pH 7.4) for cryoprotection. Leave tissue in this solution until it sinks to the bottom of the vial (at least 24 h) before histological processing.
(9) Freeze tissue in dry ice and cut sections (30–60 μm) using a freezing microtome or a cryostat. Collect sections in four parallel series. Mount one series on gelatine-coated slides and counterstain with cresyl violet to determine cytoarchitectonic boundaries and virus-induced gross pathology. Collect the other three series free-floating in PBS, and use for detection of HSV-1 using immunoperoxidase or immunofluorescence.
(10) For long-term storage before processing keep free-floating sections at 4°C in PBS containing 0.05% sodium azide.

Protocol #144: Immunoperoxidase Detection of HSV-1 in Light Microscopy—Peroxidase-Antiperoxidase Method (PAP)

(1) Incubate free-floating sections at room temperature with gentle agitation in a solution of primary antibody (rabbit antiserum to HSV-1). Dilute the primary antiserum 1:50 in PBS for 3 h incubation, or 1:2000 for overnight incubation (Ugolini, 1992). Example of 1:2000

dilution: 10 μl primary antibody in 20 ml buffer.

(2) Wash sections in ten changes of PBS (3 min each change, total time 30 min).
(3) Incubate sections in the secondary antibody—an antibody directed against the species of the primary antibody. For example, if the primary antibody is rabbit anti-HSV-1, a suitable secondary antibody is swine anti-rabbit IgG, diluted 1:50 in PBS for 30 min incubation or 1:200 for 2 h incubation.
(4) Wash sections in PBS as in Step 2.
(5) Incubate sections in a peroxidase–antiperoxidase (PAP) complex, which must be raised in the same species as the primary antibody. For example, rabbit PAP diluted 1:200 in PBS for 2 h incubation.
(6) Wash sections in PBS as in Step 2.
(7) Incubate for 15 min in a solution of DAB (0.05% in PBS) or DAB–$NiSO_4$ (DAB 0.03%, $NiSO_4$ 0.04–2.5%). To visualize peroxidase activity add H_2O_2 (0.01%) and incubate for 2–12 min with constant agitation—the optimal incubation time will depend on the quantity of virus antigen present in the sections. Dispose safely of all solutions and materials containing, or which have been in contact with, DAB.
(8) Stop the peroxidase–DAB reaction by washing the sections in PBS as in Step 2.
(9) Mount sections on gelatine-coated slides, leave to air-dry for 24–48 h, and coverslip.

Protocol #145: Immunoperoxidase Detection of HSV-1 in Light Microscopy—Avidin-Biotin Method

(1) Incubate free-floating sections at room temperature with gentle agitation in a solution of primary antibody (e.g. rabbit antiserum to HSV-1). Dilute the primary antiserum 1:50 in PBS for 3 h incubation, or 1:2000 for overnight incubation (Ugolini, 1992).
(2) Wash sections in ten changes of PBS (3 min each change, total time 30 min).
(3) Incubate sections for 60–90 min in biotinylated secondary antibody, e.g. biotinylated goat anti-rabbit IgG diluted 1:200 in PBS.
(4) During Step 3 prepare the avidin–biotin–peroxidase complex (ABC); it must settle for at least 30 min before use. Using the Vectastain Elite Kit (Vector Labs, USA), the complex is prepared by adding 100 μl reagent A and 100 μl reagent B to 5 ml buffer.
(5) Wash sections in PBS as in Step 2.
(6) Incubate sections in the ABC complex for 1 h at room temperature.
(7) Wash sections in PBS as in Step 2.
(8) Incubate for 15 min in a solution of DAB or DAB-$NiSO_4$, stop the reaction and mount sections as in Steps 7–9 of Protocol #144.

Protocol #146: Two-color Immunoperoxidase Labeling of Pha-L Fibers and Terminals Impinging onto HSV-1 Infected Neurons

First part: immunoperoxidase detection of PHA-L (ABC method: Li et al., 1992b).

(1) Incubate the sections overnight at 4°C in goat anti-PHA-L serum, diluted 1:5000 in 0.1 M Tris buffer containing 1% normal horse serum (1% NHS-TBS) (pH 7.4).
(2) Wash the sections in 1% NHS-TBS.
(3) Incubate overnight at 4°C in biotinylated anti-goat IgG diluted 1:200 in 1% NHS-TBS.
(4) Wash the sections in several changes of 1% NHS-TBS (time 30 min).
(5) Incubate for 1 h in ABC, diluted 1:50 in 1% NHS-TBS. Prepare the ABC complex at least 30 min before use.
(6) Rinse briefly in 0.1 M acetate buffer (pH 6.0).
(7) Detect PHA-L immunoperoxidase staining by incubating the sections for 20 min in a solution containing 0.03% DAB, 2.5% nickel ammonium sulfate and 0.01% H_2O_2 in Tris buffer. Reaction product must become black.
(8) Wash in Tris buffer.

Second part: immunoperoxidase detection of HSV-1 infected neurons (ABC method).

(9) Incubate the sections overnight at 4°C in goat anti-HSV-1, diluted 1:5000 in 1% NHS-TBS.
(10) Repeat Steps 2–6.
(11) Detect HSV-1 immunoperoxidase labeling by incubating the sections for 10 min in a solution of 0.05% DAB and 0.01% H_2O_2 in Tris buffer. Reaction product should be brown.

Protocol #147: Colocalization of HSV-1 and Another Antigen with Double Immunofluorescence

(1) Dilute the primary antibodies (e.g. 1:500, see Gieroba et al., 1991; Li et al., 1992b) and incubate overnight at 4°C. Sections may be incubated simultaneously with both primary antibodies.
(2) Wash sections in several changes of buffer (e.g. 1% NHS-TBS).
(3) Incubate in secondary antibodies at the appropriate dilution, e.g. 1:80 for 1 h at room temperature (see Gieroba et al., 1991; Li et al., 1992b). Establish empirically the optimal dilutions and incubation times for first and second antibody for each antigen.
(4) Wash sections in several changes of buffer, mount and coverslip immediately with bicarbonate-buffered glycerol (pH 8.6) or other mounting medium for immunofluorescence.

4 NOTES AND TROUBLESHOOTING

4.1 On Protocol #142: Inoculation of HSV-1 into Peripheral Nerves

Leakage of virus from the injection site should be avoided, because it may result in unwanted uptake from neighboring structures. Measures for minimizing leakage of the virus are essentially the same as for conventional tracers: inoculate the smallest possible amount and leave the injection needle in place for a few minutes after the injection to minimize any reflux of virus along the needle track. If the virus is inoculated into a peripheral nerve, addition of a small amount of dye (e.g. pontamine sky blue, see Gieroba et al., 1991) to the virus will help to visualize the diffusion of the inoculum, but the dye must not interfere with viral replication.

4.1.1 Fragility of HSV-1

The titer of infectious virus, measured in plaque-forming units (p.f.u.) per milliliter, exerts a crucial role in HSV-1 infectivity. The ability of HSV-1 to infect neurons depends on the integrity of the viral envelope, which carries several glycoproteins involved in viral attachment and penetration (Roizman and Sears, 1990; Mettenleiter, 1994; Wildy, 1986). The envelope is very fragile and can be destroyed by alcohol, bleach, detergents, ultraviolet light, heat, desiccation, repeated freeze/thaw cycles and storage at −20°C. Microsyringes and surgical instruments used for the inoculations must be free of alcohol or detergents. Even the condition of storage of the virus stock is crucial: the virus must be kept at −70°C and the temperature of the freezer carefully monitored. The virus stock should be divided in small aliquots before freezing. Each aliquot must be thawed just before use and kept on ice during the time required to complete the inoculations. Unused virus must be discarded and not refrozen, because repeated freezing/thawing will affect the titer.

4.1.2 Safety Precautions

HSV-1 is a human pathogen and must be handled according to Biosafety level 2 (BSL 2) regulations. The main safety aspects are summarized below, but investigators should seek further advice from their local Biosafety Officer, because individual institutions may impose additional restrictions.

Experimental Facilities

The rooms for virus culture and storage, inoculations and animal housing should be used only for HSV-1 work. The doors should be labeled with biohazard signs and access to the rooms must be restricted to experienced personnel. The freezer used to store the virus should be locked and labeled with a biohazard sign. Infected animals should be housed individually and their cages labeled to identify the nature of the experiments. Infected primates must be housed in a squeeze cage. If infected animals are kept in the same room as stock animals, their cages should be distanced to avoid contact. It is best to keep infected and stock rodents in separate housing cabinets equipped with air filters.

Precautions

HSV-1 may be transmitted by aerosol, direct contact with oral and ocular mucosae and inoculation. Measures for avoiding contamination are straightforward and very effective: use of laboratory coat, gloves, goggles and a mask. All of these must be left in the BSL 2 facility at the end of the experiment. These protective garments should be worn when inoculating the virus, cleaning the cages of infected animals and carrying out the perfusion-fixation of infected animals. Histological handling is safe once the tissue is fixed with 4% paraformaldehyde, because the virus is inactivated by the fixative. When working in these conditions, the only risk of contamination is by autoinoculation: contaminated needles, microsyringes and sharp instruments should be handled with caution, and used needles should be promptly discarded in puncture-resistant containers. In the event of needle puncture, it is sufficient to make the wound bleed and clean it with detergent and 70% alcohol—these inactivate the virus.

Decontamination Procedures and Waste Disposal

HSV-1 is easily inactivated by detergents, alcohol, heat and fixatives. Surgical instruments, work surfaces and cages are usually decontaminated with bleach, quaternary ammonium disinfectant or strong detergents. Surgical instruments and cages should also be autoclaved. Unused virus is inactivated with bleach or 70% ethanol and discarded by incineration. All solid waste (surgical dressing, cage bedding, animal carcasses) should be double-bagged, labeled with a biohazard sign and incinerated.

4.2 Notes on the Choice of Animal Model: Species, Strain and Age

The choice of a suitable animal model is crucial for the success of transneuronal labeling with HSV-1. Not all species are equally susceptible to the virus, and great differences in susceptibility exist even between individuals of the same species, depending on genetic factors and age. In humans, for example, 80% of the population has been exposed to HSV-1 during childhood and has anti-HSV-1 antibodies, but only a few individuals develop recurrent HSV-1 infections (Wildy, 1986). Genetic differences in susceptibility to HSV-1 within the same species have been most clearly documented in inbred mice strains on the basis of median lethal dose tests: AKR and A/J strains are very susceptible to HSV-1; CBA and Balb/c are moderately susceptible and C57BL mice are resistant (Lopez, 1975, 1985). The genetic resistance to HSV-1 is transmitted as a dominant trait governed by at least two loci, and is mediated by natural defense mechanisms that do not require previous exposure to the virus (Lopez, 1985). These genetic differences are correlated with great differences in the extent of transneuronal transfer of HSV-1. Inoculation of a high dose of HSV-1 into the hypoglossal (XII) nerve of "resistant" C57BL mice (8 weeks old) produces infection of only a few XII motoneurons and transneuronal transfer does not occur (Ugolini, unpublished observations). In contrast, if the same dose of virus is inoculated into the XII nerve of "susceptible" Balb/c mice of the same age, the infection involves a great number of XII motoneurons and retrograde transneuronal labeling can extend to all groups of second-order neurons (Ugolini et al., 1987).

Within a given species and strain, the susceptibility to HSV-1 is also age-dependent. For example, C57BL mice are resistant to HSV-1 as adults, but susceptible as neonates, resistance developing at about 3 weeks of age (Zawatzky et al., 1982). Even in a susceptible mouse strain (such as Balb/c), susceptibility to HSV-1 is greatest in neonates and progressively decreases with age: a first drop occurs by the fourth week of age, an intermediate stage of susceptibility is observed between the fourth and eighth weeks and resistance is reached by 15–20 weeks (Hirsch et al., 1970; Nash and Wildy, 1983). This reflects maturation of natural defense mechanisms.

Therefore the animal species, the strain and even the age of the animals used must be carefully chosen when designing the experiments. We have obtained very extensive transneuronal labeling using the SC16 strain of HSV-1 in Balb/c mice (Ugolini et al., 1987) and Wistar rats (Ugolini et al., 1989; Ugolini, 1992) 8 weeks of age. Successful results have also been obtained in ICR mice (Margolis et al., 1989), Fisher rats (Blessing et al., 1991), Sprague-Dawley and Long-Evans rats (McLean et al., 1989), golden hamsters (Norgren et al., 1992) and New Zealand White rabbits (Gieroba et al., 1991; Li et al., 1992a, b). Transfer of HSV-1 has never been tested in cats. Transneuronal labeling may be obtained in experimental primates with HSV-1, but it is not always successful, and could depend on the primate species, the virus strain and/or the route of inoculation. We have obtained negative results after inoculating HSV-1 (strain SC16) into peripheral nerves of *Macaca fascicularis*, although we had attempted to maximize infectivity by using young animals and inoculating a very high dose of a virus stock that was cultured in primate (Vero) cells (Ugolini, unpublished observations). In contrast, transneuronal transfer of HSV-1 (strains McIntyre-B and H129) is successful after intracortical injections in cebus monkey (Zemanick et al., 1991; Hoover and Strick, 1993; Middleton and Strick, 1994). The possibility of applying the methodology to primates, at least after cortical inoculation, is an advantage of HSV-1 over PRV, which does not infect primates even by the intracortical route (Strick and Card, 1992).

4.3 Choice of HSV-1 Strain

Different strains of HSV-1 may not be equally suitable as transneuronal tracers, because they exhibit dramatic differences in neuroinvasiveness (see Dix et al., 1983). The transneuronal transfer properties of only a few HSV-1 strains have so far been characterized.

Strain SC16 is very effective in Wistar rats and Balb/c mice (Ugolini et al., 1987, 1989; Ugolini, 1992). After administration of high doses, transfer of this strain is extensive both in the anterograde and retrograde directions and can involve all groups of first- and second-order neurons as well as third-order neurons (Ugolini et al., 1987, 1989; Ugolini, 1992) (Fig. 25.1). Strain HFEM is also very effective (Ugolini, unpublished results). In rodents HSV-1 transneuronal labeling has also been obtained with the F strain and the McKrea strain in Balb/c and ICR mice (Margolis et al., 1989; La Vail et al., 1990, 1993), the FMC-1 and FMC-134 strains in rats and rabbits (Blessing et al., 1991; Li et al., 1992a) and the McIntyre strain in Sprague-Dawley rats and golden hamsters (McLean et al., 1989; Norgren et al., 1992).

After intracortical inoculation in primates, strains H129 and McIntyre-B differ greatly in preferential direction of transfer: H129 is transferred especially in the anterograde direction, McIntyre-B almost exclusively in the retrograde direction (Zemanick et al., 1991). The preferential retrograde transfer of the McIntyre strain can be exploited in primates for tracing second-order neurons that provide cortical input (Hoover and Strick, 1993; Middleton and Strick, 1994). However, this property may not hold in all systems and species: in rats and hamsters, for example, McIntyre is transferred anterogradely in visual pathways (Norgren et al., 1992) and bidirectionally in the olfactory system (McLean et al., 1989). After inoculation into the vitreous body, anterograde transneuronal transfer of the McIntyre strain leaves unlabeled specific subsets of retinorecipient neurons (Norgren et al., 1992) that can be infected by other strains of alpha-herpesviruses (Card et al., 1991; Norgren et al., 1992). The same deficit is produced by the attenuated Bartha strain of PRV (Card et al., 1991, 1992). For Bartha PRV, this is due to mutation of the genes encoding the viral envelope glycoproteins gE and gI (previously designated gI and gp63) (Card et al., 1992; Whealy et al., 1993; Standish et al., 1994), which also affect retrograde transneuronal transfer of Bartha PRV to specific subsets of autonomic neurons (Standish et al., 1994). Regardless of the precise location of gene mutations responsible for the similarity in the behavior of McIntyre (HSV-1) and Bartha (PRV), these two strains can fail to label some groups of neurons; therefore they may not be the viral tracers of choice if the aim is to map all groups of neurons that are part of a given neuronal circuit. For this purpose it may be better to use strains such as SC16.

A well characterized strain of virus should be used. Even if one strain is able to infect all categories of neurons in a given neuronal system, other neuronal types may not have the same permissiveness to the virus. For example, viral uptake and transneuronal transfer may be delayed, or may not occur at all in some categories of neurons, and the picture of the circuit provided by viral tracing may be incomplete. Thus, the results of viral transneuronal tracing should be always correlated with data obtained with conventional tracing methods, regardless of the virus strain used.

4.4 Importance of Virus Dose

Successful infection of first-order neurons and transneuronal transfer require high doses of virus: for example, the minimal dose for inoculation into the hypoglossal nerve of mice is 10^4 p.f.u. (as contained in 0.8 μl stock with a titer of 10^7 p.f.u./ml) (Ugolini et al., 1987). Even when the titer of the HSV-1 stock is very high (e.g. 10^9 p.f.u./ml), small variations in the amount given (0.2–0.8 microliters) can cause variability of results (Ugolini et al., 1987). If the dose is kept constant and very high (e.g. 10^7 p.f.u.) results are highly reproducible (Ugolini et al., 1989; Ugolini, 1992). In these conditions infectivity is obtained in 100% of the animals, transneuronal transfer is strictly time-dependent and can involve all groups of second-order neurons as well as third-order neurons (Ugolini et al., 1989; Ugolini, 1992). The same considerations apply to the use of PRV: high-titer stocks (5×10^8 p.f.u./ml) and inoculation of high doses (10^6 p.f.u.) result in 100% infectivity and extensive transneuronal transfer (Card et al., 1991; Loewy et al., 1991; Strick and Card, 1992), whereas lower titers (2×10^5 p.f.u./ml) and/or administration of low doses (e.g. 10^3 p.f.u.) result in low infectivity rates (20%) and variability of results (Strack et al., 1989a, b; Strack and Loewy, 1990; Loewy et al., 1991).

To obtain highly reproducible results and maximize the extent of transneuronal transfer to second- and third-order neurons, we recommend choosing a high-titer virus stock, using the same stock for a series of experiments and injecting a high, constant, dose (10^7–10^8 p.f.u.) (Ugolini, 1992). However, high doses may also increase the chance of local (non-specific) spread of virus from first-order neurons to nearby cells. Local spread may be minimized by monitoring the time following inoculation, because local spread is time dependent and partially delayed relative to transneuronal transfer (Ugolini et al., 1987; Kuypers and Ugolini, 1990; Ugolini, 1992, 1995). Another measure for minimizing local spread is to inoculate small doses, as for PRV (Loewy et al., 1991; Jansen et al., 1993). However, the optimal dose should be determined empirically for each system. The problem with administering low doses is that the efficiency of transneuronal transfer is reduced because it is dose-dependent: some groups of second-order neurons and all third-order neurons are likely to be left unlabeled (Strack et al., 1989a, b; Strack and Loewy, 1990).

4.5 On Protocols #144 and 145: Immunohistochemical Methods for Detection of HSV-1 in Light Microscopy

HSV-1 can be detected easily with standard immunohistochemical methods—immunofluorescence and immunoperoxidase (peroxidase–antiperoxidase and avidin–biotin complex) (La Vail et al., 1990; Li et al., 1992b; Ugolini, 1992). The sensitivity of the immunolabeling depends on the fixative, the histological processing and the primary antibodies used. Paraformaldehyde (4%) is a good fixative but glutaraldehyde should be avoided, even in small amounts, because it inactivates most HSV-1 antigens. The best immunolabeling results are obtained using frozen sections and reacting free-floating the sections. Immunoperoxidase staining can also be carried out on paraffin-embedded sections (Ugolini et al., 1987), but sensitivity is lower. It is better to use polyclonal antibodies generated against the entire virus as a primary antibody, because they can recognize all major antigenic determinants and produce intense, often Golgi-like, staining of neuronal cell bodies, nuclei, dendrites and axons (Ugolini, 1992) (Fig. 25.1). Antibodies directed against individual viral glycoproteins are generally less suitable because they produce weak labeling. When carrying out immunohistochemistry, the specificity and sensitivity of the staining should be checked by reacting the first series of sections from a new case together with negative and positive controls. As positive control we routinely use the second and third series of sections from a case that has shown HSV-1 immunolabeling in the first series. In all immunolabeling protocols, primary and secondary antibodies can be used several times if 0.02% sodium azide is added to the diluted samples and the samples are stored at 4°C. Never add sodium azide to the PAP complex used for immunoperoxidase detection because sodium azide blocks peroxidase activity and ruins the reaction.

Immunoperoxidase staining is our method of choice, because it provides permanent staining. The labeling in immunofluorescence fades very quickly. However, the advantage of immunofluorescence is that it is possible to colocalize HSV-1 and another antigen in the same neurons with double immunofluorescence, by tagging the secondary antibodies to the two antigens with two different fluorescent chromophores.

4.6 On Protocol #147: Colocalization of HSV-1 and Another Antigen with Double Immunofluorescence

With double immunofluorescence, HSV-1 can be colocalized with several neurotransmitter-related antigens and specific glial cell markers (Blessing et al., 1991; Gieroba et al., 1991; Li et al., 1992b). However, care must be taken if the results of colocalization are negative: HSV-1 replication blocks protein synthesis of the host cell so it can also affect neurotransmitter turnover, especially if it is rapid, and produce false negative results. To maximize the chances of successful colocalization in a given neuronal cell group, double immunofluorescence should be carried out at early times of infection. The optimal time may be defined by studying the kinetics of the infection of the neuronal cell group in question.

Immunofluorescence can be carried out on free-floating sections or on sections mounted on slides. Slide-mounted sections should be stored at −20°C if they are not processed immediately, because antigenicity is lost during prolonged storage at higher temperatures.

The primary antibodies to the two antigens must be raised in two different species. For example, for colocalization of HSV-1 and neurotransmitters, Blessing and collaborators have used goat anti-HSV-1 antiserum in combination with rabbit anti-tyrosine hydroxylase, rat monoclonal anti-5-hydroxytryptamine (5HT) or mouse monoclonal anti-PH8 (a marker for serotonin synthesis) (Gieroba et al., 1991; Li et al., 1992b).

The two secondary antibodies must be directed against the species of the corresponding primary antibody and tagged with a different fluorophor, e.g. fluorescein and tetramethyl-rhodamine, which produce green and red fluorescence respectively. For example, if goat anti-HSV-1 and rabbit anti-TH are used as primary antibodies, secondary antibodies may be a combination of fluorescein-labeled swine anti-goat IgG (for green fluorescent labeling of HSV-1 infected neurons) and rhodamine-labeled swine anti-rabbit IgG (for red fluorescent labeling of TH-positive neurons) (Gieroba et al., 1991; Li et al., 1992b).

4.7 Notes on Combination of HSV-1 Immunostaining with Other Methodologies

A two-color immunoperoxidase protocol has been developed to combine HSV-1 labeling of neurons (brown) with PHA-L labeling of fibers and terminals (black) (Li et al., 1992b; See Protocol #146). This is useful for studying synaptic contacts between PHA-L-labeled terminals and HSV-1-labeled neurons. An advantage of this over immunofluorescence is that the staining is permanent.

Immunofluorescence labeling of first-order neurons infected with HSV-1 (and PRV) can be combined with retrograde labeling of the same or other neurons using a conventional tracer. This can serve to study the efficiency of viral uptake or to check whether the virus can spread locally from infected first-order neurons to nearby neurons that supply a different site. For this combination to be valuable, it is crucial that the second tracer does not interfere with replication of the virus. The fluorescent tracer Fluorogold is unsuitable because it impairs HSV-1 replication and can produce false-negative results (La Vail et al., 1993). Other fluorescent probes that bind to DNA and/or RNA are also likely to interfere with viral replication. In contrast, the Wheatgerm agglutinin–horseradish peroxidase conjugate (WGA–HRP) (2.5% in saline) appears to be suitable: after sequential injection of virus and WGA–HRP (1 day later) at the same site, most neurons are double labeled (Strack and Loewy, 1990), suggesting that WGA–HRP does not affect viral uptake or replication. The cholera toxin–horseradish peroxidase conjugate (CT–HRP) (0.25%) can also be used (Card et al., 1993). Double labeling of infected neurons with WGA–HRP or CT–HRP is visualized with double immunofluorescence (Strack and Loewy, 1990; Card et al., 1993). HSV-1 infected neurons can also be double-labeled with the tracer DiI (Li et al., 1992a), but the amount of colocalization is not as good as for the combination of virus and WGA–HRP: when DiI is injected into the adrenal gland immediately before the virus only approximately 45% of HSV-1-positive first-order neurons also contain DiI and only 60% of DiI-labeled neurons also contain HSV-1 (Li et al., 1992a). Since DiI is dissolved in ethanol (Li et al., 1992a), it may be that the presence of ethanol at the injection site may affect the virus.

4.8 Notes on Other Methods for Detection of HSV-1 in Light Microscopy

A new method for detecting alpha-herpesviruses is based on the insertion into the viral genome of the marker *lacZ* gene encoding β-galactosidase, which is expressed during viral replication. This can be convenient for rapid screening of infected neurons, because β-galactosidase labeling may be detected with a simple histochemical reaction (Loewy et al., 1991; Babic et al., 1993), but it may be less satisfactory than immunohistochemistry because the labeling may diffuse from heavily infected cells (Babic et al., 1993). A potential problem of viral constructs carrying foreign genes as markers is the fact that the gene insertion may modify the pattern of transfer of the virus. This should not occur if the gene is inserted into a region of the viral genome that does not play a role in replication or transneuronal transfer, such as the gene encoding the non-essential viral glycoprotein gG of PRV (previously designated gX) (Loewy et al., 1991; Babic et al., 1993). However, it is always preferable to check whether a viral construct can produce the same pattern of transfer as the viral strain of origin.

Another technique for detecting HSV-1 is based on systemic administration of tritiated thymidine, which is incorporated by infected cells during virus replication (Margolis et al, 1987, 1989). However, this method is not recommended because it is time-consuming and insensitive. Detection requires at least 4 weeks of autoradiographic exposure and the labeling is weak and largely confined to cell nuclei.

4.9 Interpretation of Results

4.9.1 Kinetics of Neuronal Infection and Virus-induced Neuronal Degeneration

Immunolabeling in HSV-1 infected neurons is initially restricted to the sites of assembly and packaging of replicated virus: the nucleus, cytoplasm, and proximal dendrites. Later, when replicated virus is transported centrifugally and begins to be transferred transneuronally, the labeling extends to distal dendrites and axons (Fig. 25.1). Infected neurons initially show normal morphology (Fig. 25.1) (Ugolini et al., 1987; Ugolini, 1992) but later degenerate, showing a great increase in cell size and loss of Nissl staining (Ugolini et al., 1987; Ugolini, 1992; Babic et al., 1993). Neuronal degeneration is unavoidable with all strains of alpha-herpesviruses that function as transneuronal tracers, because replication of the virus causes a complete shut-off of the metabolism of the host cell (Roizman and Sears, 1990). Virus-induced degeneration of first-order neurons is inevitably obtained at the times required for visualization of transneuronal labeling (Ugolini et al., 1987; Ugolini, 1992).

4.9.2 Bidirectional Transfer

The transneuronal transfer of HSV-1 can occur both anterogradely (from afferent fibers to post-synaptic (second-order) neurons) and retrogradely (from the cell bodies and dendrites of first-order neurons to presynaptic terminals of second-order neurons and then from these terminals to their parent cell bodies). Retrograde transneuronal transfer is always very effective, even over long distances (Ugolini et al., 1989), whereas the efficiency of anterograde transneuronal transfer depends on the distance between the first- and second-order neurons: transfer is extensive over short distances, e.g. from primary sensory neurons in dorsal root ganglia to connected spinal regions (Fig. 25.2), but does not occur over long distances, e.g. from dorsal root ganglion neurons to dorsal column nuclei (Ugolini et al., 1989; Ugolini, 1992). This phenomenon has a simple explanation: the neurons that transport the virus anterogradely are affected by viral replication in their cell bodies, and this impairs anterograde axonal transport of the virus over long distances. In contrast, the neurons infected by retrograde transneuronal transfer are still healthy when they transport the virus retrogradely through their axons because this transport precedes replication of the virus in their cell body (Ugolini et al., 1989).

4.9.3 Possibility of Local Spread

Although most of the propagation of alpha-herpesviruses is mediated by transneuronal transfer, a small amount of local spread may also occur (Ugolini et al., 1987; Loewy et al., 1991; Li et al., 1992a; Ugolini, 1992; Babic et al., 1993; Jansen et al., 1993). At the times required for transneuronal labeling the "problem area" of local spread is the immediate proximity of the cell bodies and axons of first-order neurons, i.e. neurons that are affected by long-standing infection (Ugolini et al., 1987; Loewy et al., 1991; Li et al., 1992a; Ugolini, 1992; Babic et al., 1993). The extent of local spread in this region is variable: it may involve only glial cells, where viral replication is abortive (Card et al., 1993), or may also extend to local neurons, but it does not cause uptake by fibers of passage (Ugolini et al., 1987, 1989; Loewy et al., 1991; Li et al., 1992a; Ugolini, 1992; Card et al., 1993). Spurious neuronal labeling resulting from local spread may be a problem, because it may be difficult to distinguish from transneuronal labeling of local interneurons. Moreover, the neurons infected by local spread may transfer the virus transneuronally to connected neurons (Ugolini et al., 1987). For example, local spread from hypoglossal axons can produce spurious labeling of neurons in the inferior olive, which can be followed by anterograde transneuronal transfer through olivocerebellar fibers to the cerebellar cortex (Ugolini et al., 1987).

The possibility of a small amount of local spread should always be considered at long times after inoculation, because no strain of alpha-herpesvirus without the potential to produce local spread has been found. The ideal strain may not exist, because both transneuronal transfer and local spread depend upon the same viral envelope glycoprotein (gB, previously called gII for PRV) (Babic et al., 1993). Local spread is, like transneuronal transfer, dose- and time-dependent but is less likely to occur. It is therefore possible to obtain transneuronal transfer in the absence of local spread by monitoring the time or by inoculating small doses of virus. The optimal parameters should be determined empirically for each system. Administering small doses is also likely to reduce the efficiency of transneuronal transfer. In contrast, injecting high doses will maximize transneuronal transfer, but in these conditions a small amount of local spread may be unavoidable, especially at the long times required for transneuronal labeling of third-order neurons (SEE SECTION 4.4, PAGE 358).

4.9.4 Kinetics of Transneuronal Transfer and the Possibility of Asynchronous Labeling of Different Groups of Second-order Neurons

The intense labeling of first-, second- and even third-order neurons is a unique advantage of transneuronal tracing with alpha-herpesviruses. A practical problem is that first-, second- and third-order neurons cannot be distinguished on the basis of differences in the intensity of labeling (Fig. 25.1). To make this distinction the propagation of the viruses must be studied at sequential intervals after injection of a constant dose. In this manner first-, second- and third-order neurons can be identified on the basis of their sequential appearance (Ugolini et al., 1987; Margolis et al., 1989; Card et al., 1991; Ugolini, 1992) because transneuronal transfer is strictly time-dependent.

Interpretation of the kinetics of transfer may be complicated by the fact that different groups of second-order neurons are not always labeled in synchrony (Ugolini et al., 1987; Ugolini, 1992). The different speed of visualization of these cell groups may be determined by differences in synaptic density, receptor differences and the route of inoculation. Take, for example, the transfer of HSV-1 after inoculation into forelimb mixed nerves (Fig. 25.2): the virus is transferred through all classes of infected axons, but this transfer does not occur in synchrony (Ugolini, 1992). The speed of viral transneuronal transfer in this system is inversely correlated with the diameter of the axons of first-order neurons (Fig. 25.2) (Ugolini, 1992). Thus, anterograde transneuronal transfer through small diameter (unmyelinated or small myelinated) sensory afferents to superficial dorsal horn laminae precedes transfer via large (myelinated) sensory afferents to deeper laminae (Fig. 25.2). Similarly, retrograde transneuronal transfer from small (largely unmyelinated) sympathetic axons to sympathetic preganglionic neurons precedes transfer from large (myelinated) motor axons (Fig. 25.2) (Ugolini, 1992). In this model the greater speed of transfer through small relative to large axons may be determined by the route of inoculation: the myelin sheet of Schwann cells may delay uptake from large (myelinated) axons (Ugolini, 1992).

Asynchronous labeling of different groups of second neurons may also occur during retrograde transneuronal transfer of the virus from the same group of first-order neurons—e.g. sympathetic neurons or motoneurons (Ugolini et al., 1987; Ugolini, 1992). The speed of transfer to the various groups of second-order neurons may depend on the strength of connection with the transferring (first-order) neurons. For example, in the transneuronal transfer of HSV-1 from the stellate ganglion to sympathetic preganglionic cell groups initially the labeling involves only the cell groups containing the greatest number of neurons that supply the stellate ganglion (Fig. 25.2); later, it also extends to cell groups with only a few connections to the stellate ganglion (Ugolini, 1992). Asynchronous labeling of different groups of second-order neurons can also occur with PRV (Card et al., 1991).

In view of this, the possibility of non-synchronous labeling of different groups of second-order neurons should always be considered. This phenomenon will not mislead the interpretation of the results obtained at short times because all neurons labeled at the onset of transneuronal transfer can be regarded as second order, although the labeling at these times may not comprise all second-order neurons (Card et al., 1991; Ugolini, 1992). At later times, however, it may be difficult to distinguish the delayed labeling of the last groups of second-order neurons from early labeling of third-order neurons (and eventual spurious labeling that might be produced by local spread at these times) (Ugolini, 1992). Therefore the study of transneuronal labeling should never be limited to only one time point, and the results should always be cross-referenced with other methods (Ugolini, 1992, 1995). If these aspects of the behavior of HSV-1 are carefully taken into account, transneuronal tracing with HSV-1 is a very powerful tool for unraveling neuronal connections.

ACKNOWLEDGMENTS

I wish to thank S. Brasiles for assistance with photography. This work was supported by the CNRS (UPR 2431).

REFERENCES

Babic, N., Mettenleiter, T.C., Flamand, A., and Ugolini, G. (1993) "Role of essential glycoproteins gII and gp50 in transneuronal transfer of Pseudorabies virus from the hypoglossal nerve of mice", *J. Virol.* **67,** 4421–4426.

Blessing, W.W., Li, Y.-W., and Wesselingh, S.L. (1991) "Transneuronal transport of herpes simplex virus from the cervical vagus to brain neurons with axonal input to central vagal sensory nuclei in the rat", *Neuroscience* **42,** 261–274.

Card, J.P., Rinaman, L., Lynn, R.B., Lee, B.-H., Meade, R.P., Miselis, R.R., and Enquist, L.W. (1993) "Pseudorabies virus infection of the rat central nervous system: ultrastructural characterization of viral replication, transport and pathogenesis", *J. Neurosci.* **13,** 2515–2539.

Card, J.P., Whealy, M.E., Robbins, A.K., and Enquist, L.W. (1992) "Pseudorabies virus envelope glycoprotein gI influences both neurotropism and virulence during infection of the rat visual system", *J. Virol.* **66,** 3032–3041.

Card, J.P., Whealy, M.E., Robbins, A.K., Moore, R.Y., and Enquist, L.W. (1991) "Two α-herpesvirus strains are transported differentially in the rodent visual system", *Neuron* **6,** 957–969.

Dix, R.D., McKendall, R.R., and Baringer, J.R. (1983) "Comparative neurovirulence of herpes simplex virus type 1 strains after peripheral or intracerebral inoculation of Balb/c mice", *Infect. Immun.* **40,** 103–112.

Gieroba, Z.J., Li, Y.-W., Wesselingh, S.L., and Blessing, W.W. (1991) "Transneuronal labeling of neurons in rabbit brain after injection of herpes simplex virus type 1 into the aortic depressor nerve", *Brain Res.* **558,**

264–272.

Gosztonyi, G., Falke, D., and Ludwig, H. (1992) "Axonal and transsynaptic (transneuronal) spread of Herpesvirus simiae (B virus) in experimentally infected mice", *Histol. Histopathol.* **7,** 63–74.

Hirsch, M.S., Zisman, B., and Allison, A.C. (1970) "Macrophage and age-dependent resistance to herpes simplex virus in mice", *J. Immunol.* **104,** 1160–1165.

Hoover, J.E., and Strick, P.L. (1993) "Multiple output channels in the basal ganglia", *Science* **259,** 819–821.

Jansen, A.S.P., Farwell, D.G., and Loewy, A.D. (1993) "Specificity of pseudorabies virus as a retrograde marker of sympathetic preganglionic neurons: implications for transneuronal labeling studies", *Brain Res.* **617,** 103–112.

Kuypers, H.G.J.M., and Ugolini, G. (1990) "Viruses as transneuronal tracers", *Trends Neurosci.* **13,** 71–75.

La Vail, J.H., Carter, S.R., and Topp, K.S. (1993) "The retrograde tracer Fluoro-Gold interferes with the infectivity of Herpes Simplex Virus", *Brain Res.* **625,** 57–62.

La Vail, J.H., Zhan, J., and Margolis, T.P. (1990) "HSV (type 1) infection of the trigeminal complex", *Brain Res.* **514,** 181–188.

Li, Y.-W., Ding, Z-Q., Wesselingh, S.L., and Blessing, W.W. (1992a) "Renal and adrenal sympathetic preganglionic neurons in rabbit spinal cord: tracing with Herpes simplex virus", *Brain Res.* **573,** 147–152.

Li, Y.-W., Wesselingh, S.L., and Blessing, W.W. (1992b) "Projections from rabbit caudal medulla to C1 and A5 sympathetic premotor neurons, demonstrated with phaseolus agglutinin and herpes simplex virus", *J. Comp. Neurol.* **317,** 379–395.

Loewy, A.D., Bridgman, P.C., and Mettenleiter, T.C. (1991) "β-galactosidase expressing recombinant pseudorabies virus for light and electron microscopic study of transneuronally labeled CNS neurons", *Brain Res.* **555,** 346–352.

Lopez, C. (1975) "Genetics of natural resistance to herpesvirus infections in mice", *Nature* **258,** 152–153.

Lopez, C. (1985) "Natural resistance mechanisms in herpes simplex virus infection", in *The Herpesviruses* (Ed. B. Roizman), Vol. 4, pp. 37–68, Plenum Press, New York.

Margolis, T.P., La Vail, J.H., Setzer, P.Y., and Dawson, C.R. (1989) "Selective spread of herpes simplex virus in the central nervous system after ocular inoculation", *J. Virol.* **63,** 4756–4761.

Margolis, T.P., Togni, B., La Vail, J.H., and Dawson, C.R. (1987) "Identifying HSV infected neurons after ocular inoculation", *Curr. Eye Res.* **6,** 119–126.

Martin, X., and Dolivo, M. (1983) "Neuronal and transneuronal tracing in the trigeminal system of the rat using the Herpes Virus Suis", *Brain Res.* **273,** 253–276.

McLean, J.H., Shipley, M.T., and Bernstein, D.I. (1989) "Golgi-like, transneuronal retrograde labelling with CNS injections of Herpes Simplex Virus type 1", *Brain Res. Bull.* **22,** 867–881.

Mettenleiter, T.C. (1994) "Initiation and spread of α-herpesvirus infections", *Trends Microbiol.* **2,** 2–4.

Middleton, F.A., and Strick, P.L. (1994) "Anatomical evidence for cerebellar and basal ganglia involvement in higher cognitive function", *Science* **266,** 458–461.

Nash, A.A., and Wildy, P. (1983) "Immunity in relation to the pathogenesis of herpes simplex virus", in *Human Immunity to Viruses* (Ed. F. Ennis), pp. 179–192, Academic Press, New York.

Norgren, R.B. Jr., McLean, J.H., Bubel, H.C., Wander, A. Bernstein, D.I., and Lehman, M.N. (1992) "Anterograde transport of HSV-1 and HSV-2 in the visual system", *Brain Res. Bull.* **28,** 393–399.

Paxinos, G., and Watson, C. (1986) *The Rat Brain in Stereotaxic coordinates*, 2nd edition, Academic Press, New York.

Roizman, B., and Sears, A.E. (1990) "Herpes simplex viruses and their replication", in *Fields Virology*, second edition (Eds. B.N. Fields and D.M. Knipe), pp. 1795–1841, Raven Press, New York.

Standish, A., Enquist, L.W., and Schwaber, J.S. (1994) "Innervation of the heart and its central medullary origin defined by viral tracing", *Science* **263,** 232–234.

Strack, A.M., and Loewy, A.D. (1990) "Pseudorabies virus: a highly specific transneuronal cell body marker in the sympathetic nervous system", *J. Neurosci.* **10,** 2139–2147.

Strack, A.M., Sawyer, W.B., Hughes, J.H., Platt, K.B., and Loewy, A.D. (1989a) "A general pattern of CNS innervation of the sympathetic outflow demonstrated by transneuronal pseudorabies viral infections", *Brain Res.* **491,** 156–162.

Strack, A.M., Sawyer, W.B., Platt, K.B., and Loewy, A.D. (1989b) "CNS cell groups regulating the sympathetic outflow to adrenal gland as revealed by transneuronal cell body labeling with pseudorabies virus", *Brain Res.* **491,** 274–296.

Strick, P.L., and Card, J.P. (1992) "Transneuronal mapping of neural circuits with alpha herpesviruses", in *Experimental Neuroanatomy. A practical approach* (Ed. J.P. Bolam), pp. 81–101, IRL Press, Oxford.

Ugolini, G. (1992) "Transneuronal transfer of Herpes Simplex Virus type 1 (HSV-1) from mixed limb nerves to the CNS. I. Sequence of transfer from sensory, motor and sympathetic nerve fibres to the spinal cord", *J. Comp. Neurol.* **326,** 527–548.

Ugolini, G. (1995) "Transneuronal tracing with alpha-herpesviruses: a review of the methodology", in *Viral*

Vectors: Gene Therapy and Neuroscience Applications (Eds M.G. Kaplitt and A.D. Loewy), pp.293–317. Academic Press, New York.

Ugolini, G., Kuypers, H.G.J.M., and Simmons, A. (1987) "Retrograde transneuronal transfer of Herpes Simplex Virus type 1 (HSV-1) from motoneurones", *Brain Research* **422,** 242–256.

Ugolini, G., Kuypers, H.G.J.M., and Strick, P.L. (1989) "Transneuronal transfer of Herpes Virus from peripheral nerves to cortex and brainstem", *Science* **243,** 89–91.

Whealy, M.E., Card, J.P., Robbins, A.K., Dubin, J.R., Rziha, H.-J., and Enquist, L.W. (1993) "Specific pseudorabies virus infection of the rat visual system requires both gI and gp63 glycoproteins", *J. Virol.* **67,** 3786–3797.

Wildy, P. (1986) "Herpesvirus", in *Portraits of viruses, Intervirology Vol.* 25 (Ed. F. Rapp), pp. 117–140, S. Karger AG, Basel.

Zawatzky, R., Engler, H., and Kirchner, H. (1982) "Experimental infection of inbred mice with herpes simplex virus. III. Comparison between newborn and adult C57BL/6 mice", *J. Gen. Virol.* **60,** 25–29.

Zemanick, M.C., Strick, P.L., and Dix, R.D. (1991) "Direction of transneuronal transport of herpes simplex virus 1 in the primate motor system is strain-dependent", *Proc. Natl Acad. Sci. USA,* **88,** 8048–8051.

CHAPTER 26

Immune Responses to Viruses: Practical Implications for the Use of Viruses as Vectors for Experimental and Clinical Gene Therapy

Matthew J.A. Wood, Andrew P. Byrnes, Mary McMenamin, Koji Kajiwara, Alison Vine, Ian Gordon, Jill Lang, Kathryn J. Wood* and Harry M. Charlton

Department of Human Anatomy, South Parks Road, Oxford OX1 3QX, UK. Tel: 01865 272 145; Fax: 01865 272 420; Email: mjwood@vax.ox.ac.uk

**Nuffield Department of Surgery, University of Oxford, John Radcliffe Hospital, Oxford, OX3 9DU, UK. Tel: 01865 221 300; Fax: 01865 63545; Email: kathryn.wood@nds.ox.ac.uk*

1 INTRODUCTION

There is considerable interest in gene therapy as a treatment for human neurogenetic and neurodegenerative disease and as a tool for research (Friedmann, 1994). The only current method for transfecting appreciable numbers of adult central nervous system (CNS) cells *in vivo* is to use a non-replicating virus as a vector. Herpes simplex virus type I (HSV-1) (Chiocca et al., 1990; Kaplitt et al., 1991), adenovirus (Akli et al., 1993; Bajocchi et al., 1993; Davidson et al., 1993; Le Gal La Salle et al., 1993) and adeno-associated virus (AAV) (Kaplitt et al., 1994) have all been successfully exploited, but their possible toxic effects on brain cells or harmful interactions with the immune system have yet to be fully evaluated. Neurotoxic or immune effects, in addition to their potential damaging consequences for cells of the CNS, seem to play a significant role in limiting vector-driven gene expression. The construction of non-replicating DNA viral vectors is described elsewhere in this volume, and has recently been reviewed (Ali et al., 1994). In this chapter we briefly outline the nature of the immune response to viruses and non-replicating viral vectors in the CNS, and give a detailed discussion of the experimental approaches that can be used to investigate immune responses in the brain.

The CNS was originally thought to be an immunologically privileged site but it is now known to have only relative protection from the potentially deleterious effects of the immune system, and complex regulatory mechanisms are thought to control immune function in the CNS (Sloan et al., 1991; Perry et al., 1993). Cytokines (low molecular weight soluble proteins) are known to mediate and regulate the local pro- and anti-inflammatory effects of the immune system within the brain. Microglia and astrocytes, quiescent immunocompetent cells within the brain, can be activated by a variety of stimuli to secrete and respond to cytokines, express major histocompatibility complex (MHC) class I and class II antigens (essential for antigen presentation to and activation of T lymphocytes), and present peptide antigens to T lymphocytes (Perry et al., 1993). Stimuli include

Protocols for Gene Transfer in Neuroscience: Towards Gene Therapy of Neurological Disorders
Edited by P.R. Lowenstein and L.W. Enquist

brain trauma (such as that associated with stereotaxic injections of viral vector into the CNS using a micropipette) and viral infection. Brain trauma stimulates glia and neurons to produce pro-inflammatory cytokines interleukin 1 (IL-1) α and β, tumor necrosis factor (TNF)α and IL-6 (Kiefer et al., 1993). Viral infection of astrocytes and microglia in culture stimulates IL-6 and TNFα production (Frei et al., 1989). Viral infection of the CNS *in vivo* stimulates the early production of mRNA for IL-1α and β, IL-6, TNFα, IL-4, IL-10 and TGFβ, suggesting that these molecules are expressed by intrinsic cells of the CNS as an immediate and direct response to the virus infection (Wesselingh et al., 1994). Pro-inflammatory cytokines (such as IL-1α and β, TNFα and IL-6) recruit monocytes and leukocytes into the CNS to process and present antigens, kill virus infected cells, and induce further production of cytokines. In contrast, the cytokines IL-4, IL-10 and TGFβ are all thought to have broadly inhibitory effects upon monocytes, microglia and astrocytes (Wahl et al., 1989; Chao et al., 1993; Frei et al., 1994). It is likely therefore that the interactions between these factors regulate the balance of immune activity within the brain.

Although the neuropathology of naturally occurring viral infections of the CNS is well understood, very little is known about the behavior in the brain under experimental conditions of wild-type viruses which do not normally infect the brain. The neuropathologic effects of non-replicating viral vectors from these two broad groups have yet to be studied in detail. The natural course of wild-type HSV-1 infection of the nervous system involves replication in the periphery followed by latent infection of peripheral sensory neurons (Stevens 1989). However, experimental infection of the CNS with wild-type HSV-1 (by direct intracranial infection) results in a lethal encephalitis. The characteristic neuropathologic features of this encephalitis are MHC antigen induction (both class I and class II) on intrinsic brain cells (Weinstein et al., 1990), followed by the heavy infiltration of T lymphocytes and macrophages into the CNS (Chan et al., 1989; Lewandowski et al., 1993). The neuropathologic effects of a related virus, the swine alpha herpes virus pseudorabies virus (PRV), have also been studied in detail using wild-type and attenuated strains (Rinaman et al., 1993; and see Chapter 24). Detailed *in vivo* investigations of the immune responses to non-replicating recombinant HSV vectors are currently in progress, but an indication of what might be expected in these cases can been gained from earlier immunocytochemical studies of the neuropathology associated with the direct injection of defective HSV-1 amplicon vectors into the CNS (Wood et al., 1994b). In this study, expression of a reporter gene *lacZ* was correlated with an immunocytochemical analysis of the inflammatory response following the defective HSV-1 injection. Experiments with amplicon vectors are complicated by the fact that contaminating membrane fragments and helper virus (in this case HSV strain 17 tsK) are always present in the vector preparation. A number of important principles emerged from this study. Defective HSV-1 vectors elicited a strong host immune response in the CNS, comprising an early inflammatory component (characterized by MHC class I and II induction and microglial activation), followed by the infiltration of activated T lymphocytes and macrophages. This was similar to that previously reported in HSV encephalitis but of lower intensity. Importantly, inflammation in response to the defective HSV inoculation was found not only at the primary injection site (the dentate gyrus of the hippocampus) but also at secondary sites in the hypothalamic supramammillary nuclei (Wood et al., 1994a). These observations correlated closely with the expression of the reporter gene at the secondary sites, which was probably a consequence of the retrograde axonal transport of virus vector from the primary injection site (SEE CHAPTER 24).

Of the group of viruses that do not display natural neuropathologic effects or neurotropism adenovirus is perhaps the most relevant to CNS gene therapy. Studies on other organ systems show that the immune system is important in determining the duration of expression from adenovirus vectors (Kass-Eisler et al., 1994; Yang et al., 1994). In normal mouse liver, marker gene expression declines and then disappears a few weeks after viral injection. Young animals with immature immune systems or T-cell deficient animals, however, express the marker gene much longer. In addition, an intense inflammatory response to the virus is present in normal mice but not in immunodeficient mice (Kass-Eisler et al., 1994; Yang et al., 1994). A similar immunocytochemical study to that of Wood et al. (1994b) was undertaken to examine the immune response to non-replicating, E1-deleted, human adenovirus type 5 vectors in the CNS (Byrnes et al., 1995). The inflammatory response was found to be triggered mostly by the virion particles themselves rather than through expression of new proteins from the vector, because ultraviolet irradiation of the virus did not substantially diminish the inflammation. Within 48 h there was strong upregulation of MHC class I expression and infiltration of leukocytes (mainly T cells and macrophages) at the primary injection site (the caudate nucleus of the striatum). Retrograde transport of adenovirus to neurons of the substantia nigra (predominantly the pars compacta) was associated with a delayed and less intense inflammation. In spite of this inflammatory response, vector-driven expression of the marker protein β-galactosidase and an adenovirus early protein (E2A gene product) was seen for at least 2 months after injection, although expression declined with time. This inflammatory response comprised a late T-cell mediated phase, and the severity of inflammation depended on the strain of rat used.

These experiments indicate very clearly that inflammatory/immune responses are associated with the injection of viral vectors into the CNS. The important questions to be answered are whether such immune responses have deleterious effects on cells of the CNS, and whether they compromise the expression of vector-driven genes. To answer this requires more sophisticated investigation of the immunology (by studying infiltrating immune cell function and cytokine expression within the brain) and the use of various strategies to modulate the effects of the immune system (such as immunosuppression induced by drugs or monoclonal antibodies). If the inflammatory response elicited by viral vectors is a major obstacle to successful gene transfer and long-term gene expression then strategies to modulate these responses will assume greater importance in future research.

2 MATERIALS AND EQUIPMENT

2.1 X-gal Histochemistry

(1) Phosphate-buffered saline (PBS).
(2) Paraformaldehyde.
(3) EGTA, $MgCl_2$.
(4) Sucrose.
(5) OCT embedding compound.
(6) Potassium ferricyanide, potassium ferrocyanide, sodium deoxycholate, nonidet P-40.
(7) X-gal.
(8) Dimethylsulfoxide (DMSO).
(9) Xylene, histological clearing agent, ethanol, glass coverslips.

2.2 Immune Marker Immunocytochemistry

(1) Primary monoclonal antibodies (MAb) of use for following immune processes in the rat and mouse central nervous systems (Tables 26.1 and 26.2).
(2) PBS, pH 7.6.
(3) Blocking serum for the species to be studied (rat or mouse).
(4) Humidification chamber.
(5) Secondary anti-mouse (or anti-rat) HRP-conjugated polyclonal antibody.
(6) OCT embedding compound.
(7) Isopentane (2-methylbutane).
(8) Liquid nitrogen.
(9) Ethanol.
(10) Hydrogen peroxide.
(11) Diaminobenzidine (DAB).
(12) Tris buffer.
(13) Toluidine blue, or cresyl violet counterstain.
(14) Acetic acid (glacial).
(15) Histoclear, histological clearing agent (National Diagnostics, USA).
(16) Glass coverslips.
(17) DPX mountant.

Table 26.1 Monoclonal antibodies recognizing rat cell-surface antigens

Antibody	*Specificity*	*Reference*
OX-1	CD45, Leukocyte common antigen (LCA)	(Woolett et al., 1985)
OX-6	MHC class II (I-A)	(McMaster and Williams, 1979)
OX-8	CD8 T cell subset	(Brideau et al., 1980)
OX-18	MHC class I	(Fukumoto et al., 1982)
OX-19	CD5, T cells	(Dallman et al., 1982)
OX-30	CD45 LCA, non-competitive with OX-1	(Woolett et al., 1985)
OX-33	Isoform of CD45, B cells	(Woolett et al., 1985)
OX-35	CD4 T cell subset	(Jefferies et al., 1985)
OX-39	CD25, IL-2 receptor, T blasts	(Paterson et al., 1987)
OX-40	Activated CD4+ T cells	(Mallett et al., 1990)
OX-42	Complement receptor type 3, microglia/macrophages	(Robinson et al., 1986)
OX-62	Dendritic cells, $\gamma\delta$ T cells	(Brenan and Puklavec, 1992)
R73	$\alpha\beta$ T cell receptor	(Hunig et al., 1989)
ED1	Activated macrophages/microglia	(Dijkstra et al., 1985)
3.2.3	NKR-P1, NK cells, polymorphs	(Chambers et al., 1989)

Commercial sources for the above monoclonal antibodies include Serotec (Oxford, UK) and Pharmingen (Cambridge, UK)

Table 26.2 Monoclonal antibodies recognizing mouse cell-surface antigens

Antibody	*Specificity*	*Reference*
M1.42	MHC class I	(Kennett, 1980)
TIB122	CD45 LCA	(Springer et al., 1978)
KT3	$\alpha\beta$ TCR	(Tomonari, 1988)
YTA3.1	CD4 T cell subset	(Qin et al., 1987)
YTS191.1	CD4 T cell subset	(Cobbold et al., 1984)
YTS169.4	CD8 T cell subset	(Cobbold et al., 1984)
TIB222	CD25, mouse IL-2R	(Zubler et al., 1984)
F4/80	Macrophage; microglia	(Austyn and Gordon, 1981)
2F8	Sialoadhesin; macrophage; microglia	(Rabinowitz and Gordon, 1991)
P7/7	MHC class II (Ia)	(Momburg et al., 1986)

Commercial sources for the above monoclonal antibodies include Serotec (Oxford, UK) and Pharmingen (Cambridge, UK)

2.3 Cytokine Gene Expression in Brain

(1) Water treated with diethylpyrocarbonate (DEPC water): add 0.1% DEPC to double-distilled water. Incubate at 37°C for 3 h and then autoclave to denature the DEPC.
(2) RNAsin water: add RNAase inhibitor 40 U/μl to a final concentration of 0.1 U/μl in DEPC water.
(3) Ethanol/RNAsin water (80%/20%): 40 ml filtered ethanol + 10 ml DEPC water + 25 μl RNAsin at 40U/μl.
(4) RNAzol B, commercial preparation for RNA extraction (Biogenesis Ltd, Poole, England).
(5) Cloned Moloney Murine Leukemia Virus (M-MLV) reverse transcriptase (RT), 200 U/μl.
(6) 5 × RT buffer (supplied with the enzyme).
(7) Primer: pd$(T)_{12-18}$ (Pharmacia), 1 mg/ml in RNAsin water.
(8) Dithiothreitol (DTT), 0.1 M (supplied with the reverse transcriptase enzyme).
(9) Ultrapure dNTP set. Make a 10mM mix by adding 20 μl of each to 120 μl RNAsin water.
(10) G3PDH oligonucleotide primers, and relevant species cytokine oligonucleotide primers (Table 26.3).
(11) Taq polymerase.
(12) The above reagents should all be stored at −20°C.
(13) Mineral oil.

Table 26.3 Sequences for rat oligonucleotide primers

Primer	*Sequence*	*Fragment size (base pairs)*
G3PDH	5′5′ TGAAGGTCGGTGTGAACGGATTTGGC 3′ 3′5′ CATGTAGGCCATGAGGTCCACCAC 3′	483
IL-1α	5′5′ CTAAGAACTACTTCACATCCGCAGC 3′ 3′5′ CTGGAATAAAACCCACTGAGGTAGG 3′	623
IL-1β	5′5′ ATGGCAACTGTTCCTGAACTCAACT 3′ 3′5′ CAGGACAGGTATAGATTCTTTCCTTT 3′	380
IL-2	5′5′ AACAGCGCACCCACTTCAA 3′ 3′5′ TTGAGATGATGCTTTGACA 3′	400
IL-2 receptor	5′5′ TCCTGGAGCAGCAACTGCCAGTGCACCAGCA 3′ 3′5′ CTTATACTCCATTGTGAGCACAAATGTCT 3′	501
IL-6	5′5′ CAAGAGACTTCCAGCCAGTTGC 3′ 3′5′ TTGCCGAGTAGACCTCATAGTGACC 3′	614
IL-10	5′5′ ATGCAGGACTTTAAGGGTTACTTGGGTT 3′ 3′5′ ATTTCGGAGAGAGGTACAAACGAGGTTT 3′	455
TNFα	5′5′ TACTGAACTTCGGGGTGATTGGTCC 3′ 3′5′ CAGCCTTGTCCCTTGAAGAGAACC 3′	295
TGFβ1	5′5′ CTTCAGCTCCACAGAGAAGAACTGC 3′ 3′5′ CACGATCATGTTGGACAACTGCTCC 3′	298
IFNγ	5′5′ GGAGGAACTGGCAAAAGGACG 3′ 3′5′ AGGCTAGATTCTGGTGACAGC 3′	288

Primer sequences are given for the 5′ primer and 3′ primer, reading 5′–3′ for each cytokine

(14) Ethanol (molecular biology grade).
(15) Chloroform.
(16) Isopropanol.
(17) TEB buffer (10× stock: 108 g Tris, 9.3 g EDTA, 55 g Boric acid per liter of water).
(18) 1.5% TEB agarose gels in minigel apparatus.
(19) 5× Sample buffer (5 ml 10× TEB, 1 g Ficoll Type 400, 4 ml 0.1% bromophenol blue, distilled water to 10 ml).
(20) Ethidium bromide (1 mg/ml aqueous solution).

2.4 Isolation of Lymphocytes from Brain

(1) Hanks' balanced salt solution (HBSS).
(2) Collagenase D.
(3) Trypsin inhibitor.
(4) DNAase I.
(5) Hepes buffer, pH 7.4.
(6) Ca^{++}/Mg^{++}-free HBSS.
(7) Dulbecco's modified Eagle's medium (DMEM).
(8) Fetal calf serum (FCS).
(9) Gentamicin.
(10) Ficoll-paque 1077.
(11) PBS/2% FCS.

3 THE PROTOCOLS

Protocol #148: X-gal Histochemistry

(1) Anesthetize experimental animal and perfuse with 100 ml ice-cold PBS (pH 7.3) transcardially.
(2) Perfuse with 200–400 ml fixative containing 2% paraformaldehyde/5 mM EGTA/2 mM $MgCl_2$.

(3) Remove brain and place in fixative for 1 h.
(4) Immerse brain overnight in 30% sucrose/2 mM $MgCl_2$ in PBS.
(5) Embed brain in OCT embedding compound and freeze on dry ice. Cut 50–75 μm sections on cryostat and float in PBS/2 mM $MgCl_2$ at 4°C. (Alternatively, sections may be cut on a vibratome, in which case overnight immersion in sucrose and embedding are not required.)
(6) Prepare stock solution of X-gal containing 40 mg X-gal in 1 ml DMSO.
(7) Transfer sections to X-gal substrate containing 1 mg/ml X-gal/5 mM potassium ferricyanide/5 mM potassium ferrocyanide/2 mM $MgCl_2$/0.01% sodium deoxycholate/0.02% nonidet P-40 in PBS, pH 7.2. Stain for 3 h at 32°C.
(8) Wash sections for 30 s in water at room temperature.
(9) Wash sections for 15 min in PBS at 32°C.
(10) Wash sections for 5 min in water at room temperature.
(11) Wash sections in PBS at 4°C to allow tissue to solidify.
(12) Float sections onto gelatinized slides, counterstain if necessary.
(13) Dehydrate in ethanol, 70% for 2 min, 90% for 2 min and 100% for 2 min.
(14) Treat with xylene by inversion, and coverslip.

Protocol #149: Immune Marker Immunocytochemistry

(1) Anesthetize experimental animal and flush transcardially with saline. Remove brain for frozen section immunocytochemistry, and place in OCT embedding medium in aluminum foil containers. Freeze brains in 2-methylbutane (isopentane), cooled in liquid nitrogen.
(2) Store blocks at −20°C, if necessary, before immunocytochemical analysis.
(3) Prepare tissue sections on a cryostat. Cut serial 10 μm sections at rostral, mid and caudal positions throughout the virus injection site.
(4) Air dry sections for 1 h.
(5) Ring tissue sections with a hydrophobic material such as nail polish or a commercially available 'PAP' pen.
(6) Fix tissue sections in cold 100% ethanol for 10 min.
(7) Wash sections twice (10 min each wash) in PBS.
(8) Place tissue sections in 1% hydrogen peroxide in PBS for 10 min to quench endogenous peroxidase, and wash sections again as before.
(9) Primary MAb may be either a tissue culture supernatant (TCS) or purified. Appropriate concentrations (prepared in PBS) must be optimized before use. Place 100 μl primary MAB (50 μl for mouse sections) on each section in a humidity chamber at room temperature for at least 1 h.
(10) Wash tissue sections twice (5 min each wash) in PBS.
(11) Secondary antibody is polyclonal HRP-conjugated rabbit anti-rat or rabbit anti-mouse. Dilute secondary antibody 1:50 (2%) with PBS, and with 5% rat or mouse serum as appropriate. The required concentration is source-dependent and must be optimized before use. Place 100 μl on each section.
(12) Place sections in a humidity chamber at room temperature for 1 h.
(13) Wash sections three times (15 min each wash) in PBS.
(14) The chromogenic substrate is prepared by dissolving 150 mg DAB in 300 ml 0.1 M Tris (pH 7.6), and adding 100 μl hydrogen peroxide per 150 ml.
(15) Allow sections to develop in DAB for 5–10 min at room temperature.
(16) Wash tissue sections (three times, 10 min each) in PBS.
(17) Counterstain sections if necessary using toluidine blue.
(18) Place sections in a 0.5% toluidine blue/0.5% acetic acid solution for 10–30 min.
(19) Place sections successively in 70%, 90% and 100% ethanol (2 min each) to dehydrate tissue.
(20) Transfer sections to Histoclear for 30 min.
(21) Coverslip sections using DPX mounting medium.

Protocol #150: Analysis of Cytokine Gene Expression in CNS

Extraction and Purification of Total RNA from Brain Tissue

(1) Anesthetize experimental animal and flush transcardially with saline. Remove brain and freeze on dry ice. Punch out relevant area of CNS tissue for analysis. Place 200 μl RNAzol solution in a 1.5 ml tube. Weigh frozen tissue, then tip in no more than 100 mg.
(2) Homogenize tissue. Add RNAzol to 800 μl (up to 1400 μl may be added if a large tissue sample is used), so that RNAzol remains blue. Mix well.
(3) Add 80 μl chloroform (10% of the volume of RNAzol extract). Vortex for 15 s. Stand on ice for 5 min. Centrifuge at 10 000 *g* for 15 min at 4°C. Collect upper aqueous layer (about 400 μl).
(4) Add equal volume of isopropanol. Precipitate overnight at −20°C.
(5) Centrifuge at 10 000 *g* for 40 min at 4°C. Aspirate supernatant. Dissolve pellet in 100 μl 2.5 M ammonium acetate. Add 300 μl chilled absolute ethanol. Precipitate overnight at −20°C.
(6) Wash pellet. Centrifuge at 10 000 *g* 30 min at 4°C. Remove ethanol by aspiration. Wash pellet with 80% ethanol/RNAsin water. Centrifuge and wash again, then spin for a third time. Remove ethanol by aspiration and dry under vacuum.
(7) Dissolve RNA in 20 μl RNAsin water. Take 2 μl for spectrophotometric quantitation. Make up to 130 μl with water and scan at 324–224 nm. One absorbency unit is equivalent to 40 ng/μl RNA. Proceed immediately with cDNA synthesis using 1 μg RNA as template.

Reverse Transcriptase Polymerase Chain Reaction, Electrophoresis and Ethidium Bromide Staining of Gel

(1) Anneal primer and RNA. Take a volume of RNA containing 1 μg, add oligodT (4 μl of 1 mg/ml), make up to 20 μl with RNAsin water. Incubate at 65°C for 5 min. Cool to room temperature over 10 min to anneal primer and RNA.
(2) Transcribe cDNA. Make up a mix containing 5 × RT buffer (8 μl), DTT 0.1 M (4 μl), RNAsin 40 U/μl (0.125 μl), dNTPs 10 mM (4 μl) and RT 200 U/μl (2 μl). Add 18 μl to annealed primer and RNA. Incubate at 37°C for 40 min. Add another 2 μl RT. Incubate for 40 min.
(3) Heat at 98°C for 5 min. Quench on ice for 5 min. Mix.
(4) Store 1μl aliquots at −70°C ready for PCR.
(5) cDNA is checked for comparability by PCR using 1 μl of cDNA with G3PDH primers. G3PDH is a housekeeping gene and therefore an indicator of the quantity of cDNA.
(6) PCR. Mix buffer, $MgCl_2$ (1.5–2.5 mM; the optimum concentration needs to be determined for each pair of primers), dNTPs 200 μM each, oligonucleotide primers 2 μM each, Taq polymerase 0.5 U/50 μl. Pipette 49 μl of mix into each PCR tube containing 1 μl template cDNA. Add 1 drop mineral oil. Spin briefly. Place tubes in a thermal cycler.
(7) After an initial 2 min 45 s at 93°C, an iterative cycle of 15 s melt (92°C), 1 min anneal (60°C; but depends on primer), 1 min extension, is followed for the required number of cycles. Cool to 4°C. Sample, and then if necessary run additional segment again (93°C for 15 s), followed by the iterative cycle. Cool to 4°C and repeat sample. Samples can be stored at −20°C.
(8) Add 5 μl loading buffer to 15 μl sample of PCR reaction and load all the samples to be compared in the same row on a 1.5% agarose TEB minigel. Run gel and post-stain for 15 min with ethidium bromide (20 μl of 1 mg/ml into the gel tank). Visualize the bands on a UV transillumiator. After checking the uniformity of cDNA the mRNAs of interest may be studied.
(9) Interrupted PCR. The relative amounts of specific cDNA, hence mRNA, in the samples, is related to the cycle in which the PCR product can be detected: the smaller the cycle number the more message there is. The cycle number is found by sampling the reaction three times.

Evaluation of PCR Product

All samples taken at 30 cycles are run in one row on a minigel, as are those taken at 40 cycles, 50 cycles, etc. to see at which cycle a band is obtained. The PCR is then repeated and sampled at the appropriate cycle. This method does not show absolute amounts of mRNA but traces the change in level of a given cytokine.

Protocol #151: Isolation of Lymphocytes from Brain

(1) Anesthetize experimental animal. Flush transcardially with saline and remove brain.
(2) Mince brain gently through a fine mesh screen using a syringe plunger.
(3) Collect tissue into 10 ml HBSS containing 0.05% collagenase D, 0.1 μg/ml trypsin inhibitor TLCK, 10 μg/ml DNAase I, 10 mM Hepes buffer pH 7.4.
(4) Mix at room temperature for 60 min.
(5) Allow to settle for 30 min.
(6) Deplete any undigested debris by withdrawing supernatant.
(7) Centrifuge supernatant at 200*g* for 5 min and collect pellet.
(8) Resuspend in 10 ml Ca^{++}/Mg^{++}-free HBSS.
(9) Layer 5 ml of this suspension carefully onto 10 ml of modified density separation medium prepared by mixing 25% DMEM (containing 10% FCS, 10 mM Hepes, 50 μg/ml gentamicin), and 75% Ficoll-paque in a 50 ml conical centrifuge tube.
(10) Centrifuge at 500*g* for 30 min.
(11) Remove the overlying medium and tissue debris interface.
(12) Dilute entire 10 ml of gradient medium tenfold with HBSS.
(13) Centrifuge at 300*g* for 10 min.
(14) Count cells and resuspend at 1×10^6 cells/ml in PBS/2% FCS ready for further analysis.

4 NOTES AND TROUBLESHOOTING

4.1 On Protocol #148: X-gal Histochemistry

This method enables the expression of the *E. coli lacZ* reporter gene by CNS cells transfected *in vivo* to be examined in fixed sections. The reaction is highly sensitive but often so vigorous that determination of the precise cellular localization of the reaction product is difficult. Important features of this method allow elimination of endogenous enzyme activity within the CNS so that only bacterial enzyme activity is detectable (Kaplitt et al., 1991). An example is given in Fig. 26.1.

The pH and magnesium concentrations of the various solutions are crucial. Variations in these concentrations are probably the most common cause of non-specific background staining. A frequent site of non-specific background staining is the choroid plexus.

The other major variable factors are the duration of staining and the temperature at which this is performed. It is important to standardize these for any given set of experiments. Staining for too long at too high a temperature is likely to cause non-specific staining.

Always perform negative controls.

4.2 On Protocol #149: Immune Marker Immunocytochemistry

This immunocytochemical method allows the detailed analysis of immune system activity by the identification, through cell-specific surface markers, of immunologically active cells in fixed or frozen sections of brain tissue. In addition, various cellular markers of immune activation (expressed by intrinsic CNS cells as well as by infiltrating extrinsic immune cells) can be detected. This method has been adapted from Barclay (Barclay 1981) as previously described (Wood et al., 1992). Examples of this immunocytochemical staining are given in Fig. 26.1.

The most common problem is background or non-specific tissue staining. The following important factors should be considered if background staining is problematic: (1) an adequate saline flush is necessary to clear the cerebral vasculature before staining; (2) tissue sections should be treated adequately with hydrogen peroxide to remove endogenous peroxidase enzyme activity; (3) primary and secondary antibodies should be used at the lowest possible concentrations, with adequate blocking serum of the appropriate species. The optimum concentration of the MRC OX

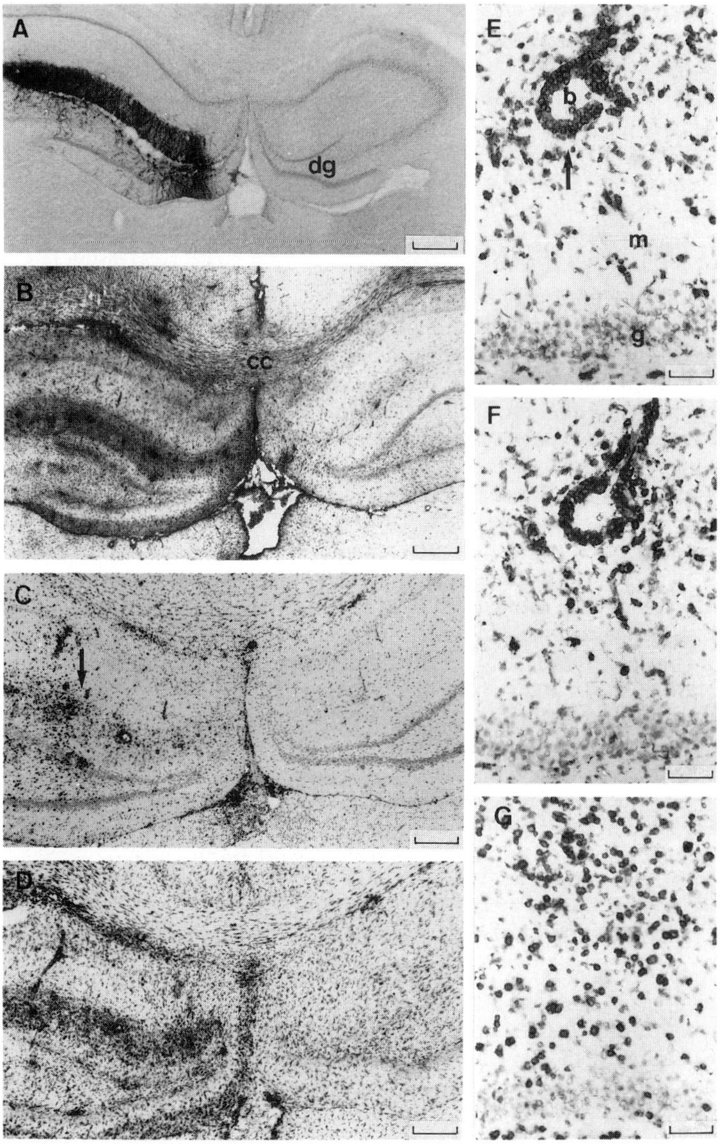

Figure 26.1 X-gal histochemistry and immunocytochemistry for immune markers, at 2 and 10 days respectively, after injection of HSV-1 amplicon vector expressing the reporter gene *lacZ* into the rat dentate gyrus. (A) X-gal positive cells detectable in the rat dentate gyrus (dg). Many of these are dentate granule neurons. (B) Induction of MHC class I antigen expression (MRC OX-18) in the rat dentate gyrus and contiguous brain areas. Most notable microglial cells are in the corpus callosum (cc). (C) CD45/Leukocyte common antigen expression (MRC OX-1) on intrinsic and extrinsic cells in the rat dentate gyrus (arrow), and corpus callosum. Very few positive cells are detectable in the contralateral hemisphere. (D) Upregulated complement receptor type 3 expression (MRC OX-42) on infiltrating macrophages and intrinsic microglia in the rat dentate gyrus and corpus callosum. There is considerable upregulation of this antigen on microglia in the contralateral dentate gyrus. (E) CD45 expression (MRC OX-1) in the dentate gyrus 10 days after the injection of HSV-1 vector. CD45 positive cells are prominent in a perivascular cuff (arrow) around a blood vessel (b) in the molecular layer (m) of the dentate gyrus, located above the granule cell layer (g). (F) Detection of CD25 expression (IL-2 receptor, MRC OX-39) on infiltrating T cells in the molecular layer (predominantly) of the rat dentate gyrus. (G) Infiltration of $\alpha\beta$ T cell receptor-positive (R73) cells into the rat dentate gyrus 10 days after the injection of HSV-1 amplicon vector. Cells are present throughout the molecular and granule cell layers. Scale bars: A–D = 350 μm; E–G = 75 μm

primary antibodies will depend on whether they are supplied as tissue culture supernatant (TCS) or in a more concentrated purified form. The appropriate concentrations need to be established before staining; (4) sections must be watched carefully during the DAB reaction, and the reaction halted as soon as adequate staining is obtained; (5) sections should be washed thoroughly at all stages.

Negative controls should always be performed, ideally with an isotype-matched mouse (or rat) primary MAb against an irrelevant antigen of another species (e.g. human).

4.3 On Protocol #150: Analysis of Cytokine Gene Expression in CNS

In order to study the regulation of immune responses to viral vectors in the CNS methods for the analysis of cytokine activity in the brain are essential. Because of their very low concentrations these molecules are difficult to detect reliably using immunocytochemistry. Methods have been developed based on those described by Dallman et al. (1991) in order to identify and analyse cytokine mRNA expression in the CNS in response to viral vector inoculation. This involves the use of reverse transcriptase-polymerase chain reaction (RT-PCR).

The procedure takes three phases: (1) extraction of total RNA from brain using RNAzol; (2) RT-PCR followed by electrophoresis and ethidium bromide staining of gel; (3) evaluation of the PCR product.

For a comparison of gene expression between samples to be valid all the samples must contain a similar amount of cDNA. This is achieved by synthesizing the cDNA from a measured quantity (1 μg) of RNA. Comparability is indicated by a similar level of G3PDH expression.

RNAzol works best with small amounts of tissue, ideally less than 10 mg. The optimum extract depends on the kind of tissue used: brain yields less RNA, and has a high lipid content, so two 4 mg samples are routinely used and pooled at the isopropanol stage.

The quantity of RNA extracted is variable, even between replicates of the same tissue. However 1 μg of RNA yields a very constant amount of cDNA, which is essential for the comparative method.

For the cDNAs to be of use for comparative analysis, the intensity of the bands obtained with G3PDH must be similar. In addition, the sample must be taken during the linear phase of the PCR (and not the plateau phase). This phase has to be found empirically.

4.4 On Protocol #151: Isolation of Lymphocytes from Brain

The first step necessary to making functional measurements of the infiltrating lymphocytes within the brain is a reliable method for isolating these cells from brain tissue. This will allow quantitative measurements of the numbers of specific subsets of infiltrating cells using fluorescent activated cell sorting (FACS) analysis, as well as the functional analysis of these cells. The method describes the isolation of lymphocytes from brain tissue, based on that of Irani and Griffin (1991). Methods of FACS analysis and further functional analysis of these isolated cells are beyond the scope of this chapter, but can be found in standard immunology texts and laboratory manuals.

REFERENCES

Akli, S., Caillaud, C., Vigne, E., Stratford-Perricaudet, L. D., Poenaru, L., Perricaudet, M., Kahn, A. and Pechanski, M. R. (1993) Transfer of a foreign gene into the brain using adenovirus vectors. *Nature Genet.*, **3**, 224–228.

Ali, M., Lemoine, N. R. and Ring, C. J. A. (1994) The use of DNA viruses as vectors for gene therapy. *Gene Ther.*, **1**, 367–384.

Austyn, J. M. and Gordon, S. (1981) F4/80, a monoclonal antibody directed specifically against the mouse macrophage. *Eur. J. Immunol.*, **11**, 805–815.

Bajocchi, G., Feldman, S. H., Crystal, R. G. and Mastrangeli, A. (1993) Direct *in vivo* gene transfer to ependymal cells in the central nervous system using recombinant adenovirus vectors. *Nature Genet.*, **3**, 229–234.

Barclay, A. N. (1981) The localisation of populations of lymphocytes defined by monoclonal antibodies in rat lymphoid tissue. *Immunology*, **42,** 593–600.

Brenan, M. and Puklavec, M. (1992) The MRC OX-62 antigen: A useful marker in the purification of rat veiled cells with the biochemical properties of an integrin. *J. Exp. Med.*, **175,** 1457–1465.

Brideau, R. J., Carter, P. B., McMaster, W. R., Mason, D. W. and Williams, A. F. (1980) Two subsets of rat T lymphocytes defined with monoclonal antibodies. *Eur. J. Immunol.*, **10,** 609–615.

Byrnes, A., Rusby, J. E., Wood, M. J. A. and Charlton, H. M. (1995) Adenovirus gene transfer causes inflammation in the brain. *Neuroscience* (In Press).

Chambers, W. H., Vujanovic, N. L., DeLeo, A. B., Olszowy, M. W., Herberman, R. B. and Hiserodt, J. C. (1989) Monoclonal antibody to a triggering structure expressed on rat natural killer cells and adherent lymphokine-activated killer cells. *J. Exp. Med.*, **169,** 1373–1389.

Chan, W. L., Javanovic, T. and Lukie, M. L. (1989) Infiltration of immune T cells in the brain of mice with herpes simplex virus-induced encephalitis. *J. Neuroimmunol.*, **23,** 195–201.

Chao, C. C., Molitor, T. W. and Hu, S. (1993) Neuroprotective role of IL-4 against activated microglia. *J. Immunol.*, **151,** 1473–1481.

Chiocca, E. A., Choi, B. B., Cai, W., DeLuca, N. A., Schaffer, P. A., DiFiglia, M., Breakefield, X. O. and Martuza, R. L. (1990) Transfer and expression of the *lacZ* gene in rat brain neurons mediated by herpes simplex virus mutants. *New Biol.*, **2,** 739–746.

Cobbold, S. P., Jayasuriya, A., Nash, A., Prospero, T. D. and Waldmann, H. (1984) Therapy with monoclonal antibodies by elimination of T-cell subsets *in vivo*. *Nature*, **312,** 548–551.

Dallman, M. J., Mason, D. W. and Webb, M. (1982) The roles of host and donor cells in the rejection of skin allografts by T cell-deprived rats injected with syngeneic T cells. *Eur. J. Immunol.*, **12,** 511–518.

Dallman, M. J., Larsen, C. P. and Morris, P. J. (1991) Cytokine gene transcription in vascularised organ grafts: analysis using semiquantitative polymerase chain reaction. *J. Exp. Med.*, **174,** 493–496.

Davidson, B. L., Allen, E. D., Kozarsky, K. F., Wilson, J. M. and Roessler, B. J. (1993) A model system for *in vivo* gene transfer into the central nervous system using an adenoviral vector. *Nature Genet.*, **3,** 219–223.

Dijkstra, C. D., Dopp, E. A., Joling, P. and Kraal, G. (1985) The heterogeneity of mononuclear phagocytes in lymphoid organs: distinct macrophage sub-populations in the rat recognised by monoclonal antibodies ED1, ED2 and ED3. *Immunology*, **54,** 589–599.

Frei, K., Malipiero, U. V., Leist, T. P., Zinkernagel, R. M., Schwab, M. E. and Fontana, A. (1989) On the cellular source and function of interleukin 6 produced in the central nervous system in viral diseases. *Eur. J. Immunol.*, **19,** 689–694.

Frei, K., Lins, H., Schwerdel, C. and Fontana, A. (1994) Antigen presentation in the central nervous system: The inhibitory effect of IL-10 on MHC class II expression and the production of cytokines depends on the inducing signals and the type of cell analyzed. *J. Immunol.*, **152,** 2720–2728.

Friedmann, T. (1994) Gene therapy for neurological disorders. *Trends Genet.*, **10,** 210–214.

Fukumoto, T., McMaster, W. R. and Williams, A. F. (1982) Mouse monoclonal antibodies against rat major histocompatibility antigens. Two Ia antigens and expression of Ia and class I antigens in rat thymus. *Eur. J. Immunol.*, **12,** 237–243.

Hunig, T., Wallny, H. J., Hartley, J. K., Lawetzky, A. and Tiefenthaler, G. (1989) A monoclonal antibody to a constant determinant of the rat T cell antigen receptor that induces T cell activation. Differential reactivity with subsets of immature and mature T lymphocytes. *J. Exp. Med.*, **169,** 73–86.

Irani, D. N. and Griffin, D. E. (1991) Isolation of brain parenchymal lymphocytes for flow cytometric analysis. Application to acute viral encephalitis. *J. Immunol. Methods*, **139,** 223–231.

Jefferies, W. A., Green, J. R. and Williams, A. F. (1985) Authentic T helper CD4 (W3/25) antigen on rat peritoneal macrophages. *J. Exp. Med.*, **162,** 117–127.

Kaplitt, M. G., Pfaus, J. G., Kleopoulos, S. P., Hanlon, B. A., Rabkin, S. D. and Pfaff, D. W. (1991) Expression of a functional foreign gene in adult mammalian brain following *in vivo* transfer via a herpes simplex virus type 1 defective viral vector. *Mol. Cell. Neurosci.*, **2,** 320–330.

Kaplitt, M. G., Leone, P., Samulski, R. J., Xiao, X., Pfaff, D. W., O'Malley, K. L. and During, M. J. (1994) Long-term gene expression and phenotypic correction using adeno-associated virus vectors in the mammalian brain. *Nature Genet.*, **8,** 148–154.

Kass-Eisler, A., Falck-Pedersen, E., Elfenbein, D. H., Alvira, M., Buttrick, P. M. and Leinwand, L. A. (1994) The impact of developmental stage, route of administration and the immune system on adenovirus-mediated gene transfer. *Gene Ther.*, **1,** 395–402.

Kennett, M. (1980) Rat IgG2a and anti H-2 haplotypes. In M. Kennett (ed.), *Monoclonal antibodies*. Plenum Press, New York, pp. 185–217.

Kiefer, R., Lindholm, D. and Kreutzberg, G. W. (1993) Interleukin-6 and transforming growth factor-β1 mRNAs are induced in rat facial nucleus following motoneuron axotomy. *Eur. J. Neurosci.*, **5,** 775–781.

Le Gal La Salle, G., Robert, J. J., Berrard, S., Ridoux, V., Stratford-Perricaudet, L. D., Perricaudet, M. and Mallet, J. (1993) An adenovirus vector for gene transfer into neurons and glia in the brain. *Science*, **259,**

988–990.

Lewandowski, G. A., Lo, D. and Bloom, F. E. (1993) Interference with major histocompatibility complex class II-restricted antigen presentation in the brain by herpes simplex virus type I: a possible mechanism of evasion of the immune response. *Proc. Natl Acad. Sci. U.S.A.*, **90,** 2005–2009.

Mallett, S., Fossum, S. and Barclay, A. N. (1990) Characterisation of the MRC OX40 antigen of activated CD4 positive T-lymphocytes: a molecule related to nerve growth factor receptor. *EMBO J.*, **9,** 1063–1068.

McMaster, W. R. and Williams, A. F. (1979) Identification of Ia glycoproteins in rat thymus and purification from rat spleen. *Eur. J. Immunol.*, **9,** 426–433.

Momburg, F., Koch, N., Möller, P., Moldenhauer, G., Butcher, G. W. and Hammerling, G. J. (1986) Differential expression of Ia and Ia-associated invariant chain in mouse tissues after *in vivo* treatment with IFN-γ. *J. Immunol.*, **136,** 940–948.

Paterson, D. J., Jefferies, W. A., Green, J. R., Brandon, M. R., Corthesy, P., Puklavec, M. and Williams, A. F. (1987) Antigens of activated rat T lymphocytes including a molecule of 50,000 Mr detected only on CD4 positive T blasts. *Mol. Immunol.*, **24,** 1281–1290.

Perry, V. H., Andersson, P.-B. and Gordon, S. (1993) Macrophages and inflammation in the central nervous system. *Trends Neurosci.*, **16,** 268–273.

Qin, S., Cobbold, S., Tighe, H., Benjamin, R. and Waldmann, H. (1987) CD4 monoclonal antibody pairs for immunosuppression and tolerance induction. *Eur. J. Immunol.*, **17,** 1159–1165.

Rabinowitz, S. S. and Gordon, S. (1991) Macrosialin: a macrophage-restricted membrane sialoprotein differentially glycosylated in response to inflammatory stimuli. *J. Exp. Med.*, **174,** 827–831.

Rinaman, L., Card, J. P. and Enquist, L. W. (1993) Spatiotemporal responses of astrocytes, ramified microglia, and brain macrophages to central neuronal infection with pseudorabies virus. *J. Neurosci.*, **13,** 685–702.

Robinson, A. P., White, T. M. and Mason, D. W. (1986) Macrophage heterogeneity in the rat as delineated by two monoclonal antibodies MRC OX-41 and MRC OX-42, the latter recognising complement receptor type 3. *Immunology*, **57,** 239–247.

Sloan, D. J., Wood, M. J. and Charlton, H. M. (1991) The immune response to intracerebral neural grafts. *Trends Neurosci.*, **14,** 341–346.

Springer, T., Galfre, G., Secher, D. S. and Milstein, C. (1978) Monoclonal xenogeneic antibodies to murine cell surface antigens: identification of novel leukocyte differentiation antigens. *Eur. J. Immunol.*, **8,** 539–551.

Stevens, J. G. (1989) Human herpesviruses: a consideration of the latent state. *Microbiol. Rev.*, **53,** 318–332.

Tomonari, K. (1988) A rat antibody against a structure functionally related to the mouse T cell receptor/CD3 complex. *Immunogenetics*, **28,** 455–458.

Wahl, S. M., McCartney-Francis, N. and Mergenhagen, S. E. (1989) Inflammatory and immunomodulatory roles of TGF-β. *Immunol. Today*, **10,** 258–261.

Weinstein, D. L., Walker, D. G., Akiyama, H. and McGeer, P. L. (1990) Herpes simplex virus type I infection of the CNS induces major histocompatibility complex antigen expression on rat microglia. *J. Neurosci. Res.*, **26,** 55–65.

Wesselingh, S. L., Levine, B., Fox, R. J., Choi, S. and Griffin, D. E. (1994) Intracerebral cytokine mRNA expression during fatal and nonfatal alphavirus encephalitis suggests a predominant type 2 T cell response. *J. Immunol.*, **152,** 1289–1297.

Wood, M. J. A., Sloan, D. J., Dallman, M. J. and Charlton, H. M. (1992) A monoclonal antibody to the interleukin-2 receptor enhances the survival of neural allografts: a time-course study. *Neuroscience*, **49,** 409–418.

Wood, M. J. A., Byrnes, A. P., Kaplitt, M. G., Pfaff, D. W., Rabkin, S. D. and Charlton, H. M. (1994a) Specific patterns of defective HSV-1 gene transfer in the adult central nervous system: Implications for gene targeting. *Exp. Neurol.*, **130,** 127–140.

Wood, M. J. A., Byrnes, A. P., Pfaff, D. W., Rabkin, S. D. and Charlton, H. M. (1994b) Inflammatory effects of gene transfer into the CNS with defective HSV-1 vectors. *Gene Ther.*, **1,** 283–291.

Woolett, G. R., Barclay, A. N., Puklavec, M. and Williams, A. F. (1985) Molecular and antigenic heterogeneity of the rat leukocyte-common antigen from thymocytes and T and B lymphocytes. *Eur. J. Immunol.*, **15,** 168–173.

Yang, Y., Nunes, F. A., Berencsi, K., Furth, E. E., Gönczöl, E. and Wilson, J. M. (1994) Cellular immunity to viral antigens limits E1 deleted adenoviruses for gene therapy. *Proc. Natl Acad. Sci. U.S.A.*, **91,** 4407–4411.

Zubler, R. H., Lowenthal, J. W., Erard, F., Hashimoto, N., Devos, R. and MacDonald, H. R. (1984) Activated B cells express receptors for, and proliferate in response to, pure interleukin-2. *J. Exp. Med.*, **160,** 1170–1183.

SECTION 7

Prospects and Shortcomings of Neurological Gene Therapy

CHAPTER 27

Gene Therapy Approaches to the Treatment of Human Neurological Disease: The Future of Neurological Therapies?

J.C. MacMillan and P.R. Lowenstein*

MRC Clinician Scientist, Institute of Medical Genetics, Cardiff, UK. Currently: Queensland Clinical Genetics Service, Royal Children's Hospital, Herston 4029, Brisbane, Australia. Tel: 61 7 3253 1686; Fax: 61 7 3253 1987

**University of Manchester, School of Medicine, Department of Medicine, Molecular Medicine Unit, Room 1.302, Stopford Building, Oxford Road, Manchester M13 9PT, UK. Tel: 0161 275 5672; Fax: 0161 274 5672; Email: lowenstein@man.ac.uk*

1 INTRODUCTION

The vast majority of diseases of the human nervous system have been, and to some extent still are, perceived as "untreatable". This is understandable, given our lack of knowledge of the underlying fundamental pathophysiological basis of many of them. The only clear exceptions to this are the infectious diseases of the nervous system, although even here we lack effective therapy for all but the bacterial infections. The past decade has seen a revolution in our understanding of the molecular basis for the inherited neurological diseases (Martin, 1993; MacMillan and Harper, 1994) but to date this has not been accompanied by effective strategies for their treatment.

There is, however, an expectation, not only in the medical/scientific fields but also in the public arena, that "gene therapy" may offer the ultimate "cure" for some inherited and acquired human neurological diseases. Nevertheless, only very few gene therapy protocols are designed to treat neurological diseases, and so far these experimental neurological therapies are limited to the brain tumors (Anderson, 1995). Is this confidence in "gene therapy" misplaced? We believe not, despite our reservations about their applicability in the short term, especially in relation to the treatment of dominantly inherited neurodegenerative diseases.

This chapter addresses the following questions:

- which diseases would we like to "treat"?
- which diseases should we "treat"?
- what strategies are available or could be developed for gene therapy of human neurological diseases?
- for which diseases do we think it feasible that "gene therapy" will offer an effective treatment?

We will not consider in this chapter the place of gene therapy in the treatment of non-inherited neoplastic disease of the CNS; this is addressed elsewhere in this volume (See Chapter 22). We will also limit discussion on the treatment of metabolic disorders affecting the CNS (See Chapters 20

Protocols for Gene Transfer in Neuroscience: Towards Gene Therapy of Neurological Disorders
Edited by P.R. Lowenstein and L.W. Enquist

AND 21) and the specific use of viral vectors in the treatment of genetic disorders of the CNS, these topics are addressed by many other authors in this volume.

2 WHICH DISORDERS SHOULD WE TARGET?

Is it reasonable to expect some ethical and public health policy guidance on the nature of the disorders for which we should aim to develop treatment? The Committee on the Ethics of Gene Therapy (UK) (Committee on the Ethics of Gene Therapy, 1992) addressed many topics relevant to this issue and their report provides a framework around which we can build some principles. Of primary importance, the disease should be life threatening or cause serious handicap and current treatment should be unavailable or unsatisfactory. These basic criteria should be mandatory given the lack of knowledge concerning the long-term effects of the manipulations proposed. Where these requirements have been met we can then examine other practical issues.

The protocols used in any trial of gene therapy in the UK need approval by a variety of local and government agencies, including local research ethics committees, the Gene Therapy Advisory Committee (GTAC), the Medicines Control Agency (MCA) and the Health and Safety Executive (HSE). Guidelines on making clinical gene therapy research proposals have been published (Lloyd and Taylor, 1994).

The scientific requirements to be met are not insubstantial, as will be clear to readers of the other chapters in the volume: the gene encoding the desired function, or which contains the disease-causing mutation, must have been isolated and available for therapeutic use; the function of the gene or gene product should be known so that treatment can be sensibly designed; the cell types and tissues and the stage of development at which gene expression is required should be known because a requirement for activity in embryonic/fetal development is likely to preclude gene therapy as an option. Suitable methods should be available for effectively delivering the gene, including its transcription-regulating elements, into the appropriate cells, and for obtaining adequate levels of expression of its product. Finally, the means must be available for monitoring in the long term the efficacy and safety of the treatment.

Further criteria by which the effectiveness of a therapy is gauged are dictated by the contingencies of health care economics. Commercial ventures are unlikely to make gene therapy a priority if its applications appear to be limited to rare inherited conditions or terminal malignancies unresponsive to other treatments. At present most protocols are funded by research agencies and charities and this situation is likely to continue for the foreseeable future. Researchers and clinicians need, however, to consider whether there is a commercial future for their proposals, although this should not limit the scope of the clinical trials of neurological gene therapy (Lowenstein, 1994).

3 WHAT STRATEGIES ARE AVAILABLE OR COULD BE DEVELOPED FOR NEUROLOGICAL GENE THERAPY?

It will become imperative, both from a basic scientific tenet and from a clinical viewpoint, to determine whether most benefit is likely to be gained from targeting cells *in situ* or from genetic manipulation of cells *in vitro* with subsequent transplantation back into the nervous system. Situations are possible in which one or other option is the more appropriate or practicable.

For example, in treating a diffuse disease of the adult central nervous system such as Alzheimer's disease several options must be evaluated. There are essentially three basic methods by which genes can be delivered to the brain:

(1) Transplantation into the brain of "native" or engineered cells (SEE CHAPTERS 19–21).
(2) The use of viral or non-viral vectors to introduce genes into the cells of the CNS either by direct injection or peripherally after disruption of the blood–brain barrier (SEE CHAPTERS 7, 12, 13, 16, 23; Akli et al., 1993; Bajocchi et al., 1993; Davidson et al., 1993; Le Gal La Salle et al, 1993; Lowenstein, 1994, 1995a,c).
(3) Transplantation of "native" or engineered bone marrow precursor cells and subsequent migration into the CNS (SEE CHAPTERS 20 AND 21).

4 TRANSPLANTATION OF GENETICALLY MODIFIED CELLS

Grafts of genetically modified fibroblasts secreting nerve growth factor (NGF) can, when placed into surgical lesions, prevent degeneration of lesioned septohippocampal cholinergic neurons in rats (Rosenberg et al., 1988). Sustained delivery of physiological (or pharmacological) levels of NGF using such cells introduced into one or several sites in the brain may offer a means by which we can rescue cholinergic neurons in patients with Alzheimer's disease. An alternative strategy may be to transplant genetically modified (using retroviral constructs) CNS progenitor cells which retain the ability to divide, migrate extensively throughout the brain and differentiate into several CNS cell types. The cell types that will develop from grafts of CNS progenitor cells depend on the age of the brain into which they are being transplanted (Snyder, 1994): whereas neurons, astrocytes and glial cells arise in an immature brain, only glial cells arise in a mature adult brain. If specific cell types are to be targeted (especially neurons in humans) this technique may be appropriate only where intrapartum access to the developing brain is possible and acceptable.

The recent identification and isolation from mature adult brain tissue of pluripotential progenitor cells (Reynolds and Weiss, 1992; Ray et al., 1993) raises the possibility of genetic modification of such autologous cells for subsequent retransplantation. Again, however, the question of what cell lineages will differentiate on retransplantation from these cells remains to be answered. We do know that cells transplanted into the CNS stably express transgenes for long periods, migratory astrocyte grafts having been shown to express a reporter gene in specific brain areas for up to 1 year (Mucke and Rockenstein, 1993). Prolonged transgene expression, perhaps in some cases for up to 50 years, will be a prerequisite for successful treatment of the diseases under discussion but has not yet been achieved in *in situ* gene therapy experiments. At present, second-generation adenovirus vectors have been shown to maintain transgene expression for up to 70 days (Engelhardt et al, 1994), new herpesvirus vectors are able to express for more than 6 months in both peripheral spinal ganglia and hippocampus (Lokensgard, et al., 1994), and adeno-associated virus vectors have been expressed for several months (Kaplitt et al., 1994).

The migratory potential of glial cells derived from neuronal progenitors transplanted into the adult brain, coupled with their ability to synthesize and release a protein such as NGF, makes this an interesting therapeutic possibility. It may be that focal replacement of genetically modified cells, even those such as astrocytes and oligodendrocytes that migrate long distances in the host, will not be sufficient and a strategy which effectively targets cells across a wider area may be more effective.

5 INTRODUCTION OF GENES INTO CNS CELLS *IN SITU*

Neuwelt et al. (1994) have shown that it is possible to deliver virus-sized particles to the brain parenchyma after temporary disruption of the blood–brain barrier. Adenovirus or herpes virus-mediated expression of NGF in cells *in vivo* after blood–brain barrier disruption may offer a means of achieving widespread delivery. Once again, however, we need to consider which cell types will express transgenes by this procedure and the areas (a function of the vessel used for introducing the vectors) most likely to be successfully targeted. Other avenues might include introducing the vectors via the cerebrospinal fluid, preferably using a spinal rather than a ventricular approach, although again the question of the location and type of cells that will be successfully targeted is unanswered. Whether enough protein product could be produced by ependymal cells (easily infectable by intra-CSF vector administration), to cross into the brain in a significant quantity remains to be determined.

6 BONE MARROW TRANSPLANTATION FOR NEUROLOGICAL DISORDERS

Krall et al. (1994) have recently shown in a murine system that up to 20% of brain microglia can be replaced with cells expressing a transgene (human glucocerebrosidase) after bone marrow transplantation. This system, if it could be applied to Alzheimer's disease, would obviate the need for either direct CNS inoculation or disruption of the blood–brain barrier to deliver the therapeutic constructs. Its efficacy in other conditions would, however, depend on the ability of transduced microglial cells to correct a defect which may be primarily neuronal (Krivit and Shapiro, 1991; SEE CHAPTER 21). Strategies that target the brain may not directly affect neurons, which may be a limiting factor in some conditions such as Huntington's disease where the cell population affected is relatively specific (Ferrante et al., 1994).

For gene therapy to be effective it will be necessary to maintain transgene function for a considerable length of time. Although this is valid for the neurodegenerative conditions under discussion in this chapter, it may not necessarily be so for conditions such as non-inherited CNS malignancies (SEE CHAPTER 22) or for possible neuroprotective therapies following acute vascular events.

7 DOES A COMMON PATHOPHYSIOLOGY/ETIOLOGY MEAN A COMMON STRATEGY FOR THERAPY?

The title of this chapter implies that it is possible to develop strategies for treating groups of neurological diseases rather than addressing each disorder individually. The premise that diseases that share a mechanism of origin are likely to be amenable to a common approach to therapy remains to be validated. If we are to attempt to devise strategies based on our understanding of the pathophysiological and molecular basis of these disorders we must identify these common features.

There are two fundamental mechanisms by which a pathological phenotype can emerge: loss of the normal function of the gene product and gain of a novel deleterious function. The exact mechanisms by which gains of function arise vary and include increased gene dosage due to duplications, disruption of a structural protein and direct toxicity of the altered protein (see review by Wilkie, 1994).

From a therapeutic perspective it is self-evident that diseases arising from a loss of normal function are likely to be more amenable to treatment than those arising from the gain of a novel function, particularly as most strategies are designed to replace the function of mutated genes within diseased cells/tissues by introducing extra copies of wild-type alleles. We begin, therefore, by considering some neurological diseases in which such loss of function is responsible for the disease phenotype.

7.1 Disorders Caused by Loss of Normal Function

Traditionally these comprise the autosomal and X-linked recessive genetic diseases of the nervous system. They include the metabolic diseases affecting the CNS, most spinal muscular atrophies, some ataxias and a number of retinal degenerations. The fact that the heterozygous parents of an affected child (or the carrier mothers of affected hemizygous males) are, with few exceptions (which can be explained by factors such as skewed X-chromosome inactivation in heterozygous females carrying X-chromosome mutations), clinically normal indicates that it is possible to maintain normal function on reduced amounts of gene product. Where the gene has been cloned and its product known (e.g. HPRT in Lesch–Nyhan syndrome, glucocerebrosidase in Gaucher disease, dystrophin in Duchenne/Becker muscular dystrophy) it might be possible to introduce into appropriate cells at least one extra functional gene sequence and obtain a clinically significant level of biological activity. The strategy most effective for each disease remains to be elucidated but some considerations are independent of the particular disease.

What cell type and what proportion of the cells must be transduced for the modifications to result in optimal benefit? At present we do not know which lineage and proportion of cells we must transduce and the level of functional activity that must be restored in order to ameliorate the clinical manifestations of recessive genetic disorders. Krall et al. (1994) have shown (in a murine system) that 20% of the brain microglial cell population had been replaced with donor cells expressing human glucocerebrosidase (deficient in Gaucher disease) 3 months after reconstitution of hematopoietic tissues with retrovirally transduced vector-marked cells. Whether such a

Table 27.1 Phenotype of HPRT deficiency

Disease	*Symptoms*	*HPRT activity (% of control)*
Classical Lesch–Nyhan	Mental retardation, self-mutilation, choreoathetosis, hyperuricemia	1.4
Intelligent Lesch–Nyhan	Self-mutilation, choreoathetosis hyperuricemia	1.4–1.6
Neurological Lesch–Nyhan	Choreoathetosis, hyperuricemia	1.6–8
Neurologically normal individuals	Hyperuricemia	8–60
	Normal uricemia	≥60

Modified from Sege-Peterson et al., 1993

level of microglial replacement would have a clinical effect in humans remains unanswered. Table 27.1 gives some indication of the complex relationships between functional enzyme levels and clinical manifestations in Lesch–Nyhan syndrome. If it were possible to augment the level of the enzyme in question in 10% of cells we still could not answer the question of whether only those cells benefit or whether adjacent cells will be affected (bystander effect), perhaps by export of protein from the transduced cells and uptake by non-transduced cells.

The amount of augmentation possible in an individual cell is another unknown variable. Optimal therapy at a cellular level would mean restoration of normal levels of missing gene product, whereas a clinically effective therapy may require only 10% of the normal activity for that cell. However, levels acceptable for therapy appearing in only 10% of cells may mean that a clinically valuable threshold is not attained, whereas optimal levels in this proportion may do so if a "bystander" effect occurs. If it can be shown that supraoptimal levels of expression are not deleterious to an individual cell, overexpression may also be clinically useful; Duchenne muscular dystrophy may be one such case. Overexpression might also be of some use in releasing high levels of enzyme into the extracellular space. In other disorders, particularly the lysosomal enzyme disorders, the level of transgene product is likely to need close regulation to avoid deleterious effects. For example, overexpression of alpha-L-iduronidase (IDUA) in fibroblasts from individuals with mucopolysaccharidosis type I (Hurler's disease) produces less correction of the phenotype, as measured by the intracellular accumulation of glycosaminoglycans, than lower levels of expression (Anson et al., 1992). This effect might have been caused by the high levels of IDUA saturating the lysosomal mannose-6-phosphate targeting pathway, with a concomitant reduction in the amounts of other enzymes dependent on this pathway reaching the lysosome, producing a phenotype similar to I-cell disease. If this phenomenon is more widespread it will place significant constraints on the design of vectors for use in the gene therapy of lysosomal storage diseases.

7.1.1 Duchenne Muscular Dystrophy

The gene associated with Duchenne/Becker muscular dystrophies was cloned in 1986 (Monaco et al., 1986) and shown to encode a 400 kDa cytoskeletal protein, dystrophin. Individuals with Duchenne muscular dystrophy (DMD) have mutations which result in little or no functional dystrophin reaching the subsarcolemmal region; in those with Becker dystrophy it is present but abnormal (in amount, structure or both) (see review by Hoffman, 1993). Experimental approaches to replace the dystrophin in DMD provide examples of how basic strategies have been applied to striated muscle (rather than the brain). The methods have included transplantation of donor myoblasts (Gussoni et al., 1992) and retroviral and adenovirus-mediated delivery of dystrophin minigenes by direct inoculation into muscle (Ragot et al., 1993; reviewed by Morgan, 1994). Direct inoculation of "naked" DNA has been tried but results in a level of expression too low to be of clinical use in DMD; only 1–2% of myofibers are dystrophin-positive after focal injection (Ascadi et al., 1991).

The cause of death in most cases of DMD is cardiorespiratory failure. Effective gene therapy for the disease cannot therefore be limited to the transduction of skeletal muscle. Cardiac tissue can be transduced with adenovirus vectors *in vivo* but both the extent and the duration of transgene expression remains problematic (see review by Leiden and Barr, 1994). In addition, a significant proportion of affected boys display some level of cognitive impairment and the dystrophin gene in brain tissue uses a promoter distinct from that in muscle cells. The issue of which promoter to use is not simple, even in striated muscle. Lee et al. (1993), using a dystrophin transgene controlled by a mouse muscle creatine kinase (CK) promoter and two CK gene enhancer elements, found wide variation in the degree of expression in different striated muscles, with minimal expression in the diaphragm.

Ascadi et al. (1994) have shown that an adenovirus vector in high titer can efficiently transduce (with reporter genes) only immature normal muscle cells, and not mature normal muscle fibers, *in vivo*, whereas regenerating normal adult mouse and mdx mouse muscle fibers are transduced. Muscle fibers from boys with DMD (for which the mdx mouse is a model) do not regenerate to any significant extent and it remains to be demonstrated that transduction of these cells is possible. Whether upregulation of the expression of adenovirus internalization receptors, to a state analogous to that found in immature muscle fibers, would result in higher efficiency of transduction is also unknown.

Mature muscle fibers are mutlinucleate and the translation product from any one gene can, in appropriate situations, be found at a distance from the nucleus in which it was encoded. Overexpression of dystrophin is not a problem for individual cells (Cox et al., 1993) and it might be possible to devise a vector system which constitutively overexpresses the dystrophin gene in myocytes. The probability that this vector will not be effective in the CNS means that multiple therapeutic protocols may be needed to achieve maximum benefit in a single individual. The demonstration that intravenous injection of a recombinant adenovirus vector can result in prolonged expression (up to 12 months) of a reporter gene in various tissues in neonatal rodents (Stratford-Perricaudet et al., 1992) raises the possibility that systemic treatment with a cocktail of such vectors, where the dystrophin gene is driven by different tissue-specific promoters, may be the most effective strategy. The issues raised by the immunogenicity of adenovirus and other vectors are addressed in Chapter 26.

At the time of writing the molecular bases for the most common spinal muscular atrophies, the autosomal recessive childhood forms, have only just been elucidated. It would seem that the crucial gene (SMN) is deleted in over 98% of cases and mutated in the rest (Lefebvre et al., 1995). There is no correlation between the size of the deletion or type of mutation and severity of disease but it is possible that severity may be determined by additional deletions in a nearby gene which encodes a neuronal apoptosis inhibitory protein (Roy et al., 1995). If mutations in more than one gene underlie this phenotype then major difficulty is likely to be encountered in designing an effective gene therapy paradigm for its treatment. The other form of spinal muscular atrophy for which the mutational basis is understood is Kennedy's disease (discussed below, along with the other trinucleotide expansions).

Autosomal recessive forms of retinitis pigmentosa are associated with mutations in the rhodopsin and phospodiesterase-β genes. The recent report of the successful delivery using adenovirus vectors of reporter genes to the retina (Mashhour et al., 1994) may encourage optimism in the development of successful treatments of these disorders.

7.1.2 Inherited Tumors of the CNS

Genetic diseases associated with tumor formation in the CNS (neurofibromatosis types 1 and 2, tuberous sclerosis, von Hippel Lindau disease, retinoblastoma) are dominant at a clinical level: that is, the offspring of an affected individual are each at 50% risk of inheriting a germline mutation in the appropriate gene. At a cellular level, however, the development of malignant potential depends on the occurrence of an additional somatic event mutating the remaining normal copy of the relevant gene. This "two-hit" mechanism defines these disorders as recessive at the cellular level and implies that replacing a functional copy of the appropriate tumor suppressor gene in the malignant cell should revert such cells to a normal growth pattern. There appears, however, to be little advantage in using such local therapy rather than surgical excision of the tumor as it does not address the problem of the germinal mutation present in every cell.

There is no way to predict when and in what cell a second hit will occur and it remains to be clarified what effect additional (more than two) functional copies of these genes would have on a transduced cell. It is not possible with present protocols to prevent a cell from being transduced with more than one copy of a transgene. Would, for instance, additional copies of the Rb gene introduced into the retinal cells of an individual with a germline Rb mutation induce spontaneous apoptotic cell death? We know that one normal function of the products of such tumor suppressor genes is to facilitate an apoptotic response to DNA damaging agents (an altruistic cell suicide mechanism which prevents the clonal expansion of modified cells) as the apoptotic cell death in response to DNA damaging agents is abolished in cells where both copies of the p53 tumor suppressor gene have been inactivated.

Conversely, overexpressing p53 protein results either in apoptosis or arrest of the cell cycle in G1 (Levine et al., 1994). Maintenance of the intracellular balance between the products of such tumor suppressor genes and proto-oncogenes such as bcl-2 appears essential for control of proliferation and it may be naive to believe that increasing the functional level of a tumor suppressor gene will solely revert to normal the growth characteristics of a clonal population of malignant cells.

7.1.3 Non-genetic Diseases Caused by loss of Normal Function

Of the non-genetic neurodegenerative diseases Parkinson's disease is the archetype. It is thought to arise as a result of a loss of normal function and which might therefore be amenable to replacement protocols using the strategies outlined earlier. Alzheimer's disease, whose ultimate cause remains elusive, is the condition causing the largest socioeconomic burden.

7.1.3.1 Parkinson's Disease

Parkinson's disease is a degenerative CNS disease with onset in mid–late life characterized by rigidity, tremor and bradykinesia. The symptoms arise from a reduction in the dopaminergic input to the striatum due to loss of the dopaminergic neurons in the pars compacta of the substantia nigra and neurodegeneration of the mesostriatal pathway. Most affected individuals gain significant benefit from peripheral administration of L-dopa, which replaces dopamine in the basal ganglia. Eventually most individuals lose the ability to respond to this drug and, although temporary benefit is sometimes obtained from a change in medication regimen, such as continuous infusion of dopaminergic agonists (Obeso et al., 1988), alternate treatment strategies, in particular neural transplantation, have been proposed (Kopin, 1993).

The first tissue transplanted into the striatum was autologous adrenal medulla (Madrazo et al, 1987) but with results varied (see review by Lindvall, 1994). More recently, transplantation of fetal mesencephalic grafts (containing substantia nigra) into the caudate nucleus and/or putamen of individuals with Parkinson's disease resistant to drug therapy resulted in minor to moderate alleviation of motor symptoms in most cases (Freed et al., 1992). The most consistent benefit has been seen for rigidity and bradykinesia with little improvement in tremor (Lindvall, 1994). There are difficulties, however, in obtaining suitable tissue for engraftment and in maintaining graft viability.

Recent work has examined the role of grafting genetically modified cells into the brains of Parkinson's disease patients. Cells such as fibroblasts (which secrete L-dopa; SEE CHAPTER 19), myocytes (Jiao et al., 1993) and neuronal progenitors (both of which secrete dopamine as they naturally express dopa decarboxylase enzyme activity), transfected with retroviruses containing the gene for tyrosine hydroxylase, have been used in animal experiments with varying degrees of success. Difficulties have been found in obtaining prolonged synthesis of dopamine in some transduced cells. It is also not clear whether such cells can be made to release the dopamine at a physiologically appropriate time and in the correct amounts (Horellou et al., 1991). What is clear is that the cell type producing the L-dopa or dopamine is immaterial to the efficacy of the protocol; even transduced astroglial cells or endothelial cells should be able to provide the missing neurotransmitter to the extracellular space.

The success of transplantation in relieving symptoms of Parkinson's disease is tempered by the knowledge that the graft does not alter the disease process in the host brain (as shown where unilateral grafting is performed), the benefit being confined to the contralateral limbs and loss of the contralateral nigrostriatal pathway continues (as shown by PET scanning). Different procedures will have to be compared to determine whether targeting surviving neurons or glia *in situ* using virally delivered transgenes, for example, will have a clinically significant advantage over bilateral grafting.

Kaplitt et al. (1994) have obtained some phenotype correction in unilateral 6-hydroxydopamine lesioned rats treated with direct intrastriatal inoculation of adeno-associated viral vectors expressing tyrosine hydroxylase. At 10 weeks after injection a 36% reduction (from approximately 66 to 44 rotations per 5 min) in apomorphine-induced rotations was seen compared with controls and immunoreactivity noted at 4 months after treatment (although they made no comment on whether there was any functional benefit at this time point). Similar results have been reported by During and colleagues (Geller et al., 1995) using amplicon vectors derived from herpes simplex virus 1. Vectors or genetically engineered cells could be used to deliver specific growth factors to dopamine neurons, and thus halt their degeneration (Tomac et al., 1995).

7.1.3.2 Alzheimer's Disease

This diffuse neurodegeneration affects 3% of the population over the age of 70 and 10% over the age of 80 worldwide. The clinical manifestations of early memory loss, progressive cognitive decline and additional neurological sequelae are accompanied pathologically by the presence of intraneuronal neurofibrillary tangles and extracellular neuritic plaques associated with deposition of amyloid peptide. A multitude of biochemical abnormalities have been reported including a depletion of acetylcholine, leading to suggestions that augmentation of acetylcholine levels may be a therapeutic option. The activity of the brain cholinergic systems has been correlated with memory in experimental animals (see review by Sinden et al., 1994) and there is circumstantial evidence that cholinergic agents may have similar effects in humans. Approximately 5% of cases of Alzheimer's disease are genetically determined, at least five loci being involved in the pathogenesis of these familial cases. Mutations in the amyloid precursor protein (APP) gene on chromosome 21q have been identified in a number of families where the disease has onset in the 50s and 60s (Goate et al., 1991). Such mutations are dominant in their expression and it has been suggested that they result in the accumulation of a form of β-amyloid which is resistant to intracellular degradation (Mayer et al., 1994). The neuropathological hallmarks of AD (neurofibrillary plaques and tangles) are also seen in cases of Down's syndrome where, commonly, an extra chromosome 21 is present. An additional gene on chromosome 14, Presenilin-1, is associated with onset of symptoms before the age of 50 years and accounts for less than 70% of early-onset familial cases. Presenilin-2 on chromosome 1 accounts for a small proportion of inherited cases of AD.

The E4 allele of the gene for apolipoprotein E (ApoE, chromosome 19q) has been identified as a predisposing factor for the development of both familial and sporadic late-onset Alzheimer's disease (Corder et al., 1993; Saunders et al., 1993). ApoE binds to amyloid and is deposited along with it and neurofibrillary tangles in the brain. The mechanism by which this association with the E4 allele predisposes to disease is unknown, although the E4 protein isoform of A*B*1-42 has been shown to stimulate the rate of formation and number of amyloid fibrils more than the E3 or E2 isoforms. If the E4 allele is directly related to the development of late-onset Alzheimer's disease the question arises (as it does with any late-onset untreatable disease) of whether identification of individuals at risk by molecular analysis while they are asymptomatic has any relevance to this discussion. We believe that, at present and in the absence of any proven therapy, such presymptomatic testing is inappropriate, particularly in Alzheimer's disease where the phenotype is not fully penetrant. The first clinical trials will almost certainly be directed towards treating individuals with well delineated clinical manifestations.

Where a phenotype arises from such a variety of causes strategies designed to retard the neuronal loss, such as delivery of nerve growth factor directly to the brain as described earlier, or prevent accumulation of amyloid and the resulting inflammation (Schehr, 1994) may offer a more realistic option for treatment than attempts to target specific causes such as APP mutations or

ApoE haplotype. New transgenic animal models (Games et al., 1995; Lamb, 1995; LaFerla et al., 1995) will allow exploration of novel therapeutic approaches.

7.2 Disorders Caused by a Gain of Function

The discussion on the etiology of Alzheimer's disease noted that, although the memory deficit in this disorder is associated with an apparent reduction of brain cholinergic activity, at least one of the primary mechanisms responsible is likely to be a gain of toxic function through disruptive interaction; the accumulation of β-amyloid. Where gain of function is the underlying basis for a disorder we can foresee major difficulties in developing effective strategies to directly target the primary abnormality. It is likely that a gain of function is responsible for a significant proportion of dominant genetic diseases (Wilkie, 1994); some examples of these are outlined below.

The genetic neuropathies associated with alterations in the peripheral myelin protein 22 (PMP22) gene show how separate disease phenotypes can depend on gene dosage. Charcot–Marie–Tooth disease type 1 is most commonly due to the duplication of a 1.1 Mb segment of chromosome 17p11.2 containing the PMP22 gene. Haploinsufficiency of the same gene leads to the development of hereditary neuropathy with liability to pressure palsies due to the deletion of the same 1.1 Mb segment (reviewed by Patel and Lupski, 1994). It is clear therefore that two active copies of PMP22 are needed to allow normal peripheral nerve myelination.

This may give us some insight into, perhaps even a warning of, what may occur if we attempt to modify the levels of expression of this or other genes. Strategies for downregulating the expression of a gene include the use of antisense RNA (Murray and Crockett, 1992), allele-specific ribozymes (Beaudry and Joyce, 1992) and genetic suppressor elements (GSEs) (Holzmayer et al., 1992). It is critical that reduction in expression of three copies of the PMP22 gene in an individual with Charcot–Marie–Tooth type 1A using such techniques was only by 33%: "overcorrection" (by 66%) would result in a different disorder. This issue of achieving adequate transcriptional regulation was also mentioned in our discussion on the pseudo I-cell disease associated with over-production of alpha-L-iduronidase in "corrected" Hurler fibroblasts and requires careful consideration in trials of human gene therapy. Nevertheless, newer vector systems able to include large genomic regulatory and coding sequences might allow for adequate levels of transgene expression, in a tissue-specific, developmentally regulated manner (Huxley, 1994).

One dominant disease originally thought to be caused by loss of function of the gene product is that form of familial motor neuron disease associated with mutations in the superoxide dismutase (SOD) gene (Rosen et al., 1993). This enzyme is a free radical scavenger. Heterozygotes with SOD mutations have only 50% of normal enzyme activity in their brains (Deng et al., 1993). Recently doubt has been cast on whether the reduction in enzyme activity is responsible for the anterior horn cell death. Gurney et al. (1994) have demonstrated that transgenic mice expressing high levels of mutant human SOD develop a motor neuron disorder in the absence of any significant change in enzyme activity. It may well be that SOD mutations cause familial amyotropic lateral sclerosis (ALS) through a dominant gain of function. If this is confirmed it means that strategies aimed at restoring a normal enzyme level would have no effect on the disease phenotype.

Although it might be expected that a similar mutation of different genes would result in a disease phenotype through the same mechanism, this may not be the case. The group of neurological disorders in which the molecular genetic abnormality is an unstable expanded trinucleotide repeat shows us that this is not necessarily so: in some disorders the pathophysiology is due to a gain of function (Huntington's disease), while others clearly result from a loss of function (FraX-A, Kennedy's disease).

7.2.1 Diseases Caused by Expansions of Unstable Trinucleotide Repeats

The molecular basis for a growing number of currently untreatable genetic neurological diseases has been identified as the expansion of an unstable trinucleotide repeat sequence within, or immediately adjacent to, a gene (Table 27.2). It is intriguing that, although the genes are ubiquitously expressed, such expansions are associated with pathological features largely confined to the central nervous system, particularly where the repeat sequence is a CAG triplet.

Table 27.2 Unstable trinucleotide repeat sequences and neurological disease

Condition	*Inheritance*	*Repeat sequence*	*Intragenic location*	*Repeat expansion (bp)*
Unstable trinucleotide repeat sequences with associated neurological disease				
Fragile X-A	X-linked	CGG	5′ Untranslated region	200–>1000
Fragile X-E	X-linked	CGG	Unknown	200–>1000
Myotonic dystrophy	Autosomal dominant	CTG	3′ Untranslated region	50–>4000
X-Linked bulbospinal neuronopathy	X-linked	CAG	Open reading frame	39–>50
Huntington's disease	Autosomal dominant	CAG	Open reading frame	38–>100
Spinocerebellar ataxia type 1	Autosomal dominant	CAG	Open reading frame	43–<100
Dentatorubral pallidoluysian atrophy	Autosomal dominant	CAG	Open reading frame	54–<100
Machado–Joseph disease	Autosomal dominant	CAG	Open reading frame	68–<100
Unstable trinucleotide repeat sequences without associated neurological disease				
Fragile X-F	X-linked	CGG	Unknown	300–>500
Fragile X-16A	Autosomal dominant	CGG	Unknown	1000–>2000

For further details on the diseases see Appendix 1

Five of the six dominantly inherited disorders listed in Table 27.2 are likely to result from a gain of pathogenic function whereas the X-linked trinucleotide repeat diseases are associated with loss of function of the respective gene, either a total loss, as in fragile-X type A syndrome, or a partial loss, as in bulbospinal neuronopathy (Kennedy's disease). However, not every fragile site associated with a trinucleotide repeat expansion is responsible for a clinical disorder: those associated with Fragile X-F and Fragile X-16A appear not to be.

Fragile X type A mental retardation is unlikely to be suitable for replacement therapy for a number of reasons. The cognitive defect in this disorder results, as do the accompanying dysmorphic features, from a failure of normal development rather than a decline from a previously normal level. It is likely that the crucial time for expression of the FMR1 gene is in early fetal life, a stage which is not accessible to current gene therapy proposals. It would not be possible to predict, from the size of the molecular abnormality, the severity of the mental retardation in life and therefore an appropriate baseline against which to measure clinical outcome is lacking. However, if it were to be shown that patients with Fragile X-A were to present with progressively deteriorating brain functions gene therapy might become clinically justifiable (Reiss et al., 1994).

The dominant disorders in Table 27.2 are, with the exception of myotonic dystrophy, caused by expansion of a translated CAG (polyglutamine) repeat within the coding sequence of the appropriate gene. There is heterogeneity in the length of the sequence on normal chromosomes as well as on disease-associated chromosomes and the degree of expansion is associated with the severity (measured as age at symptom onset) of disease (Huntington's Disease Collaborative Research Group, 1993; Koide et al., 1994; Harley et al., 1993; Orr et al., 1993; Kawaguchi et al., 1994). The difference between the normal and disease-associated ranges of repeat lengths are small (8–29 repeats). Cells with the expanded repeat, at least in the case of Huntington's disease, express mRNA from both the normal gene and that with the expanded sequence (Ambrose et al., 1994). The additional observation that a female carrying a balanced translocation with a breakpoint in the Huntington's gene does not display a Huntington's disease phenotype (Ambrose et al., 1994) suggests that these expanded sequences result in a disease phenotype through gain of a novel pathological function at the RNA or protein level.

Table 27.3 Comparison of some relevant features of gene therapy to a number of sporadic versus inherited CNS disorders

	Non-inherited disease		*Inherited disease*				
	Tumors	*Parkinson's*	*Huntington's*	*Charcot–Marie–Tooth*[a]	*Leukodystrophies*	*Lesch–Nyhan*	*Fragile X-A*
Outcome	Fatal	Fatal	Fatal	Non-fatal	Fatal	Fatal	Non-fatal
Distribution	Focal	Focal[b]	Diffuse	Diffuse	Diffuse	Diffuse	Diffuse
Age at manifestation	Variable	Late	Variable	Variable	Early	Early	Prenatal
Presymptomatic detection possible[c]	No	No	Yes	Yes	Yes	Yes	Yes[d]
Genotype predicts disease severity	Not known	Not known	Yes	Yes	Yes/no[e]	Yes	No
Gene cloned	Yes[f]	Yes[g]	Yes	Yes	Yes	Yes	Yes
Expression needed	Short term	Long term	Long term	Long term	Long term	Long term	Long term
Experimental gene therapy strategy	Tumor cell killing	Dopamine replacement	Reduce expression of expanded allele	Normalize PMP-22 expression	BMT expressing missing genes	Express HPRT in brain	Express FMR1 in brain
Clinically relevant therapeutic protocols available	Yes	Yes	No	No	Yes	No	No

[a]The most common genetic alteration is duplication of the region of chromosome 17p11.2 containing the PMP22 gene.
[b]The primary pathology is loss of dopaminergic neurons from the pars compacta of the substantia nigra, but other lesions are distributed throughout the brain.
[c]Even if presymptomatic detection is available, it is performed only if a positive family history causes any suspicion and is not done routinely in every pregnancy
[d]Molecular genetic diagnosis is possible in the fetus, but is it arguable whether it can be detected before pathological changes occur.
[e]Genotype predicts disease severity in metachromatic and Krabbe's leukodystrophy, but not in adrenoleukodystrophy.
[f]The genes mutated in inherited brain tumors have been cloned. However, therapeutic gene therapy is more likely to utilize the transduction of cytotoxic genes to eliminate tumor cells.
[g]The genes for tyrosine hydroxylase and dopa decarboxylase have been cloned. These are not mutated in either familial or sporadic Parkinson's disease.

These disorders may be amenable to the development of a "knockout" strategy. One difficulty is how the expanded gene/RNA/protein may be selectively targeted while leaving the normal sequence/product intact. It is not clear at present whether an antisense protocol could distinguish, for example in Huntington's disease, between 25 and 40 repeats. A more realistic option at present for treating Huntington's disease is to adopt strategies for neural transplantation similar to those already under appraisal for Parkinson's disease.

8 CONCLUSIONS

All somatic gene therapy will, even at its most successful, generate a mosaic pattern of uncorrected and corrected cells. The rare cases of clinically affected carrier females who are mosaic for Fragile X-A expansion show that "correction" of such a situation would not ensure phenotypic correction. The observation of a genetically mosaic clinically affected individual in a family with the form of Charcot–Marie–Tooth 1A associated with the 17p11.2 duplication may suggest that this has more widespread relevance to gene therapy protocols (Sorour et al., 1995).

The above discussion provides some indication of the problems that must be solved before gene therapy becomes clinically applicable to several neurological diseases. Issues such as the ability of antisense strategies to discriminate between normal and abnormal genes/RNA/proteins, the probable requirement for stringent controls on the multiplicity of infection/level of transgene expression and the lack of basic knowledge on the developmental stage at which correct gene expression is necessary have not yet been satisfactorily addressed in the context of neurological gene therapy.

Similar shortcomings are being experienced by researchers developing gene therapy for a wide range of disorders. Some authors have suggested that germline gene therapy could become an alternative to somatic gene therapy. Although practical experiments on human germline gene therapy are barred (Committee on the Ethics of Gene Therapy, 1992), several figures have urged debate on these novel horizons within gene therapy to be more widely discussed (Latchmann, 1994; Wivel and Walters, 1993).

Experimental therapeutic gene therapy protocols of clinical applicability exist only for a few of the disorders described in Table 27.3. We do not find this surprising given some of the limitations we outlined above but we do believe that for a small number of inherited neurological disorders gene therapy will offer hope in the near future. These are likely to be those recessive disorders with neurological manifestations where lack of a functioning enzyme is responsible for the phenotype, as well as those for which bone marrow transplantation has already been shown to be of clinical benefit (Krivit and Shapiro, 1991). The main obstacle for successful treatment of disorders such as the Lesch–Nyhan syndrome is the development of efficient methods for delivering functional genes, which will remain transcriptionally active indefinitely, to appropriate cells in the CNS. Until this has been achieved it is important that the hopes of families affected by these catastrophic conditions are not raised inappropriately by precipitate claims of efficacy. The goal of gene therapy must remain the provision of a "cure" for these conditions, not the substitution of one degree of chronic suffering by another.

ACKNOWLEDGMENTS

J.C.M. holds a Clinician Scientist Fellowship from the Medical Research Council, UK; P.R.L. is a Research Fellow of The Lister Institute of Preventive Medicine, UK. We wish to thank Professor Peter S. Harper for comments, discussions and support during the preparation of this manuscript.

REFERENCES

Akli, S., C. Caillaud, E. Vigne, L. D. Stratford-Perricaudet, M. Perricaudet, A. Kahn, and M. R. Peschanski. 1993. Transfer of a foreign gene into the brain using adenovirus vectors. *Nature Genet* **3**:224–228.

Ambrose, C. M., M. P. Duyao, G. Barnes, G. P. Bates, C. S. Lin, J. Srinidhi, S. Baxendale, H. Hummerich, H. Lehrach, M. Altherr, J. Wasmuth, A. Buckler, D. Church, D. Housman, M. Berks, G. Micklem, R. Durbin, A. Dodge, and A. Read. 1994. Structure and expression of the Huntington's disease gene: Evidence against simple inactivation due to an expanded CAG repeat. *Somat Cell Mol Genet* **20**:27–38.

Anderson, W. F. 1995. Human gene marker/therapy clinical protocols listing. *Hum Gene Ther* **6**.

Anson, D. S., J. Bielicki, and J. J. Hopwood. 1992. Correction of mucopolysaccharidosis type I fibroblasts by retroviral-mediated transfer of the human alpha-L-iduronidase gene. *Hum Gene Ther* **3**:371–379.

Ascadi, G., G. Dickson, D. R. Love, A. Jani, F. S. Walsh, A. Gurusinghe, J. A. Wolff, and K. E. Davies. 1991. Human dystrophin expression in mdx mice after intramuscular injection of DNA constructs. *Nature* **352**:815–818.

Ascadi, G., A. Jani, B. Massie, M. Simoneau, P. Holland, K. Blaschuk, and G. Karpati. 1994. A differential efficiency of adenovirus-mediated *in vivo* gene transfer into skeletal muscle cells of different maturity. *Hum Mol Genet* **3**:579–584.

Bajocchi, G., S. H. Feldman, R. G. Crystal, and A. Mastrangeli. 1993. Direct *in vivo* gene transfer to ependymal cells in the central nervous system using recombinant adenovirus vectors. *Nature Genet* **3**:229–234.

Beaudry, A. A. and G. F. Joyce. 1992 Directed evolution of an RNA enzyme. *Science* **257**:635–641.

Bundey, S. 1992. *Genetics and Neurology*. Churchill Livingstone, Edinburgh.

Committee on the Ethics of Gene Therapy. 1992. *Report of the Committee on the Ethics of Gene Therapy*. HMSO, London.

Corder, E. H., A. M. Saunders, W. J. Strittmatter, D. E. Schmechel, P. C. Gaskell, G. W. Small, A. D. Roses, J. L. Haines, and M. A. Pericak-Vance. 1993. Gene dose of apolipoprotein E type 4 allele and the risk of Alzheimer's disease in late onset families. *Science* **261**:921–923.

Cox, G. A., N. M. Cole, K. Matsumara, S. F. Phelps, S. D. Hauschka, K. P. Campbell, J. A. Faulkener, and J. S. Chamberlain. 1993. Overexpression of dystrophin in transgenic mdx mice eliminates dystrophic symptoms without toxicity. *Nature* **364**:725–729.

Davidson, B. L., E. D. Allen, K. F. Kozarsky, J. M. Wilson, and B. J. Roessler. 1993. A model system for *in vivo* gene transfer into the central nervous system using an adenoviral vector. *Nature Genet* **3**:219–223.

Deng, H.-X., A. Hentati, J. A. Tainer, Z. Iqbal, A. Cayabyab, W. Y. Cayabyab, W. Y. Hung, E. D. Getzoff, P. Hu, B. Herzfeldt, R. P. Roos, C. Warner, G. Deng, E. Soriano, C. Smyth, H. E. Parge, A. Ahmed, A. D. Roses, R. A. Hallewell, M. A. PericackVance, and T. Siddique. 1993. Amyotrophic lateral sclerosis and structural defects in Cu,Zn superoxide dismutase. *Science* **261**:1047–1051.

Emery, A. E. H. 1991. Population frequencies of inherited neuromuscular diseases—a world survey. *Neuromusc Dis* **1**:19–29.

Engelhardt, J. F., X. Ye, B. Doranz, and J. M. Wilson. 1994. Ablation of E2A in recombinant adenoviruses improves transgene persistence and decreases inflammatory response in mouse liver. *Proc Natl Acad Sci USA* **91**:6196–6200.

Ferrante, R. J., M. F. Beal, and N. W. Kowall. 1994. Mechanisms of neuronal degeneration in Huntington's disease. In *The Basal Ganglia IV*. Percheron, G., J. S. McKenzie and J. Feger, editors. Plenum Press, New York, 149–162.

Freed, C. R., R. E. Breeze, N. L. Rosenberg, S. A. Schneck, E. Kriek, J. X. Qi, T. Lone, Y. B. Zhang, J. A. Snyder, T. H. Wells, L. O. Ramig, L. Thompson, J. C. Mazziotta, S. C. Huang, S. T. Grafton, D. Brooks, G. Sawle, G. Schroter, and A. A. Ansari. 1992. Survival of implanted fetal dopamine cells and neurologic improvement 12 to 46 months after transplantation for Parkinson's disease. *N Engl J Med* **327**:1549–1555.

Games, D., D. Adams, R. Alessandrini, R. Barbour, P. Berthelette, C. Blackwell, T. Carr, J. Clemens, T. Donaldson, F. Gillespie, T. Guido, S. Hagopian, K. Johnsonwood, K. Khan, P. Leibowitz, I. Lieberburg, S. Little, E. Masliah, L. McConlogue, M. Montoyazavala, L. Mucke, L. Paganini, E. Penniman, M. Power, D. Schenk, P. Seubert, B. Snyder, F. Soriano, H. Tan, J. Vitale, S. Wadsworth, B. Wolozin, and J. Zhao. 1995. Alzheimer type neuropathology in transgenic mice overexpressing V717Fβ-amyloid precursor protein. *Nature* **373**:523–527.

Geller, A. I., J. R. Naegele, K. L. O'Malley, and M. J. During. 1995. Behavioral effects and gene delivery in a rat model of Parkinson's disease—response. *Science* **269**:856–857.

Goate, A., M. C. Chartier-Harlin, M. Mullan, J. Brown, F. Crawford, L. Fidani, L. Giuffra, A. Haynes, N. Irving, L. James, R. Mant, P. Newton, K. Rooke, P. Roques, C. Talbot, M. PericakVance, A. Roses, R. Williamson, J. Hardy. 1991. Segregation of a missense mutation in the amyloid precursor protein gene with familial Alzheimer's disease. *Nature* **349**:704–706.

Gurney, M. E., H. Pu, A. Y. Chui, M. C. Dal Canto, C. Y. Polchow, D. D. Alexander, J. Caliendo, A. Hentati, Y. W. Kwon, H. X. Deng, W. Chen, P. Zhai, R. L. Sufit, and T. Siddique. 1994. Motor neuron degeneration in mice that express a human Cu, Zn superoxide dismutase mutation. *Science* **264**:1772–1775.

Gussoni, E., G. K. Pavlath, A. M. Lanctot, K. R. Sharma, R. G. Miller, L. Steinman, and H. M. Blau. 1992. Normal dystrophin transcripts detected in Duchenne muscular dystrophy patients after myoblast transplantation. *Nature* **356**:435–438.

Harley, H. G., S. A. Rundle, J. C. MacMillan, J. Myring, J. D. Brook, S. Crow, W. Reardon, I. Fenton, D. J.

Shaw, and P. S Harper. 1993. Size of the unstable CTG repeat sequence in relation to phenotype and parental transmission in myotonic dystrophy. *Am J Hum Genet* **52**:1164–1174.

Hoffman, E. P. 1993. Genotype/phenotype correlations in Duchenne/Becker muscular dystrophy. In *Molecular and Cell Biology of Muscular Dystrophy*. T. A. Partridge, editor. Chapman & Hall, London, pp.12–36.

Holzmayer, T. A., D. G. Pestov, and I. B. Roninson. 1992. Isolation of dominant negative mutants and inhibitory antisense RNA sequences by expression selection of random DNA fragments. *Nucl Acids Res* **20**:711–717.

Horellou, P., C. Lundberg, B. Le Bourdelles, K. Wictorin, P. Brundin, P. Kalen, A. Bjorklund, and J. Mallet. 1991. Behavioural effects of genetically engineered cells releasing DOPA and dopamine after intracerebral grafting in a rat model of Parkinson's disease. *J Physiol* **85**:158–170.

Huntington's Disease Collaborative Research Group. 1993. A novel gene containing a trinucleotide repeat that is expanded and unstable on Huntington's disease chromosomes. *Cell* **72**:971–983.

Huxley, C. 1994. Mammalian artificial chromosomes: a new tool for gene therapy. *Gene Ther* **1**:7–12.

Jiao, S. S., V. Gurevich, and J. A. Wolff. 1993. Long term correction of a rat model of Parkinson's disease by gene therapy. *Nature* **362**:450–453.

Kaplitt, M. G., P. Leone, R. J. Samulski, X. Xiao, D. W. Pfaff, K. L. O'Malley, and M. J. During. 1994. Long term gene expression and phenotypic correction using adeno-associated virus vectors in the mammalian brain. *Nature Genet* **8**:148–154.

Kawaguchi, Y., T. Okamoto, M. Taniwaki, M. Aizawa, M. Inoue, S. Katayama, H. Kawakami, S. Nakamura, M. Nishimura, I. Akiguchi, J. Kimura, S. Narumiya, and A. Kakizuka. 1994. CAG expansions in a novel gene for Machado–Joseph disease at chromosome 14q32.1. *Nature Genet* **8**:221–228.

Koide, R., T. Ikeuchi, O. Onodera, H. Tanaka, S. Igarashi, K. Endo, H. Takahashi, R. Knodo, A. Ishikawa, T. Hayashi, M. Saito, A. Tomoda, T. Miike, H. Naito, F. Ikuta, and S. Tsuji. 1994. Unstable expansion of CAG repeat in hereditary dentatorubral-pallidoluysian atrophy (DRPLA). *Nature Genet* **6**:9–13.

Kopin, I. J. 1993. The pharmacology of Parkinson's disease therapy: an update. *Annu Rev Pharmacol Toxicol* 32:467–495.

Krall, W. J., P. M. Challita, L. S. Perlmutter, D. C. Skelton, and D. B. Kohn. 1994. Cells expressing human glucocerebrosidase from a retroviral vector repopulate macrophages and central nervous system microglia after murine bone marrow transplantation. *Blood* **83**:2737–2748.

Krivit, W. and E. G. Shapiro. 1991. Bone marrow transplantation for storage disease. In *Treatment of Genetic Disorders*. R. J. Desnick, editor. Churchill Livingstone, New York, pp.203–221.

Lamb, B. T. 1995. Making models for Alzheimer's disease. *Nature Genet* **9**:4–6.

LaFerla, F. M., B. T. Tinkle, C. J . Bieberich, C. C. Haudenschild, and G. Jay. 1995. The Alzheimer's $A\beta$ peptide induces neurodegeneration and apoptotic cell death in transgenic mice. *Nature Genet* **9**:21–29.

Latchmann, D. S. 1994. Editorial: Germline gene therapy. *Gene Ther* **1**:277–279.

Lee, C. C., F. Pons, P. G. Jones, R. D. Bies, A. M. Schland, J. J. Leger, and C. T. Caskey. 1993. Mdx transgenic mouse: restoration of recombinant dystrophin to the dystrophic muscle. *Hum Gene Ther* **4**:273–281.

Lefebvre, S., L. Burglen, S. Reboullet, O. Clermont, P. Burlet, L. Viollet, B. Benichou, C. Cruaud, P. Millasseau, M. Zeviani, D. Le Paslier, J. Frezal, D. Cohen, J. Weissenbach, A. Munnich, and J. Melki. 1995. Identification and characterisation of a spinal muscular atrophy-determining gene. *Cell* **80**:155–165.

Le Gal La Salle, G., J. J. Robert, S. Berrard, V. Ridoux, L. D. Stratford-Perricaudet, M. Perricaudet, and J. Mallet. 1993. Adenovirus as a potent vector for gene transfer in neurons and glia in the brain. *Science* **259**:988–990.

Leiden, J. M. and E. Barr, 1994. *In vivo* gene transfer into the heart. In *Gene Therapeutics: Methods and Applications of Direct Gene Transfer*, J. A. Wolff, editor. Birkhauser, Boston, pp.363–381.

Levine, A. J., M. E. Perry, A. Chang, A. Silver, D. Dittmer, M. Wu, and D. Welsh. 1994. The 1993 Walter Hubert Lecture: The role of the p53 tumour-suppressor gene in tumorigenesis. *Br J Cancer* **69**:409–416.

Lindvall, O. 1994. Neural Transplantation in Parkinson's Disease. In *Functional Neural Transplantation*, S. B. Dunnett and A. Björklund, editors. Raven Press, New York, pp.103–137.

Lloyd, J. and A. J. Taylor. 1994. Guidance on making proposals to conduct gene therapy research on human subjects. *Gene Ther* **1**:341–363.

Lokensgard, J. R., D. C. Bloom, A. T. Dobson, and L. T. Feldman. 1994. Long term promoter activity during herpes simplex virus latency. *J Virol* **68**:7148–7158.

Lowenstein, P. R. 1994. Molecular neurosurgery: mending the broken brain. *Bio/Technol* **12**:1075–1079.

Lowenstein, P. R., S. Fournel, D. Bain, P. Tomasec, P. M. Clissold, M. G. Castro, and A. L. Epstein. 1994. Herpes simplex virus 1 (HSV1) helper co-infection affects the distribution of an amplicon encoded protein in glia. *Neuroreport* **5**:1625–1630.

Lowenstein, P. R. 1995. Degenerative and inherited neurological disorders. In *Molecular and Cell Biology of Human Gene Therapeutics*, G. Dickson, editor. Chapman & Hall, London, pp.301–349.

Lowenstein, P. R., S. Fournel, D. Bain, P. Tomasec, P. M. Clissold, M. G. Castro, and A. L. Epstein. 1995a. Detection of amplicon and HSV1 helper encoded proteins reveals neurons and astrocytoma cells infected by both viral particles simultaneously: the need to monitor both particles concurrently to identify cells infected exclusively by the amplicon. *Mol Brain Res* **30**:169–175.

Lowenstein, P. R., D. Bain, A. F. Shering, G. W. G. Wilkinson, and M. G. Castro. 1995b. The cytomegalovirus major immediate early promoter within a replicon-deficient adenovirus recombinant drives transgene expression in astrocytes and fibroblasts, but not nervous Schwann cells. *J Virol*, submitted for publication.

Lowenstein, P. R., D. Bain, A. F. Shering, G. W. G. Wilkinson, and M. G. Castro. 1995c. Cell type specific expression from viral promoters within replication deficient adenovirus recombinants in primary neocortical cultures. *Restor Neurol Neurosci* **8**:37–39.

MacMillan, J. C. and P. S. Harper. 1994. Clinical genetics in neurological disease. *J Neurol Neurosurg Psychiatr* **57**:7–15.

Madrazo, I., R. Drucker-Colin, V. Diaz, J. Martinez-Marta, C. Torres, and J. J. Becerril. 1987. Open microsurgical autograft of adrenal medulla to the right caudate nucleus in two patients with intractable Parkinson's disease. *N Engl J Med* **316**:831–834.

Martin, J. B. 1993 Molecular genetics in neurology. *Ann Neurol* **34**:755–773.

Mashhour B, D. Couton, M. Perricaudet, and P. Briand. 1994. *In vivo* adenovirus-mediated gene transfer into ocular tissues. *Gene Ther* **1**:122–126.

Mayer, R. J., C. Tipler, M. Landon, and J. Lowe. 1994. Processing of membrane proteins in neurodegenerative diseases, in 205–233.

McKusick, V. A. 1995. *Genome database and online mendelian inheritance in man.* Baltimore, Johns Hopkins University and Howard Hughes Medical Institute.

Monaco, A. P., R. L. Neve, C. Colletti-Feener, C. J. Bertelson, D. M. Kurnit, and L. M. Kunkel. 1986. Isolation of candidate cDNAs for portions of the Duchenne muscular dystrophy gene. *Nature* **323**:646–650.

Morgan, J. E. 1994. Cell and gene therapy in Duchenne muscular dystrophy. *Hum Gene Ther* **5**:165–173.

Mucke, L. and E. M. Rockenstein. 1993. Prolonged delivery of transgene products to specific brain regions by migratory astrocyte grafts. *Transgene* **1**:3–9.

Murray, J. A. H. and N. Crockett. 1992. Antisense techniques: an overview. In *Antisense RNA and DNA*. J. A. H. Murray, editor. Wiley-Liss, New York, pp.1–49

Neuwelt, E. A., R. Weissleder, G. Nilaver, R. A. Kroll, S. Roman-Goldstein, J. Szumowski, M. A. Pagel, R. S. Jones, L. G. Remsen, C. I. McCormick, E. M. Shannon, and L. L. Muldoon. 1994. Delivery of virus-sized iron oxide particles to rodent CNS neurons. *Neurosurgery* **34**:777–784.

Obeso, J. A., R. Horowski, and C. D. Marsden, editors. 1988. Continuous dopaminergic stimulation in Parkinson's disease. *J Neural Transm* (Suppl. 27): 255.

Online Mendelian Inheritance in Man, OMIM™. Center for Medical Genetics, Johns Hopkins University (Baltimore, MD) and National Center for Biotechnology Information, National Library of Medicine (Bethesda, MD), 1996. World Wide Web URL:http://ww3.ucbi.nlm.uih.gov/omim/.

Orr, H. T., M. Y. Chung, S. Banfi, T. J. Kwiatkowski Jr., A. Servadio, A. L. Beaudet, A. E. McCall, L. A. Duvick, L. P. W. Ranum and H. Y. Zoghbi. 1993. Expansion of an unstable trinucleotide CAG repeat in spinocerebellar ataxia type 1. *Nature Genet* **4**:221–226.

Patel, P. I. and J. R. Lupski. 1994. Charcot–Marie–Tooth disease: a new paradigm for the mechanism of inherited disease. *Trends Genet* **10**: 128–133.

Ragot, T., N. Vincent, P. Chafey, E. Vigne, H. Gilgenkrantz, D. Couton, J. Cartaud, P. Briand, J.-C. Kaplan, M. Perricaudet, and A. Kahn. 1993. Efficient adenovirus-mediated transfer of a human minidystrophin gene to skeletal muscle of mdx mice. *Nature* **361**:647–650.

Ray, J., D. A. Peterson, M. Schinstine, and F. H. Gage. 1993. Proliferation, differentiation, and long term culture of primary hippocampal neurons. *Proc Natl Acad Sci USA* **90**:3602–3606.

Reiss, A. L., J. Lee, and L. Freund. 1994. Neuroanatomy of fragile X syndrome: the temporal lobe. *Neurology* **44**:1317–1324.

Reynolds, B. A. and S. Weiss. 1992. Generation of neurons and astrocytes from isolated cells of the adult mammalian central nervous system. *Science* **255**:1707–1710.

Rocca, W. A., A. Hofman, C. Brayne, M. M. B. Breteler, M. Clarke, J. R. M. Copeland, J. F. Dartigues, K. Engedal, O. Hagnell, T. J. Heeren, C. Jonker, J. Lindesay, A. Lobo, A. H. Mann, P. K. Molsa, K. Morgan, D. W. O'Connor, A. DaSilva Droux, R. Sulkava, D. W. K. Kay, and L. Amaducci. 1991. Frequency and distribution of Alzheimer's disease in Europe: a collaborative study of 1980–1990 prevalence findings. *Ann Neurol* **30**:381–390.

Rosen, D. R., T. Siddique, D. Patterson, D. A. Figlewicz, P. Sapp, A. Hentati, D. Donaldson, J. Goto, J. P. O'Regan, H. X. Deng, Z. Rahmani, A. Krizus, D. McKennaYasek, A. Cayabyab, S. M. Gaston, R. Berger, R. E. Tanzi, J. J. Halperin, B. Herzfeldt, R. Van den Bergh, W.Y. Hung, T. Bird, G. Deng, D. W. Mulder, C. Smyth, N. G. Laing, E. Soriano, M. Pericak-Vance, J. Haines, G. A. Rouleau, G. A. Gusella, H. R.

Horvitz and R. H. Brown Jr. 1993. Mutations in the Cu/Zn superoxide dismutase gene are associated with familial amyotrophic lateral sclerosis. *Nature* **362**:59–62.

Rosenberg, R. N., T. Friedmann, R. C. Robinson, M. Tuszynski, J. A. Wolff, X. O. Breakefield, and F. H. Gage. 1988. Grafting of genetically modified cells to the damaged brain: restorative effects of NGF expression. *Science* **242**:1575–1578.

Rosenberg, R. N., S. B. Prusiner, S. DiMauro, R. L. Barchi, and L. M. Kunkel, editors. 1993. *The Molecular and Genetic Basis of Neurological Disease.* Butterworth-Heinemann, Boston.

Roy, N., M. S. Mahadevan, M. McLean, G. Shutler, Z. Yaraghi, R. Farahani, S. Baird, A. Besner-Johnston, C. Lefebvre, X. Kang, M. Salih, H. Aubry, K. Tamai, X. Guan, P. Ioannou, T. O. Crawford, P. de Jong, L. Surh, J. E. Ikeda, R. G. Korneluk, and A. MacKenzie. 1995. The gene for neuronal apoptosis inhibitory protein is partially deleted in individuals with spinal muscular atrophy. *Cell* **80**:167–178.

Saunders, A. M., W. J. Strittmatter, D. Schmechel, P. H. St. George-Hyslop, M. A. Pericack-Vance, S. H. Joo, B. L. Rosi, J. F. Gusella, D. R. Crapper MacLachlan, M. J. Alberts, C. Hulette, B. Crain, B. Goldgaber, and A. D. Roses. 1993. Association of apolipoprotein E allele epsilon 4 with late-onset familial and sporadic Alzheimer's disease. *Neurology* **43**:1467–1472.

Schehr, R. S. 1994 Therapeutic approaches to Alzheimer's disease. An informal survey of promising drug discovery strategies. *Bio/Technol* **12**:140–144.

Sege-Peterson, K., W. L. Nyhan, and T. Page. 1993. Lesch-Nyhan disease and HPRT deficiency. In: *The Molecular and Genetic Basis of Neurological Disease*, R. N. Rosenberg, S. B. Prusiner, S. DiMauro, R. L. Barchi, and L. M. Kunkel, editors. Butterworth-Heinemann, Boston, pp.241–259.

Sinden, J. D., J. A. Gray, and H. Hodges, 1994. Cholinergic Grafts and cognitive Function. In *Functional Neural Transplantation*, S. B. Dunnett and A. Björklund, editors. Raven Press, New York, pp.253–293.

Snyder, E. Y. 1994. Grafting immortalized neurons to the CNS. *Curr Opin Neurobiol* **4**:742–751.

Snyder, E. Y., R. M. Taylor, and J. H. Wolfe. 1995. Neural progenitor-cell engraftment corrects lysosomal storage throughout the MPS-VII mouse brain. *Nature* **374**:367–370.

Sorour, E., P. Thompson, J. C. MacMillan, and M. Upadhyaya. 1995. Inheritance of CMT1A duplication from a mosaic father. *J Med Genet* **32**:483–485.

Stratford-Perricaudet, L., I. Makeh, M. Perricaudet, and P. Briand. 1992. Widespread long-term gene transfer to mouse skeletal muscles and heart. *J Clin Invest* **90**:626–630.

Tomac, A., E. Lindqvist, L. F. H. Lin, S. O. Ogren, D. Young, B.J. Hoffer, and L. Olson. 1995. Protection and repair of the nigrostriatal dopaminergic system by GDNF *in-vivo*. *Nature* **373**:335–339.

Wilkie, A. O. M. 1994. The molecular basis of genetic dominance. *J Med Genet* **31**:89–98.

Wivel, N. A. and L. Walters. 1993. Germ-line gene modification and disease prevention: some medical and ethical perspectives. *Science* **262**:533–538.

Zhang, Z. X. and G. C. Roman. 1993. Worldwide occurrence of Parkinson's disease: an updated review. *Neuroepidemiology* **12**:195–208.

Appendix 1

Notes

This table does not provide a list of all human inherited neurological disorders. For complete listings and details of these, please consult the references from which data for this table were taken.

The gene column indicates the name of the gene, and whether it has been cloned or not. The Mendelian Inheritance in Man number (McKusick, 1996) for each disease, if available, is provided after its name.

Data for this table are based on the following references: Bundey, 1992; Emery, 1991; Martin, 1993; OMIM, 1996; Rocca et al., 1991; Rosenberg et al., 1993; Zhang and Roman, 1993.

Abbreviations

y: years; AD: autosomal dominant; AR: autosomal recessive; XL: X-linked; M: mitochondrial, maternal; P: prevalence; I: incidence; microdeletions: less than 20 bp deletions; macrodeletions: more than 20bp deletions; mt: mitochondrial.

Appendix 1 Neurological disorders: overview of their pathology, molecular lesions and frequency.

Disease	*Pathology/ pathophysiology/ symptomatology*	*Gene locus*	*Gene/product*
(1) Degenerative disorders of the central nervous system, including ataxias and retinal degenerations			
Alzheimer's Disease (AZD) (all cases)	Dementia, neurodegeneration, plaques and tangles throughout the CNS	—	—
Familial AZD			
AZD Type 1, early onset (104760)	as sporadic	21q21.3-q22.05	β-amyloid precursor protein (APP)
AZD Type 2, late onset (104310)	as sporadic	19cen-q13.2	Apolipoprotein E alleles: Σ4 allele predisposes Σ2 allele protects
AZD Type 3, early onset (104311)	as sporadic	14q24.3	AD3/Presenilin 1
AZD Type 4, early onset (600759)	as sporadic	1q31-q42	AD4/Presenilin 2
AZD with mtDNA mutations	as sporadic	mitochondrial (mt)DNA	ND1 subunit of complex I of respiratory chain
Parkinson's Disease (PD) (sporadic) (168600)	Tremor, rigidity, bradikinesia. Degeneration of nigral neurons. Symptoms with ⩽80 nigral neurons	80% neurons	—
Familial PD (168600)	as sporadic	Unknown	Mitochondrial respiratory chain enzymes? Not cloned.
Familial Creutzfeld–Jakob Disease (CJD) (123400)	CNS spongy degeneration	20pter-p12	Prion protein Cloned
Huntington's Disease (143100)	Chorea, dementia, degeneration of basal ganglia, neurons.	4p16.3	IT15/huntingtin Cloned
Hereditary dentato-rubral and pallido-luysian atrophy and cortical (DRPLA) (125370)	Myoclonus, epilepsy, dementia, mental retardation, cerebellar ataxia, choreoathetosis	12p13.1-p12.3	DRPLA gene Cloned. Protein of approx. 200Kd.
Torsion dystonia-1 (128100)	Involuntary movements	9q32-q34 (50%)	DYT1 Not cloned
Ataxias (all)			
Ataxia Telangiectasia (AT) (208900)	Cerebellar ataxia, telangiectasias, immune defects, tumors	11q23	AT mutated (ATM) protein.
Spinocerebellar ataxia 1 (SCA-1) (164400)	Cerebellar ataxia, chorea	6p23	SCA1/Ataxin1
Spinocerebellar ataxia 2 (SCA2) (183090)	Cerebellar ataxia, chorea	12q2	Unknown, not cloned
Machado–Joseph Disease (109150)	Cerebellar ataxia	14q32.1	MJD1, cloned
Friedrich's Ataxia (229300)	Spinal and cerebellar ataxia	9q12-q21.1	Unknown Not cloned

Mutations	Disease mechanism	Incidence (per year) prevalence; per 100 000	Inheritance
—	Accumulation of neurotoxic products ?	30-59y: 20 [P] 60-69y: 300 [P] 70-79y: 3,200 [P] 80-89y: 10,800 [P]	
Point mutations	Mutations alter processing of APP in a way that is amyloidogenic	Rare	AD
—	Unknown Interacts with APP	Rare	AD
Point mutations	Unknown	Rare	AD
Point mutations	Unknown	Rare	AD
Point mutations at positions 4336, 3397 of mtDNA	Defects in mitochondrial respiratory chain function	Rare	M
—	—	40-59y: 100 [P] 60-69y: 400 [P] 70-79y: 800 [P] ≥80y: 1000 [P]	
Unknown	Unknown	Rare	AD
Point mutations	Conformational change in protein; neurodegeneration	0.1-0.15 [P] (10-15% of total CJD)	AD
Trinucleotide repeat expansion (CAG)	Gain of function?	8 [P]	AD
Trinucleotide repeat expansion (CAG)	Unknown	Rare Common in Japan	AD
Unknown	Unknown	6.7 [I] 16-50 in Ashkenazi Jews [P]	AD
		2 [P]	
Deletions Insertions	IP3-kinase like protein? Disruption of cell cycle regulation, mitogenic signal transduction, or meiotic recombination?	0.3 [P]	AR
Trinucleotide repeat expansion (CAG)	Unknown, gain of function?	4.5 [P] for all spino-cerebellar degenerations	AD
Unknown	Unknown, gain of function?	Rare	AD
Trinucleotide repeat expansion (CAG)	Unknown, gain of function?	Rare	AD
Unknown	Unknown	1.5 [P]	AR

Appendix 1 (*continued*)

Disease	*Pathology/ pathophysiology/ symptomatology*	*Gene locus*	*Gene/product*
Retinal degenerations			
Retinitis pigmentosa (RP); (all)	Constriction of the visual fields, night blindness, fundus changes.		
RP2 (312600)		Xp11.4-p11.2	Not cloned
RP3 (312610)		Xp21.1-p11.4	Not cloned
RP6 (312612)		Xp21.3-p21.2	Not cloned
RP1 (180100)		8p11-q21	Not cloned
RP4 (180380)		3q21-q24	Rhodopsin (cloned)
RP7 (179605)		6p21.1-cen	rds/peripherin
RP9 (180104)		7p15.1-p13	Unknown
RP10 (180105)		7q	Unknown
RP-GNGC (123825)		4p14-q13	rod cGMP channel protein
RP (180072; human homologue of mouse rd)		4p16.3	cGMP phospho-diesterase-β
(2) Tumors and infections			
Tuberous sclerosis (TSC)	Various tumors, skin lesions		
Tuberous sclerosis 1 (191100)		9q34	Unknown; not cloned.
Tuberous sclerosis 2 (191092)		16p13.3	TSC2/tuberin (homology with GTPase activating proteins). Cloned.
Neurofibromatosis type 1 (162200)	Neurofibromas, skin lesions	17q11.2	Neurofibromin (member of the GTPase activating protein family) Cloned
Neurofibromatosis type 2 (101000)	Acoustic neuromas, bilateral meningiomas	22q12.2	Merlin (cytoskeletal protein). Cloned
von Hippel Lindau Disease (193300)	Cerebellar hemangioblastomas	3p25	VHL gene. Cloned
Neuroblastoma (256700)	Tumors of the CNS	1p36.3-p36.2 14q32-qter	Unknown Not cloned
		2p23	N-myc
Glioblastoma (137800)	Glial tumors of the CNS	Many loci	Unknown
Retinoblastoma (inherited [5-10%]; sporadic [60-70%]; germline mutation [20-30%]) (180200)	Retinal and other tumors	13q14.1-q14.2	Rb gene (member of the GTPase activating protein family) Cloned
Herpes simplex virus 1 infection	Encephalitis	—	Expresses up to 80 viral genes
Acquired immunodeficiency syndrome (AIDS)	Encephalitis Opportunistic infections	—	Expresses viral genes
(3) Anterior horn (motor-neuron) diseases			
Spinal muscular atrophy (SMA)	Degeneration of anterior horn motor-neurons.		
SMA (Werding-Hoffman, SMA-1, infantile, 253300), (Kugelberg Welander, SMA-3, juvenile, 253400), (Intermediate forms, SMA-2, 253550)		5q13	Neuronal apoptosis inhibitory protein and/or Survival motor neuron protein

Mutations	*Disease mechanism*	*Incidence (per year) prevalence; per 100 000*	*Inheritance*
	Defective photoreceptor function; retinal degeneration	20-33 [P]	
Unknown	Unknown	All XL = 15% of total	XL
Unknown	Unknown		XL
Unknown	Unknown		XL
Unknown	Unknown	All AD = 50% of total	AD
Point mutations	Unknown		AD
Deletions, point mutations	Unknown		AD
Unknown	Unknown		AD
Unknown	Unknown		AD
Point mutations	Unknown	All AR = 25% of total	AR
Point mutations	Unknown		AR
		10 [I]	
Unknown	Tumor suppressor? Loss of heterozygosity?		AD
Deletions	Tumor suppressor Loss of heterozygosity		AD
Macro and microdeletions Insertions Point mutations	Tumor suppressor Loss of heterozygosity	28.6 [P]	AD
Point mutations Deletions	Tumor suppressor Loss of heterozygosity		AD
Frameshifts Deletions	Tumor suppressor Loss of heterozygosity	2.8 [P]	AD
Deletions	Loss of heterozygosity at 1p36 of possibly more than 1 tumour suppressor gene.		Sporadic
Amplification of N-myc in some tumours			
Deletions	Tumor suppressor Loss of heterozygosity		AD
Deletions	Tumor suppressor Loss of heterozygosity	7 (inherited) [I] 45 (sporadic) [I]	AD
—	—	0.5 [1]	—
—	—	Higher incidence among hemophiliacs, drug abusers, homosexuals; also heterosexuals	—
		16-66 [I] 2-40 [P]	
Small and large deletions Point mutations	Unknown	4-10 [I]	AR

Appendix 1 *(continued)*

Disease	*Pathology/ pathophysiology/ symptomatology*	*Gene locus*	*Gene/product*
SMA-4 (chronic - adult) (158590)		Unknown	Unknown Not cloned.
Familial Amyotrophic Lateral Sclerosis (ALS) (105400)	Spinal and bulbar motorneuron degeneration	21q22.1-q22.2 (some)	Cu, Zn superoxide dismutase Cloned
X-linked bulbo-spinal muscular atrophy (Kennedy's Disease) (313200)	Degeneration of bulbar and spinal motoneurons	Xq12	Androgen receptor Cloned
(4) Inherited peripheral neuropathies			
Hereditary motor and sensory neuropathy (HMSN) [all]			
Charcot–Marie–Tooth type 1A (CMT1A) [HMSN IA] (118220)	Peripheral nerve demyelination	17p11.2	Peripheral myelin protein-22 (PMP-22) Cloned
CMT1B [HMSN IB] (118200)	Peripheral nerve demyelination	1q21.2-q23	Peripheral myelin protein P0. Cloned
CMT1C [HMSN IC]	Peripheral nerve demyelination	Unknown	Unknown Not cloned
CMTX1 (302800)	Peripheral nerve demyelination	Xq13	Connexin-32 Cloned
Hereditary neuropathy with liability to pressure palsies (162500)	Peripheral nerve demyelination	17p11.2	PMP-22 Cloned
(5) Muscle disorders			
Myotonic dystrophy (DM) (160900)	Myotonia, muscle wasting, hypogonadism	19q13.3	Myotonin (DM protein kinase) Cloned
Duchenne muscular dystrophy (DMD) (310200)	Muscle weakness; mental retardation (some)	Xp21.2	Dystrophin (cytoskeletal protein) Cloned
Becker muscular dystrophy (310200)	Muscle weakness	Xp21.2	Dystrophin (cytoskeletal protein)
Facio-scapulo-humeral muscular dystrophy (158900)	Muscle weakness - wasting of face and girdle muscles	4q35	Unknown Not cloned
Periodic paralysis II (Paramyotonia congenita) (170500)	Episodic myotonic symptoms	17q23.1-25.3	Adult muscle sodium channel α subunit Cloned.
Generalized myotonia (255700)	Congenital myotonia	7q35	CLC1 / skeletal muscle chloride channel
Dominant myotonia congenita of Thomsen (160800)	Myotonia	7q35	CLC1 / skeletal muscle chloride channel
Malignant hyperthermia (145600)	Idiosyncratic reaction to anesthetics: anesthetic death; myopathy.	I: 19q13.1-q13.2 (50%) II: 17q11.2-q24 III: Unknown	I: skeletal muscle Ca^{2+} release channel (ryanodine receptor) II-III: Unknown
(6) Mitochondrial diseases			
Leber's optic atrophy (535000)	Optic atrophy, blindness, dystonia, cardiac dysrhytmias, etc.	Mitochondrial DNA	Complex I, III, IV polypeptides of respiratory chain

Mutations	*Disease mechanism*	*Incidence (per year) prevalence; per 100 000*	*Inheritance*
Unknown	Unknown	4.2 [I]	AD / AR / XL
Point mutations	Free radical mediated neurotoxicity?	0.1 [I] (10% of sporadic form)	AD
Trinucleotide repeat expansion (CAG)	Decreased androgen receptor function?	Rare	XL
		14-280 [P]	
Duplications, point mutations, 3–4 copies of PMP-22 present	Decreased myelinating capacity of Schwann cells		AD
Point mutations	Decreased myelinating capacity of Schwann cells		AD
Unknown	Decreased myelinating capacity of Schwann cells		AR/AD
Point mutations	Decreased myelinating capacity of Schwann cells		XL
Deletions, only one copy of PMP-22 present	Impaired myelinating capacity of Schwann cells		AD
Trinucleotide repeat expansion (CTG)	Unknown	9-96 [P]	AD
Frameshift mutations	Unknown	17-244 [P] 97-390 [I] (in males)	XL
Deletions, duplications, point mutations	Unknown	12-17 [P] 16-55 [I]	XL
Unknown	Unknown	2-67 [P]	AD
Point mutations	Alterations in sodium channel function	Rare	AD
Point mutations Deletions	Total loss of muscle chloride channel function leads to myotonia, recessive form	Rare	AR
Point mutations; different ones from those causing the recessive form (see above)	Partial loss of muscle chloride channel function leads to myotonia, dominant form, possibly due to a dominant negative effect	Rare	AD
I: Point mutations II-III: Unknown	Unknown	Not determined, important cause of anesthetic deaths.	AD
18 point mutations	Defect in mitochondrial respiratory chain?	Rare	M

Appendix 1 (*continued*)

Disease	*Pathology/ pathophysiology/ symptomatology*	*Gene locus*	*Gene/product*
MERFF (545000)	Myoclonus epilepsy, ataxia, myopathy, sensorineural hearing loss, ragged red muscle fibres, etc.	Mitochondrial DNA	Gene encoding for tRNA for lysine
MELAS (540000)	Mitochondrial myopathy, encephalopathy, lactic acidosis, stroke like episodes, sensorineural hearing loss, etc.	Mitochondrial DNA	Gene encoding tRNA for leucine
Kearns–Sayre (530000)	Short stature, retinal degeneration, hearing loss, ataxia, etc.	Mitochondrial DNA	Various
(7) Autonomic nervous system disorders			
Familial dysautonomia (223900)	Altered sensory and autonomic function	9q31-q33	Unknown
(8) Metabolic disorders			
Purine metabolism			
Lesch–Nyhan (308000)	Basal ganglia dysfunction	Xq2.6-q2.7	Hypoxanthine Guanine Phosphorybosyl transferase; Cloned.
Amino acid metabolism			
Phenylketonuria (PKU) (261600)	Mental retardation	12q22-q24.1	Phenylalanine hydroxylase; Cloned.
Neuronal storage diseases / Lysosomal disorders			
Gangliosidoses			
G_{M1}-gangliosidoses Infantile (230500); juvenile (230600); and adult variants (230650)	Mental retardation Neurodegeneration	3p21.33	β-galactosidase; Cloned.
G_{M2}-gangliosidoses Tay–Sachs Disease (272800)	Mental retardation Neurodegeneration	15q23-q24	Hexosaminidase A; Cloned.
G_{M2}-gangliosidoses Sandhoff's Disease (268800)	Mental retardation Neurodegeneration	5q13	Hexosaminidase A + B; β-subunit mutation. Cloned.
Lipidoses			
Gaucher's Disease, (230800); Type II: acute; subacute neuronopathic	Mental retardation Neurodegeneration	1q21	Glucocerebrosidase; Cloned.
Niemann–Pick Disease (257200)	Mental retardation Neurodegeneration	11p15	Deficiency of acid sphingomyelinase; Cloned.
Neuronal ceroid lipofuscinosis (CLN, Types 1-5)			
Batten's Disease	Mental retardation		
CLN1 (256730) Infantile		CLN1: 1p32	not cloned
CLN2 (204500) Late infantile		unknown	not cloned
CLN3 (204200) Juvenile		CLN3:16p12	Cloned; 438 AA protein of unknown function
CLN 4 (204300) Adult forms		unknown	not cloned
CLN5 (256731) variant of late infantile		13q21.1-q32	not cloned

Mutations	Disease mechanism	Incidence (per year) prevalence; per 100 000	Inheritance
Missense mutation at nucleotide 8344 in 90% of cases	Defect of translation of all mtDNA encoded genes	Rare	M
Missense mutation at nucleotide 3243 in 80% of cases	Defect of translation of all mtDNA encoded genes	Rare	M
Large rearrangements and deletions of mtDNA	Loss of mtDNA encoded proteins	Rare	M
Unknown	Unknown	5-33 (Ashkenazi Jews) [P]	AR
Point mutations Deletions	Impaired dopamine neurotransmission?	0.25-1 [P] 200/year USA [P]	XL
Point mutations	Defect in myelin formation	12.5 [P]	AR
Point mutations Duplications	Intraneuronal accumulation of G_{M1}-ganglioside	Rare	AR
4bp insertion Point mutations Deletions	Intraneuronal accumulation of G_{M2}-ganglioside	25 Jewish [I] 1 non-Jewish [I]	AR
Deletions Insertions Duplications Point mutations	Intraneuronal accumulation of G_{M2}-ganglioside	0.1 (Jewish) 0.3 (non-Jewish)	AR
Point mutations Micro-deletions	Intraneuronal accumulation of glucosyl-ceramide	Rare	AR
Micro-deletions Point mutations	Intraneuronal accumulation of sphingomyelin	Rare	AR
	Unknown for all forms of CLN	1 [I]	AR
Point mutations Deletions			

Appendix 1 (*continued*)

Disease	*Pathology/ pathophysiology/ symptomatology*	*Gene locus*	*Gene/product*
Mucopolysaccharidoses (MPS)			
MPS I (Hurler's Disease) (252800)	Mental retardation	4p16.3	α-L-iduronidase Cloned.
MPS II (Hunter's syndrome) (309900)	Mental retardation	Xq28	Idurono-sulfatase Cloned.
MPS III (Sanfilippo syndromes, type:	Mental retardation		
A (2 52900),		Unknown	A: Heparan N-sulfatase.
B (252920),		Unknown	B: N-acetyl-α-D-glucosaminidase
C (252930),		Unknown	C: acetylCoA: α-glucosaminide N-acetyl-transferase A-C: not cloned.
D (252940).		12q14	D: N-acetyl-glucosamine-6-sulfate sulfatase. Cloned.
Mucolipidoses			
I cell disease (Mucolipidosis II) (252500)	Mental retardation	4q21-q23	UDP-N-acetylglucosamine: N-acetyl-glucosaminyl-1-phosphotransferase Not cloned.
Leukodystrophies			
Metachromatic leukodystrophy (Late infantile, early juvenile, juvenile, and adult forms) (250100)	CNS demyelination; segmental demyelination in PNS	22q13-ter	Deficiency of arylsulfatase A Cloned.
Adrenoleukodystrophy (ADL) Adrenomyeloneuropathy (AMN) (300100)	CNS demyelination; adrenal insufficiency	Xq28	ALD protein (ALDP), 70Kd peroxisomal transporter protein, (member of the superfamily of ABC transporters; function: peroxisomal import of lignoceroyl-CoA synthetase?) Cloned
Krabbe's Disease (Infantile Late infantile Juvenile Adult) (245200)	CNS demyelination; segmental demyelination in PNS	14q24-q32	Galactocerebrosidase Cloned.
Canavan Disease (271900)	Neurodegeneration	17pter	Aspartoacylase. Cloned.
Pelizaeus–Merzbacher Disease (312080)	CNS demyelination	Xq22	Proteolipid protein Cloned.

Mutations	*Disease mechanism*	*Incidence (per year) prevalence; per 100 000*	*Inheritance*
Point mutations Microdeletions Deletion/insertion	Severe enzyme deficiency Intracellular accumulation of dermatan sulfate and heparan sulfate	Rare	AR
Point mutations Macro-deletions	Severe enzyme deficiency Intracellular accumulation of dermatan sulfate and heparan sulfate	1-3 [I]	XL
	Intracellular accumulation of heparan sulfate		AR
Unknown		A: 4 [I]	
Unknown		B: Rare	
Unknown		C: Rare	
Unknown		D: Rare	
Unknown	Lack of addition of mannose-6-phosphate lysosomal targeting signal onto lysosomal enzymes	Rare	AR
Point mutations Micro-deletions	Intracellular accumulation of sulphatides	1 [I]	AR
Partial deletions Point mutations Mutations in ALDP identified in only some patients	Intracellular accumulation of saturated very long chain fatty acids with C25 and C26.	1-5 [I]	XL
Unknown	Intracellular accumulation of galactosylceramide	0.5-1 [I] 600 (Druze Israelis) [I]	AR
Point mutations	Intraneuronal accumulation of N-acetyl-aspartic acid	Rare	AR
Point mutations, duplications	Decreased myelinating capacity of oligodendrocytes	Rare	XL

Appendix 1 (*continued*)

Disease	*Pathology/ pathophysiology/ symptomatology*	*Gene locus*	*Gene/product*
(9) MENTAL RETARDATION, NON-METABOLIC			
Fragile X, A (309550)	Mental retardation	Xq27	FMR1 Cloned
Fragile X, E (309548)	Mental retardation	Xq28	FMR2; not cloned
Down's syndrome	Mental retardation	21	Various genes Some cloned

Mutations	*Disease mechanism*	*Incidence (per year) prevalence; per 100 000*	*Inheritance*
Trinucleotide repeat expansion (CGG) gene and promoter deletions	Decreased expression of FMR1	57 (males) [P] 36 (females) [P]	XL
Trinucleotide repeat expansion (CGG)			XL
Gene dosage (trisomy)	Unknown	60-4100 [I] (depending on maternal age)	

Index

Note: Page references in *italics* refer to figures; those in **bold** refer to tables; the Appendix is indicated by the abbreviation App.

Index compiled by Annette J. Musker